WONG'S CLINICAL MANUAL OF Pediatric Nursing

Ninth Edition

WONG'S CLINICAL MANUAL OF Pediatric Nursing

Marilyn J. Hockenberry, PhD, RN, FAAN
Professor
Department of Pediatrics
Baylor College of Medicine;
Director
Global HOPE Nursing
Texas Children's Hospital
Houston, Texas;
Bessie Baker Professor Emerita
Duke University School of Nursing
Durham, North Carolina

EDITORS

Rosalind Bryant, PhD, RN
Clinical Instructor, Retired
Department of Pediatric Hematology and Oncology
Baylor College of Medicine
Houston, Texas

Melody Brown Hellsten, DNP, RN, MSN, MS
Assistant Professor
Department of Pediatrics
Baylor College of Medicine
Houston, Texas

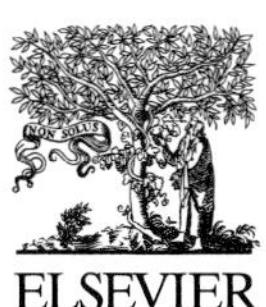

Elsevier
3251 Riverport Lane
St. Louis, Missouri 63043

WONG'S CLINICAL MANUAL OF PEDIATRIC NURSING, NINTH EDITION ISBN: 978-0-323-75476-7

Notice

Practitioners and researchers must always rely on their own experience and knowledge in evaluating and using any information, methods, compounds or experiments described herein. Because of rapid advances in the medical sciences, in particular, independent verification of diagnoses and drug dosages should be made. To the fullest extent of the law, no responsibility is assumed by Elsevier, authors, editors or contributors for any injury and/or damage to persons or property as a matter of products liability, negligence or otherwise, or from any use or operation of any methods, products, instructions, or ideas contained in the material herein.

Previous editions copyrighted 2012, 2008, 2004, 2000, 1996, 1990, 1986, and 1981.

Content Strategist: Sandra Clark
Content Development Specialist: Deborah Poulson
Publishing Services Manager: Julie Eddy
Senior Project Manager: Rachel E. McMullen
Design Direction: Maggie Reid

Printed in India

Last digit is the print number: 9 8 7 6 5 4 3 2 1

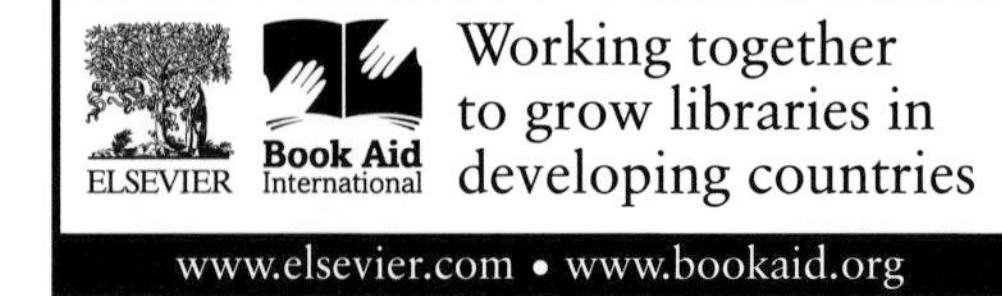

REVIEWER

Paula Silver, PharmD, MEd, BS
Pharmacist
Hampton, Virginia

PREFACE

It has been 10 years since the last edition of ***Wong's Clinical Manual of Pediatric Nursing*** was published, and this new edition brings with it extensive updates to match the significant changes in pediatric nursing practice. Like previous editions, the ***Manual*** serves a unique function in the study and practice of pediatric nursing. This new work benefits from the addition of two new editors—Dr. Rosalind Bryant and Dr. Melody Brown Hellsten, who bring their unique expertise to clinical pediatric nursing care.

The ***Manual*** is a practical guide for practicing nurses and students engaged in the care of children and their families—a compendious collection of clinical information, resources, and data packaged for convenient use and easy access. For the practicing nurse, the book is a ready resource of material that is otherwise available only in a wide array of journal articles, texts, federal publications, professional association recommendations, and brochures. Examples of current "cutting-edge" information are recommendations from the American Academy of Pediatrics, Agency for Healthcare Research and Quality, American Pain Society, National Center for Health Statistics, and Centers for Disease Control and Prevention. For the student, it is an indispensable guide to the care of children and their families.

As an adjunct to clinical practice, the ***Manual*** assumes the thorough preparation and basic theoretical knowledge only a textbook can provide. Although it is not designed to accompany any particular textbook, it serves as a valuable addition to ***Wong's Nursing Care of Infants and Children*** and ***Wong's Essentials of Pediatric Nursing.***

The ***Manual*** is authoritative and up to date. An **evidence-based practice** approach is used to present existing knowledge relevant to nursing care. Its content reflects the latest research and current clinical practice. This latest edition of the ***Manual*** has been extensively updated to include evidence-based practice nursing care as it relates to the pediatric patient and family. This unit provides Translating Evidence-Based Practice boxes, which provide the latest research information. A new unit, totally focused on the Next-Generation NCLEX® Examination–Style unfolding case studies, provides students with opportunities to critically think through real-case scenarios that are faced in the pediatric clinical setting such as providing care to the child and family facing the end of life.

The ***Manual*** is designed to ensure that specific information can be located quickly and easily when it is needed. Color tabs printed on the cover facilitate quick access to each of the six units, which have coordinating black thumbtabs. In addition to a detailed table of contents in the front of the book, a unit outline with page references is included at the beginning of each unit. A list of related topics found elsewhere in the book is included in most units. Vital reference data appear inside the front and back covers, where they can be located at a moment's notice.

Greater attention is given to **critical thinking through** the Unfolding Case Studies and by emphasizing essential nursing observations and interventions in **Safety Alert** and **Drug Alert** boxes. These call the reader's attention to considerations, which, if ignored, could lead to a deteriorating or emergency situation. Key assessment data, risk factors, and danger signs are among the kinds of information in this feature. The concept of **atraumatic care**—the provision of therapeutic care in settings by personnel and through interventions that eliminate or minimize the psychological and physical distress experienced by children and their families in the health care system—is incorporated throughout the text and highlighted as boxed material.

Unit 1 focuses on the **assessment of the child and family.** It includes history taking; assessment of present and past physical health; and a summary of developmental achievements, both general and age specific. New information to this unit includes the addition of new cultural assessment tables, and cultural behaviors related to health assessment. Updates provide the latest information on vital sign measurement including blood pressure assessment. Essential components of the assessment of the child and family are based on evidence throughout the unit.

Unit 2 emphasizes **health promotion** in the areas of preventive care, infant and childhood nutrition, immunization, safety and injury prevention, parental guidance, and play. The material on childhood immunizations and on current car restraint guidelines is completely revised to reflect current recommendations.

Unit 3 discusses neonatal, child, and adolescent pain assessment and management. Although the literature on pain assessment and management in children has grown considerably, this knowledge has not been widely applied in practice. Unit 3 outlines essential knowledge for the nurse caring for a child in pain by presenting detailed pain assessment and management strategies, including discussion of common pain states in children. This unit is a resource for all nurses caring for children in pain.

Unit 4 outlines **basic nursing procedures** adapted for the child. This section has been extensively revised and provides **Evidence-Based Practice** summaries on numerous nursing interventions. Unit 4 includes an extensive collection of skills and procedures including preparation for procedures, collection of specimens, administration of medicine, venous access devices, invasive and noninvasive oxygen monitoring, and cardiopulmonary resuscitation. The Patient and Family education guidelines have been incorporated into the skills and procedure sections of this unit. These guidelines have been revised for use by nurses as well as families in the care of a child in the acute care or home setting. The latest American Heart Association recommendations for performing cardiopulmonary resuscitation on an infant or child and for caring for a choking infant or child are included.

Unit 5 is a new unit devoted to Next-Generation NCLEX® Examination–Style Unfolding Case Studies. These unfolding cases studies require students to use critical thinking to examine the clinical evidence and make assessment and management decisions specific to the case study. Twelve unfolding cases are used to teach nurses how to care for the most common types of childhood illness; acute conditions and well as chronic diseases are represented in this Unit.

Unit 6 includes basic resource information for interpretation of **laboratory data,** including values in International Units.

Although the information in the ***Manual*** is carefully researched, references are included only when citations are required to appropriately credit the work. The reader is directed to the current editions of ***Wong's Nursing Care of Infants and Children*** and ***Wong's Essentials of Pediatric Nursing*** for additional references and discussion of material, especially for growth and development, interviewing, and health problems.

This edition of the ***Manual*** also includes a completely revised, expanded section of color photos of common pediatric dermatology conditions. This feature continues to enhance the overall quality of the ***Manual*** as a reference source for the practicing clinician and student.

Every effort has been made to ensure that the information is accurate and up to date at the time of publication. However, as new research and experience broaden our practice, standards of care change accordingly. Therefore, the reader may find some differences in local and regional practices.

The Evolve website (http://evolve.elsevier.com/Wong/clinical/) includes Emergency Treatment Guidelines, Evidence-Based Practice Guidelines, Patient Teaching Guides (and Spanish translations), Pediatric Medication Tables, and Unfolding Case Studies.

A number of people have contributed time and expertise to this edition. We are pleased to have both Dr. Rosalind Bryant and Dr. Melody Brown Hellsten as Editors on this edition. Deborah Poulson provided valuable input as part of our Elsevier team. We are so fortunate to have such an outstanding Elsevier team and thank Sandra Clark and Deborah Poulson—who make the book a reality.

Marilyn J. Hockenberry
Rosalind Bryant
Melody Brown Hellsten

Blood Pressure (BP) Levels for Boys by Age and Height Percentile

AGE (Years)	BP PERCENTILE[a]	SYSTOLIC BP (MM HG) PERCENTILE OF HEIGHT							DIASTOLIC BP (MM HG) PERCENTILE OF HEIGHT						
		5th	10th	25th	50th	75th	90th	95th	5th	10th	25th	50th	75th	90th	95th
1	50th	80	81	83	85	87	88	89	34	35	36	37	38	39	39
	90th	94	95	97	99	100	102	103	49	50	51	52	53	53	54
	95th	98	99	101	103	104	106	106	54	54	55	56	57	58	58
	99th	105	106	108	110	112	113	114	61	62	63	64	65	66	66
2	50th	84	85	87	88	90	92	92	39	40	41	42	43	44	44
	90th	97	99	100	102	104	105	106	54	55	56	57	58	58	59
	95th	101	102	104	106	108	109	110	59	59	60	61	62	63	63
	99th	109	110	111	113	115	117	117	66	67	68	69	70	71	71
3	50th	86	87	89	91	93	94	95	44	44	45	46	47	48	48
	90th	100	101	103	105	107	108	109	59	59	60	61	62	63	63
	95th	104	105	107	109	110	112	113	63	63	64	65	66	67	67
	99th	111	112	114	116	118	119	120	71	71	72	73	74	75	75
4	50th	88	89	91	93	95	96	97	47	48	49	50	51	51	52
	90th	102	103	105	107	109	110	111	62	63	64	65	66	66	67
	95th	106	107	109	111	112	114	115	66	67	68	69	70	71	71
	99th	113	114	116	118	120	121	122	74	75	76	77	78	78	79
5	50th	90	91	93	95	96	98	98	50	51	52	53	54	55	55
	90th	104	105	106	108	110	111	112	65	66	67	68	69	69	70
	95th	108	109	110	112	114	115	116	69	70	71	72	73	74	74
	99th	115	116	118	120	121	123	123	77	78	79	80	81	81	82
6	50th	91	92	94	96	98	99	100	53	53	54	55	56	57	57
	90th	105	106	108	110	111	113	113	68	68	69	70	71	72	72
	95th	109	110	112	114	115	117	117	72	72	73	74	75	76	76
	99th	116	117	119	121	123	124	125	80	80	81	82	83	84	84
7	50th	92	94	95	97	99	100	101	55	55	56	57	58	59	59
	90th	106	107	109	111	113	114	115	70	70	71	72	73	74	74
	95th	110	111	113	115	117	118	119	74	74	75	76	77	78	78
	99th	117	118	120	122	124	125	126	82	82	83	84	85	86	86
8	50th	94	95	97	99	100	102	102	56	57	58	59	60	60	61
	90th	107	109	110	112	114	115	116	71	72	72	73	74	75	76
	95th	111	112	114	116	118	119	120	75	76	77	78	79	79	80
	99th	119	120	122	123	125	127	127	83	84	85	86	87	87	88
9	50th	95	96	98	100	102	103	104	57	58	59	60	61	61	62
	90th	109	110	112	114	115	117	118	72	73	74	75	76	76	77
	95th	113	114	116	118	119	121	121	76	77	78	79	80	81	81
	99th	120	121	123	125	127	128	129	84	85	86	87	88	88	89
10	50th	97	98	100	102	103	105	106	58	59	60	61	61	62	63
	90th	111	112	114	115	117	119	119	73	73	74	75	76	77	78
	95th	115	116	117	119	121	122	123	77	78	79	80	81	81	82
	99th	122	123	125	127	128	130	130	85	86	86	88	88	89	90
11	50th	99	100	102	104	105	107	107	59	59	60	61	62	63	63
	90th	113	114	115	117	119	120	121	74	74	75	76	77	78	78
	95th	117	118	119	121	123	124	125	78	78	79	80	81	82	82
	99th	124	125	127	129	130	132	132	86	86	87	88	89	90	90
12	50th	101	102	104	106	108	109	110	59	60	61	62	63	63	64
	90th	115	116	118	120	121	123	123	74	75	75	76	77	78	79
	95th	119	120	122	123	125	127	127	78	79	80	81	82	82	83
	99th	126	127	129	131	133	134	135	86	87	88	89	90	90	91
13	50th	104	105	106	108	110	111	112	60	60	61	62	63	64	64
	90th	117	118	120	122	124	125	126	75	75	76	77	78	79	79
	95th	121	122	124	126	128	129	130	79	79	80	81	82	83	83
	99th	128	130	131	133	135	136	137	87	87	88	89	90	91	91
14	50th	106	107	109	111	113	114	115	60	61	62	63	64	65	65
	90th	120	121	123	125	126	128	128	75	76	77	78	79	79	80
	95th	124	125	127	128	130	132	132	80	80	81	82	83	84	84
	99th	131	132	134	136	138	139	140	87	88	89	90	91	92	92
15	50th	109	110	112	113	115	117	117	61	62	63	64	65	66	66
	90th	122	124	125	127	129	130	131	76	77	78	79	80	80	81
	95th	126	127	129	131	133	134	135	81	81	82	83	84	85	85
	99th	134	135	136	138	140	142	142	88	89	90	91	92	93	93
16	50th	111	112	114	116	118	119	120	63	63	64	65	66	67	67
	90th	125	126	128	130	131	133	134	78	78	79	80	81	82	82
	95th	129	130	132	134	135	137	137	82	83	83	84	85	86	87
	99th	136	137	139	141	143	144	145	90	90	91	92	93	94	94
17	50th	114	115	116	118	120	121	122	65	66	66	67	68	69	70
	90th	127	128	130	132	134	135	136	80	80	81	82	83	84	84

AGE (Years)	BP PERCENTILE[a]	SYSTOLIC BP (MM HG) PERCENTILE OF HEIGHT 5th	10th	25th	50th	75th	90th	95th	DIASTOLIC BP (MM HG) PERCENTILE OF HEIGHT 5th	10th	25th	50th	75th	90th	95th
	95th	131	132	134	136	138	139	140	84	85	86	87	87	88	89
	99th	139	140	141	143	145	146	147	92	93	93	94	95	96	97

[a]The 90th percentile is 1.28 standard deviation (SD), the 95th percentile is 1.645 SD, and the 99th percentile is 2.326 SD over the mean.
Retrieved from https://www.nhlbi.nih.gov/files/docs/guidelines/child_tbl.pdf.

Blood Pressure (BP) Levels for Girls by Age and Height Percentile

AGE (Years)	BP PERCENTILE[a]	SYSTOLIC BP (MM HG) PERCENTILE OF HEIGHT 5th	10th	25th	50th	75th	90th	95th	DIASTOLIC BP (MM HG) PERCENTILE OF HEIGHT 5th	10th	25th	50th	75th	90th	95th
1	50th	83	84	85	86	88	89	90	38	39	39	40	41	41	42
	90th	97	97	98	100	101	102	103	52	53	53	54	55	55	56
	95th	100	101	102	104	105	106	107	56	57	57	58	59	59	60
	99th	108	108	109	111	112	113	114	64	64	65	65	66	67	67
2	50th	85	85	87	88	89	91	91	43	44	44	45	46	46	47
	90th	98	99	100	101	103	104	105	57	58	58	59	60	61	61
	95th	102	103	104	105	107	108	109	61	62	62	63	64	65	65
	99th	109	110	111	112	114	115	116	69	69	70	70	71	72	72
3	50th	86	87	88	89	91	92	93	47	48	48	49	50	50	51
	90th	100	100	102	103	104	106	106	61	62	62	63	64	64	65
	95th	104	104	105	107	108	109	110	65	66	66	67	68	68	69
	99th	111	111	113	114	115	116	117	73	73	74	74	75	76	76
4	50th	88	88	90	91	92	94	94	50	50	51	52	52	53	54
	90th	101	102	103	104	106	107	108	64	64	65	66	67	67	68
	95th	105	106	107	108	110	111	112	68	68	69	70	71	71	72
	99th	112	113	114	115	117	118	119	76	76	76	77	78	79	79
5	50th	89	90	91	93	94	95	96	52	53	53	54	55	55	56
	90th	103	103	105	106	107	109	109	66	67	67	68	69	69	70
	95th	107	107	108	110	111	112	113	70	71	71	72	73	73	74
	99th	114	114	116	117	118	120	120	78	78	79	79	80	81	81
6	50th	91	92	93	94	96	97	98	54	54	55	56	56	57	58
	90th	104	105	106	108	109	110	111	68	68	69	70	70	71	72
	95th	108	109	110	111	113	114	115	72	72	73	74	74	75	76
	99th	115	116	117	119	120	121	122	80	80	80	81	82	83	83
7	50th	93	93	95	96	97	99	99	55	56	56	57	58	58	59
	90th	106	107	108	109	111	112	113	69	70	70	71	72	72	73
	95th	110	111	112	113	115	116	116	73	74	74	75	76	76	77
	99th	117	118	119	120	122	123	124	81	81	82	82	83	84	84
8	50th	95	95	96	98	99	100	101	57	57	57	58	59	60	60
	90th	108	109	110	111	113	114	114	71	71	71	72	73	74	74
	95th	112	112	114	115	116	118	118	75	75	75	76	77	78	78
	99th	119	120	121	122	123	125	125	82	82	83	83	84	85	86
9	50th	96	97	98	100	101	102	103	58	58	58	59	60	61	61
	90th	110	110	112	113	114	116	116	72	72	72	73	74	75	75
	95th	114	114	115	117	118	119	120	76	76	76	77	78	79	79
	99th	121	121	123	124	125	127	127	83	83	84	84	85	86	87
10	50th	98	99	100	102	103	104	105	59	59	59	60	61	62	62
	90th	112	112	114	115	116	118	118	73	73	73	74	75	76	76
	95th	116	116	117	119	120	121	122	77	77	77	78	79	80	80
	99th	123	123	125	126	127	129	129	84	84	85	86	86	87	88
11	50th	100	101	102	103	105	106	107	60	60	60	61	62	63	63
	90th	114	114	116	117	118	119	120	74	74	74	75	76	77	77
	95th	118	118	119	121	122	123	124	78	78	78	79	80	81	81
	99th	125	125	126	128	129	130	131	85	85	86	87	87	88	89
12	50th	102	103	104	105	107	108	109	61	61	61	62	63	64	64
	90th	116	116	117	119	120	121	122	75	75	75	76	77	78	78
	95th	119	120	121	123	124	125	126	79	79	79	80	81	82	82
	99th	127	127	128	130	131	132	133	86	86	87	88	88	89	90
13	50th	104	105	106	107	109	110	110	62	62	62	63	64	65	65
	90th	117	118	119	121	122	123	124	76	76	76	77	78	79	79
	95th	121	122	123	124	126	127	128	80	80	80	81	82	83	83
	99th	128	129	130	132	133	134	135	87	87	88	89	89	90	91
14	50th	106	106	107	109	110	111	112	63	63	63	64	65	66	66
	90th	119	120	121	122	124	125	125	77	77	77	78	79	80	80

AGE (Years)	BP PERCENTILE[a]	SYSTOLIC BP (MM HG) PERCENTILE OF HEIGHT							DIASTOLIC BP (MM HG) PERCENTILE OF HEIGHT						
		5th	10th	25th	50th	75th	90th	95th	5th	10th	25th	50th	75th	90th	95th
	95th	123	123	125	126	127	129	129	81	81	81	82	83	84	84
	99th	130	131	132	133	135	136	136	88	88	89	90	90	91	92
15	50th	107	108	109	110	111	113	113	64	64	64	65	66	67	67
	90th	120	121	122	123	125	126	127	78	78	78	79	80	81	81
	95th	124	125	126	127	129	130	131	82	82	82	83	84	85	85
	99th	131	132	133	134	136	137	138	89	89	90	91	91	92	93
16	50th	108	108	110	111	112	114	114	64	64	65	66	66	67	68
	90th	121	122	123	124	126	127	128	78	78	79	80	81	81	82
	95th	125	126	127	128	130	131	132	82	82	83	84	85	85	86
	99th	132	133	134	135	137	138	139	90	90	90	91	92	93	93
17	50th	108	109	110	111	113	114	115	64	65	65	66	67	67	68
	90th	122	122	123	125	126	127	128	78	79	79	80	81	81	82
	95th	125	126	127	129	130	131	132	82	83	83	84	85	85	86
	99th	133	133	134	136	137	138	139	90	90	91	91	92	93	93

[a]The 90th percentile is 1.28 standard deviation (SD), the 95th percentile is 1.645 SD, and the 99th percentile is 2.326 SD over the mean.
Retrieved from https://www.nhlbi.nih.gov/files/docs/guidelines/child_tbl.pdf.

Centigrade to Fahrenheit Temperature Conversions

°C	°F	°C	°F	°C	°F
35.0	95.0	37.0	98.6	39.0	102.2
35.2	95.4	37.2	99.0	39.2	102.6
35.4	95.7	37.4	99.3	39.4	102.9
35.6	96.1	37.6	99.7	39.6	103.3
35.8	96.4	37.8	100.0	39.8	103.6
36.0	96.8	38.0	100.4	40.0	104
36.2	97.2	38.2	100.8	40.2	104.4
36.4	97.5	38.4	101.1	40.4	104.7
36.6	97.9	38.6	101.5	40.6	105.1
36.8	98.2	38.8	101.8	40.8	105.4
				41.0	105.8

Conversion formulas:

°F = (°C × 9/5) + 32 or (°C × 1.8) + 32

°C = (°F − 32) + 5/9 or (°F − 32) + 0.55

Normal Body Temperature Ranges

°F	0–2 Years	3–10 Years	11–65 Years
Oral	–	95.9–99.5	97.6–99.6
Rectal	97.9–100.4	97.9–100.4	98.6–100.6
Axillary	94.5–99.1	96.6–98.0	95.3–98.4
Ear	97.5–100.4	97.0–100.0	96.6–99.7
Core	97.5–100.0	97.5–100.0	98.2–100.2

Normal Heart Rate and Respiratory Rate Ranges in Children[a]

Age	Heart Rate (Awake)	Heart Rate (Asleep)	Respiratory Rate
Newborn	85–190	80–160	30–60
3–6 months	100–190	75–150	30–40
1 year	100–140	75–130	25–35
2 years	100–140	65–100	25–35
3–5 years	80–120	65–100	25–30
6–11 years	75–120	58–90	20–25
≥12 years	60–100	50–90	15–20

[a]Numerous normal ranges exist and vary according to the reference source.

CONTENTS

Color insert can be found after p. 178.

Assessment

Symbol ▶ indicates material that may be photocopied and distributed to families.

Health History

One of the most significant aspects of a health assessment is the health history. To take a thorough history, the nurse must be well versed in communication and interviewing principles. An overview of the process is presented in terms of general guidelines for communication and interviewing, with additional specific guidelines for children. Because of the frequent need for interpreters with non–English speaking families, guidelines for using interpreters are included.

The history furnishes information about the child's physical health since birth, details the events of the present problem, and includes social and family history facts that are essential for providing comprehensive care. The objective of each assessment area is the identification of nursing diagnoses.

The summary is primarily intended for the recording of data, not the acquisition of information from the informant. Therefore, it is not meant to be used as a questionnaire. The column titled "Comments" is intended to enhance and detail sections of the history, as well as to emphasize areas of possible intervention. For a more comprehensive discussion of approaches to taking a history, see *Wong's Nursing Care of Infants and Children* or *Wong's Essentials of Pediatric Nursing.*[a]

General Guidelines for Communication and Interviewing

Assess ability to speak and understand English.

Conduct the interview in a private, quiet area.

Begin the interview with appropriate introductions.
- Address each person by name.

Clarify the purpose of the interview.

Inform the interviewees of the confidential limits of the interview.

Demonstrate interest in the interview by sitting at eye level and close to interviewees (not across a desk), leaning slightly forward, and speaking in a calm, steady voice.

Begin with a general conversation to put the interviewees at ease.
- Use comments such as, "How have things been since we talked last?" or (to the child) "What do you think is going to happen today?" to let the family express the main concern.
- Include all parties in the interview.
- Direct age-appropriate questions to children (e.g., "What grade are you in at school?" or "What do you like to eat?").

Be sensitive to instances in which family members, such as adolescents, may wish to be interviewed separately.

Recognize and respect cultural patterns of communication (see Tables 1.1 and 1.2 transcultural nursing)

Use open-ended questions or statements that begin with "What," "How," "Tell me about," or "You were saying," and reflect back key words or phrases to encourage discussion.

Encourage continued discussion with nodding and eye contact, saying "Uh-huh," "I see," or "Yes."

Use focused questions (questions that ask for a specific response, e.g., "What did you try next?") and closed-ended questions (questions that ask for a single answer, e.g., "Did you call the doctor?") to direct the focus of the interview.

Ensure mutual understanding by frequently clarifying and summarizing information.

Use active listening to attend to the verbal and nonverbal aspects of the communication.

Verbal cues to important issues include the following techniques:
- Frequent reference to a topic
- Repetition of key words
- Special reference to an event or person

Nonverbal cues to important issues include the following:
- Changes in body position (e.g., looking away or leaning forward)
- Changes in pitch, rate, intonation, and volume of speech (e.g., speaking rapidly, frequent pauses, whispering, or shouting)

Use silence to allow persons to do the following:
- Sort out thoughts and feelings
- Search for responses to questions
- Share feelings expressed by another

Break silence constructively with statements such as, "Is there anything else you wish to say?," "I see you find it difficult to continue; how may I help?," or "I don't know what this silence means. Perhaps there is something you would like to put into words but find difficult to say."

Convey empathy by attending to the verbal and nonverbal language of the interviewee and reflecting back the feeling of the communication (e.g., "I can see how upsetting that must have been for you").

Provide reassurance to acknowledge concerns and any positive efforts used to deal with problems.

Avoid the following blocks to communication (Nurse):
- Socializing
- Giving unrestricted and sometimes unsought advice
- Offering premature or inappropriate reassurance
- Giving overready encouragement
- Defending a situation or opinion
- Using stereotyped comments or clichés

[a] Hockenberry M, Wilson D, Rodgers, C *Wong's Nursing Care of Infants and Children.* 11th ed. St. Louis: Elsevier; 2019; Hockenberry M, Rodgers, C, Weilson D. *Wong's Essentials of Pediatric Nursing.* 11th ed. St. Louis: Elsevier; 2022.

TABLE 1.1 Cross-Cultural Examples of Cultural Phenomena Impacting Nursing Care

Nations of Origin	Communication	Space	Time Orientation	Social Organization	Environmental Control	Biological Variation
Asia						
China Hawaii Philippines Korea Japan Southeast Asia (Laos, Cambodia, Vietnam)	National language preference Dialects, written characters Use of silence Nonverbal and contextual cuing	Noncontact people	Present	Family: hierarchical structure, loyalty Devotion to tradition Many religions including Taoism, Buddhism, Islam, and Christianity Community social organizations	Traditional health and illness beliefs Use of traditional medicines Traditional practitioners: Chinese doctors and herbalists	Liver cancer Stomach cancer Coccidioidomycosis Hypertension Lactose intolerance
Africa						
West Coast (as slaves) Many African countries West Indian Islands Dominican Republic Haiti Jamaica	National languages Dialect: pidgin, Creole, Spanish, and French	Close personal space	Present over future	Family: many females, single parent Large, extended family networks Strong church affiliation within community Community social organizations	Traditional health and illness beliefs Folk medicine tradition Traditional healer: root-worker	Sickle cell anemia Hypertension Cancer of the esophagus Stomach cancer Coccidioidomycosis Lactose intolerance
Europe						
Germany England Italy Ireland Other European countries	National languages Many learn English immediately	Noncontact people Aloof Distant Southern countries: closer contact and touch	Future over present	Nuclear families Extended families Judeo-Christian religions Community social organizations	Primary reliance on modern health care system Traditional health and illness beliefs Some remaining folk medicine traditions	Breast cancer Heart disease Cirrhosis of the liver Diabetes mellitus
American Indian						
500 American Indian tribes Aleuts Eskimos	Tribal languages Use of silence and body language	Space very important and has no boundaries	Present	Extremely family oriented Biological and extended families Children taught to respect traditions Community social organizations	Traditional health and illness beliefs Folk medicine tradition Traditional healer: medicine man	Accidents Heart disease Cirrhosis of the liver Diabetes mellitus
Hispanic countries						
Spain Cuba Mexico Central and South America	Spanish or Portuguese primary languages	Tactile relationships Touch Handshakes Embracing Value physical presence	Present	Nuclear family Extended families Compadrazgo: godparents Community social organizations	Traditional health and illness beliefs Folk medicine traditions Traditional healers: curandero, espiritista, partera, señora	Diabetes mellitus Parasites Coccidioidomycosis Lactose intolerance

Compiled by Rachel Spector RN, In: Potter PA, Perry AG, eds. *Fundamentals of Nursing: Concepts, Process, and Practice.* 4th ed. St. Louis: Mosby; 1997.

TABLE 1.2 Cultural Behaviors Relevant to Health Assessment

Cultural Group	Cultural Variations (Common Beliefs/ Practices)	Nursing Implications
African Americans	Dialect and slang terms require careful communication to prevent error (e.g., "bad" may mean "good").	Question the client's meaning or intent.
Mexican Americans	Eye behavior is important. An individual who looks at and admires a child without touching the child has given the child the "evil eye."	Always touch the child you are examining or admiring.
American Indian	Eye contact is considered a sign of disrespect and is to be avoided.	Recognize that the client may be attentive and interested even though eye contact is avoided.
Appalachians	Eye contact is considered impolite or a sign of hostility. Verbal patter may be confusing.	Clarify statements.
American Eskimos	Body language is very important. The individual seldom disagrees publicly with others. Client may nod yes to be polite, even if not in agreement.	Monitor own body language closely as well as clients to detect meaning.
Jewish Americans	Orthodox Jews consider touching, particularly from members of the opposite sex, offensive.	Establish whether client is an Orthodox Jew and, if so, avoid excessive touch.
Chinese Americans	Individual may nod head to indicate yes or shake head to indicate no. Excessive eye contact indicates rudeness. Excessive touch is offensive.	Ask questions carefully and clarify responses. Avoid excessive eye contact and touch.
Filipino Americans	Offending people is to be avoided at all cost. Nonverbal behavior is very important.	Monitor nonverbal behaviors of self and client, being sensitive to physical and emotional discomfort or concerns of client.
Haitian Americans	Touch is used in conversation. Direct eye contact is used to gain attention and respect during communication.	Use direct eye contact when communicating.
East Indian Hindu Americans	Be aware that men may view eye contact by women as offensive. Avoid eye contact.	Women avoid eye contact as a sign of respect.
Vietnamese Americans	Avoidance of eye contact is a sign of respect. The head is considered sacred; it is not polite to pat the head. An upturned palm is offensive in communication.	Limit eye contact. Touch the head only when mandated and explain clearly before proceeding to do so. Avoid hand gesturing.

From Giger J, Davidhizar R. *Transcultural Nursing.* 2nd ed. St. Louis: Mosby; 1995; also appears in Kozier B, Erb G, Blaise K, et al. *Techniques in Clinical Nursing.* 2nd ed. Reading, MA: Addison-Wesley; 1993.

- Limiting expression of emotion by asking directed, close-ended questions
- Interrupting and finishing the person's sentence
- Talking more than the interviewee
- Forming prejudged conclusions
- Deliberately changing the focus

Watch for signs of information overload (Patient):

- Long periods of silence
- Wide eyes and fixed facial expression
- Constant fidgeting or attempting to move away
- Nervous habits (e.g., tapping, playing with hair)
- Sudden disruptions (e.g., asking to go to the bathroom)
- Looking around
- Yawning, eyes drooping
- Frequently looking at a watch or clock
- Attempting to change the topic of discussion

Close the interview with an opportunity for others to bring up overlooked or sensitive concerns with a statement such as, "Have we covered everything?"

Summarize the interview, especially if problems were identified or interventions were planned.

Discuss the need for follow-up, and schedule a time.

Express appreciation for each person's participation.

Specific Guidelines for Communicating with Children

Allow children time to feel comfortable.
Avoid sudden or rapid advances, broad smiles, extended eye contact, or other gestures that may be seen as threatening.
Talk to the parent if the child is initially shy.
Communicate through transition objects such as dolls, puppets, or stuffed animals before questioning a young child directly.
Give older children the opportunity to talk without the parents present.
Assume a position that is at the same level as the child.
Speak in a quiet, unhurried, and confident voice.
Speak clearly, be specific, and use simple words and short sentences.
State directions and suggestions positively.
Offer a choice only when one exists.
Be honest with children.
Allow children to express their concerns and fears.
Use a variety of communication techniques.

Creative Communication Techniques with Children

Verbal Techniques

"I" Messages

Relate a feeling about a behavior in terms of "I."
Describe the effect the behavior had on the person.
Avoid the use of "you."

- "You" messages are judgmental and provoke defensiveness.
  - Example: "You" message—"You are being uncooperative about doing your treatments."
  - Example: "I" message—"I am concerned about how the treatments are going because I want to see you get better."

Third-Person Technique

Express a feeling in terms of a third person ("he," "she," "they").
This is less threatening than directly asking children how they feel because it gives them an opportunity to agree or disagree without being defensive

- Example: "Sometimes when a person is sick a lot, he feels angry and sad because he cannot do what others can." Either wait silently for a response or encourage a reply with a statement such as, "Did you ever feel that way?"

This approach allows children three choices: (1) to agree and, hopefully, express how they feel; (2) to disagree; or (3) to remain silent, which means they may have such feelings but are unable to express them at this time.

Facilitative Responding

Listen carefully and reflect back to patients the feelings and content of their statements.
Responses are empathic and nonjudgmental and legitimize the person's feelings.
Formula for facilitative responses: "You feel ________ because ________."

- Example: If a child states, "I hate coming to the hospital and getting needles," a facilitative response is, "You feel unhappy because of all the things that are done to you."

Storytelling

Use the language of children to probe into areas of their thinking while bypassing conscious inhibitions or fears.
The simplest technique is asking children to relate a story about an event, such as being in the hospital.
Other approaches:

- Show children a picture of a particular event, such as a child in a hospital with other people in the room, and ask them to describe the scene.
- Cut out pictures or comic strips and have the child add statements for scenes.

Mutual Storytelling

Reveal the child's thinking and attempt to change his or her perceptions or fears by retelling a somewhat different story (more therapeutic approach than storytelling).
Begin by asking the child to tell a story about something; then tell another story that is similar to the child's tale but with differences that help the child in problem areas.

- Example: The child's story is about going to the hospital and never seeing his or her parents again. A nurse's story is also about a child (using different names but similar circumstances) in a hospital whose parents may stay with the child in the hospital or visit frequently until the child is better and goes home with them.

Bibliotherapy

Uses books in a therapeutic and supportive process.
Provide children with an opportunity to explore an event that is similar to their own but sufficiently different to allow them to distance themselves from it and remain in control.
General guidelines for using bibliotherapy are as follows:

- Assess the child's emotional and cognitive development in terms of readiness to understand the book's message.
- Be familiar with the book's content (intended message or purpose) and the age for which it is written.
- Read the book to the child if the child is unable to read.
- Explore the meaning of the book with the child by having the child:
  - Retell the story.
  - Read a special section with the nurse or parent.
  - Draw a picture related to the story and discuss the drawing.
  - Talk about the characters.
  - Summarize the moral or meaning of the story.

Dreams

Dreams often reveal unconscious and repressed thoughts and feelings.

- Ask the child to talk about a dream or nightmare.
- Explore with the child what meaning the dream could have.

"What If?" Questions

Encourage the child to explore potential situations and to consider different problem-solving options.

- Example: "What if you got sick and had to go to the hospital?" Children's responses reveal what they know already and what they are curious about, providing an opportunity for them to learn coping skills, especially in potentially dangerous situations.

Three Wishes

Ask, "If you could have any three things in the world, what would they be?"

If the child answers, "That all my wishes come true," ask the child for specific wishes.

Rating Game

Use some type of rating scale (numbers, sad to happy faces) to have the child rate an event or feeling.

- Example: Instead of asking children how they feel, ask how their day has been "on a scale of 1 to 10, with 10 being the best."

Word Association Game

State key words and ask children to say the first word they think of when they hear the word.

- Start with neutral words, and then introduce more anxiety-producing words, such as "illness," "needles," hospitals," and "operation."
- Select key words that relate to some relevant event in the child's life.

Sentence Completion

Present a partial statement and have the child complete it.

Some sample statements include the following:

- The thing I like best (least) about school is ______________________________.
- The best (worst) age to be is ______________________________.
- The most (least) fun thing I ever did was ______________________________.
- The thing I like most (least) about my parents is ______________________________.
- The one thing I would change about my family is ______________________________.
- If I could be anything I wanted, I would be ______________________________.
- The thing I like most (least) about myself is ______________________________.

Pros and Cons

Select a topic, such as "being in the hospital," and having the child list five good things and five bad things about it.

This is an exceptionally valuable technique when applied to relationships, such as things family members like and dislike about each other.

Nonverbal Techniques

Writing

Writing is an alternative communication approach for older children and adults.

Specific suggestions include the following:

- Keep a journal or diary.
- Write down feelings or thoughts that are difficult to express.
- Write letters that are never mailed (a variation is making up a pen pal to write to).
- Keep an account of the child's progress from both a physical and an emotional viewpoint.

Drawing

Drawing is one of the most valuable forms of communication- both nonverbal (from looking at the drawing) and verbal (from the child's story of the picture).

Children's drawings tell a great deal about them because they are projections of their inner selves.

Spontaneous drawing involves giving the child a variety of art supplies and providing the opportunity to draw.

Directed drawing involves a more specific direction, such as "draw a person" or the "three themes" approach (state three things about the child and ask the child to choose one and draw a picture).

Guidelines for Evaluating Drawings

Use spontaneous drawings, and evaluate more than one drawing whenever possible.

Interpret drawings in light of other available information about the child and family, including the child's age and stage of development.

Interpret drawings as a whole rather than concentrating on specific details of the drawing.

Consider individual elements of the drawings that may be significant:

- **Gender of figure drawn first:** Usually relates to child's perception of own gender role
- **Size of individual figures:** Expresses importance, power, or authority
- **Order in which figures are drawn:** Expresses priority in terms of importance
- **Child's position in relation to other family members:** Expresses feelings of status or alliance
- **Exclusion of a member:** May denote a feeling of not belonging or a desire to eliminate
- **Accentuated parts:** Usually express concern for areas of special importance (e.g., large hands may be a sign of aggression)

- **Absence of or rudimentary arms and hands:** Suggests timidity, passivity, or intellectual immaturity; tiny, unstable feet may be an expression of insecurity, and hidden hands may mean guilty feelings
- **Placement of drawing on the page and type of stroke:** Free use of paper and firm, continuous strokes express security, whereas drawings restricted to a small area and lightly drawn in broken or wavering lines may be a sign of insecurity
- **Erasures, shading, or cross-hatching:** Expresses ambivalence, concern, or anxiety with a particular area

Magic

Use simple magic tricks to help establish rapport with the child, encourage compliance with health interventions, and provide effective distraction during painful procedures.

Although the "magician" talks, no verbal response from the child is required.

Play

Play is the universal language and "work" of children.

It tells a great deal about children because they project their inner selves through the activity.

Spontaneous play involves giving the child a variety of play materials and providing the opportunity to play.

Directed play involves a more specific direction, such as providing medical equipment or a dollhouse for focused reasons, such as exploring a child's fear of injections or exploring family relationships.

Guidelines for Using an Interpreter

Explain to the interpreter the reason for the interview and the type of questions that will be asked.

Clarify whether a detailed or brief answer is required and whether the translated response can be general or literal.

Introduce the interpreter to the family, and allow some time before the interview for them to become acquainted.

Communicate directly with family members when asking questions to reinforce interest in them and to observe nonverbal expressions, but do not ignore the interpreter.

Pose questions to elicit only one answer at a time, such as "Do you have pain?" rather than "Do you have any pain, tiredness, or loss of appetite?"

Refrain from interrupting family members and interpreters while they are conversing.

Avoid commenting to the interpreter about family members, since they may understand some English.

Be aware that some medical words, such as "allergy," may have no similar word in another language; avoid medical jargon whenever possible.

Be aware that cultural differences may exist regarding views on sex, marriage, or pregnancy.

Allow time after the interview for the interpreter to share something that he or she thought could not be said earlier; ask about the interpreter's impression of nonverbal clues to communication and family members' reliability or ease in revealing information.

Arrange for the family to speak with the same interpreter on subsequent visits whenever possible.

Outline of a Health History

A. **Identifying information**
   1. Name
   2. Address
   3. Telephone number
   4. Birth date
   5. Birthplace
   6. Race or ethnic group
   7. Gender
   8. Religion
   9. Nationality
   10. Date of interview
   11. Informant

B. **Chief complaint (CC): To establish the major specific reason for the child's and parents' seeking of health care**

C. **Present illness (PI): To obtain all details related to the chief complaint**
   1. Details of present illness onset
   2. Complete interval history
   3. Present illness status
   4. Reason for seeking health care now

D. **Past history (PH): To elicit a profile of the child's previous illnesses, injuries, or surgeries**
   1. Birth history (pregnancy, labor and delivery, perinatal history)
   2. Previous illnesses, injuries, or surgeries
   3. Allergies
   4. Current medications
   5. Immunizations
   6. Growth and development
   7. Habits

E. **Review of systems (ROS): To elicit information concerning any potential health problem**
   1. Constitutional
   2. Integument
   3. Head
   4. Eyes
   5. Nose
   6. Ears
   7. Mouth
   8. Throat

9. Neck
10. Chest
11. Respiratory
12. Cardiovascular
13. Gastrointestinal
14. Genitourinary
15. Gynecologic
16. Musculoskeletal
17. Neurologic
18. Endocrine
19. Hematologic/lymphatic
20. Allergic/ immunologic
21. Psychiatric

F. Family medical history: To identify genetic traits or diseases that have familial tendencies and to assess exposure to a communicable disease in a family member and family habits (such as smoking and chemical use) that may affect the child's health

G. Psychosocial history: To elicit information about the child's self-concept

H. Sexual history: To elicit information concerning the child's sexual concerns or activities and any pertinent data regarding an adult's sexual activity that influences the child

I. Family assessment[b]: To develop an understanding of the child as an individual and as a member of the family and community

1. Family composition
2. Home and community environment
3. Occupation and education of family members
4. Cultural and religious traditions
5. Family function and relationships

J. Nutrition assessment[b]: To elicit information on the adequacy of the child's nutritional intake and needs

1. Dietary intake
2. Clinical examination

K. Patient profile (summary)

1. Health status
2. Psychologic status
3. Socioeconomic status[b]

[b] Because of the importance of Nutritional Assessment and Family Assessment, separate sections are devoted to these two topics.

Summary of a Health History

Information	Comments
Identifying Information	
1. Name 2. Address 3. Telephone number 4. Birth date 5. Birthplace 6. Race or ethnic group 7. Gender 8. Religion 9. Date of interview 10. Informant	Additional information appropriate to older adolescent may include occupation, marital status, and temporary and permanent addresses. Under "informant," include subjective impression of reliability, general attitude, willingness to communicate, overall accuracy of data, and any special circumstances, such as use of an interpreter. Informants should include parent and child, as well as others who may be primary caregivers, such as a grandparent.
Chief Complaint (CC)	
To establish the major specific reason for the child and parents seeking professional health attention	Record in patient's own words; include duration of symptoms. If informant has difficulty isolating one problem, ask which problem or symptom led person to seek help now. In case of routine physical examination, state CC as reason for visit.
Present Illness (PI)	
To obtain all details related to the chief complaint 1. Onset a. Date of onset b. Manner of onset (gradual or sudden) c. Precipitating and predisposing factors related to onset (emotional disturbance, physical exertion, fatigue, bodily function, pregnancy, environment, injury, infection, toxins and allergens, therapeutic agents)	In its broadest sense, illness denotes any problem of a physical, emotional, or psychosocial nature. Present information in chronological order; may be referenced according to one point in time, such as prior to admission (PTA). Concentrate on reason for seeking help now, especially if problem has existed for some time.

Summary of a Health History—cont'd

Information	Comments
2. Characteristics a. Character (e.g., quality, quantity, consistency) b. Location and radiation (e.g., pain) c. Intensity or severity d. Timing (continuous or intermittent, duration, temporal relationship to other events) e. Aggravating and relieving factors f. Associated symptoms	
3. Course since onset a. Incidence: single or recurrent acute attack(s), daily or periodic occurrences, continuous chronic episode b. Progress (better, worse, unchanged) c. Effect of therapy	
Past History (PH)	
To elicit a profile of the child's previous illnesses, injuries, or surgeries	Importance of perinatal history depends on child's age; the younger the child, the more important the perinatal history.
1. Birth history a. Pregnancy number (gravida) and delivery dates b. Outcome (parity) Gestation (full-term, preterm, postterm) Stillbirths, Abortions c. Health during pregnancy d. Medications taken	Explain relevance of birth history in revealing important factors relating to the child's health. Assess parents' emotional attitudes toward the pregnancy and birth.
2. Labor and delivery a. Duration of labor b. Type and place of delivery c. Medications	Assess parents' feelings regarding delivery; investigate factors that may affect bonding, such as separation from infant.
3. Perinatal period a. Weight and length at birth b. Condition of health immediately after birth d. Apgar score e. Presence of problems, including congenital anomalies f. Date of discharge from nursery g. Time of regaining birth weight	If birth problems are reported, inquire about treatment, such as use of oxygen, phototherapy, and surgery, and parents' emotional response to the event.
4. Previous illnesses, injuries, or surgeries a. Onset, symptoms, course, termination b. Occurrence of complications c. Incidence of disease in other family members or in community d. Emotional response to previous hospitalization e. Circumstances and nature of injuries	Ask about colds, earaches, and childhood diseases (e.g., diphtheria, tuberculosis, scarlet fever, measles, rubella (German measles), chickenpox, mumps, tonsillitis, strep throat, pertussis, or allergic manifestations). Elicit a description of disease to verify the diagnosis. Be alert to areas of injury prevention.
5. Allergies a. Hay fever, asthma, or eczema b. Unusual reactions to foods, drugs, animals, plants, latex products, or household products	Have parent describe the type of allergic reaction and its severity.
6. Current medications a. Name, dose, schedule, duration, and reason for administration	Assess parents' knowledge of correct dosage of common drugs, such as acetaminophen; note underuse or overuse.
7. Cultural remedies[a] a. Herbs, natural products, special foods, drinks	Ask about names of the products used, frequency given, and dosages.
8. Pain a. Previous experiences b. Reactions c. Effective management d. Cultural influences	When age-appropriate, elicit information from child as well as parent. Does the child tend to be stoic or expressive with pain? What is the family's attitude about taking pain medications?

Continued

Summary of a Health History—cont'd

Information	Comments
9. Immunizations a. Name, number of doses, age when given b. Occurrence of reaction c. Administration of horse or other foreign serum, gamma-globulin, or blood transfusion	Since parents may be unaware of name and date of each immunization, whenever possible, confirm information by checking medical or school records. **NURSING ALERT** Information about allergic reactions to drugs or other products is essential. Failure to document a serious reaction places the child at risk if the agent is given.
10. Growth and development a. Weight at birth, 6 months, 1 year, and present b. Dentition: age of eruption/shedding, number, problems with teething c. Age of head control, sitting unsupported, walking, first words	Compare parents' responses with your own observations of child's achievement and results from objective tests, such as Developmental screening (see Assessment of Development).
d. Present grade in school, scholastic achievement e. Interaction with peers and adults f. Participation in organized activities, such as Scouting, sports	School and social history can be more thoroughly explored under Family Assessment.
11. Habits a. Behavior patterns: nail biting, tumb sucking, pica, unusual movements	Assess for any habits and behavioral patterns such as nail biting, thumb sucking, pica (habitual ingestion of nonfood substances) rituals (e.g., security blanket or special toy), unusual movements (e.g., head banging, rocking), temper tantrums
b. Activities of daily living: sleep patterns (e.g., hour of sleep and arising, duration of nighttime sleep or naps), elimination patterns (e.g., age of toilet training, daytime or nighttime bedwetting or stool incontinence) Exercise (type and duration)	Assess for sleep problems (e.g., trouble falling asleep or staying asleep, any sleep terrors, sleepwalking, or nightmares. Record child's terms for urination and defecation.
c. Use or abuse of drugs, alcohol, caffeine drinks, energy drinks, tobacco, vaping, vitamins, supplements, or alternative therapies. d. Usual disposition; response to frustration	With adolescents, ask about quantity and frequency of smoking, alcohol and chemicals used or any past experimentation
Review of Systems (ROS)	
The ROS is a specific review of each body system, following an order similar to that of the physical examination (Box 1.1)	Explain relevance of questioning to parents (similar to the explanation concerning the relevance of the birth history) in composing total health history of child. Make positive statements about each system (e.g., "Mother denies headaches, bumping into objects, or squinting").
Nutrition Assessment	
To elicit information about adequacy of child's dietary intake and eating patterns (see Nutrition-Focused Clinical Findings p. 121)	After collecting the data needed for a thorough nutritional assessment, evaluate the findings (e.g., malnourished, well-nourished, risk of malnourished, overweight, obese) and plan appropriate counseling.
Family Health History	
To discover any genetic or chronic diseases affecting the child's family members; to assess family habits and exposure to a communicable disease that may affect family members	Choose terms wisely when asking about child's parentage: for example, inquire about paternal history by referring to the child's "father" rather than mother's husband; use the term "partner" rather than "spouse."
1. Family pedigree and guidelines for construction	A pedigree is a pictorial representation or diagram of a family tree to visualize patterns of disease transmission.

BOX 1.1 Review of Systems

General—Overall state of health, fatigue, recent and/or unexplained weight gain or loss (period of time for either), contributing factors (change of diet, illness, altered appetite), exercise tolerance, fevers (time of day), chills, night sweats (unrelated to climatic conditions), frequent infections, general ability to carry out activities of daily living

Integument—Pruritus, pigment or other color changes, acne, moles, discoloration, eruptions, rashes (location), tendency toward bruising, petechiae, excessive dryness, general texture, disorders or deformities of nails, hair growth or loss, hair color change (for adolescent, use of hair dyes or other potentially toxic substances such as hair straighteners)

Head—Headaches, dizziness, injury (specific details)

Eyes—Visual problems (ask about behaviors indicative of blurred vision, such as bumping into objects, clumsiness, sitting very close to the television, holding a book close to the face, writing with head near the desk, squinting, rubbing the eyes, bending the head in an awkward position), cross-eye (strabismus), eye infections, edema of lids, excessive tearing, use of glasses or contact lenses, date of last optic examination

Nose—Nosebleeds (epistaxis), constant or frequent running or stuffy nose, nasal obstruction (difficulty breathing), alteration or loss of sense of smell

Ears—Earaches, discharge, evidence of hearing loss (ask about behaviors such as the need to repeat requests, loud speech, inattentive behavior), results of any previous auditory testing, pulling or rubbing the ear

Mouth—Mouth breathing, gum bleeding, toothaches, toothbrushing, use of fluoride, difficulty with teething (symptoms), last visit to the dentist (especially if temporary dentition is complete), response to dentist

Throat—Sore throats, difficulty in swallowing, choking (especially when chewing food—may be from poor chewing habits), hoarseness, or other voice irregularities

Neck—Pain, limitation of movement, stiffness, difficulty in holding head straight (torticollis), thyroid enlargement, enlarged nodes or other masses

Chest—Breast enlargement, discharge, masses, enlarged axillary nodes (for adolescent female, ask about breast self-examination)

Respiratory—Chronic cough, frequent colds (number per year), wheezing, shortness of breath at rest or on exertion, difficulty in breathing, sputum production, infections (pneumonia, tuberculosis), date of last chest x-ray examination, and skin reaction from tuberculin testing

Cardiovascular—Cyanosis or fatigue on exertion, history of a heart murmur or rheumatic fever, anemia, date of last blood count, blood type, recent transfusion

Gastrointestinal—Nausea, vomiting (not associated with eating, may be indicative of brain tumor or increased intracranial pressure), jaundice or yellowing skin or sclera, belching, flatulence, a recent change in bowel habits (blood in stools, change in color, diarrhea, and constipation)

Genitourinary—Pain on urination, frequency, hesitancy, urgency, hematuria, nocturia, polyuria, unpleasant odor to urine, the force of stream, discharge, change in the size of the scrotum, date of last urinalysis (for adolescent, sexually transmitted disease, type of treatment; for male adolescent, ask about testicular self-examination)

Gynecologic—Menarche, date of last menstrual period, regularity or problems with menstruation, vaginal discharge, pruritus, date and result of last Pap smear (include obstetric history as discussed under birth history when applicable); if sexually active, type of contraception

Musculoskeletal—Weakness, clumsiness, lack of coordination, unusual movements, back or joint stiffness, muscle pains or cramps, abnormal gait, deformity, fractures, serious sprains, activity level, redness, swelling, tenderness

Neurologic—Seizures, tremors, dizziness, loss of memory, general affect, fears, nightmares, speech problems, any unusual habit

Endocrine—Intolerance to weather changes, excessive thirst and urination, excessive sweating, salty taste to skin, signs of early puberty

Lymphatic—History of frequent infections, enlarged lymph nodes in any region, swelling, tenderness, red streaks

Summary of a Health History—cont'd

Information	Comments
2. Information includes any evidence of conditions such as early heart disease, stroke, sudden death from unknown cause, hypertension, cancer, diabetes mellitus, obesity, congenital anomalies, allergy, asthma, tuberculosis, seizures, abnormal bleeding, sickle cell disease, cognitive impairment, hearing or visual deficits, psychiatric disorders (e.g., depression, emotional problems). Confirm the accuracy of reported disorders by inquiring about the symptoms, course, treatment, and sequelae of each diagnosis.	
3. Family habits, such as smoking or chemical use	
4. Geographic location, including birthplace, present location, and travel (domestic or international) or contact with foreign visitors	Important for identification of possible exposure to any diseases

Continued

Summary of a Health History—cont'd

Information	Comments
Alternative Therapies[a]	
The American Academy of Pediatrics (2017) has the following recommendations when discussing alternative and complementary therapies: 1. Obtain reliable, evidence-based information and be prepared to share it with families. 2. Evaluate the scientific merits of specific therapeutic approaches. 3. Identify risks or potential harmful effects. 4. Provide families with information on treatment options. 5. Educate families to evaluate information and treatment options. 6. Discuss complementary and alternative therapies (CAM) maintaining a respect for the family's culture and values. 7. Ask about all therapies in use to reduce any potential supplement-drug interactions. 8. Monitor and evaluate the patient's response to treatment and outcome. 9. Actively listen to the family and child.	These recommendations should be used by nurses when discussing CAM with families. Remember, introducing the subject of CAM requires tactful communication skills. Rather than asking whether a patient is using any alternative therapies, the nurse may ask whether the patient uses any vitamins, herbs, supplements, teas, massage, acupuncture, or other services to enhance the patient's health. When families are using an unfamiliar intervention, ask for their sources of information and review them before giving advice. In general, if a therapy produces no adverse effect, including significant financial burden, do not discourage its use. Maintain a trusting, supportive relationship with the family using ongoing communication centered on the patient's well-being.
Family Personal and Social History	
To gain an understanding of the family's structure and function (see Family Assessment p. 111)	
Sexual History	
To elicit information concerning young person's concerns and/or activities and any pertinent data regarding adult's sexual activity that influence child 1. Sexual concerns and activity of child 2. Sexual concerns and activity of adults if warranted	Sexual history is an essential component of preadolescents' and adolescents' health assessments. Degree of investigation into parents' sexual history depends on its relevance to the child's health. It may be limited to family planning concerns, or it may be more detailed if overt sexual activity or abuse is suspected. Investigate toward end of history when rapport is greatest. Respect sensitive and complex nature of questioning. Give parents and child the option of discussing sexual matters alone with nurse. Ensure confidentiality. Clarify terms such as "sexually active" or "having sex." Refer to sexual contacts as "partners" not "girlfriends" or "boyfriends." Discussion may flow easily after review of genitourinary tract, such as asking female about menstruation or male about urinary problems. Suggestions for beginning discussion include the following: "Tell me about your social life." "Who are your closest friends?" "Is there one very special friend?" Take detailed history of all contacts if sexually transmitted disease is suspected or diagnosed.
Patient Profile (Summary)	
To summarize the interviewer's overall impression of the child's and family's physical, psychological, and socioeconomic background 1. Health status 2. Psychologic status 3. Socioeconomic status	A comprehensive summary often identifies nursing diagnoses based on subjective and objective findings.

[a]McClafferty H, Vohra S, Bailey M, et al. Pediatric integrative medicine. *Pediatrics*. 2017;140(3):e20171961.

Habits to Explore During a Health Interview

Behavior patterns such as nail biting, thumb sucking, pica (habitual ingestion of nonfood substances), rituals ("security" blanket or toy), and unusual movements (head banging, rocking, overt masturbation, and walking on toes)

Activities of daily living, such as hours of sleep and arising, duration of nighttime sleep and naps, type and duration of exercise, regularity of stools and urination, age of toilet training, and daytime or nighttime bed-wetting

Unusual disposition; response to frustration

Use or abuse of alcohol, drugs, caffeine drinks, or tobacco

Taking an Allergy History

Identifying a Medication Allergy

Has your child ever taken any prescription or over-the-counter medications that have disagreed with him or her or caused an allergic reaction? If yes, can you remember the name(s) of the medication(s)?

Can you describe the reaction?

Was the medication taken by mouth (as a tablet or syrup), or was it an injection?

How soon after starting the medication did the reaction happen?

How long ago did this happen?

Did anyone tell you it was an allergic reaction, or did you decide for yourself?

Has your child ever taken this medication, or a similar one, again? If yes, did your child experience the same problems?

Have you told the physicians or nurses about your child's reaction or allergy?

Has the child's medication reaction been confirmed by laboratory evidence?

Identifying Food Allergy

Has your child taken any foods/fluids that caused an allergic reaction? If yes, do you remember the food or liquid? (Nuts, eggs, wheat, soy, and dairy products are the most common allogenic sources.)

Describe the reaction.

Did the reaction occur immediately (within minutes to hours) or was the reaction delayed (2 to 48 hours)?

How long ago did this reaction occur?

Have you informed the physician or nurse about your child's reaction or allergy?

Identifying Latex Allergy

Does the child have any symptoms (e.g., sneezing, coughing, rashes, wheezing) when handling rubber products (balloons, tennis balls, adhesive bandage strips) or when in contact with rubber hospital products, such as gloves and catheters?

Has your child ever had an allergic reaction during surgery?

How would you identify or recognize an allergic reaction in your child?

What would you do if an allergic reaction occurred?

Has anyone ever discussed latex or rubber allergy or sensitivity with you?

Has the child had any allergy testing?

When did the child last come in contact with any type of rubber product? Were you present?

Cultural Assessment

Cultural assessment helps identify the family's understanding of the health-related problem in relation to how their culture may affect the plan of care. The cultural assessment identifies the family beliefs, values, norms, and practices that may facilitate or interfere with health care. Careful assessment can assist the nurse in better understanding the patient and family.

Strategies for Gathering Cultural Information

Listen to the patient and family's understanding of the health problem.

Use cultural resources to promote understanding of different ethnic and religious cultures.

Assess cultural influences throughout the comprehensive nursing assessment.

Culturally Sensitive Interactions

Nonverbal Strategies

Invite family members to choose where they would like to sit or stand, allowing them to select a comfortable distance.

Observe interactions with others to determine which body gestures (e.g., shaking hands) are acceptable and appropriate. Ask when in doubt. Know when physical contact is prohibited.

Avoid appearing rushed.

Be an active listener.

Observe for cues regarding appropriate eye contact.

Avoiding eye contact may be a sign of respect.

Learn the appropriate use of pauses or interruptions for different cultures.

Ask for clarification if the nonverbal meaning is unclear.

Learn if smiling indicates friendliness.

Verbal Strategies

Learn proper terms of address.

Use a positive tone of voice to convey interest.

Speak slowly and carefully, not loudly, when families have poor language comprehension.

Encourage questions.

Learn basic words and sentences of the family's language, if possible.

Avoid professional terms.

When asking questions, tell the family why the questions are being asked, the way the information they provide will be used, and how it might benefit their child.

Repeat important information more than once.

Always give the reason or purpose for a treatment or prescription.

Use the information written in the family's language if possible.

Arrange for the services of an interpreter when necessary.

Learn from families and representatives about their cultural methods of communicating information without creating discomfort.

Address intergenerational needs (e.g., family's need to consult with others).

Be sincere, open, and honest to establish rapport and trust.

Cultural Assessment Outline

Communication

What language is spoken at home?

How does the family demonstrate respect or disrespect?

How well does the family understand English (spoken and written)?

Is an interpreter needed?

Health Beliefs

How are health and illness defined by the family?

How are feelings expressed regarding illness or death?

What are the attitudes toward sickness?

Who makes the decisions regarding health practices in the family?

Are there cultural practices that would restrict the type of care needed?

Is a health professional of the same gender or ethnic background an issue for the family?

Religious Practices and Rituals

What is the family's religious preference?

Who does the family turn to for support and counseling?

Are there special practices or rituals that may affect care?

Are there special rituals or ceremonies when a patient is ill or dying?

Are special rituals or ceremonies attached to birth, baptism, puberty, or death?

Dietary Practices

Are some foods restricted by the family's culture?

Are there cultural practices in observance of certain occasions or events?

How is food prepared?

Who is responsible for food preparation?

Do certain foods have special meaning to the family or child?

Are special foods believed to cause or cure an illness or disease?

Are there times of required food fasting?

How are the periods of fasting defined, and who fasts in the family?

Family Characteristics

Who makes the decisions in the family?

How many generations are considered to be a single family?

Which relatives compose the family unit?

When are children disciplined or punished?

How is affection demonstrated in the family?

How are emotions exhibited in the family?

What is the attitude toward children?

Sources of Support

To what ethnic or cultural organizations does the family belong?

How do the organizations influence the family's approach to health care?

Who is most responsible for influencing the family's health beliefs?

Is there a specific cultural group with which the family identifies?

Is the specific cultural group identified by where the child was born and has lived?

Resources for Cultural Information

Clarke S. Cultural congruent care: a reflection on patient outcome. *J Healthc Commun.* 2017;2(4):51.

Dibble SL, Hayre-Kwan S, Lipson JG, eds. *Culture & Clinical Care.* 3rd ed. UCSF Nursing Press, San Francisco. 2019.

Giger JN, Haddah LG. *Transcultural Nursing: Assessment and Intervention.* 8th ed. St. Louis: Elsevier; 2021.

Marion L, Douglas M, Lavin MA, et al. Implementing the new ANA standard 8: culturally congruent practice. *Online J Issues Nurs.* 2017;22(1):9.

McFarland MR, Wehbe-Akamahm HB. Leininger's theory of culture care diversity and universality: a overview with a historical retrospective and a view toward the future. *J Transcult Nurs.* 2019;30(6):540–557.

Pacquiao DF, Katz JR, Sattler V, et al. Development of the clients' perceptions of providers' culture competency instrument. *J Transcult Nurs.* 2021;32(5):539–550.

Physical Assessment

Physical assessment is a continuous process that begins during the interview, primarily by using inspection or observation. During the more formal examination, the tools of percussion, palpation, and auscultation are added to enhance and refine the assessment of body systems. Like the health history, the objective of the physical assessment is to formulate nursing diagnoses and evaluate the effectiveness of therapeutic interventions.

Because of important differences in the physical assessment of the child and newborn, separate guidelines and summaries for conducting the physical examination of each age group are presented.

The summary of the physical assessment of the newborn is also presented according to the area to be assessed, usual findings, common variations and minor abnormalities, and potential signs of distress or major abnormalities. Common variations and minor abnormalities should be recorded but generally do not require further evaluation. Potential signs of distress or major abnormalities are recorded and need to be reported for further evaluation. The procedures for assessment are not presented here but in the summary of the physical assessment of the child. In addition to the newborn summary, an assessment of clinical gestational age is also described.

The summary of the physical assessment of the child is presented according to the area to be assessed, the procedure for assessment, usual findings, and comments. The comments column includes findings that deviate from the normal and should be reported, the special significance of certain findings, and areas for nursing intervention. This section includes detailed instructions for various assessment procedures.

For a more comprehensive discussion of performing a physical assessment, see *Wong's Nursing Care of Infants and Children 11e*, or *Wong's Essentials of Pediatric Nursing 11e*.

General Guidelines for Physical Examination of the Newborn

Provide a comfortably normothermic and nonstimulating examination area.

- To prevent heat loss, undress only the body area to be examined unless the newborn is already under a heat source, such as a radiant warmer.
- Proceed quickly to avoid stressing the infant.
- Check that equipment and supplies are working properly and are accessible
- Proceed in an orderly sequence (usually head to toe) with the following exceptions:
- Observe the infant's attitude and position of flexion first to avoid disturbing him or her.
- Perform all procedures that require quiet observation (such as auscultating the lungs, heart, and abdomen).
- Perform disturbing procedures, such as testing reflexes, last.
- Measure head, crown-to-rump, and head-to-heel length at the same time to compare results.
- Comfort the infant during and after the examination; involve a parent in the following:
- Talking softly.
- Hold the infant's hands against the chest.
- Swaddling and holding the infant.
- Providing nonnutritive sucking such as a pacifier if needed.

Summary of Physical Assessment of the Newborn

Usual Findings	Common Variations and Minor Abnormalities	Potential Signs of Distress or Major Abnormalities
General Measurements		
Head circumference—33 to 35 cm (13–14 inches); equal or up to 2 cm (0.8 inches) larger than crown-to-rump length	Molding after birth may alter head circumference.	Head circumference <10th or >90th percentile
Crown-to-rump length—31 to 35 cm (12.5–14 inches); approximately equal to head circumference		
Head-to-heel length—48 to 53 cm (19–21 inches)		
Birth weight—2700 to 4000 g (6–9 pounds)	Loss of 10% of birth weight in first week; regained in 10–14 days, depending on feeding method	Birth weight <10th or >90th percentile Loss of >10% of birth weight in the first week

Continued

Summary of Physical Assessment of the Newborn—cont'd

Usual Findings	Common Variations and Minor Abnormalities	Potential Signs of Distress or Major Abnormalities
Vital Signs		
Temperature (axillary)—36.5°C to 37°C (97.9°F–98°F)	Crying may increase body temperature slightly. Radiant warmer may falsely increase axillary temperature.	Hypothermia Hyperthermia
Heart rate (apical)—120 to 140 beats/min	Crying will increase heart rate; sleep will decrease heart rate. During first period of reactivity (6–8 h), rate can reach 180 beats/min.	Bradycardia—Resting rate <80–100 beats/min Tachycardia—Rate >160–180 beats/min Irregular rhythm
Respirations—30 to 60 breaths/min	Crying will increase respiratory rate; sleep will decrease respiratory rate. During first period of reactivity (6–8 h), rate can reach 80 breaths/min.	Irregular rhythm Apnea >15 s
Blood pressure (oscillometric)—65/41 mm Hg in arm and calf	Crying and activity will increase blood pressure. Placing cuff on thigh may agitate infant; thigh blood pressure may be higher than arm or calf blood pressure by 4–8 mm Hg and is least preferred method. See Guidelines box.	Oscillometric systolic pressure in calf 6–9 mm Hg less than in upper extremity (possible sign of coarctation of aorta). Systolic pressure >90 mm Hg is considered hypertension.
General Appearance		
Posture—Flexion of head and extremities, which rest on chest and abdomen	*Frank breech*—Extended legs, abducted and fully rotated thighs, flattened occiput, extended neck	Limp posture, extension of extremities
Skin		
At birth, bright red, puffy, smooth Second to third day, pink, flaky, dry Vernix caseosa Lanugo Edema around eyes, face, legs, dorsa of hands, feet, and scrotum or labia *Acrocyanosis*—Cyanosis of hands and feet *Cutis marmorata*—Transient mottling when infant is exposed to stress, decreased temperature	Neonatal jaundice after first 24 h Ecchymoses or petechiae caused by birth trauma *Milia*—Distended sebaceous glands that appear as tiny white papules on cheeks, chin, and nose *Miliaria* or *sudamina*—Distended sweat (eccrine) glands that appear as minute vesicles, especially on face *Erythema toxicum*—Pink papular rash with vesicles superimposed on thorax, back, buttocks, and abdomen; may appear in 24–48 h and resolve after several days *Harlequin color change*—Clearly outlined color change as infant lies on side; lower half of body becomes pink and upper half is pale *Mongolian spots*—Irregular areas of deep blue pigmentation, usually in sacral and gluteal regions; seen predominantly in newborns of African, Native American, Asian, or Hispanic descent *Telangiectatic nevi* (stork bite or salmon patch)—Flat, deep pink, localized areas usually seen on nape of neck, upper eyelid, glabella, or on the upper lip; blanches with pressure and frequently becomes more prominent with crying	Progressive jaundice, especially in first 24 h after birth Generalized cyanosis Pallor Mottling Grayness Plethora Hemorrhage, ecchymoses, or petechiae that persist *Sclerema*—Hard and stiff skin Poor skin turgor (tenting) Rashes, pustules, or blisters *Café-au-lait spots*—Light brown spots *Nevus flammeus*—Port-wine stain Herpetic blister(s) Capillary hemangiomas-Bright red, raised, soft, lobulated tumor occurring on the head, neck, trunk, or extremities; does not blanch with pressure

Summary of Physical Assessment of the Newborn—cont'd

Usual Findings	Common Variations and Minor Abnormalities	Potential Signs of Distress or Major Abnormalities
Head		
Anterior fontanel—Diamond shaped, size varies from barely palpable to 4–5 cm (0.5–2 inches) (Fig. 1.1) *Posterior fontanel*—Triangular, 0.5–1 cm (0.2–0.4 inches) Fontanels should be flat and firm. Widest part of fontanel measured from bone to bone, not suture to suture	Molding following vaginal delivery Third sagittal (parietal) fontanel Bulging fontanel because of crying or coughing *Caput succedaneum*—Edema of soft scalp tissue *Cephalhematoma (uncomplicated)*— Hematoma between periosteum and skull bone	Fused sutures Bulging or depressed fontanels when quiet Widened sutures and fontanels. *Craniotabes*—Snapping sensation along lambdoidal suture that resembles indentation of Ping-Pong ball
Eyes		
Lids usually edematous Iris color—Slate gray, dark blue, brown Absence of tears Presence of red reflex Corneal reflex in response to touch Pupillary reflex in response to light Blink reflex in response to light or touch Rudimentary fixation on objects and ability to follow to midline	Epicanthal folds in Asian infants Searching nystagmus or strabismus *Subconjunctival (scleral) hemorrhages*—Ruptured capillaries, usually at limbus	Pink color of iris Purulent discharge Upward slant in non-Asians Hypertelorism (3 cm [1.8 inches] or greater) Hypotelorism *Congenital cataracts*(unilateral or bilateral) Constricted or dilated fixed pupil Absence of red reflex Absence of pupillary or corneal reflex Inability to follow object or bright light to midline Yellow sclera Leukocoria (white pupil)- possible retinoblastoma
Ears		
Position—Top of pinna on horizontal line with outer canthus of eye Startle (Moro) reflex elicited by a loud, sudden noise or stimulus Pinna flexible, cartilage present	Inability to visualize tympanic membrane because of filled aural canals Pinna flat against head Irregular shape or size Pits or skin tags	Low placement of ears Absence of startle (Moro)reflex in response to loud, sudden noise or stimulus Minor abnormalities possible signs of various syndromes, especially renal
Nose		
Nasal patency Nasal discharge—Thin, white mucus Sneezing	**Flattened and bruised**	**Nonpatent canals** Thick, bloody nasal discharge Flaring of nares *(alae nasi)* Single nasal canal Copious nasal secretions or stuffiness (may be minor)

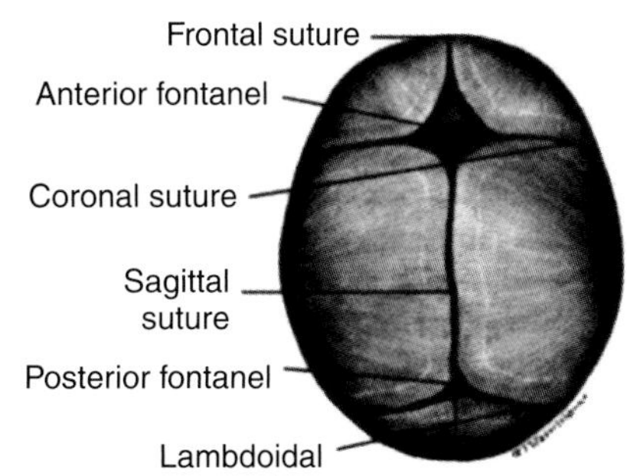

FIG. **1.1** Locations of sutures and fontanels.

Continued

Summary of Physical Assessment of the Newborn—cont'd

Usual Findings	Common Variations and Minor Abnormalities	Potential Signs of Distress or Major Abnormalities
Mouth and Throat		
Intact, high-arched palate Uvula in midline Frenulum of tongue Frenulum of upper lip Sucking reflex—Strong and coordinated Rooting reflex Gag reflex Extrusion reflex Absent or minimal salivation Vigorous cry	*Natal teeth*—Teeth present at birth; benign but may be associated with congenital defects *Epstein pearls*—Small, white epithelial cysts along midline of hard palate	Cleft lip Cleft palate Large, protruding tongue or posterior displacement of tongue Profuse salivation or drooling *Candidiasis (thrush)*—White, adherent patches on tongue, palate, and buccal surfaces Inability to pass nasogastric tube to stomach Hoarse, high-pitched, weak, absent, or other abnormal cry Stridor Micrognathia-small lower jaw seen in Pierre-Robin sequence (see *Wong's Nursing Care of Infants and Children* or *Wong's Essentials of Pediatric Nursing*)
Neck		
Short, thick, usually surrounded by skinfolds Tonic neck reflex	*Torticollis (wry neck)*—Head held to one side with chin pointing to opposite side	Excessive skinfolds or webbing Resistance to flexion Absence of tonic neck reflex Fractured clavicle; crepitus
Chest		
Anteroposterior and lateral diameters equal Slight sternal retractions evident during inspiration Xiphoid process evident Breast enlargement	Funnel chest (pectus excavatum) Pigeon chest (pectus carinatum) Supernumerary nipples Secretion of milky substance from breasts ("witch's milk")	Depressed sternum Marked retractions of chest and intercostal spaces during respiration Asymmetric chest expansion Redness and firmness around nipples Wide-spaced nipples
Lungs		
Respirations chiefly abdominal Cough reflex absent at birth, present by 1–2 days Bilateral, equal bronchial breath sounds	Rate and depth of respirations may be irregular; periodic breathing. Crackles shortly after birth	Inspiratory stridor Expiratory grunt Retractions Persistent irregular breathing Periodic breathing with repeated apneic spells Seesaw respirations (paradoxic) Apnea Unequal breath sounds Persistent fine, medium, or course crackles Wheezing Diminished breath sounds Peristaltic bowel sounds on one side with diminished breath sounds on same side

Summary of Physical Assessment of the Newborn—cont'd

Usual Findings	Common Variations and Minor Abnormalities	Potential Signs of Distress or Major Abnormalities
Heart		
Apex—Fourth to fifth intercostal space, lateral to left sternal border S2 slightly sharper and higher in pitch than S1	*Sinus arrhythmia*—Heart rate increasing with inspiration and decreasing with expiration. Transient cyanosis on crying or straining	*Dextrocardia*—Heart on right side Displacement of apex, muffled heart sound Cardiomegaly Abdominal shunts Murmur Thrill Persistent central cyanosis Hyperactive precordium
Abdomen		
Cylindric (rounded) in shape *Liver*—Palpable 2–3 cm (0.8–1.8 inches) below right costal margin *Spleen*—Tip palpable at end of first week of age *Kidneys*—Palpable 1–2 cm (0.4–0.8 inches) above umbilicus *Umbilical cord*—Bluish white at birth with two arteries and one vein *Femoral pulses*—Equal bilaterally	Umbilical hernia *Diastasis recti*—Midline gap between recti muscles *Wharton's jelly*—Unusually thick umbilical cord	Abdominal distension Localized bulging Distended veins Absent bowel sounds Enlarged liver and spleen Ascites Visible peristaltic waves Scaphoid or concave abdomen (possible congenital diaphragmatic hernia) Moist umbilical cord Presence of only one artery in cord Urine, stool or pus leaking from cord or cord insertion site Periumbilical erythema Palpable bladder distention after scant voiding Absent femoral pulses Cord bleeding or hematoma Omphalocele or gastroschisis-protrusion of abdominal contents through umbilical cord or abdominal wall *Bladder exstrophy* (exteriorized bladder; also associated with epispadias or cloaca)
Female Genitalia		
Labia and clitoris usually edematous Urethral meatus behind clitoris Vernix caseosa between labia Urination within 24 h	*Pseudomenstruation*—Blood-tinged or mucoid discharge Hymenal tag	Enlarged clitoris with urethral meatus at tip Fused labia Absence of vaginal opening Meconium from vaginal opening No urination within 24 h Masses in labia Ambiguous genitalia Bladder exstrophy
Male Genitalia		
Urethral opening at tip of glans penis Testes palpable in each scrotum Scrotum usually large, edematous, pendulous, and covered with rugae; usually deeply pigmented in dark-skinned ethnic groups	Urethral opening covered by prepuce Inability to retract foreskin *Epithelial pearls*—Small, firm, white lesions at tip of prepuce Erection or priapism Testes palpable in inguinal canal	*Hypospadias*—Urethral opening on ventral surface of penis *Epispadias*—Urethral opening on dorsal surface of penis *Chordee*—Ventral curvature of penis

Continued

Summary of Physical Assessment of the Newborn—cont'd

Usual Findings	Common Variations and Minor Abnormalities	Potential Signs of Distress or Major Abnormalities
Smegma Urination within 24 h	Scrotum small	Testes not palpable in scrotum or inguinal canal No urination within 24 h Inguinal hernia Hypoplastic scrotum *Hydrocele*—Fluid in scrotum Masses in scrotum Meconium from scrotum, raphe, or perineum Discoloration of testes Ambiguous genitalia Bladder exstrophy
Back and Rectum		
Spine intact; no openings, masses, or prominent curves Trunk incurvation reflex Anal reflex Patent anal opening Passage of meconium within 48 h	Green liquid stools in infant under phototherapy Delayed passage of meconium in very low–birth-weight neonates	Anal fissures or fistulas Imperforate anus Absence of anal reflex No meconium within 36–48 h Pilonidal cyst or sinus Tuft of hair along spine Spina bifida (any degree)
Extremities		
Ten fingers and 10 toes Full range of motion Nail beds pink, with transient cyanosis immediately after birth Creases on anterior two-thirds of sole Sole usually flat Symmetry of extremities Equal muscle tone bilaterally, especially resistance to opposing flexion Equal bilateral brachial and femoral pulses	Partial syndactyly between second and third toes Second toe overlapping third toe Wide gap between first (hallux) and second toes Deep crease on plantar surface of foot between first and second toes Asymmetric length of toes Dorsiflexion and shortness of hallux	*Polydactyly*—Extra digits *Syndactyly*—Fused or webbed digits *Phocomelia*—Hands or feet attached close to trunk *Hemimelia*—Absence of distal part of extremity Hyperflexibility of joints Persistent cyanosis of nail beds Yellowing of nail beds Sole covered with creases Transverse palmar (simian) crease Fractures Decreased or absent range of motion (ROM) Dislocated or subluxated hip Limitation in hip abduction Unequal gluteal or leg folds Unequal knee height (Allis or Galeazzi sign) Audible clunk on abduction (Ortolani sign) Asymmetry of extremities Unequal muscle tone or ROM
Neuromuscular System		
Extremities usually in some degree of flexion. Extension of an extremity followed by previous position of flexion Head lag while sitting, but momentary ability to hold head erect Able to turn head from side to side when prone Able to hold head in horizontal line with back when held prone	Quivering or momentary tremors	*Hypotonia*—Floppy, poor head control, extremities limp *Hypertonia*—Jittery, arms and hands tightly flexed, legs stiffly extended, startles easily Asymmetric posturing (except tonic neck reflex) *Opisthotonic posturing*—Arched back Signs of paralysis Tremors, twitches, and myoclonic jerks Marked head lag in all positions

GUIDELINES

Using the Blood Pressure Screening Tables

1. Use the standard height charts to determine the height percentile.
2. Measure and record the child's systolic blood pressure (SBP) and diastolic blood pressure (DBP) annually beginning at 3 years of age or at every visit if risk factors (e.g., obesity, diabetes, kidney disease, aortic arch obstruction, coarctation) are present.
3. Use the correct gender table for SBP and DBP.
4. Locate the child's age on the left side of the table. Follow the age row horizontally across the table to the intersection of the line for the height percentile (vertical column).
5. Locate the 50th, 90th, and 95th percentile (%) for SBP in the left columns and for DBP in the right columns.
   - Normal blood pressure (BP): <90th % (aged 1–13 years). In adolescents (aged ≥13 years) normal BP: <120/<80 mm Hg (mercury)
   - Elevated BP: ≥90th % to <95th % or 120/80 mm Hg to <95% (whichever is lower). In adolescents, elevated BP: 120/<80 mm Hg to 129/<80 mm Hg.
   - Stage 1 hypertension (HTN): ≥95th % to <95% + 12 mm Hg, or 130/80 to 139/89 mm Hg (whichever is lower). In adolescents, stage 1 HTN: 130/80 to 139/89 mm Hg.
   - Stage 2 HTN: ≥95% + 12 mmHg or ≥140/90 mm Hg (whichever is lower). In adolescent, stage 2 HTN: ≥140/90 mmHg.
6. If the BP is ≥90th percentile in children <13 years or in children ≥13: ≥120 mm Hg SBP or ≥80 mm Hg DBP, the BP should be remeasured twice at the same office visit, and use the averaged SBP and DBP values. If averaged oscillometric (validated calibrated machine) reading is >90%, 2 auscultatory (Hg or aneroid sphygmomanometer) measurements should be taken and averaged to define the BP stage. Therapeutic lifestyle changes (e.g., healthy diet, regular physical activity) are recommended.[a]
7. In stage 1, recommend therapeutic lifestyle changes and BP measurements should be repeated on two more occasions within 3 months. If HTN is confirmed, evaluation should proceed. If BP is stage 2, prompt referral should be made for evaluation and therapy. If the patient is symptomatic, immediate referral and treatment are indicated[a]

[a]Flynn JT, Kaelber DC, Baker-Smith CM, et al. Clinical practice guideline for screening and management of high blood pressure in children and adolescents. *Pediatrics.* 2017;140(6):e20173035.

Assessment of Reflexes

Reflexes	Expected Behavioral Responses
Localized	
Eyes	
Blinking or corneal reflex	Infant blinks at sudden appearance of a bright light or at approach of an object toward cornea; persists throughout life.
Pupillary	Pupil constricts when a bright light shines toward it; persists throughout life.
Doll's eye	As head is moved slowly to right or left, eyes lag behind and do not immediately adjust to new position of head; disappears as fixation develops; if persists, indicates neurologic damage.
Nose	
Sneeze	Spontaneous response of nasal passages to irritation or obstruction; persists throughout life.
Glabellar	Tapping briskly on glabella (bridge of nose) causes eyes to close tightly; usually disappears in infancy.
Mouth and Throat	
Sucking	Infant begins strong sucking movements of circumoral area in response to stimulation; persists throughout infancy, even without stimulation, such as during sleep.
Gag	Stimulation of posterior pharynx by food, suction, or passage of a tube causes infant to gag; persists throughout life.
Rooting	Touching or stroking the cheek along side of mouth causes infant to turn head toward that side and begin to suck; should disappear at about age 3–4 months but may persist for up to 12 months.
Extrusion	When tongue is touched or depressed, infant responds by forcing it outward; disappears by age 4 months.
Yawn	Spontaneous response to decreased oxygen by increasing amount of inspired air; persists throughout life.
Cough	Irritation of mucous membranes of larynx or tracheobronchial tree causes coughing; persists throughout life; usually present after first day of birth.
Extremities	
Grasp	Touching palms of hands or soles near base of digits causes flexion of hands and toes; palmar grasp lessens after age 3 months, to be replaced by voluntary movement; plantar grasp lessens by 8 months of age.
Babinski	Stroking outer sole of foot upward from heel and across ball of foot causes toes to hyperextend and hallux to dorsiflex; disappears after age 1 year.

Continued

Assessment of Reflexes—cont'd

Reflexes	Expected Behavioral Responses
Ankle clonus	Briskly dorsiflexing foot while supporting knee in partially flexed position results in one or two oscillating movements ("beats"); eventually, no beats should be felt.
Mass (Body)	
Moro[a]	Sudden jarring or change in equilibrium causes sudden extension and abduction of extremities and fanning of fingers, with index finger and thumb forming a *C* shape, followed by flexion and adduction of extremities; legs may weakly flex; infant may cry; disappears after age 3–4 months, usually strongest during first 2 months.
Startle[a]	A sudden loud noise causes abduction of the arms with flexion of elbows; hands remain clenched; disappears by age 4 months.
Perez	While infant is prone on a firm surface, thumb is pressed along spine from sacrum to neck; infant responds by crying, flexing extremities, and elevating pelvis and head; lordosis of the spine, defecation and urination, may occur; disappears by age 4–6 months.
Asymmetric tonic neck	When infant's head is turned to one side, arm and leg extend on that side, and opposite arm and leg flex; disappears by age 3–4 months, to be replaced by symmetric positioning of both sides of body.
Trunk incurvation (Galant)	Stroking infant's back alongside spine causes hips to move toward stimulated side; disappears by age 4 weeks.
Dance or step	If infant is held so that sole of foot touches a hard surface, there is a reciprocal flexion and extension of the leg, simulating walking; disappears after age 3–4 weeks, to be replaced by deliberate movement.
Crawl	When placed on abdomen, infant makes crawling movements with arms and legs; disappears at about age 6 weeks.
Placing	When infant is held upright under arms and dorsal side of foot is briskly placed against hard object, such as table, leg lifts as if foot is stepping on table; age of disappearance varies.

[a]Some authorities consider Moro and startle reflexes to be the same response.

Assessment of Gestational Age

Assessment of gestational age is an important criterion because perinatal morbidity and mortality are related to gestational age and birth weight. A frequently used method of determining gestational age based on physical and neurologic findings is the New Ballard Score (NBS) by Ballard and colleagues (1991). A research study that compared the NBS to the Dubowitz gestational scoring system proved the NBS scoring system is equally effective in assessing gestational age as the Dubowitz scoring system, although, it has the added advantage of having a smaller number of criteria (Singhal et al., 2017). In Fig. 1.2A assesses six external physical and six neuromuscular signs. Each sign has a number score, and the cumulative score correlates with a maturity rating from 20 to 44 weeks (see Fig. 1.2A maturity rating).

The NBS scores reflect signs of extremely premature infants, such as fused eyelids; imperceptible breast tissue; sticky, friable, transparent skin; no lanugo; and square-window (flexion of the wrist) angle of greater than 90 degrees (see Fig. 1.2A and description of gestational assessment tests section). For infants with a gestational age of at least 26 weeks, the examination can be performed up to 96 hours after birth; however, it is recommended that the initial examination be performed within the first 48 hours of life. In a study published in 2017, the researchers found that the NBS overestimated the physical component scores of the small for gestational age (SGA) infants. However, reanalysis after reducing skin and plantar crease physical parameter scores, the NBS scores were more consistent with the infants' gestational age (Singhal et al., 2017).[e]

Classification of infants at birth by both weight and gestational age provides a more accurate method for predicting morbidity and mortality risks and providing guidelines for the management of the neonate than estimating gestational age or birth weight alone. The infant's birth weight, length, and head circumference are plotted on standardized graphs with normal values for gestational age. Fig. 1.2B denotes the classification of newborns based on intrauterine growth. Infants whose weight is appropriate for gestational age (AGA) (between the 10th and 90th percentiles) are classified as having grown at a normal rate regardless of the time of birth—preterm, term, or postterm. Infants who are large for gestational age (LGA) (above the 90th percentile) are considered to have grown at an accelerated rate during fetal life; the small-for-gestational-age (SGA) infants (below the 10th percentile) are classified as having experienced intrauterine growth restriction or delay. When gestational age is determined according to the NBS, the newborn will fall into one of the following nine possible categories for birth weight and gestational age: AGA—term, preterm, postterm; SGA—term, preterm, postterm; or LGA—term, preterm, postterm.

To facilitate the use of Fig. 1.2A, the following tests are described:

[e] Singhal S, Bawa S, Bansal S. Comparison of Dubowitz scoring versus Ballard scoring for assessment of fetal maturation of newly born infants setting. *Int J Reprod Contracept Obstet Gynecol.* 2017;6:3096–3102.

NEUROMUSCULAR MATURITY

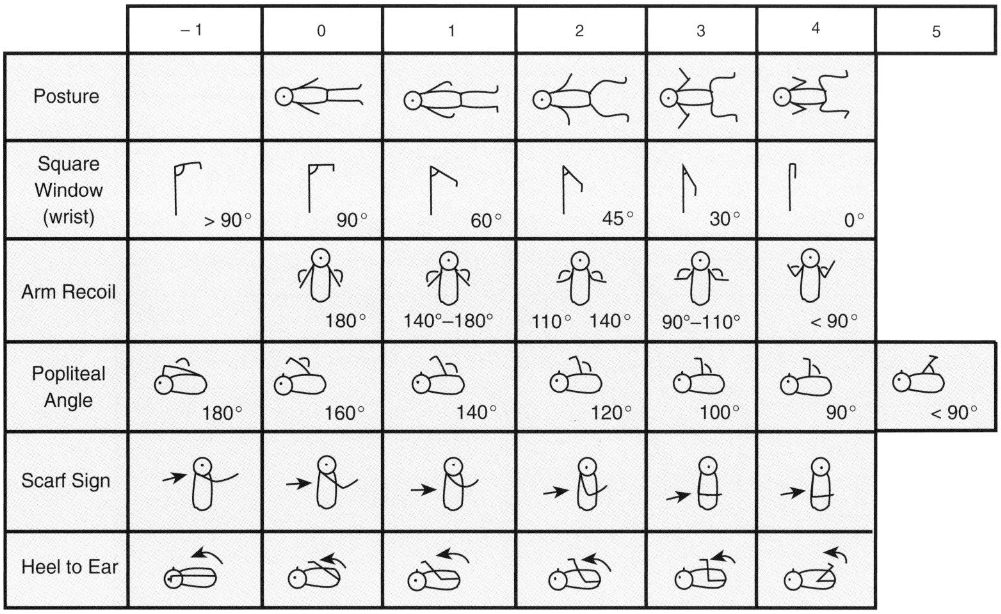

	−1	0	1	2	3	4	5
Posture							
Square Window (wrist)	> 90°	90°	60°	45°	30°	0°	
Arm Recoil		180°	140°–180°	110° 140°	90°–110°	< 90°	
Popliteal Angle	180°	160°	140°	120°	100°	90°	< 90°
Scarf Sign							
Heel to Ear							

PHYSICAL MATURITY

Skin	sticky friable transparent	gelatinous red, translucent	smooth pink, visible veins	superficial peeling &/or rash, few veins	cracking pale areas rare veins	parchment deep cracking no vessels	leathery cracked wrinkled
Lanugo	none	sparse	abundant	thinning	bald areas	mostly bald	
Plantar Surface	heel-toe 40–50 mm: –1 <40 mm: –2	>50 mm no crease	faint red marks	anterior transverse crease only	creases ant. 2/3	creases over entire sole	
Breast	imperceptible	barely perceptible	flat areola no bud	stippled areola 1–2 mm bud	raised areola 3–4 mm bud	full areola 5–10 mm bud	
Eye/Ear	lids fused loosely: –1 tightly: –2	lids open pinna flat stays folded	sl. curved pinna; soft; slow recoil	well-curved pinna; soft but ready recoil	formed & firm instant recoil	thick cartilage ear stiff	
Genitals (male)	scrotum flat, smooth	scrotum empty faint rugae	testes in upper canal rare rugae	testes descending few rugae	testes down good rugae	testes pendulous deep rugae	
Genitals (female)	clitoris prominent labia flat	prominent clitoris small labia minora	prominent clitoris enlarging minora	majora & minora equally prominent	majora large minora small	majora cover clitoris & minora	

MATURITY RATING

score	weeks
−10	20
−5	22
0	24
5	26
10	28
15	30
20	32
25	34
30	36
35	38
40	40
45	42
50	44

A

FIG. **1.2** (A) New Ballard Score for newborn maturity rating. Expanded score includes extremely premature infants and has been refined to improve accuracy in more mature infants.

Continued

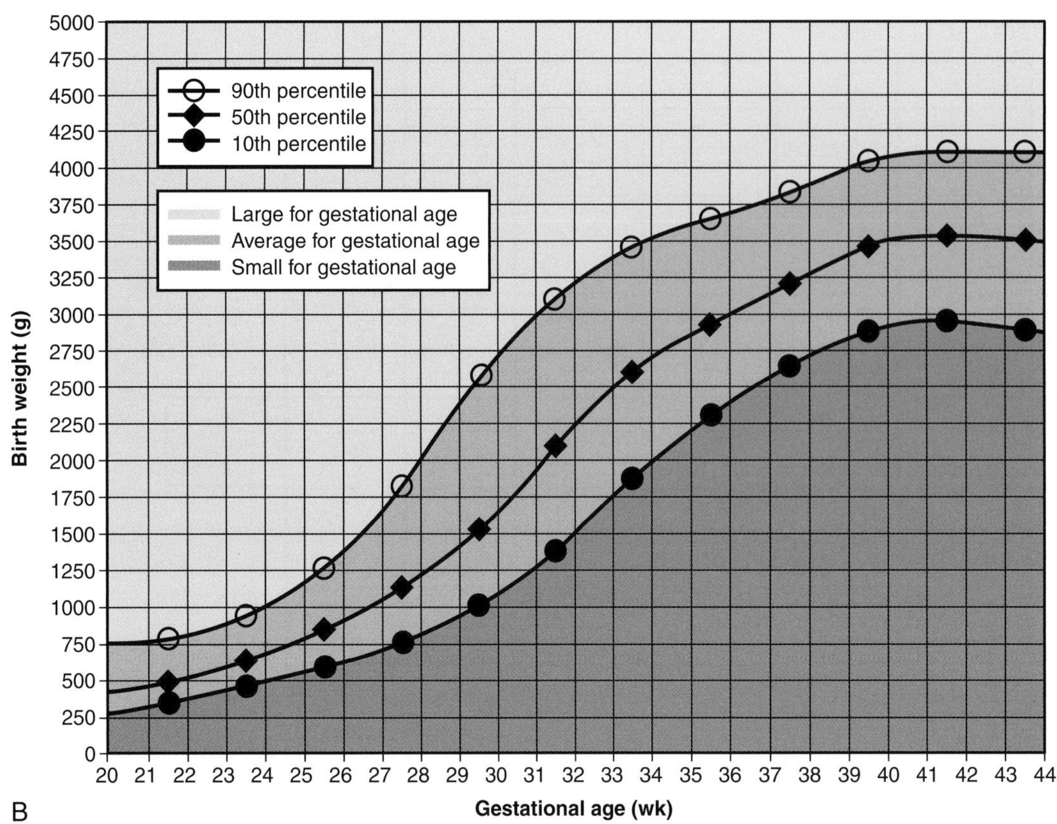

FIG. **1.2, cont'd** (B) Intrauterine growth: birth weight percentiles based on live single births at gestational ages 20 to 44 weeks. (Adapted from Ballard JL, Khoury JC, Wedig K, et al. New Ballard score expanded to include extremely premature infants. J Pediatr. 1991;119[3]:417–423; Sasidharan K, Dutta S, Narang A. Validity of New Ballard score until 7th day of postnatal life in moderately preterm neonates. Arch Dis Child Fetal Neonatal Ed. 2009;94[1]:F39–F44. Data from Alexander GR, Himes JH, Kaufman RB, et al. A United States national reference for fetal growth. Obstet Gynecol. 1996;87(2):163–168.)

Test	Assessment of Gestational Age
Posture	With the infant quiet and in a supine position, observe the degree of flexion in the arms and legs. Muscle tone and degree of flexion increase with maturity. Full flexion of the arms and legs = 4.
Square window	With the thumb supporting the back of the arm below the wrist, apply gentle pressure with index and third fingers on dorsum of hand without rotating the infant's wrist. Measure the angle between the base of the thumb and forearm. Full flexion (hand lies flat on ventral surface of forearm) = 4.
Arm recoil	With the infant supine, fully flex both forearms on upper arms, hold for 5 s; pull down on hands to fully extend and rapidly release arms. Observe the rapidity and intensity of recoil to a state of flexion. A brisk return to full flexion = 4.
Popliteal angle	With the infant supine and the pelvis flat on a firm surface, flex lower leg on thigh, then flex thigh on abdomen. While holding knee with thumb and index finger, extend lower leg with index finger of other hand. Measure the degree of the angle behind the knee (popliteal angle). An angle <90 degrees = 5.
Scarf sign	With the infant supine, support the head in the midline with one hand; use other hand to pull infant's arm across the shoulder so that infant's hand touches the opposite shoulder. Determine location of elbow in relation to midline. Elbow does not reach midline—4.
Heel to ear	With the infant supine and the pelvis flat on a firm surface, pull the foot as far as possible up toward the ear on the same side. Measure the degree of knee flexion (same as popliteal angle). Knees flexed with a popliteal angle <90 degrees—4.

Estimation of Gestational Age by Maturity Rating

Fig. 1.2.

Assessment of Newborn Bilirubin

Hour-specific serum bilirubin levels to predict newborns at risk for rapidly rising levels may be used as a screening tool before discharge from the hospital. Using a nomogram with three designated risk levels (high, intermediate, and low risk) for hour-specific total serum bilirubin values assists in the determination of which newborns might need further evaluation before and after discharge. Risk factors recognized to place infants in the high-risk category include gestational age of younger than 38 weeks, breastfeeding, a sibling who had significant jaundice, and jaundice appearing before discharge.

General Guidelines for Performing a Pediatric Physical Examination

Perform examination in an appropriate, nonthreatening area:
- Have the room well-lit and decorated with neutral colors.
- Have room temperature comfortably warm.
- Place all strange and potentially frightening equipment out of sight.
- Have some toys, dolls, and games available for the child.
- If possible, have rooms decorated and equipped for different-age children.

Provide privacy, especially for school-age children and adolescents.

Provide time for play and becoming acquainted.

Observe behaviors that signal the child's readiness to cooperate:
- Talking to the nurse
- Making eye contact
- Accepting the offered equipment
- Allowing physical touching
- Choosing to sit on the examining table rather than the parent's lap

If signs of readiness are not observed, use the following techniques:
- Talk to the parent while essentially "ignoring" the child; gradually focus on the child or a favorite object, such as a doll.
- Make complimentary remarks about the child, such as about his or her appearance, dress, or a favorite object.
- Tell a funny story, or play a simple magic trick.
- Have a non-threatening "friend," such as a hand puppet to "talk" to the child for the nurse.

If the child refuses to cooperate, use the following techniques:
- Assess the reason for uncooperative behavior; consider that a child who is unduly afraid may have had a previous traumatic experience.
- Try to involve the child and parent in the process.
- Avoid prolonged explanations about the examining procedure.
- Use a firm, direct approach regarding expected behavior.
- Perform examination as quickly as possible.
- Have the attendant gently restrain the child.
- Minimize any disruptions or stimulation:

Limit the number of people in the room.

Use an isolated room.

Use a quiet, calm, confident voice.

Begin the examination in a non-threatening manner for young children or children who are fearful (see Atraumatic Care)

ATRAUMATIC CARE

Reducing Young Children's Fears

Young children, especially preschoolers, fear intrusive procedures because of their poorly defined body boundaries. Therefore, avoid invasive procedures, such as measuring rectal temperature, whenever possible. Also, avoid using the word "take" when measuring vital signs, because young children interpret words literally and may think that their temperature or other function will be taken away. Instead, say, "I want to know how warm you are."

- Use activities that can be presented as games, such as tests for cranial nerves (see Creative Communication Techniques with Children p. 5).
- Use approaches such as "Simon says" to encourage the child to make a face, squeeze a hand, stand on one foot, and so on.
- Use the paper-doll technique:
- Lay the child supine on an examining table or floor that is covered with a large sheet of paper.
- Trace around the child's body outline.
- Use a body outline to demonstrate what will be examined, such as drawing a heart and listening with the stethoscope before performing the activity on the child.

If several children in the family will be examined, begin with the most cooperative child to model desired behavior.

Involve the child in the examination process:
- Provide choices, such as sitting on the examination table or in the parent's lap.
- Allow the child to handle or hold equipment.
- Encourage the child to use the equipment on a doll, family member, or examiner.
- Explain each step of the procedure in simple language.

Examine the child in a comfortable and secure position:
- Sitting in parent's lap
- Sitting upright if in respiratory distress

Proceed to examine the body in an organized sequence (usually head to toe) with the following exceptions:
- Alter sequence to accommodate the needs of different-age children (see Age-Specific Approaches to Physical Examination During Childhood p. 26).
- Examine painful areas last.
- In an emergency, examine vital functions (airway, breathing, circulation) and the injured area first.

Reassure the child throughout the examination, especially about bodily concerns that arise during puberty.

Discuss the findings with the family at the end of the examination.

Praise the child for cooperation during the examination; give a reward such as a toy from a toy box or sticker.

Age-Specific Approaches to Physical Examination During Childhood

Position	Sequence	Preparation
Infant		
Before able to sit alone: supine or prone, preferably in parent's lap; before 4–6 months: can place on examining table After able to sit alone: sit in parent's lap whenever possible; if on table, place with parent in full view	If quiet, auscultate heart, lungs, abdomen. Record heart and respiratory rates. Palpate and percuss same areas. Proceed in usual head-to-toe direction. Perform traumatic procedures last (eyes, ears, mouth [while crying]). Elicit reflexes as body part is examined. Elicit Moro reflex last.	Completely undress infant if room temperature permits. Leave diaper on male. Gain cooperation with distraction, bright objects, rattles, and talking. Smile at infant; use soft, gentle voice. Use pacifier (if used) or bottle with feeding (if bottle feeding). Enlist parent's aid for restraining to examine ears, mouth. Avoid abrupt, jerky movements.
Toddler		
Sitting on parent's lap or standing by parent Prone or supine in parent's lap	Inspect body area through play: count fingers, tickle toes. Use minimal physical contact initially. Introduce equipment slowly. Auscultate, percuss, palpate whenever quiet. Perform traumatic procedures last (same as for infant).	Have parent remove toddler's outer clothing. Remove underwear as body part is examined. Allow toddler to inspect equipment; demonstrating use of equipment is usually ineffective. If uncooperative, perform procedures quickly. Use restraint when appropriate; request parent's assistance. Talk about examination if cooperative; use short phrases. Praise for cooperative behavior.
Preschool Child		
Prefer standing or sitting Usually cooperative prone or supine Prefer parent's closeness	If cooperative, proceed in head-to-toe direction. If uncooperative, proceed as with toddler.	Request self-undressing. Allow to wear underpants. Offer equipment for inspection; briefly demonstrate use. Make up story about procedure (e.g., "I'm seeing how strong your muscles are" [blood pressure]). Use paper-doll technique. Give choices when possible. Expect cooperation; use positive statements (e.g., "Open your mouth").

Age-Specific Approaches to Physical Examination During Childhood—cont'd

Position	Sequence	Preparation
School-Age Child		
Prefer sitting Cooperative in most positions Younger child prefers parent's presence. Older child may prefer privacy.	Proceed in head-to-toe direction. May examine genitalia last in older child.	Respect need for privacy Request self-undressing. Allow to wear underpants. Give gown to wear. Explain purpose of equipment and significance of procedure, such as otoscope to see eardrum, which is necessary for hearing. Teach about body function and care.
Adolescent		
Same as for school-age child Offer option of parent's presence.	Same as for older school-age child. May examine genitalia last	Respect need for privacy. Allow to undress in private. Give gown. Expose only area to be examined. Explain findings during examination (e.g., "Your muscles are firm and strong"). Matter-of-factly comment about sexual development (e.g., "Your breasts are developing as they should be"). Emphasize normalcy of development. Examine genitalia as any other body part; may leave for end.

Outline of a Physical Assessment

A. Growth measurements
1. Height or recumbent length
2. Crown-to-rump length or sitting height
3. Weight
4. Head circumference

B. Physiologic measurements
1. Temperature
2. Pulse
3. Respiration
4. Blood pressure
5. Pain assessment
6. Pulse oximetry as needed

C. General appearance
D. Skin
E. Accessory structures
F. Lymph nodes
G. Head
H. Neck
I. Eyes
J. Ears
K. Nose
L. Mouth and throat
M. Chest
N. Lungs
O. Heart
P. Abdomen
Q. Genitalia
1. Male
2. Female

R. Anus
S. Back and extremities
T. Neurologic assessment
1. Mental status
2. Motor functioning
3. Sensory functioning
4. Reflexes (deep tendons)
5. Cranial nerves

Summary of Physical Assessment of the Child

Assessment	Procedure
Growth Measurements	
See Fig. 1.3A and B.	Plot length, weight, and head circumference on standard percentile charts. Charts for 0–36 months and 2–20 years both include children ages 24–36 months; record only recumbent length on 0- to 36-month chart and only stature on 2- to 20-year chart. The prepubescent charts are appropriate only for plotting values for prepubescent boys and girls, regardless of chronologic age, and not for any child showing signs of pubescence, such as breast budding, testicular enlargement, or growth of axillary or pubic hair.

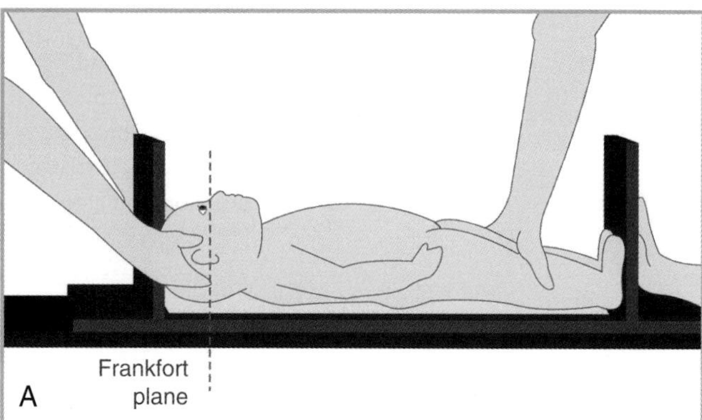

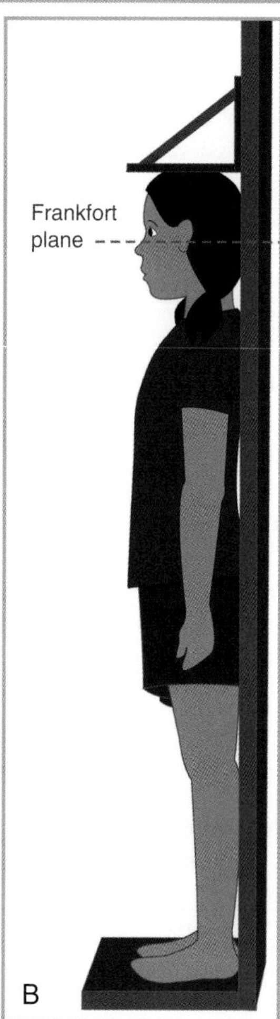

FIG. **1.3** Measurement of linear growth. (A) Infant. (B) Child. (Courtesy Jan M. Foote, Blank Children's Hospital, Des Moines, IA.)

Usual Findings	Comments
Measurements of length, weight, and head circumference between the 25th and 75th percentiles are likely to represent normal growth (see Nursing Alert). **NURSING ALERT** The 50th percentile represents the median growth (or midpoint of all the growth measurements for each age). The 5th percentile represents the lowest 5%, and the 95th percentile represents the highest 5% of growth measurements for each age.	Questionable results may include the following: 1. Children whose height and weight percentiles are widely disparate, for example, height in the 10th percentile and weight in the 90th percentile, especially with above-average skinfold thickness 2. Children who fail to show the expected gain in height and weight, especially during the rapid growth periods of infancy and adolescence 3. Children who show a sudden increase, except during puberty, or decrease in a previously steady growth pattern
Measurements between the 10th and 25th and between the 75th and 90th percentiles may or may not be normal, depending on previous and subsequent measurements and on genetic and environmental factors. Growth curve remains generally within the same percentile, except during rapid growth periods.	Compare findings with growth patterns of other family members: consider genetic influence on growth determination Compare children's growth trends (height and weight) with midparental height (MPH). Most children with normal birth weights and heights and normal childhood growth will achieve an adult height within ±2 inches of MPH. Special charts are available for parent-specific adjustments for evaluation of the child's height. To calculate MPH, use the following formulas: For girls: Father's height − 13 cm or 5 inches + Mother's height/2 For boys: Father's height − 13 cm or 5 inches + Mother's height/2

Summary of Physical Assessment of the Child—cont'd

Assessment	Procedure
Length and Height	Recumbent length in children below 24–36 months (see Fig. 1.3A): Place supine with head in midline. Grasp knees and push gently toward table to *fully* extend legs. Measure from vertex (top) of head to heels of feet (toes pointing upward). Standing height (stature) in children over 24–36 months: Remove socks and shoes. Have child stand as tall as possible, back straight, head in midline, and eyes looking straight ahead (see Fig. 1.3B.) Check for flexion of knees, slumping shoulders, and raising of heels. Measure from top of head to standing surface. Measure to the nearest cm or ⅛ inch.
Weight	Weigh infants and young children nude on platform-type scale; protect infant by placing hand above body to prevent falling off scale. Weigh older children in underwear (and gown if privacy is a concern; no shoes) on standing-type upright scale. Check that scale is balanced before weighing. Cover scale with clean sheet of paper for each child. Measure to the nearest 10 g or ½ ounce for infants and 100 g or ½ pound for children.
Head Circumference	Measure with paper or non-stretchable tape at greatest circumference, from top of the eyebrows and pinna of the ear to around occipital prominence at back of the skull.
Chest Circumference	Measure around chest at nipple line. Ideally, take measurements during inhalation and expiration; record the average of the two values.
Pulse	Auscultate an apical pulse in infants and young children because it is more reliable. Point of maximum intensity located lateral to nipple at fourth to fifth interspace at or near midclavicular line. Palpate a radial pulse in children older than 2 years to obtain satisfactory pulse rate. Count pulse for 1 full minute, because of possible irregularities in rhythm. For repeated measurement, count pulse for 15 or 30 s and multiply by 4 or 2, respectively.
Respiration	Count the respiratory rate for 1 full minute for accuracy. In infants and young children, observe abdominal movement. In older children, observe thoracic movement.

<table>
<tr><th>Usual Findings</th><th>Comments</th></tr>
<tr><td>Plot on growth chart.
Compare value with percentile for weight.
Expected Growth Rates at Various Ages[a]
<table>
<tr><th>Age</th><th>Expected Growth Rate (cm/year)</th></tr>
<tr><td>1–6 months</td><td>18–22</td></tr>
<tr><td>6–12 months</td><td>14–18</td></tr>
<tr><td>Second year</td><td>11</td></tr>
<tr><td>Third year</td><td>8</td></tr>
<tr><td>Fourth year</td><td>7</td></tr>
<tr><td>Fifth to tenth years</td><td>5–6</td></tr>
</table></td><td>For accurate measurements, use infant-measuring device for recumbent length and stadiometer for standing height.
Normally height is less if measured in the afternoon than in the morning. To minimize this variation, apply modest upward pressure under the jaw or the mastoid processes.</td></tr>
<tr><td>Plot on growth chart.
Compare value with percentile for length.</td><td>Compare weight with appearance, for example, excessive fat; well-developed musculature; flabby, loose skin; bony prominences (for skinfold measurement, see below).
Assess nutritional status; compare with weight.</td></tr>
<tr><td>Plot on growth chart.
Compare percentile with those of height and weight.
Compare with chest circumference:
At birth, head circumference exceeds chest circumference by 2–3 cm (1 inch).
At 1–2 years, head circumference equals chest circumference.
During childhood, chest circumference exceeds head circumference by about 5–7 cm (2–3 inches).</td><td>Usually taken in children under 36 months of age
Taken in any child whose head size appears abnormal</td></tr>
<tr><td>Compare with head circumference (see earlier in table).</td><td>May be measured during examination of chest</td></tr>
<tr><td>(For average pulse rates at rest, see inside front cover.)</td><td>Pulse rate normally may increase with inspiration and decrease with expiration (sinus arrhythmia) (see also Box 1.2.)
May grade pulses:
Grade 0—Not palpable
Grade +1—Difficult to palpate; thready, weak, easily obliterated with pressure
Grade +2—Difficult to palpate; may be obliterated with pressure
Grade +3—Easy to palpate; not easily obliterated with pressure (normal)
Grade +4—Strong, bounding; not obliterated with pressure</td></tr>
<tr><td>(For average respiratory rates at rest, see inside front cover.)</td><td></td></tr>
</table>

Continued

Summary of Physical Assessment of the Child—cont'd

Assessment	Procedure

Blood Pressure

BOX 1.2 Various Patterns of Respiration

Tachypnea—Increased rate
Bradypnea—Decreased rate
Dyspnea—Distress during breathing
Apnea—Cessation of breathing
Hyperpnea—Increased depth
Hypoventilation—Decreased depth (shallow) and irregular rhythm
Hyperventilation—Increased rate and depth
Kussmaul breathing—Hyperventilation, gasping, and labored respiration, usually seen in respiratory acidosis (e.g., diabetic coma)
Cheyne-Stokes respiration—Gradually increasing rate and depth with periods of apnea
Biot breathing—Periods of hyperpnea alternating (similar to Cheyne-Stokes except that the depth remains constant)
Seesaw (paradoxic) respirations—Chest falls on inspiration and rises on expiration
Agonal breathing—Last gasping breaths before death

Selection of Cuff

No matter what type of noninvasive technique is used, the most important factor in accurately measuring blood pressure is the use of an appropriately sized cuff (cuff size refers only to the inner inflatable bladder, not the cloth covering) (Table 1.3). A technique to establish an appropriate cuff size is to choose a cuff having a bladder width that is approximately 40% of the arm circumference midway between the olecranon and the acromion (Fig. 1.4A). This will usually be a cuff bladder that covers 80%–100% of the circumference of the arm (see Fig. 1.4B). BP should be measured with the cubital fossa at the heart level (see Fig. 1.4C). Researchers have found that selection of a cuff with a bladder width equal to 40% of the upper arm circumference most accurately reflects directly measured radial arterial pressure.

Cuffs that are either too narrow or too wide affect the accuracy of blood pressure measurements. If the cuff size is too small, the reading on the device is falsely high. If the cuff size is too large, the reading is falsely low.

When using a site other than the arm, blood pressure measurements using noninvasive techniques may differ. Generally, systolic blood pressure in the lower extremities (thigh or calf) is greater than pressure in the upper extremities, and systolic blood pressure in the calf is higher than that in the thigh (Fig. 1.5).

TABLE 1.3 Recommended Dimensions for Blood Pressure Cuff Bladders

Age Range	Width (cm)	Length (cm)	Maximum Arm Circumference (cm)[a]
Newborn	4	8	10
Infant	6	12	15
Child	9	18	22
Small adult	10	24	26
Adult	13	30	34
Large adult	16	38	44
Thigh	20	42	52

[a]Calculated so that the largest arm would still allow the bladder to encircle arm by at least 80%.

From National High Blood Pressure Education Program Working Group on High Blood Pressure in Children and Adolescents: The fourth report on the diagnosis, evaluation, and treatment of high blood pressure in children and adolescents. *Pediatrics.* 2004;114(2 Suppl 4th Report):555–576.

[a]Riley M, Hernandez AK, Kuznia AL. High blood pressure in children and adolescents. *Am Fam Physician.* 2018;98(8):486–494.

[b]Dionne JM, Bremner SA, Baygani S, et al. Method of blood pressure measurement in neonates and infants: a systematic review and analysis. *J Pediatr.* 2020;221:23–31; Eliasdottir SB, Steinhorsdottir SD, Indridason OS, et al. Comparison of aneroid and oscillometric blood pressure measurements in children. *J Clin Hypertens.* 2013;15(11):776–783.

Usual Findings	Comments
NURSING ALERT Published norms for blood pressure are valid only if the same method of measurement (auscultation and cuff size determination) is used in clinical practice. **NURSING ALERT** When taking blood pressure, use an appropriately sized cuff. When the correct size is not available, use an oversized cuff rather than an undersized one, or use another site that more appropriately fits the cuff size. **NURSING ALERT** Compare blood pressure (BP) in the upper and lower extremities to detect abnormalities, such as coarctation of aorta, in which the lower extremity pressure is less than the upper extremity pressure.	Repeat measurements above 95th percentile later during initial visit when child is least anxious; if a high reading persists, repeat measurements at least three times during subsequent visits to detect hypertension. *Significant hypertension*—Blood pressure persistently between 95th and 99th percentile for age, gender, and height *Severe hypertension*—Blood pressure persistently at or above 99th percentile for age, gender, and height Refer children with repeated elevated blood pressure readings or significant differences in pressure between upper and lower extremities for further evaluation.[a] Blood pressure readings using oscillometric (automated) devices are generally higher than those using auscultation therefore further research is recommended.[b]

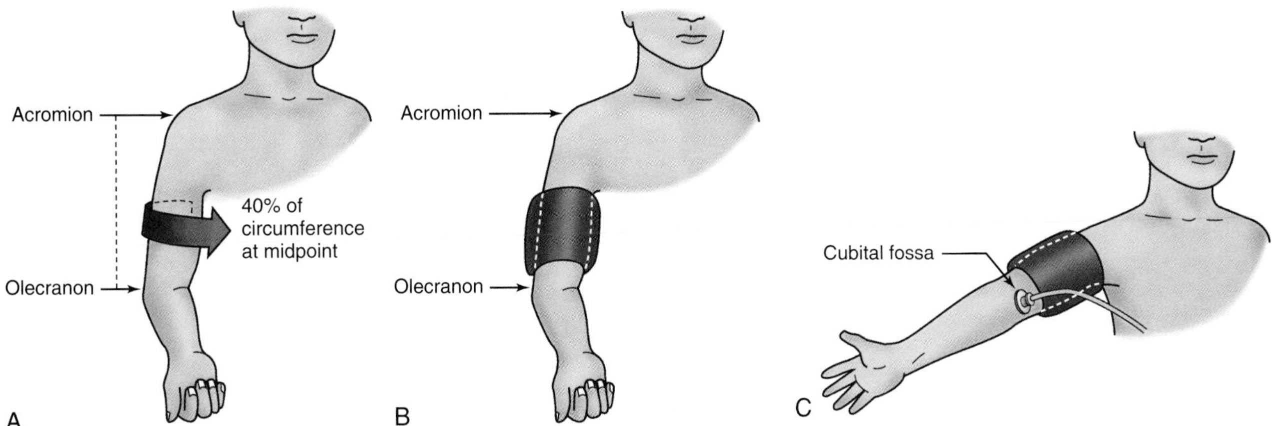

FIG. **1.4** Determination of proper cuff size. (A) Cuff bladder width should be approximately 40% of circumference of arm measured at a point midway between olecranon and acromion. (B) Cuff bladder length should cover 80% to 100% of arm circumference. (C) Blood pressure should be measured with the cubital fossa at the heart level. (From National Institutes of Health, National Heart, Lung, and Blood Institute. [1996]. Update on the Task Force Report [1987] on high blood pressure in children and adolescents: A working group report from the National High Blood Pressure Education Program. NIH Pub No 96-3790. Bethesda, MD: Author.)

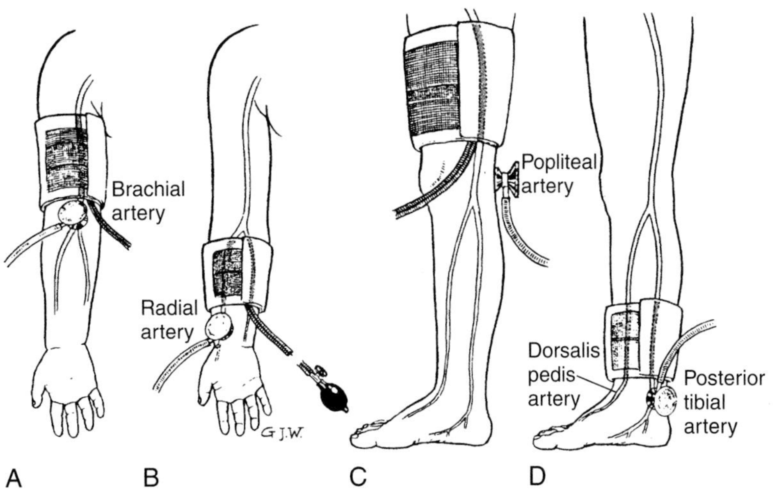

FIG. **1.5** Sites for measuring blood pressure. (A) Upper arm. (B) Lower arm or forearm. (C) Thigh. (D) Calf or ankle.

Continued

Summary of Physical Assessment of the Child—cont'd

Assessment	Procedure
General Appearance	
	Observe the following: Facies Posture Body movement Hygiene Nutrition Behavior Development State of awareness
Skin	
	Observe skin in natural daylight or neutral artificial light. *Color*—Most reliably assessed in sclera, conjunctiva, nail beds, tongue, buccal mucosa, palms, and soles. *Texture*—Note moisture, smoothness, roughness, integrity of skin, and temperature. *Temperature*—Compare each part of body for even temperature. *Turgor*—Grasp skin on abdomen between thumb and index finger, pull taut, and release quickly. Indent skin with finger.

Usual Findings	Comments
Evaluated in terms of a comprehensive assessment, including the child's physical appearance, nutrition status, behavior, personality, posture, development, and speech.	Record general appearance at beginning of physical exam encompassing all observations of child during interview and physical assessment.
	Reveals significant observation of the skin and its accessory organs involving both inspection and palpation.
Genetically determined: Light-skinned—From milky white and rose to deeply hued pink. Dark-skinned—Various shades of brown, red, yellow, olive, and bluish tones	Observe for abnormalities such as pallor, cyanosis, erythema, ecchymosis, petechiae, and jaundice (Table 1.4). Factors that tend to affect skin color include natural skin tone, melanin, edema, hygiene, hemoglobin levels, amount of room lighting, atmospheric temperature, and use of cosmetics.
Smooth, slightly dry to touch, with even temperature	Note obvious changes, such as clammy skin, oily skin, excessive dryness, and obvious lesions (Boxes on primary skin lesions at end of Unit 1).
Usually same all over body, although exposed parts, such as hands, may be cooler	Note any differences in skin temperature with symmetrical skin palpation and comparing body areas, such as noting warm upper extremities and cold lower extremities.
Resumes shape immediately with no tenting, wrinkling, prolonged depression, residual marks or creases.	Elastic skin turgor indicates adequate hydration and possibly nutrition. Inelastic (poor) skin turgor is that skin remains suspended or tented for a few seconds before slowly falling back on the abdomen (sign of dehydration and/or malnutrition). Evaluate for signs of pitting of skin on indentation or other signs of swelling (signs of edema).

TABLE 1.4 Differences in Color Changes of Racial Groups

Color Change	Appearance in Light Skin	Appearance in Dark Skin
Cyanosis	Bluish tinge, especially in palpebral conjunctiva (lower eyelid), nail beds, earlobes, lips, oral membranes, soles, and palms	Ashen gray lips and tongue
Pallor	Loss of rosy glow in skin, especially face	Ashen gray appearance in black skin; more yellowish brown color in brown skin
Erythema	Redness easily seen anywhere on body	Much more difficult to assess; palpate for warmth or edema
Ecchymoses	Purplish to yellow-green areas; may be seen anywhere on skin	Very difficult to see unless in mouth or conjunctiva
Petechiae	Purplish pinpoints most easily seen on buttocks, abdomen, and inner surfaces of the arms or legs	Usually invisible except in oral mucosa, conjunctiva of eyelids, and conjunctiva covering eyeball
Jaundice	Yellow staining seen in sclera of eyes, skin, fingernails, soles, palms, and oral mucosa	Most reliably assessed in sclera, hard palate, palms, and soles

Continued

Summary of Physical Assessment of the Child—cont'd

Assessment	Procedure
Accessory Structures	
	Hair—Note color, texture, quality, distribution, elasticity, and hygiene.
	Nails—Inspect color, shape, texture, quality, and hygiene.
	Dermatoglyphics—Observe flexion creases of palm.
Lymph Nodes	
Fig. 1.6.	Palpate using distal portion of fingers. Press gently but firmly in a circular motion. Note size, mobility, temperature, tenderness, and any change in enlarged nodes. *Submaxillary*—Tilt head slightly downward. *Cervical*—Tilt head slightly upward. *Axillary*—Have arms relaxed at side but slightly abducted. *Inguinal*—Place child supine.

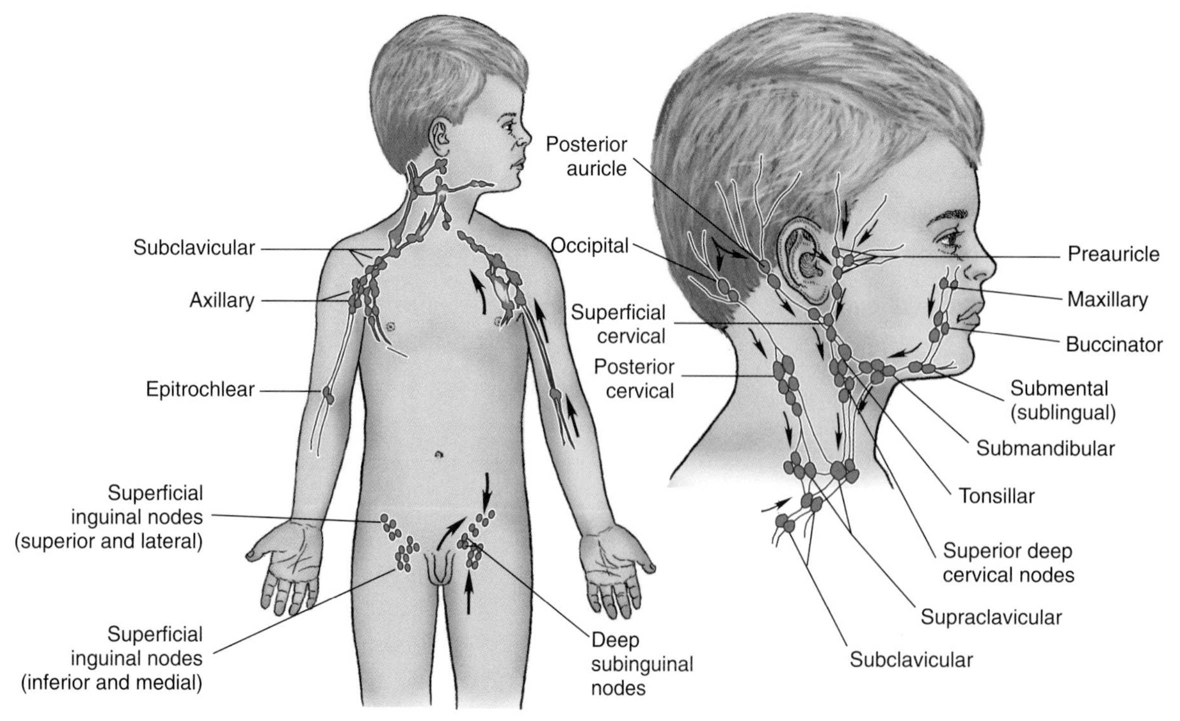

FIG. **1.6** Locations of superficial lymph nodes. *Arrows* indicate directional flow of lymph.

Usual Findings	Comments
Lustrous, silky, strong, elastic hair Genetic factors influence appearance; for example, an African American child's hair is usually curlier and coarser than Caucasian children.	Inspect hair for color, texture, quality, distribution elasticity, lesions, cleanliness, signs of infestations (e.g., lice, ticks), or trauma (e.g., scars, masses, ecchymosis). Hair that is stringy, dull, friable, brittle, dry, depigmented may suggest inadequate nutrition. Record any bald or thinning areas. During puberty, secondary hair growth indicates normal pubertal changes.
Pink, convex, smooth, hard and flexible; not brittle Dark-skinned child may have more deeply pigmented nail beds.	Note color changes, such as blueness or yellow tint. Observe for uncut or short, ragged nails (nail biting). Report any signs of clubbing (base of the nail becomes swollen and feels springy or floating when palpated), a sign of serious respiratory or cardiac dysfunction.
Three flexion creases	If pattern differs, describe it. Observe for transpalmar crease (one horizontal crease), a characteristic of children with Down syndrome.
Generally not palpable, although small, nontender, movable nodes are normal.	Observe size, mobility, temperature, tenderness, and any change in nodes. Note tender, enlarged, warm nodes that usually indicate infection or inflammation close to their location.

Continued

Summary of Physical Assessment of the Child—cont'd

Assessment	Procedure
Head	
	Note head for shape and symmetry.
	Note head control in infants and head posture in older children.
	Assess range of motion (ROM).
	Note skull for irregularity or obvious swellings and note if fontanels are bulging or fused.
	Transilluminate skull in darkened room; firmly place rubber-collared flashlight against skull at various points.
	Examine scalp for hygiene, lesions, infestation, signs of trauma, loss of hair, and discoloration.
	Percuss frontal sinuses in children older than 7 years.
Neck	
	Observe neck size.
	Trachea—Palpate for deviation; place thumb and index finger on each side, and slide fingers back and forth.
	Thyroid— Palpate, noting size, shape, symmetry, tenderness, nodules; place index and middle fingers below cricoid cartilage; feel for isthmus (tissue connecting lobes) rising during swallowing; feel each lobe laterally and posteriorly.
	Carotid arteries-Palpate on both sides.
Eyes	
	Observe placement and alignment.
	If abnormality is suspected, measure inner canthal distance.
	Palpebral slant—Draw imaginary line through two points of medial (inner) canthi and across outer orbit of eyes aligning each eye on the line (Fig. 1.7).

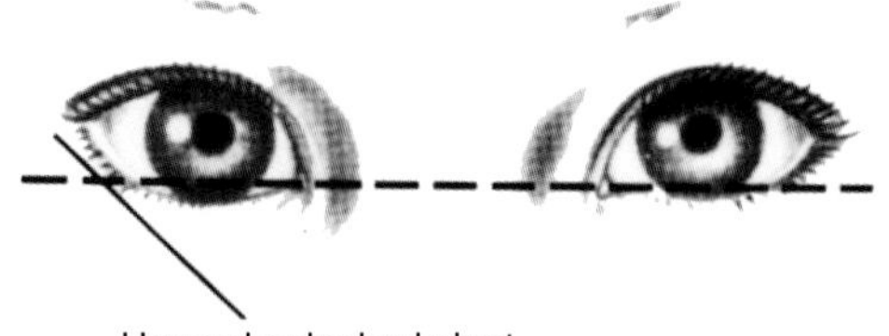

FIG. **1.7** Upward palpebral slant.

Usual Findings	Comments
Even molding of head, occipital prominence	Report any marked skull asymmetry as may indicate premature closure of the sutures.
Symmetric facial features	Observe facial general appearance for signs of movement **and** *asymmetry* that may indicate paralysis
In most infants, head control well established by 4 months of age with head erect and in midline when in a vertical position.	Observe head control for any signs of *head lag*—(may indicate cerebral injury) or *Head tilt* (may indicate vision abnormality)
Moves head up, down, and from side to side	Evaluate for signs of *limited ROM*—Torticollis (wry neck)
Smooth, fused except for fontanels (see Fig. 1.1) Posterior fontanel closes by 2 months Anterior fontanel closes by 12–18 months	Palpate the skull for patent sutures, fontanels, swelling. Observe skull movement for any *resistance or signs of pain* (e.g., meningeal irritation)
Absence of halo around rubber collar	*Halo of light through skull*—Loss of cortex (hydrocephaly)
Clean, pink (more deeply pigmented in dark-skinned children)	*Ecchymotic areas on scalp*—Trauma (possibly abuse) *Loss of hair*—Trauma (hair pulling), lack of stimulation (lying in same position) *Painful sinuses*—Infection
During infancy, normally short with skinfolds between the head and shoulders During early childhood, lengthens	Inspect neck for any masses or webbing and report abnormal findings for further investigation.
In midline; rises with swallowing	Note any deviation, masses, or nodules when palpating neck structures.
In midline; rises with swallowing; lobes equal but often are not palpable	Thyroid is often difficult to palpate.
Equal bilaterally	Note any unequal pulses and protruding neck veins.
Placement is symmetric. Inner canthal distance averages 3 cm (1.2 inches).	Note asymmetry, abnormal spacing (hypertelorism).
Usually palpebral fissures lie horizontally on imaginary line; in Asians, there may be an upward slant.	Presence of upward slant and epicanthal folds may indicate finding in Down syndrome.

Continued

Summary of Physical Assessment of the Child—cont'd

Assessment	Procedure
	Epicanthal fold—Observe for excess fold from roof of nose to inner termination of eyebrow (Fig. 1.8).
	Lids—Observe placement, movement, and color (Fig. 1.9).

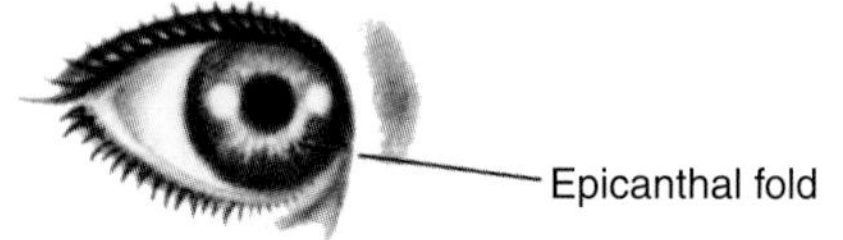

FIG. **1.8** Epicanthal fold.

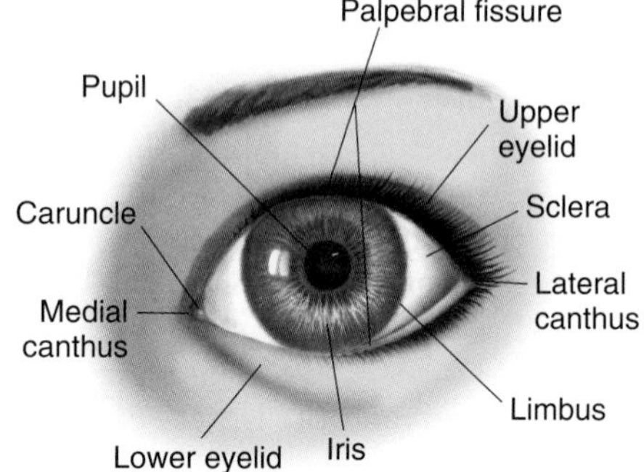

FIG. **1.9** External structures of the eye.

Palpebral conjunctiva

Inspect conjunctive by pulling lower lid down while child looks up.

Evert upper lid by holding lashes and pulling down and forward.

Observe color.

Bulbar conjunctiva—Observe color.

Lacrimal punctum—Observe color, drainage, swelling and discomfort.

Eyelashes and eyebrows—Observe distribution and direction of growth.

Sclera—Observe color (see Fig. 1.9).

Cornea—Observe color and clarity. Check for opacities by shining light toward eye.

Pupils (see Fig. 1.9)

Compare size, shape, and movement.

Test reaction to light; shine light source toward and away from eye.

Test accommodation; have child focus on bright, shiny object at a distance, and quickly moving the object toward the face and the pupils should constrict.

Iris—Observe shape, color, size, and clarity (see Fig. 1.9).

Lens—Inspect lens for transparency. Practice ophthalmoscope use to determine the lens setting that produces the clearest image.

Usual Findings	Comments
Often present in Asian children	Observe epicanthal fold, however, may give false impression of strabismus
When eye is open, lids fall between upper iris and pupil When lid is closed, sclera, cornea, and palpebral conjunctiva are completely covered. Symmetric blink Color is same as surrounding skin.	Inspect lid for symmetry, color and movement Observe for lid deviations: Ptosis (upper lid covers part of pupil or lower iris) Setting sun sign (upper lid above iris) Inability to completely close eye Entropion (turning in) Asymmetric, excessive, or infrequent blinking Signs of inflammation along lid margin or on lid
Pink and glossy Sebaceous glands appear as vertical yellow striations along edge near hair follicle	Note any signs of pallor (may indicate anemia), inflammation, and drainage.
Covers the eye up to the limbus or junction of cornea and sclera and is transparent. Sclera is white in color	Inspect bulbar conjunctiva for color. A reddened conjunctiva may indicate eye strain, fatigue, infection, or irritation such as from excessive rubbing or exposure to environmental irritants.
Tiny opening located in the inner or medial canthus and situated on the upper and lower lids. Same color as lid	Note any excessive discharge, tearing, pain, redness, or swelling that may indicate dacryocystitis.
Eyelashes curl away from eye. Eyebrows are above eye.	Note inward growth of lashes and any unusual hairiness of brows.
White	Observe color as indicate conditions. A yellowish color may indicate jaundice and bluish color may indicate osteogenesis imperfecta.
Cornea is covering of iris and pupil and is clear and transparent. Tiny black marks normal in heavily pigmented children	Note any opacities or ulcerations as may be signs of scarring or ulceration.
Round, clear, and equal Pupils constrict when light approaches, dilate when light fades. Pupils constrict as object is brought near face.	Test reaction to light; record normal findings as *PERRLA* is common notation for pupils equal, round, react to light, and accommodation. Note any asymmetry in size and movement.
Round, equal, clear Color varies from shades of brown, green, or blue and usually established by 6–12 months of age.	Note asymmetry in size, lack of clarity, an iris defect (coloboma) that appears as a black notch at pupil edge giving an irregular shape to pupil. Observe for absence of color (a pinkish glow seen in albinism), or black- and-white speckling (Brushfield spots commonly found in Down syndrome).
Normally not visible through the pupil. Lens permit clear visualization of eye structures with clearest image per ophthalmoscope.	Inspect lens for any opacities.

Continued

Summary of Physical Assessment of the Child—cont'd

Assessment

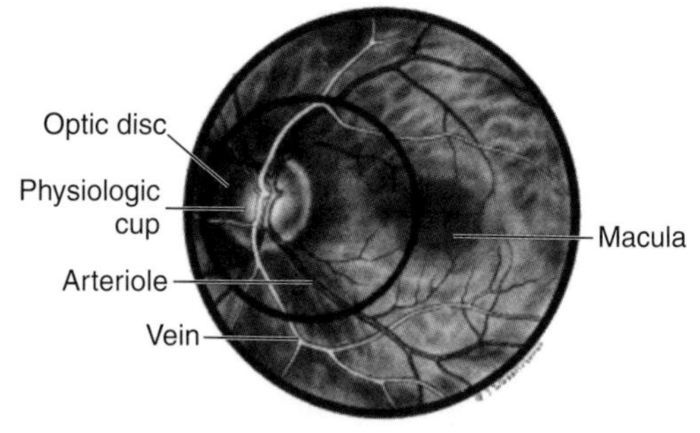

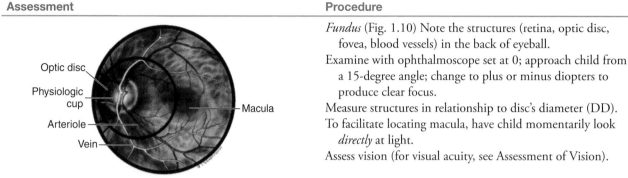

FIG. **1.10** Structures of the fundus. *Interior circle* represents approximate size of area seen with ophthalmoscope.

Procedure

Fundus (Fig. 1.10) Note the structures (retina, optic disc, fovea, blood vessels) in the back of eyeball.

Examine with ophthalmoscope set at 0; approach child from a 15-degree angle; change to plus or minus diopters to produce clear focus.

Measure structures in relationship to disc's diameter (DD).

To facilitate locating macula, have child momentarily look *directly* at light.

Assess vision (for visual acuity, see Assessment of Vision).

STRABISMUS

Normal eyes

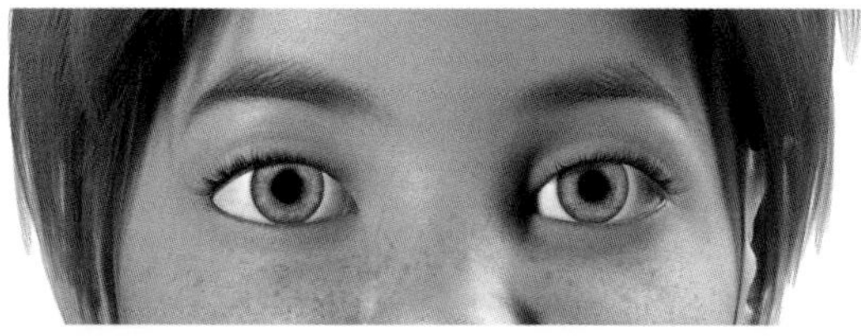

Esotropia

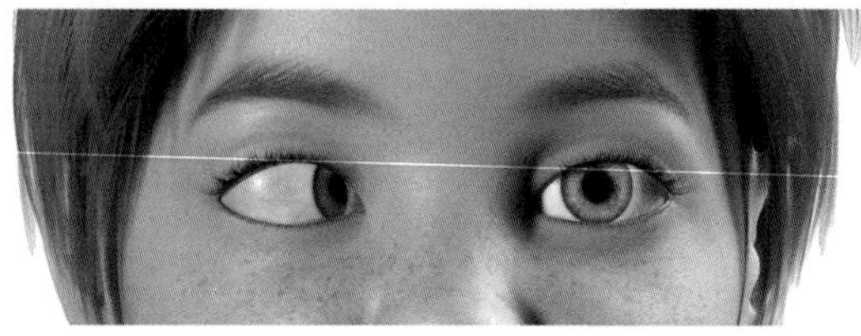

Exotropia

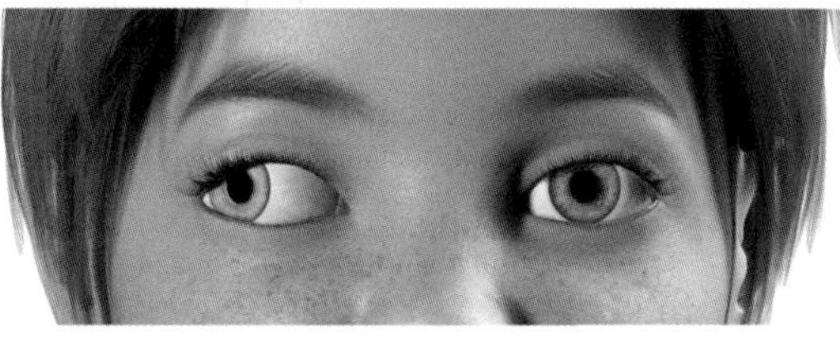

Hypertropia

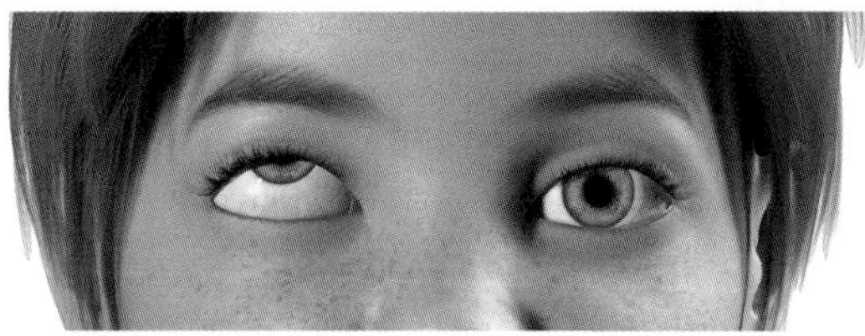

Hypotropia

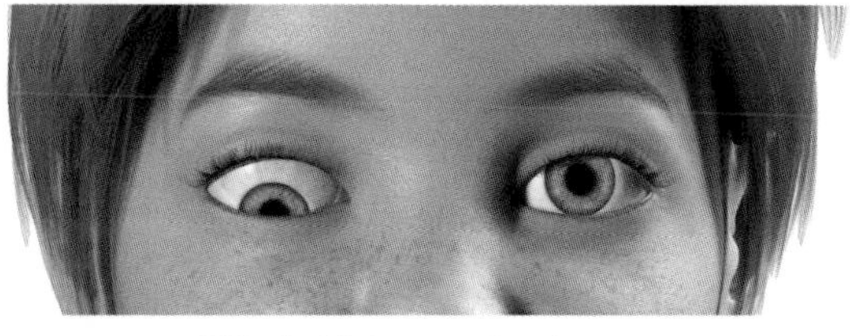

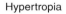

FIG. **1.11** Types of strabismus.

Use following tests for binocular vision:

> **NURSING ALERT**
> The cover test is usually easier to perform if the examiner uses a hand. Attractive occluders in shape of lollipop or Disney characters tend to be used for young children.

Corneal light reflex test (also called *red reflex gemini* or *Hirschberg test*); detects misalignment. Shine flashlight or ophthalmoscope light directly into the eyes from a distance of about 40.5 cm (16 inches).

Cover–uncover test—detect misalignment. Have child fixate on near (33 cm [13 inches]) or distant (50 cm [20 inches]) object; cover one eye, and observe movement of the uncovered eye. (Fig. 1.11 for types of strabismus)

Alternate cover test—detect misalignment. Perform same as cover test, except rapidly cover one eye then the other eye several times; observe movement of covered eye when it is uncovered.

Peripheral vision—visual field of each eye. Instruct child look straight ahead; move an object, such as your finger, from beyond child's field of vision into view; ask child to signal as soon as the object is seen; estimate the angle from straight line of vision to first detection of peripheral vision.

Usual Findings	Comments
Red reflex—Brilliant, uniform reflection of red; appears darker color in deeply pigmented children, lighter in infants	Visualization of red reflex virtually rules out most serious defects of cornea, lens, and aqueous and vitreous chambers.
Optic disc—Orange to creamy pink with pale center but lighter than surrounding fundus; it is normally round or vertically oval	Observe for abnormalities such as partial red or white reflex, blurring of disc margins, bulging of disc, dilated blood vessels, tortuous vessels, hemorrhages
Physiologic cup—Small, pale depression in center of optic disc through which blood vessels pass.	Absence of pulsations
Blood vessels—Emanate from disc; veins are darker and about one-fourth larger than arteries; narrow band of light, the arteriolar light reflex, is reflected from center of arteries, not veins; branches cross each other; may see obvious pulsations	Notching or indenting at crossing of vessels
Macula—1 DD in size, darker in color than disc or surrounding fundus, located 2 DD temporal to the disc	
Fovea centralis—Minute, glistening spot of reflected light in center of macula	
Normally by 3–4 months of age, children are able to fixate on visual field with both eyes simultaneously (binocularity).	Assess vision for visual acuity using binocular test (corneal light reflex test, cover tests, peripheral, color test) and use charts (tumbling E, LEA chart, HOTV test, Snellen screening). Refer any child with nonbinocular vision for further evaluation.
Normally, the light falls symmetrically within each pupil.	Abnormal if the light falls off-center in one eye, the eyes are misaligned.
If uncovered eye does not move, it is aligned.	Abnormal if uncovered eye moves when the other eye is covered
Normal alignment is present if neither eye moves when covered or uncovered.	Abnormal if covered eye moves as soon as cover is removed
In each quadrant, normally the child sees object at 50 degrees upward, 70 degrees downward, 60 degrees nasalward, and 90 degrees temporally	Inability to see object until it is brought closer to straight line of vision indicates need for further evaluation

Continued

Summary of Physical Assessment of the Child—cont'd

Assessment	Procedure
	Color vision—test color vision. Visual screening test: test for measuring visual acuity. Perform visual acuity test with one eye covered with child standing or sitting 10–20 feet away from chart depending on the child's age. Instruct child to keep both eyes open during examination.
Ears	
	Pinnae or auricle—outer portion of the ear located on each side of the head. Inspect placement and alignment (Fig. 1.12). 1.Measure height of pinna by drawing an imaginary line from outer orbit of eye to occiput of skull. 2.Measure angle of pinna by drawing a perpendicular line from the imaginary horizontal line and aligning pinna next to this mark.
	Inspect skin around the ear for presence of any openings, skin tags, earlobe creases, sinuses, or discharge.
	Inspect hygiene (odor, discharge, color).

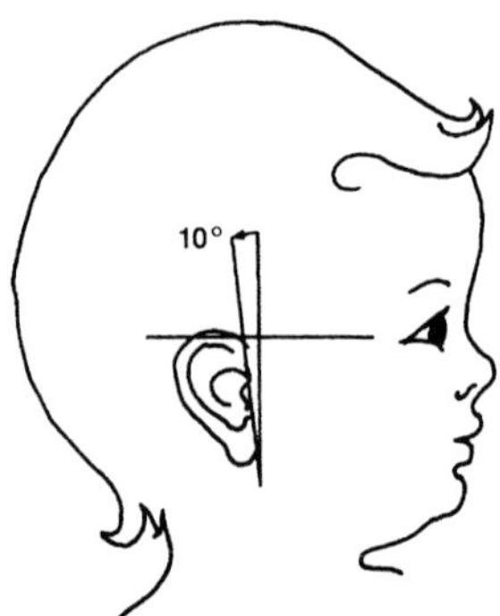

FIG. **1.12** Placement and alignment of pinna.

Usual Findings	Comments
Using Ishihara or Hardy-Rand-Rittler test, child is able to see a letter or figure within the colored dots. All of the following tests are performed with uncovered eyes, then one eye covered in young children (usually 5–6 years or less) standing 10 feet from chart. Older children stand 20 feet from the chart. Snellen chart consists of letters or numbers that child must identify 4 of 6 symbols correctly on each line with progressively smaller symbols displayed as each line is completed. Tumbling E chart displays capital E pointing in 4 directions that is normal if the child points in the correct direction the E is facing, HOTV chart displays H, O, T, V and child has a board with same letters as examiner points to letter on board, if the child matches the correct letter on the board then results are normal. LEA symbols chart displays symbols that the child must identify verbally or point to same symbol on key card. Identifying at least 4 out of 5 symbols on each line is a normal result. Red reflex checks light perception and elicits pupillary light reflex that indicates the anterior half of visual apparatus is intact, it does not confirm the infant can see.	Each test consists of cards on which a color field composed of spots of a certain "confusion" color is printed; against the field is a number (Ishihara) or symbol (Hardy-Rand-Rittler) similarly printed in dots but of a color likely to be confused with the field color by the person with a color vision deficit. Counsel the affected child and parents about the practical inconveniences. Perform red reflex examination in newborns by shining a light into eyes and noting responses (e.g., blinking, pupillary constriction). In newborns, even though little evidence exists to support red reflex exam, it is a widely accepted practice to identify congenital cataract and retinoblastoma.
Pinnae normally slightly crosses or meets this line (see Fig. 1.12).	
Normally, the pinna lies within a 10-degree angle of the vertical line	
Normally the pinna extends slightly forward from the skull Pinna normally prominent and symmetrical	Inspect pinna landmarks (prominences, symmetrical) and report abnormal landmarks. Flattened ears may suggest a frequent side-lying position, and masses or swelling may make the pinna protrude from scalp. Abnormal landmarks are often signs of possible middle ear anomalies.
Normally, the skin is without earlobe creases, sinuses, or drainage. Adherent lobule (normal variation). Tags represent no serious condition.	Note abnormalities (e.g., opening, any discharge, low-set ears).
Normally cerumen is a waxy, soft, yellow substance located in the outer portion of ear canal and produced by ceruminous glands.	If ear needs cleaning, discuss hygiene with parent and child; advise against the use of cotton-tipped applicators or sharp or pointed objects in the canal.

Continued

Summary of Physical Assessment of the Child—cont'd

Assessment	Procedure
ATRAUMATIC CARE Reducing Distress From Otoscopy in Young Children Make examining the ear a game by explaining that you are looking for an "animal" such as an elephant in the ear. This make-believe game is a distraction and usually elicits cooperation. After examining the ear, clarify that "looking for elephants" was only pretend and thank the child for letting you examine the ear.	Internal ear structures include external canal and middle ear structures that are viewed using an otoscope. Otoscope permits visualization of tympanic membrane by use of bright light, magnifying glass and speculum (see Atraumatic Care): Before beginning the otoscopic exam, position the young child properly and gently restrain by the child sitting on parent's lap with parent holding head and body or another position involves placing the child on side, prone or supine with ear to be examined toward ceiling; lean over child, using upper body to restrain arms and trunk and the examining hand stabilizing head. Older children usually cooperate. *Child younger than 3 years*: Introduce speculum between 3 o'clock and 9 o'clock position in a *downward* and *forward* slant. Pull pinna *down* and *back* to the 6 o'clock to 9 o'clock range (Fig. 1.13A). *Child over 3 years* Examine while seated with head tilted slightly away from examiner (if child needs restraining, use one of the previously mentioned positions). Pull pinna *up* and *back* toward a 10 o'clock position (see Fig. 1.13B). Insert speculum ¼ to ½ inch; use widest speculum that diameter of canal easily accommodates. Insert the speculum and inspect the external canal walls, color of tympanic membrane, light reflex, middle ear bony landmarks.

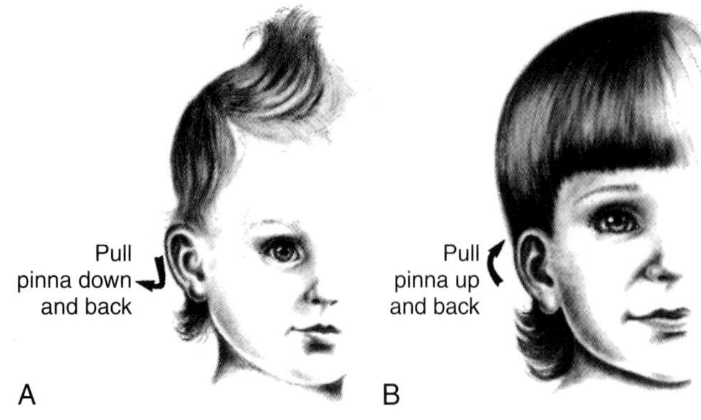

FIG. **1.13** Positions of eardrum. (A) Infant. (B) Child over 3 years of age.

Usual Findings	Comments
External canal—Pink (more deeply colored in dark-skinned child); outermost portion lined with minute hairs, some soft yellow cerumen	Note signs of irritation, discharge, foreign body, and packed cerumen (may interfere with hearing). Helpful suggestion is to let child see you first examine the parent's ear.
Tympanic membrane (Fig. 1.14) is translucent, light pearly pink or gray color. Slight redness seen normally in infants and children as a result of crying *Light reflex*—Cone-shaped reflection, normally points away from face at 5 o'clock or 7 o'clock position Bony landmarks present	Note the following: Red, tense, bulging drum (may indicate suppurative otitis media) Dull, transparent gray color (may indicate serous otitis media) Black areas (may indicate unhealed perforation) Absence of light reflex or bony prominences Retraction of drum with abnormal prominence of landmarks

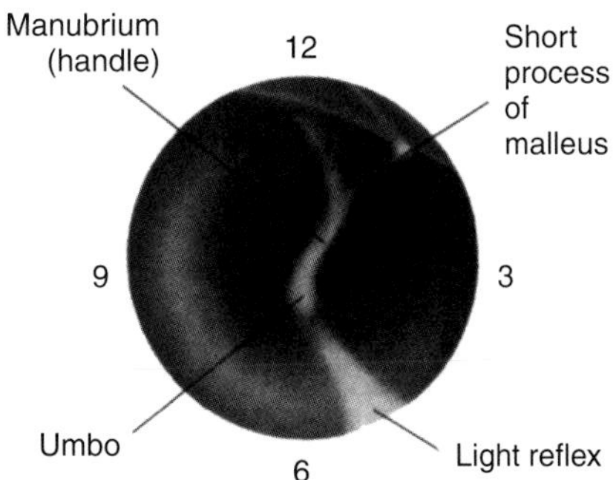

FIG. **1.14** Landmarks of tympanic membrane with clock superimposed.

Continued

Summary of Physical Assessment of the Child—cont'd

Assessment	Procedure
	Auditory screening using auditory test based on age (see Auditory test for infants and children table)

Nose

See Fig. 1.15.	Inspect size, compare nose placement, and alignment by drawing an imaginary vertical line from center point between eyes to notch of upper lip. The nose should lie exactly vertical to the line with each side symmetric. *Anterior vestibule*—Tilt head backward; push tip of nose up and illuminate cavity with flashlight or otoscope without the attached ear speculum; to detect perforated septum, shine light into one naris and observe for admittance of light through perforation.

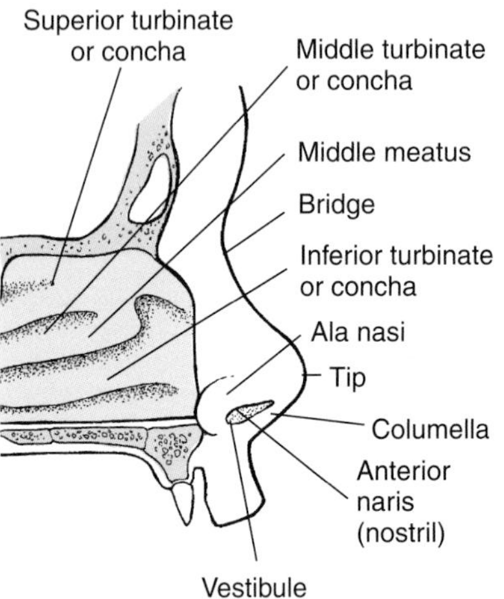

FIG. **1.15** External landmarks and internal structures of the nose.

Mouth and Throat

Lips—Note color, texture, and any obvious lesions.

Internal structures (Fig. 1.16)

Ask cooperative child to open mouth wide and say "Ahh"; which depresses the tongue for full view of the back of the mouth (tonsils, uvula, oropharynx) (Atraumatic Care box).

With young child, place supine with both arms extended alongside of head; have parent maintain arm position to immobilize head; may be necessary to use a tongue blade but avoid eliciting gag reflex by depressing only toward the side of the tongue; use flashlight for good illumination.

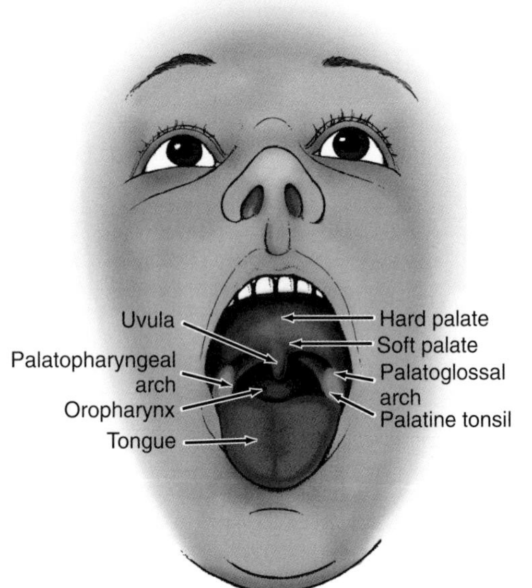

FIG. **1.16** Internal structures of the mouth.

Usual Findings	Comments
Elicit normal hearing results from each type of hearing test (see Auditory test for infants and children table)	Observe for abnormal response to auditory stimuli in neonate (e.g., lack startle reflex, head turning, eye blink, or body movement); infant (e.g., lack of startle or blink reflex to loud sound, absence of babble) children (e.g., use gestures rather than verbalization, intelligible speech, irritability when not understood), then refer for auditory testing.
Both nostrils equal in size Bridge of nose is sometimes flattened in African American or Asian children	Note any deviation to one side, inequality in size of nostrils, or flaring of alae nasi (sign of respiratory difficulty).
Mucosal lining—Redder than oral membranes; moist, but no discharge	Note the following: Abnormally pale, grayish pink, swollen, and boggy membranes Red, swollen membranes
Turbinate and meatus—Same color as mucosal lining Septum—In midline	Any discharge or bleeding Foreign object in nose Deviated septum Perforated septum
More deeply pigmented than surrounding skin; smooth, moist *Mucous membranes*—Bright pink, glistening, smooth, uniform, and moist	Note cyanosis, pallor, lesions, or cracks, especially at corners. Note lesions, bleeding, sensitivity, or odor.
Gingiva—Firm, coral pink, and stippled; margins are "knife-edged" *Teeth*—Number appropriate for age, white, good occlusion of upper and lower jaws General rule for estimating number of teeth in children: Under 2 years: Age (in months) minus 6 (e.g., 12 months minus 6 = 6 teeth)	Note redness, puffiness (especially at margin), or tendency to bleed. Note loss of teeth, delayed eruption, malocclusion, or obvious discoloration. Compare dental findings with parental report of dental hygiene. Assess need for further dental counseling: Eating habits, such as bottle-feeding or prolonged breast-feeding during day for use as "pacifier" or at bedtime, excessive sugar Toothbrushing Sources of fluoride, need for supplementation Periodic, regular examinations by dentist
Tongue—Rough texture, freely movable, tip extends to lips, no lesions or masses under tongue	Note smoothness, fissuring, coating on the tongue, excessive redness, swelling, or inability to move the tongue forward to lips; can interfere with speech.
Palate—Intact, slightly arched	Note presence of any clefts.

Continued

Summary of Physical Assessment of the Child—cont'd

Assessment	Procedure
Chest	
See Fig. 1.17.	Inspect size, shape, symmetry, movement, breast development and bony landmarks formed by ribs and sternum. Describe findings according to geographic and imaginary landmarks (Fig. 1.18). Locate intercostal space (ICS), the space directly below rib, by palpating chest inferiorly from second rib. Other landmarks: Nipples usually at fourth ICS Tip of eleventh rib felt laterally Tip of twelfth rib felt posteriorly Tip of scapula at eighth rib or ICS
	Inspect breast development.

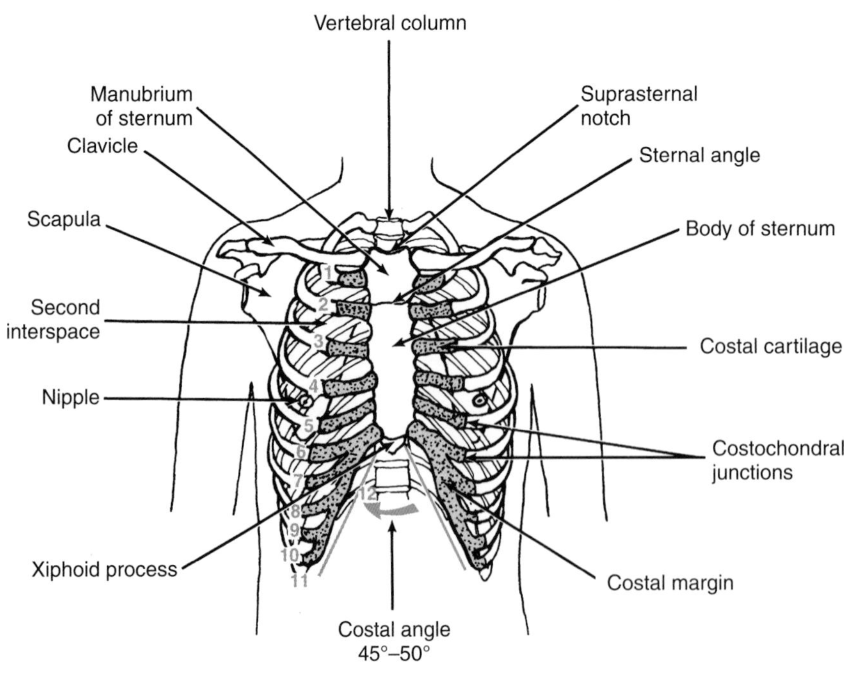

FIG. **1.17** Structures of the rib cage.

Usual Findings	Comments
Uvula—Protrudes from back of soft palate, moves upward during gag reflex	Note if a bifid (divided in midline) uvula is present.
Palatine tonsils—Same color as surrounding mucosa, glandular rather than smooth, size varies during childhood.	Note exudate and enlargement that could become obstructive.
Posterior pharynx—Same color as surrounding mucosa, smooth, moist	Assess for signs of infection (erythema, edema, white lesions, or exudate).
In infants, shape is almost circular; with growth, lateral diameter increases in proportion to anteroposterior diameter.	Measurement of chest and palpation of axillary nodes may be done here.
Both sides of chest symmetric Points of attachment between ribs and costal cartilage smooth Movement—During inspiration, chest rises and expands, costal angle increases, and diaphragm descends; during expiration, reverse occurs Nipples—Darker pigmentation, located slightly lateral to midclavicular line between fourth and fifth ribs	Note deviations: Barrel-shaped chest (round chest) Asymmetry Wide or narrow costal angle Bony prominences *Pectus carinatum (pigeon breast)*—Sternum protrudes outward. *Pectus excavatum (funnel chest)*—Lower portion of sternum is depressed. Retraction Asymmetric or decreased movement
Breast development depends on age; no masses.	Compare breast development with expected stage for age (see Fig. 1.50). Discuss importance of monthly breast self-examination with female adolescents.

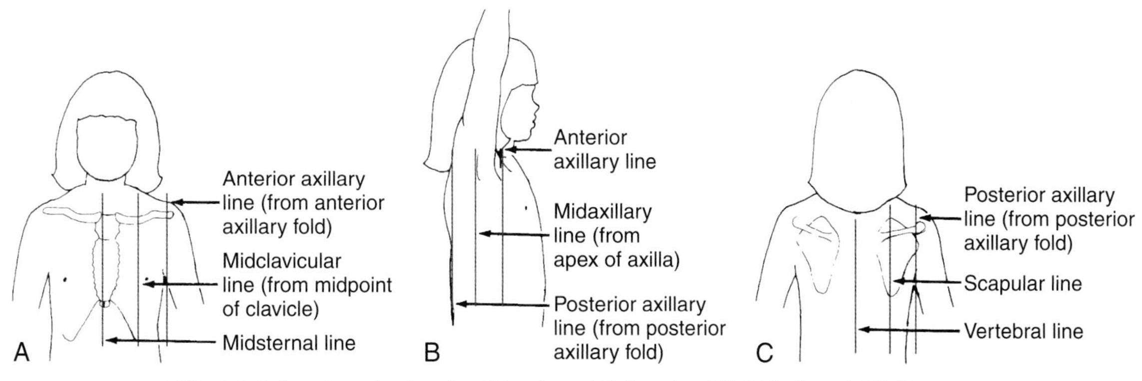

FIG. **1.18** Imaginary landmarks of the chest. (A) Anterior. (B) Right lateral. (C) Posterior.

Continued

Summary of Physical Assessment of the Child—cont'd

Assessment	Procedure
Lungs	
Figs. 1.19 and 1.20.	Evaluate respiratory movements for rate, rhythm, depth, quality, and character. (See Atraumatic Care below) With child sitting, place each hand flat against back or chest with thumbs in midline along lower costal margins of lungs. The child should be sitting during procedure, if cooperative should take several deep breathes. *Vocal fremitus*—Palpate as above, and have child say "99," "eee." Percuss each side of chest in sequence from apex to base (see Fig. 1.20): For anterior aspects of lungs, child sitting or supine For posterior aspects of lungs, child sitting Auscultate breath and voice sounds for intensity, pitch, quality, and relative duration of inspiration and expiration.

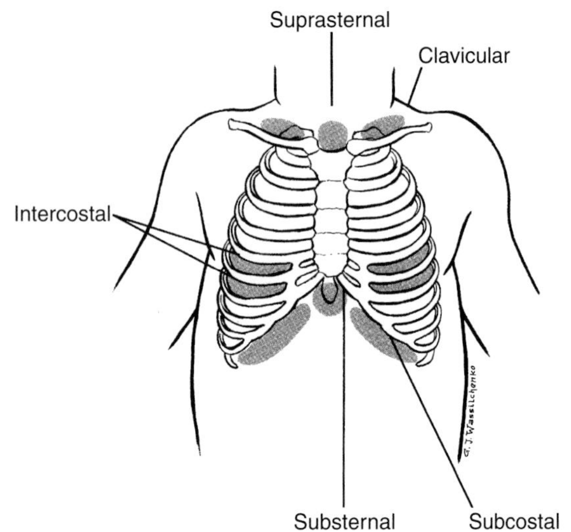

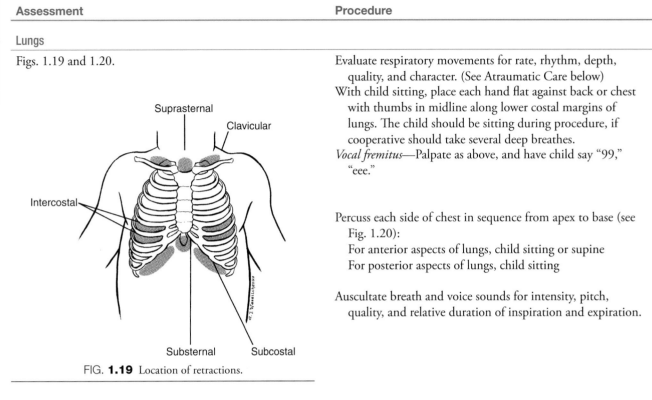

FIG. **1.19** Location of retractions.

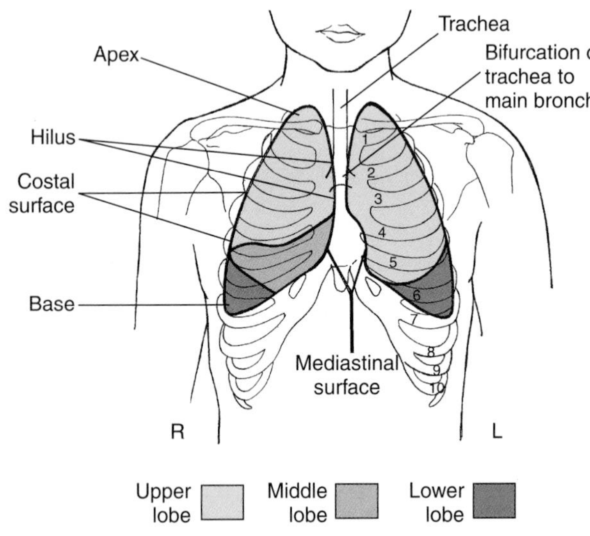

FIG. **1.20** Location of anterior lobes of lungs within thoracic cavity.

Usual Findings	Comments
Rate expected for age (see inside front cover); regular, effortless, and quiet	Note abnormal rate; irregular rhythm; shallow depth; difficult breathing; or noisy, grunting respirations (see Box 1.2).
Moves symmetrically with each breath; posterior base descends 5–6 cm (2–2.3 inches) during deep inspiration	Note asymmetric breaths
Vibrations are symmetric and most intense in thoracic area and least intense at base.	Note asymmetric vibrations or sudden absence or decrease in intensity. Note abnormal vibrations, such as pleural friction rub or crepitation.
Lobes are resonant except for (Fig. 1.21): Dullness at fifth interspace right midclavicular line (liver) Dullness from second to fifth interspace over left sternal border to midclavicular line (heart) Tympany below left fifth interspace (stomach)	Note deviation from expected sounds.
Vesicular breath sounds—Heard over entire surface of lungs except upper intrascapular area and beneath manubrium; inspiration louder, longer, and of higher pitch than expiration Sound is soft, swishing noise.	Note deviations from expected breath sounds, particularly if diminished; note absence of sounds. Note adventitious sounds.
Bronchovesicular breath sounds—Heard in upper intrascapular area and over the manubrium; inspiration is louder and higher pitched than in vesicular breathing.	*Crackles*—Discrete, noncontinuous crackling sound, heard primarily during inspiration from passage of air through fluid or moisture; if crackles clear with deep breathing, they are not pathologic
Bronchial breath sounds—Heard only over trachea near suprasternal notch; expiration longer, louder, and of higher pitch than inspiration	*Wheezes*—Continuous musical sounds; caused by air passing through narrowed passages, regardless of cause (e.g., exudate, inflammation, foreign body, spasm, tumor) *Audible inspiratory wheeze (stridor)*—Sonorous, musical wheeze heard without a stethoscope; indicates a high obstruction (e.g., epiglottitis) *Audible expiratory wheeze*—Whistling, sighing wheeze heard without a stethoscope; indicates a low obstruction *Pleural friction rub*—Crackling, grating sound during inspiration and expiration; occurs from inflamed pleural surfaces; not affected by coughing
Voice sounds—Heard, but syllables are indistinct	Consolidation of lung tissue produces three types of abnormal voice sounds: *Whispered pectoriloquy*—The child whispers words, and the nurse hears the syllables. *Bronchophony*—The child speaks words that are not distinguishable, but the vocal resonance is increased in intensity and clarity. *Egophony*—The child says "ee," which is heard as the nasal sound "ay" through the stethoscope.

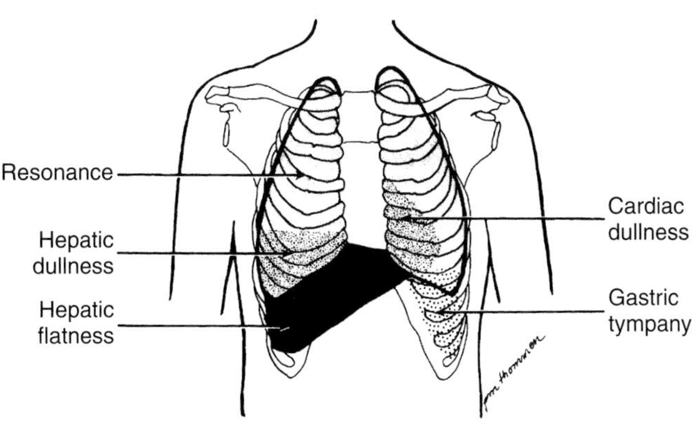

FIG. **1.21** Percussion sounds in thorax.

Continued

Summary of Physical Assessment of the Child—cont'd

Assessment	Procedure
Heart	
Fig. 1.22.	*General Instructions* Begin with inspection, followed by palpation, then auscultation. Percussion is not done because it is of limited value in defining the borders or the size of the heart. Palpate to determine the location of the apical impulse, the most lateral cardiac impulse that may correspond to the apex.

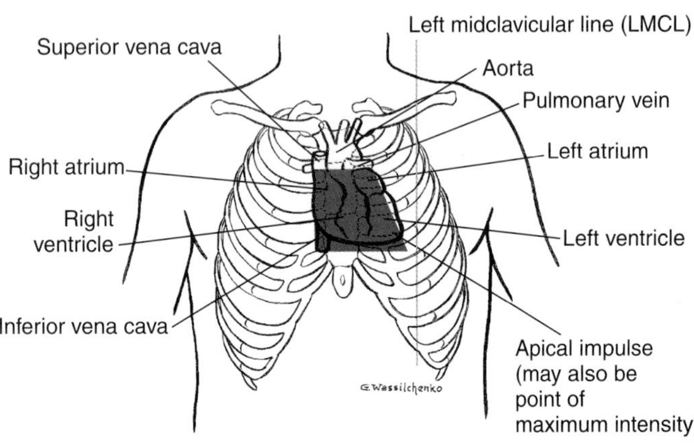

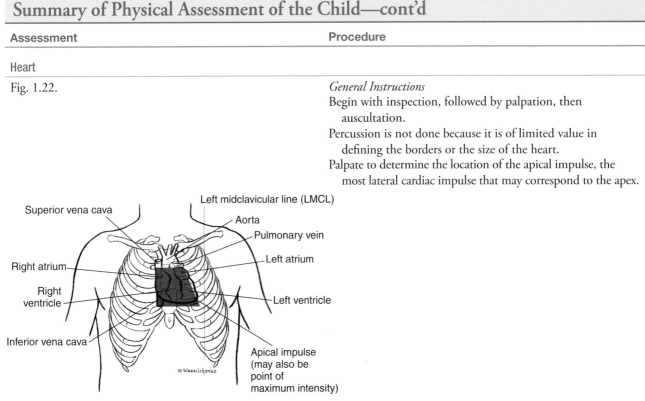

FIG. **1.22** Position of heart within thorax.

Palpate skin for capillary filling time as is an important test for circulation and hydration:

- Lightly press skin on central site, such as forehead, and peripheral site, such as top of hand or foot, to produce slight blanching.
- Assess time it takes for blanched area to return to original color. Auscultate for heart sounds:
- Listen with child in sitting and reclining positions.
- Use both diaphragm and bell chest pieces.
- Evaluate sounds for quality, intensity, rate, and rhythm (Box 1.3).Follow sequence (Fig. 1.23):

Aortic area—Second right intercostal space close to sternum
Pulmonic area—Second left intercostal space close to sternum
Erb point—Second and third left intercostal spaces close to sternum
Tricuspid area—Fifth right and left intercostal spaces close to sternum
Mitral or apical area—Fifth intercostal space, left midclavicular line (third to fourth intercostal space and lateral to left midclavicular line [MCL] in infants)

BOX 1.3 Various Patterns of Heart Rate or Pulse

Tachycardia—Increased rate
Bradycardia—Decreased rate
Pulsus alternans—Strong beat followed by a weak beat
Pulsus bigeminus—Coupled rhythm in which beat is felt in pairs because of premature beat
Pulsus paradoxus—Intensity or force of pulse decreases with inspiration
Sinus arrhythmia—Rate increases with inspiration, decreases with expiration
Water-hammer or Corrigan's pulse—Especially forceful beat caused by a very wide pulse pressure (systolic blood pressure minus diastolic blood pressure)
Dicrotic pulse—Double radial pulse for every apical beat
Thready pulse—Rapid, weak pulse that seems to appear and disappear

Usual Findings	Comments
Symmetric chest wall apical impulse (AI) sometimes apparent (in thin children)	Note obvious bulging. Infant's heart is larger in proportion to chest size and lies more centrally.
AI is found in the following: Just lateral to the left MCL and fourth ICS in children >7 years of age At the left MCL and fifth ICS in children >7 years of age	Although the apical impulse gives a general idea of the size of the heart (with enlargement, the apex is lower and more lateral), its normal location is quite variable, making it a rather unreliable indicator of heart size; **point of maximum intensity (PMI)**, area of most intense pulsation, usually is located at same site as apical impulse but it can occur elsewhere. For this reason, the two terms should not be used synonymously. During palpation, may feel abnormal vibrations called **thrills** that are similar to cat's purring; they are produced by blood flowing through narrowed or abnormal opening, such as stenotic valve or septal defect.
Capillary refilling in 1–2 s	Refilling taking longer than 2 s is abnormal and indicates impaired skin perfusion; cool temperature prolongs capillary refill time.
S_1 to S_2—Clear, distinct, rate equal to radial pulse; rhythm regular and even Aortic area—S_2 louder than S_1 Pulmonic area—Splitting of S_2 heard best (normally widens on inspiration) Erb point—Frequent site of innocent murmurs Tricuspid area—S_1 louder sound preceding S_2 Mitral or apical area—S_1 heard loudest; splitting of S_1 may be audible Quality—Clear and distinct Intensity—Strong, but not pounding Rate—Same as radial pulse Rhythm—Regular and even	To distinguish S_1 from S_2, palpate for carotid pulse, which is synchronous with S_1. A normal arrhythmia is **sinus arrhythmia**, in which heart rate increases with inspiration and decreases with expiration. Identify abnormal sounds; note presence of adventitious sounds such as pericardial friction rubs (similar to pleural friction rubs but not affected by change in respiration). Record murmurs in relation to the following: Area best heard Timing within S_1–S_2 cycle Change with position Loudness and quality

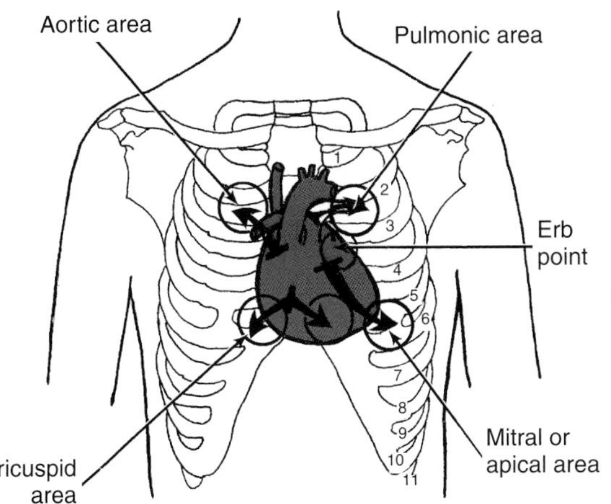

FIG. **1.23** Directions of heart sounds from anatomic valve sites.

Continued

Summary of Physical Assessment of the Child—cont'd

Assessment	Procedure
Abdomen	
	General Instructions Inspection is followed by auscultation, percussion, then perform palpation last as may distort the normal abdominal sounds. Palpation may be uncomfortable for the child; deep palpation causes a feeling of pressure, and superficial palpation causes a tickling sensation. To minimize any discomfort and encourage cooperation, use the following: Position child supine with legs flexed at hips and knees. Distract child with stories or talking. Have child "help" with palpation by placing own hand over examiner's palpating warm hand or have child place own hand on abdomen with fingers spread wide apart and palpate between the fingers. Inspect contour, size, and tone in erect and supine positions.
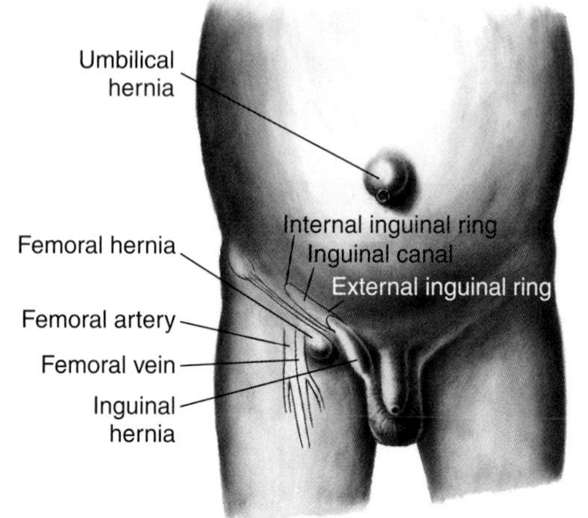 FIG. **1.24** Locations of hernias.	Note condition of skin. Note movement. Inspect umbilicus for size, hygiene, and any abnormalities (herniation, fistulas, and discharge). Observe for hernias (Fig. 1.24): *Inguinal*—Slide little finger into external inguinal ring at base of scrotum; ask child to cough. If hernia present, it will hit the finger tip. *Femoral*—Place finger over femoral canal (located by placing index finger over femoral pulse and middle finger against skin toward midline). Auscultate for bowel sounds and aortic pulsations. Listen up to 5 min before determining bowel sounds are absent.

Usual Findings	Comments
Usual findings of innocent murmurs: Timing within ***S1-S2 cycle***—Systolic, that is, they occur with or after S1 Quality—Usually of a low-pitched, musical, or groaning quality Loudness—Grade III or less in intensity and do not increase over time Area best heard—Usually loudest in the pulmonic area, with no transmission to other areas of the heart Change with position—Audible in the supine position but absent in the sitting position Other physical signs—Not associated with any physical signs of cardiac disease	Grading of the intensity of heart murmurs: I—Very faint, frequently not heard if child sits up II—Usually readily heard, slightly louder than grade I, audible in all positions III—Loud but not accompanied by a thrill IV—Loud, accompanied by a thrill V—Loud enough to be heard with the stethoscope barely on the chest, accompanied by a thrill VI—Loud enough to be heard with the stethoscope not touching the chest, often heard with the human ear close to the chest, accompanied by a thrill
Infants and young children—Cylindric and prominent in erect position, flat when supine *Adolescents*—Characteristic adult curves, fairly flat when erect Circumference decreases in relation to chest size with age. Firm tone	Contour, size, and tone are indicators of nutritional status and muscular development. Note deviations: Prominent, flabby Distention Concave Tense, boardlike Loose, wrinkled Midline protrusion Silvery, whitish striae Distended veins
Smooth, uniformly taut In children under 7 or 8 years, rises with inspiration and synchronous with chest movement In older children, less respiratory movement In thin children, visible pulsations from descending aorta sometimes seen in epigastric region	Paradoxic respirations (chest rises while abdomen falls) Visible peristaltic waves
Flat to slight protrusion; no herniation or discharge	If herniation is present, palpate sac for abdominal contents and estimate size of opening.
No herniation present	
Bowel sounds—Short, metallic, tinkling sounds like gurgles, clicks, or growls heard every 10–30 s	Bowel sounds may be stimulated by stroking abdominal wall with a fingertip.

Continued

Summary of Physical Assessment of the Child—cont'd

Assessment	Procedure
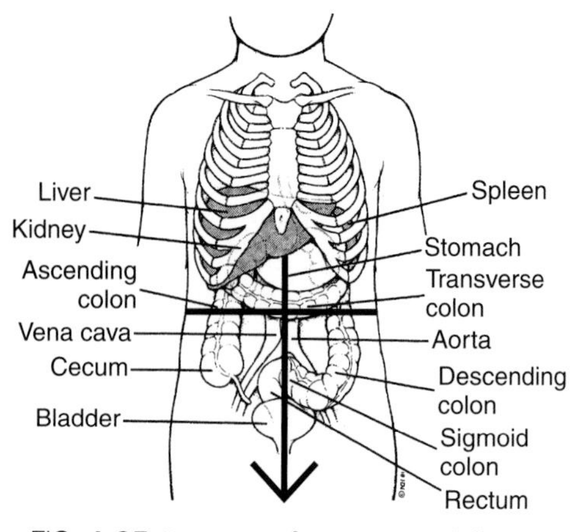 FIG. **1.25** Locations of structures in abdomen.	Percuss the abdomen. Palpate abdominal organs (Fig. 1.25): Place one hand flat against back, and use palpating hand to "feel" organs between both hands. Proceed from lower quadrants *upward* to avoid missing edge of enlarged organ.
	For descriptive purpose, the abdominal cavity is divided into four quadrants by drawing an imaginary vertical line midway from sternum to the symphysis pubis and horizontal line across the abdomen at umbilicus (see Fig. 1.25): Right upper quadrant (RUQ) Right lower quadrant (RLQ) Left upper quadrant (LUQ) Left lower quadrant (LLQ) Palpate femoral pulses simultaneously—Place tips of two or three fingers along the inguinal ligament about midway between iliac crest and pubic symphysis. Elicit abdominal reflex—Scratch skin from side to midline in each quadrant.
Genitalia	
Male Fig. 1.26. 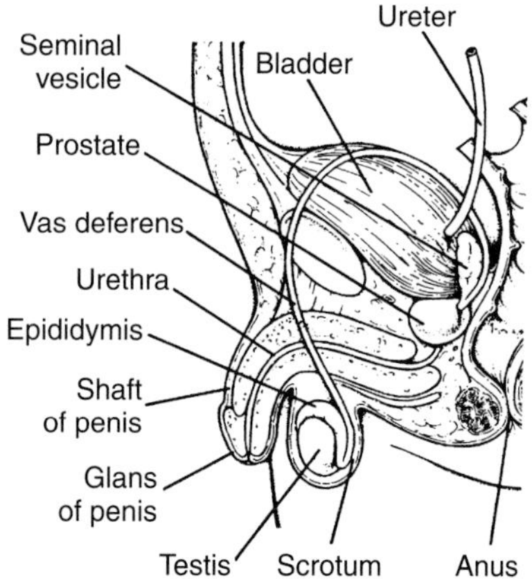 FIG. **1.26** Major structures of genitalia in circumcised prepubertal male.	*General Instructions* Proceed in same manner as examination of other areas; explain procedure and its significance prior to exam, such as palpating for testes. Respect privacy at all times. Use opportunity to discuss concerns or questions about sexual development or sexual activity with older child and adolescent. Use opportunity to discuss sexual safety with young children. If in contact with body substances, wear gloves. *Penis*—Inspect size. *Glans and shaft*—Inspect for signs of swelling, skin lesions, inflammation, or other irregularities. *Prepuce*—Inspect in uncircumcised male.

Usual Findings	Comments
Aortic pulsations—Heard in epigastrium, slightly left of midline	Note hyperperistalsis or absence of bowel sounds.
Tympany over stomach on left side and most of abdomen, except for dullness or flatness just below right costal margin (liver)	Note percussion sounds other than those expected.
Liver—1 to 2 cm below right costal margin in infants and young children	Usually not palpable in older children Considered enlarged if 3 cm below costal margin Normally descends with inspiration; should not be considered a sign of enlargement
Spleen—Sometimes 1 to 2 cm below left costal margin in infants and young children	Usually not palpable in older children Considered enlarged if more than 2 cm below left costal margin; also descends with inspiration Other structures that sometimes are palpable include kidneys, bladder, cecum, and sigmoid colon; know their location to avoid mistaking them for abnormal masses; most common palpable mass is feces. In sexually active females, consider a palpable mass in the lower abdomen a pregnant uterus.
Equal and strong bilaterally	Note absence of femoral pulse. Normally may be absent in children under 1 year of age
Umbilicus moves toward quadrant that was stroked.	Examination may be anxiety producing for older children and adolescents; may be left for end of physical examination.
Generally, size is insignificant in prepubescent male. Compare growth with expected sexual development during puberty (see Fig. 1.49). None	Note large penis, possible sign of precocious puberty. In obese child, penis may be obscured by fat pad over pubic symphysis.
Easily retracted to expose glans and urethral meatus	In infants, prepuce is tight for up to 3 years and should not be retracted.

Continued

Summary of Physical Assessment of the Child—cont'd

Assessment	Procedure
	Urethral meatus—Inspect location, and note any discharge.
	Scrotum—Inspect size, location, skin, and hair distribution.
	Testes—Palpate each scrotal sac using thumb and index finger of a warm hand.
Female Fig. 1.27.	*External genitalia*—Inspect structures; place young child in semireclining position in parent's lap with knees bent and soles of feet in apposition.
	Labia—Palpate for any masses.
	Urethral meatus—Inspect for location; identified as *V*-shaped slit by wiping downward from clitoris to perineum. *Skene glands*—Palpate or inspect
	Vaginal orifice—Internal examination usually not performed; inspect for obvious opening.
	Bartholin glands—Palpate or inspect

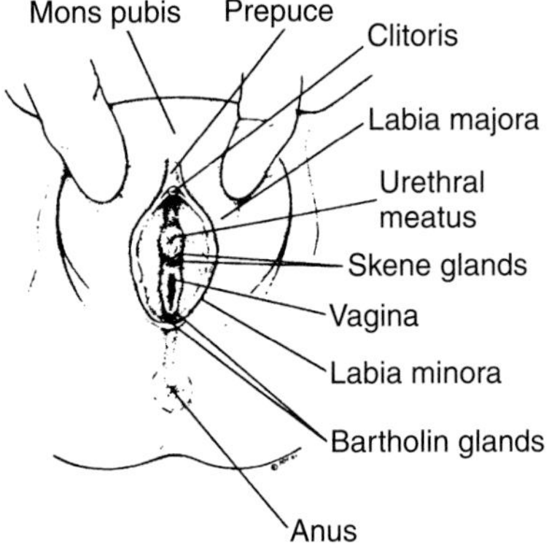

FIG. **1.27** External structures of genitalia in prepubertal female. Labia are spread to reveal deep structures.

Anus	
	Anal area—Inspect for general firmness, condition of skin, preferably with child placed on abdomen. *Anal reflex (anal wink)*—Elicit by gently scratching perianal area.

Usual Findings	Comments
Centered at tip of glans	Discuss importance of hygiene.
No discharge	Note location on ventral or dorsal surface of penis, possible sign of ambiguous genitalia, hypospadias, or epispadias. Whenever possible, note strength and direction of urinary stream.
May appear large in infants Hangs freely from perineum behind penis One sac hangs lower than other.	Note scrota that are small, close to perineum, with any degree of midline separation.
Loose, wrinkled skin, usually redder and coarser in adolescents	Well-formed rugae indicate descent of testes.
Compare hair distribution with that expected for pubertal stage; typical mature male pattern forms a diamond shape from umbilicus to anus (see Fig. 1.49).	
Small ovoid bodies about 1.5–2 cm long Double in size during puberty	Prevent cremasteric reflex that retracts testes by: Warming hands Having child sit in tailor fashion or squat Blocking pathway of ascent by placing thumb and index finger over upper part of scrotal sac along inguinal canal Note and report any failure to palpate testes after taking these precautions. Discuss testicular self-examination with adolescent male.
Mons pubis—pad of adipose tissue over symphysis pubis; covered with hair in adolescence; usual hair distribution is triangular (see Fig. 1.51)	Note hair distribution as an early sign of sexual maturation in pre-pubescent girl.
Clitoris—Located at anterior end of labia minora; covered by small flap of skin (prepuce)	Note evidence of enlargement (may be small phallus).
Labia majora—Two thick folds of skin from mons to posterior commissure; inner surface pink and moist	Note any palpable masses, evidence of fusion, enlargement, or signs of female circumcision.
Labia minora—Two folds of skin interior to labia majora, usually invisible until puberty; prominent in newborn	
Located posterior to clitoris and anterior to vagina	Note opening from clitoris or inside vagina.
Surround meatus; no lesions	Common sites of cysts and venereal warts (condyloma acuminata)
Located posterior to urethral meatus; may be covered by crescent-shaped or circular membrane (**hymen**); discharge usually clear or whitish	Note excessive, foul-smelling, or colored discharge.
Surround vaginal opening; no lesions, secrete clear mucoid fluid	
Buttocks—Firm; gluteal folds symmetric	Note evidence of diaper rash; inquire about hygiene and type of diaper (cloth or disposable).
Quick contraction of external anal sphincter; no protrusion of rectum	Note: Fissures Polyps Rectal prolapse Hemorrhoids Warts

Continued

Summary of Physical Assessment of the Child—cont'd

Assessment	Procedure
Back and Extremities	
	Inspect curvature and symmetry of spine (Fig. 1.28).
	Test for scoliosis: Have child stand erect; observe from behind, and note asymmetry of shoulders and hips. Have child bend forward at the waist until back is parallel to floor; observe from side, and note asymmetry or prominence of rib cage. Note mobility of spine.
	Inspect each extremity joint for symmetry, size, temperature, color, tenderness, and mobility. Test for developmental dysplasia of the hip.
	Assess shape of bones: Measure distance between the knees when child stands with malleoli in apposition. Measure distance between the malleoli when child stands with knees together. Inspect position of feet; test if foot deformity at birth is result of fetal position or development by scratching outer, then inner, side of sole; if self-correctable, foot assumes right angle to leg.

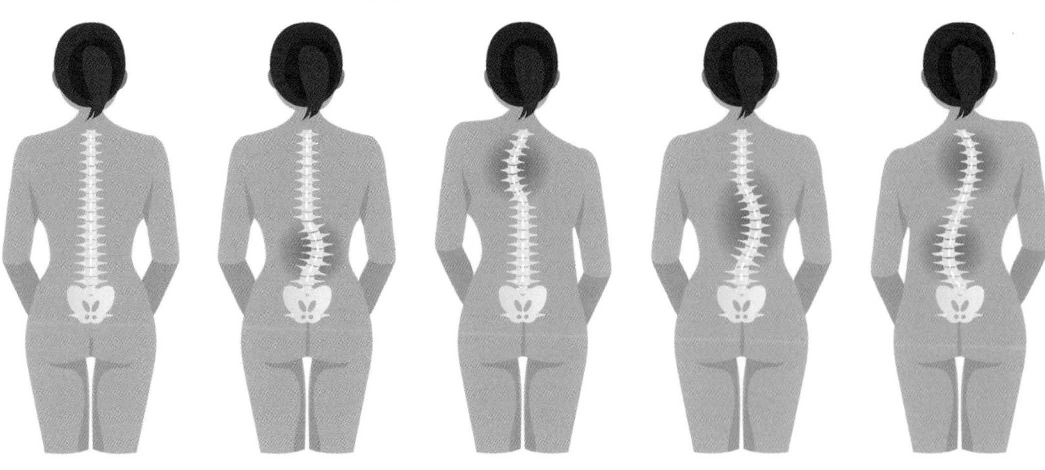

FIG. **1.28** Defects of spinal column. (A) Normal spine. (B) Kyphosis. (C) Lordosis. (D) Normal spine in balance. (E) Mild scoliosis in balance. (F) Severe scoliosis not in balance. (G) Rib hump and flank asymmetry seen in flexion caused by rotary component.

Usual Findings	Comments
Rounded or C-shaped in the newborn from the thoracic and pelvic curves. Older children have the typical double-S curve Cervical secondary curve forms at about 3 months of age. Lumbar secondary curve forms at about 12–18 months, resulting in typical double-S curve Lordosis normal in young children but decreases with age Shoulders, scapula, and iliac crests symmetric	Note any abnormal curvatures and presence of masses or lesions. Other signs and symptoms of scoliosis: Slight limp, crooked hem or complaint of backache
Flexible, full range of motion, no pain or stiffness	Note stiffness and pain on movement of neck or back; requires immediate evaluation.
Symmetric length Equal size Correct number of digits Nails pink Temperature equal, although feet may be cooler than hands Full range of motion	Note any deviations (e.g., extra digit or fused digit). Note warmth, swelling, color, tenderness, and immobility of joints.
Less than 5 cm (2 inches) in children over 2 years of age	Greater distance indicates **genu varum (bowleg)** (Fig. 1.29A).
Less than 7.5 cm (3 inches) in children over 7 years of age	Greater distance indicates **genu valgum (knock knee)** (see Fig. 1.29B).
Held at right angle to leg; pointed straight ahead or turned slightly outward when standing Fat pads on sole give appearance of flat feet; arch develops after child is walking.	Note foot and ankle deformities (Box 1.4).

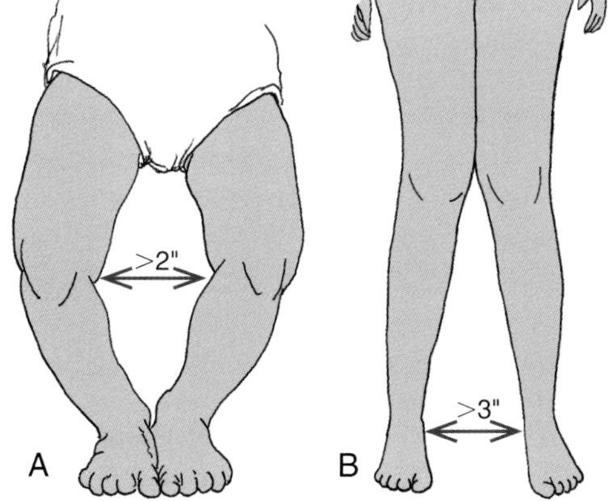

FIG. **1.29** (A) Genu varum (bowleg). (B) Genu valgum (knock knee).

BOX 1.4 Types of Foot and Ankle Deformities

Pes planus (flatfoot)—Normal finding in infancy; may be the result of muscular weakness in an older child
Pes valgus—Eversion (turning outward) of the entire foot, but the sole rests on the ground
Pes varus—Inversion (turning inward) of the entire foot, but the sole rests on the ground
Metatarsus valgus—Eversion of forefoot while the heel remains straight; also called toeing out or duck walk
Talipes valgus—Eversion of the foot so that only the inner side of the foot rests on the ground
Talipes varus—Inversion of the foot so that only the outer sole of the foot rests on the ground
Talipes equinus—Extension or plantar flexion of the foot so that only ball and toes rest on the ground; commonly combined with talipes varus (most common of clubfoot deformities)
Talipes calcaneus—Dorsal flexion of the foot so that only the heel rests on the ground

Continued

Summary of Physical Assessment of the Child—cont'd

Assessment	Procedure
	Inspect gait: Have child walk in straight line. Estimate angle of gait by drawing imaginary line through center of foot and line of progression.
	Plantar reflex—Elicit by stroking lateral sole from heel upward to little toe across to hallux. Babinski reflex is elicited by stroking outer sole upward from heel and across ball of foot causes toes to fan and big toe to dorsiflex Inspect symmetry and quality of muscle development and tone and strength of muscles. Test strength: *Arms*—Have child hold arms outstretched in front of body and tries to raise arms while downward pressure is applied. *Legs*—Have child sit with legs dangling; proceed as with arms. *Hands*—Have child squeeze 1 or 2 fingers of nurse's hand as tightly as possible. *Feet*—Have child plantar flex (push soles toward floor) while applying counterpressure to soles.
Neurologic Assessment	
Mental Status	Observe behavior, mood, affect, general orientation to surroundings, and level of consciousness (see Box 1.23).
Motor Functioning	Test muscle strength, tone, and development. Test cerebellar functioning: *Finger-to-nose test*—With child's arm extended, have child touch nose with the index finger. *Heel-to-shin test*—With child standing, have child run the heel of one foot down the shin of the other leg. During heel-to-shin and Romberg tests, stand close to child to prevent falls. *Romberg test*—Have child stand erect with feet together and eyes closed. Have child touch tip of each finger to thumb in rapid succession. Have child pat leg with first one side, then the other side of hand in rapid sequence. Have child tap your hand with ball of foot as quickly as possible.
Sensory Functioning	Test vision and hearing (see Assessment of Hearing [see p. 138] and Assessment of Vision [see p. 134]). *Sensory intactness*—Touch skin lightly with an object, and have child point to stimulated area while keeping eyes closed. Sensory discrimination: Touch skin with pin and cotton; have child describe the sensation as sharp or dull. Touch skin with cold and warm object (e.g., metal and rubber heads of reflex hammer); have child differentiate between temperatures. Using two pins, touch skin simultaneously with both or only one pin; have child discriminate when one or two pins are used.

Usual Findings	Comments
"Toddling" or broad-based gait normal in young children; gradually assumes graceful gait with feet close together. Feet turn outward less than 30 degrees and inward less than 10 degrees.	Note abnormal gait: Waddling Scissor Toeing-in Broad-based in older children
Flexion of toes in children older than 1 year Babinski reflex disappears after age 1 year.	Babinski reflex seen in children over 2 years is considered abnormal and may denote nervous system or brain disorder (see Assessment of Reflexes)
Symmetric Increase in tone during muscle contraction Equal bilaterally	Note and report any signs of atrophy, hypertrophy, spasticity, flaccidity, rigidity, or weakness.
	Subjective impressions are based on observation throughout the examination. Objective findings can be attained through developmental testing.
Performs each test successfully with eyes opened and closed	May be difficult to test in children younger than preschool age
	Note any awkwardness or lack of coordination in performance.
Romberg test—Does not lean to side or fall	Falling or leaning to one side is abnormal and is called the **Romberg sign**.
Localizes object	Abnormal if unable to localize object on skin. Compare sensation in symmetric areas at both distal and proximal points.
Able to distinguish types of sensation and temperature	Note difficulty in performing test, especially in older child.
Minimal distance for discrimination on finger is about 2–3 mm.	

Continued

Summary of Physical Assessment of the Child—cont'd

Assessment	Procedure
Reflexes (Deep Tendon)	**Biceps**—Hold child's arm by placing the partially flexed elbow in your hand with the thumb over the antecubital space; strike your thumbnail with the hammer (Fig. 1.30A).

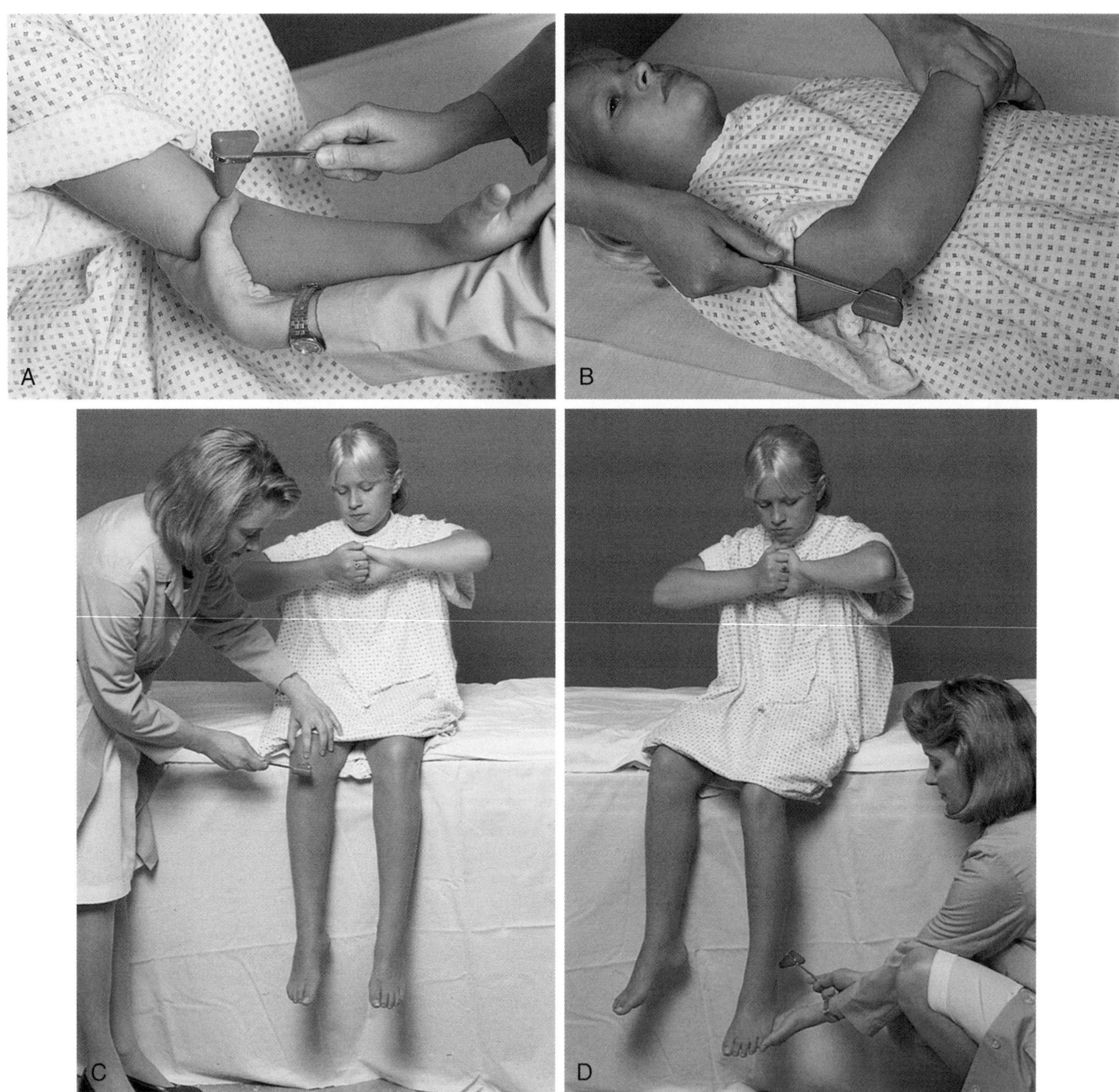

FIG. **1.30** (A) Testing for the biceps reflex (from Fig. 4.43). (B) Testing for the triceps reflex (from Fig. 4.42). (C) Testing for the patellar reflex (from Fig. 4.44). (D) Testing for the Achilles reflex. (From Fig. 4.45). (All Added from Essentials 11th ed, Chapter 4, p. 109.)

Usual Findings	Comments
Biceps—Partial flexion of forearm	Use distraction techniques to prevent child from inhibiting reflex activity: For upper extremity reflexes, ask child to clench teeth or to squeeze thigh with the hand on the side not being tested. Rest upper arm in palm of hand. For lower extremity reflexes, have child lock fingers and pull one hand against the other or grip hands together. Usual grading of reflexes: **Grade 0**—Absent **Grade 1**— Diminished **Grade 2**—Normal, average **Grade 3**—Brisker than normal **Grade 4**—Hyperactive (clonus) Note asymmetric, absent, diminished, or hyperactive reflexes.

Continued

Summary of Physical Assessment of the Child—cont'd

Assessment	Procedure
	Triceps—Bend the arm at the elbow, and rest the palm in your hand; strike the triceps tendon (see Fig. 1.30B). *Alternate procedure*—If child is supine, rest arm over chest and strike the triceps tendon (see Fig. 1.30B). *Brachioradialis*—Rest forearm on the lap or abdomen, with the arm flexed at the elbow and palm down; strike the radius about 1 inch (depending on child's size) above the wrist. *Knee jerk or patellar reflex*—Sit child on the edge of the examining table or on parent's lap with the lower legs flexed at the knee and dangling freely; tap the patellar tendon just below the knee cap (see Fig. 1.30C). *Achilles*—Use the same position as for the knee jerk; support the foot lightly in your hand, and strike the Achilles tendon (see Fig. 1.30D). *Ankle clonus*—See Ankle clonus in Assessment of Reflexes (see p. 22). *Kernig sign*—Flex child's leg at hip and knee while supine; note pain or resistance. *Brudzinski sign*—With child supine, flex the head; note pain and involuntary flexion of hip and knees.
Cranial Nerves	See Assessment of Cranial Nerves on Table 1.5.

Usual Findings	Comments
Triceps—Partial extension of forearm	
Brachioradialis—Flexion of the forearm and supination (turning upward) of the palm	
Patellar—Partial extension of lower leg	
Achilles—Plantar flexion of foot (foot pointing downward)	
Ankle clonus—Absence of beats	
Kernig—Absence of pain or resistance	These special reflexes are elicited when meningeal irritation is suspected.
Brudzinski—Absence of pain or associated movements	Signs of pain, resistance, or associated movements require immediate referral. Testing of cranial nerves (Fig. 1.31) may be done as part of the neurologic examination or integrated into assessment of each system, such as cranial nerves II, III, IV, and VI with the eye (Fig. 1.32). Cranial nerves can usually be tested in children of preschool age and older. Note inability to perform any of the items correctly.

Continued

TABLE 1.5 Assessment of Cranial Nerves

Description and Function	Tests
I—Olfactory Nerve	
Olfactory mucosa of nasal cavity Smell	With eyes closed, have child identify odors such as coffee, alcohol from a swab, or other smells; test each nostril separately.
II—Optic Nerve	
Rods and cones of retina, optic nerve Vision	Check for perception of light, visual acuity, peripheral vision, color vision, and normal optic disc.
III—Oculomotor Nerve	
Extraocular muscles of eye: • Superior rectus—moves eyeball up and in • Inferior rectus—moves eyeball down and in • Medial rectus—moves eyeball nasally • Inferior oblique—moves eyeball up and out	Have child follow an object (toy) or light in six cardinal positions of gaze (see Fig. 4.47).
Pupil constriction and accommodation	Perform PERRLA (Pupils Equal, Round, React to Light, and Accommodation).
Eyelid closing	Check for proper placement of lid.
IV—Trochlear Nerve	
Superior oblique muscle (SO)—moves eye down and out	Have child look down and in (see Fig. 4.47).
V—Trigeminal Nerve	
Muscles of mastication	Have child bite down hard and open jaw; test symmetry and strength.
Sensory—face, scalp, nasal and buccal mucosa	With child's eyes closed, see if child can detect light touch in mandibular and maxillary regions. Test corneal and blink reflex by touching cornea lightly with a whisk of cotton ball twisted into a point (approach from side so that child does not blink before cornea is touched).
VI—Abducens Nerve	
Lateral rectus (LR) muscle—moves eye temporally	Have child look toward temporal side (see Fig. 4.47).
VII—Facial Nerve	
Muscles for facial expression	Have child smile, make funny face, or show teeth to see symmetry of expression.
Anterior two-thirds of tongue (sensory)	Have child identify sweet or salty solution; place each taste on anterior section and sides of protruding tongue; if child retracts tongue, solution will dissolve toward posterior part of tongue.
VIII—Auditory, Acoustic, or Vestibulocochlear Nerve	
Internal ear Hearing and balance	Test hearing; note any loss of equilibrium or presence of vertigo.
IX—Glossopharyngeal Nerve	
Pharynx, tongue	Stimulate posterior pharynx with a tongue blade; child should gag.
Posterior third of tongue Sensory	Test sense of sour or bitter taste on posterior segment of tongue.
X—Vagus Nerve	
Muscles of larynx, pharynx, some organs of gastrointestinal system, sensory fibers of root of tongue, heart, and lung	Note hoarseness of voice, gag reflex, and ability to swallow. Check that uvula is in midline; when stimulated with tongue blade, it should deviate upward and to stimulated side.
XI—Accessory Nerve	
Sternocleidomastoid and trapezius muscles of shoulder	Have child shrug shoulders while applying mild pressure; with examiner's hands placed on shoulders, have child turn head against opposing pressure on either side; note symmetry and strength.
XII—Hypoglossal Nerve	
Muscles of tongue	Have child move tongue in all directions; have child protrude tongue as far as possible; note any midline deviation. Test strength by placing tongue blade on one side of tongue and having child move it away.

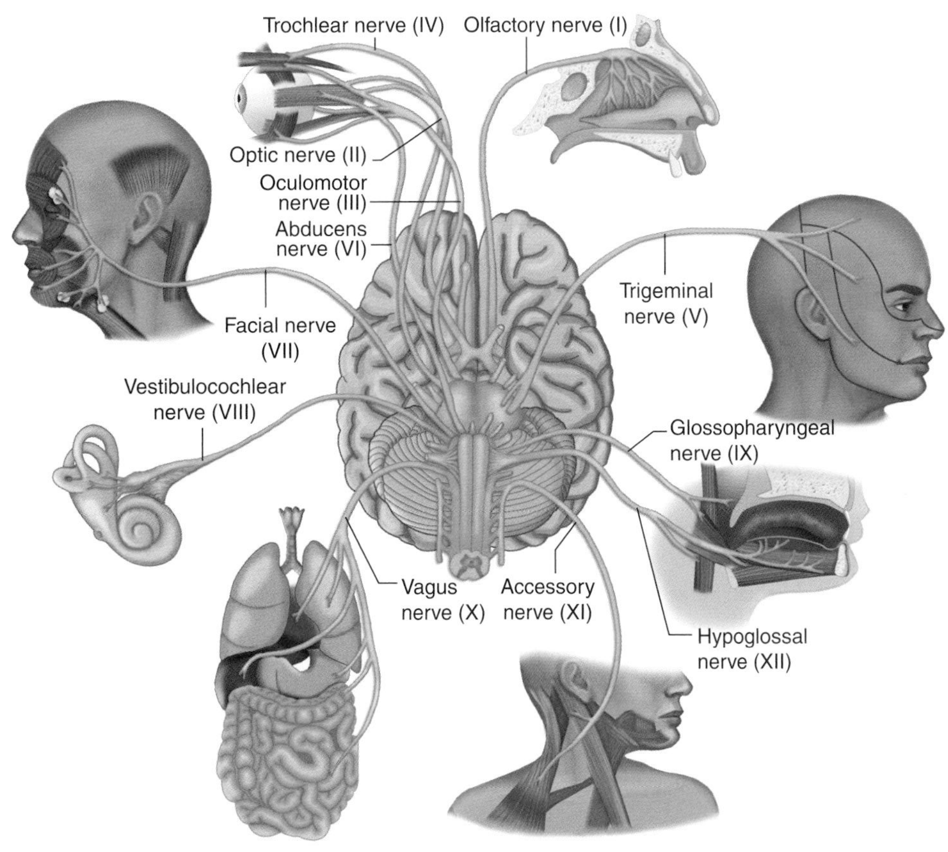

FIG. **1.31** Cranial nerves. (From Patton, K. T., & Thibodeau, G. A. [2013]. *Anatomy and physiology* [8th ed.]. St Louis: Mosby.)

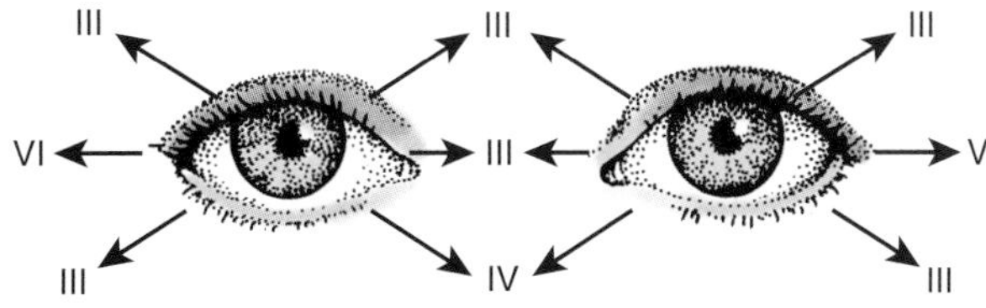

FIG. **1.32** Checking extraocular movements in the six cardinal positions indicates the functioning of cranial nerves III, IV, and VI. (From Ignatavicius DD, Workman ML: Medical-Surgical Nursing: Patient-Centered Collaborative Care. 6th ed. St. Louis: Saunders; 2009.)

Temperature Measurement Locations for Infants and Children

Oral

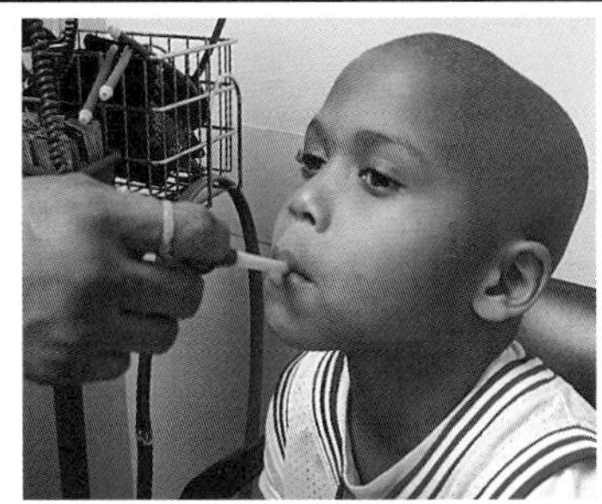

Place tip under tongue in right or left posterior sublingual pocket, not in front of tongue. Have child keep mouth closed, without biting on thermometer.

Continued

Pacifier thermometers measure intraoral or supralingual temperature and are available but lack support in the literature.
Several factors affect mouth temperature: Eating and mastication, hot and cold beverages, open-mouth breathing, ambient temperature.

Axillary

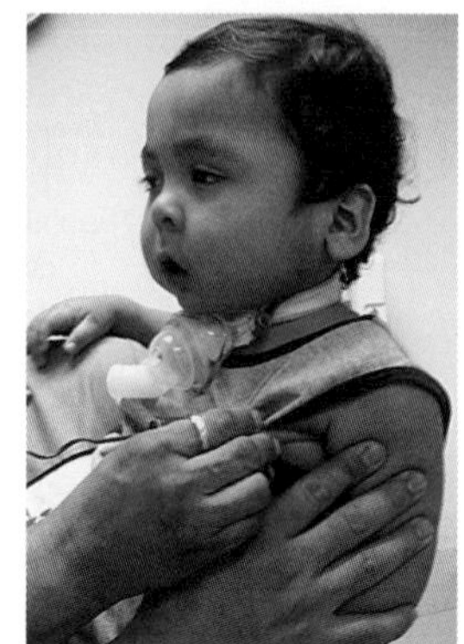

Place tip under arm in center of axilla and keep close to skin, not clothing. Hold child's arm firmly against side.
Temperature may be affected by poor peripheral perfusion (results in lower value), clothing or swaddling, use of radiant warmer, or amount of brown fat in cold-stressed neonate (results in higher value).
Advantage: avoids intrusive procedure and eliminates risk of rectal perforation.

Ear Based (Aural)

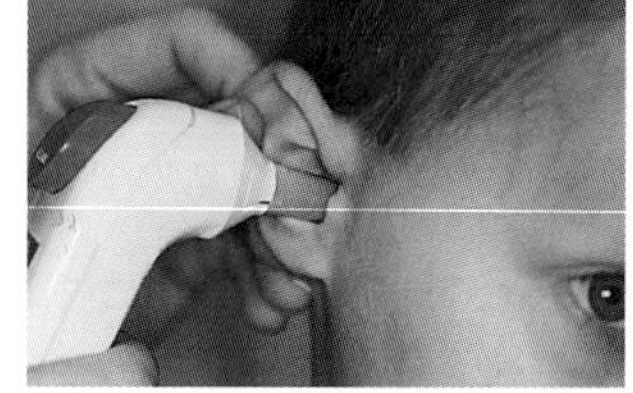

Insert small infrared probe deeply into the canal to allow the sensor to obtain the measurement from tympanic membrane. Size of the probe (most are 8 mm) may influence accuracy of result. In young children, this may be a problem because of the small diameter of the canal. Proper placement of the ear is controversial to whether the pinna should be pulled in manner similar to that used during otoscopy.

Rectal

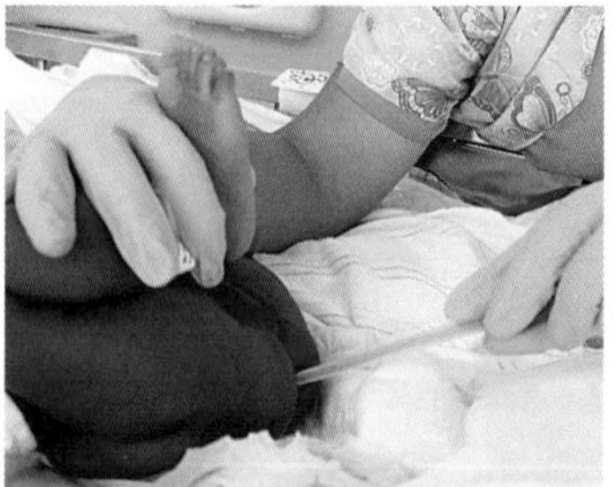

Place well-lubricated tip at maximum 2.5 cm (1 inch) into rectum for children and 1.5 cm (0.6 inch) for infants; securely hold thermometer close to anus.
Child may be placed in side-lying, supine, or prone position (i.e., supine with knees flexed toward abdomen); cover penis because procedure may stimulate urination. A small child may be placed prone across parent's lap.

Temporal Artery

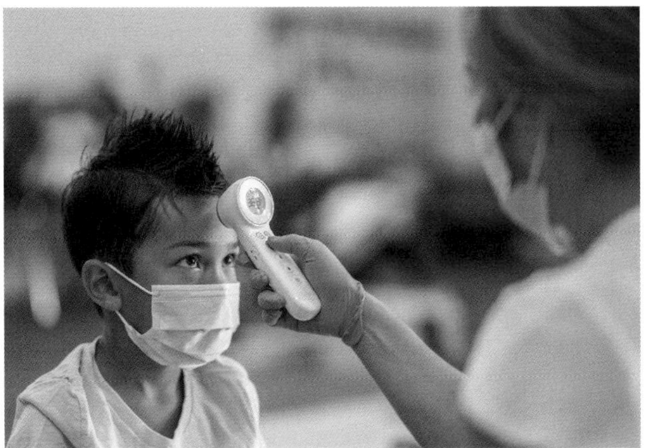

An infrared sensor probe scans across the forehead, capturing heat from the arterial blood flow. Temporal artery is the only artery close enough to the skin's surface to provide access for accurate temperature measurement.

Data from Martin SA, Kline AM. Can there be a standard for temperature measurement in the pediatric intensive care unit? *AACN Clin Issues.* 2004;15(2):254–266; Falzon A, Grech V, Caruana B, et al. How reliable is axillary temperature measurement? *Acta Paediatr.* 2003;92(3):309–313. Oral, axillary, rectal, and temporal artery images courtesy Paul Vincent Kuntz, Texas Children's Hospital, Houston, TX.

Nursing Assessment of Specific Health Problems

The Child with Acute Respiratory Infection

Assessment—The Child with Acute Respiratory Infection

Acute respiratory infection—An inflammatory process caused by viral, bacterial, or atypical (mycoplasma) infection or aspiration of foreign substances, which involves any or all parts of the respiratory tract

Lower respiratory tract—Consists of the bronchi and bronchioles (which constitute the reactive portion of the airway because of their smooth muscle content and ability to constrict) and the alveoli

Croup syndromes—Consist of the epiglottis, larynx, and trachea (the structurally stable, nonreactive portion of the airway)

Upper respiratory tract (upper airway)—Consists of the oronasopharynx, pharynx, larynx, and upper part of the trachea

Assessment

Assist with diagnostic procedures and tests (e.g., radiography, throat culture, thoracentesis, venipuncture for blood analysis).

Observe for general clinical manifestations of acute respiratory tract infection (Box 1.5).

Identify factors affecting the type of illness and response to acute respiratory infection (e.g., age and size of the child, ability to resist infection, contact with infected children, and coexisting disorders affecting the respiratory tract).

Assess respiratory status.

Monitor respirations for rate, depth, pattern, presence of retractions, and flaring nares.

Auscultate lungs.

- Evaluate breath sounds (type and location).
- Detect the presence of crackles or wheezes or the absence of breath sounds (movement of air).
- Detect areas of consolidation.
- Evaluate the effectiveness of chest physiotherapy.

Observe for the presence or absence of retractions, and nasal flaring.

Observe the color of skin and mucous membranes for pallor and cyanosis.

Observe for the presence of hoarseness, stridor, and cough.

Monitor heart rate and regularity.

Observe behavior.

- Restlessness
- Irritability
- Apprehension

Observe for components of the respiratory function listed in Box 1.6 for assessing respiratory function

- The pattern of respirations (rate, depth, ease, rhythm, labored breathing)
- Other observations (chest pain, cough, wheeze, cyanosis, sputum, halitosis)

Observe for clinical manifestations of respiratory infection

Upper Respiratory Tract Infections

Nasopharyngitis—Viral infection, acute rhinitis or coryza, equivalent of the common cold. Symptoms are more severe in infants and children and typically last 4 to 14 days. The diameter of the airways is smaller in young children and subject to considerable narrowing from edematous mucus membranes and increased production of secretions.

BOX 1.5 Components for Assessing Respiratory Function

Pattern of Respirations

Rate: Rapid (tachypnea), normal, or slow for the particular child

Depth: Normal depth, too shallow (hypopnea), too deep (hyperpnea); usually estimated from the amplitude of thoracic and abdominal excursion (age dependent)

Ease: Effortless, labored (dyspnea), orthopnea (difficult breathing except in an upright position), associated with intercostal or substernal retractions (inspiratory "sinking in" of soft tissues in relation to the cartilaginous and bony thorax), pulsus paradoxus (blood pressure falling with inspiration and rising with expiration), nasal flaring, head bobbing (head of sleeping child with suboccipital area supported on caregiver's forearm bobbing forward in synchrony with each inspiration), grunting, wheezing, or stridor

Labored breathing: Continuous, intermittent, becoming steadily worse, sudden onset, at rest or on exertion, associated with wheezing, grunting, and/or chest pain

Rhythm: Variation in rate and depth of respirations

Other Observations

In addition to respirations, particular attention is addressed to:

Evidence of infection: Check for elevated temperature; enlarged cervical lymph nodes; inflamed mucous membranes; and purulent discharges from the nose, ears, or lungs (sputum).

Cough: Observe the characteristics of the cough (if present), when the cough is heard (e.g., night only, on arising), the nature of the cough (paroxysmal with or without wheeze, "croupy" or "brassy"), frequency of the cough, association with swallowing or other activity, character of the cough (moist or dry), productivity.

Wheeze: Note whether it is with expiration or inspiration, high pitched or musical, prolonged, slowly progressive or sudden, or associated with labored breathing.

Cyanosis: Note distribution (peripheral, perioral, facial, trunk, and face), degree, duration, and association with activity.

Chest pain: Older children tend to have this complaint. Note location and circumstances: localized or generalized; referral to the base of neck or abdomen; dull or sharp; deep or superficial; association with rapid, shallow respirations or grunting.

Sputum: Older children may provide a sputum sample by coughing, whereas young children may need the use of a bulb suction or early-morning gastric lavage to provide a sample. Note volume, color, viscosity, and odor.

Bad breath (halitosis): May be associated with some throat and lung infections.

Assessment

Younger child

- Fever
- Irritability, restlessness
- Decrease oral intake
- Sneezing
- Nasal mucus (may cause mouth breathing)
- Vomiting and/or diarrhea, sometimes
- Decreased appetite
- Decreased activity

Older child

- Low-grade fever
- Dryness and irritation of nose and throat initially
- Sneezing, chilling
- Muscular aches
- Nasal discharge
- Cough, sometimes

Pharyngitis—Throat (including the tonsils) is the principal anatomic site of pharyngitis (sore throat) caused by bacteria or viruses (Box.1.7). Most common causative organism is group A beta-hemolytic streptococci (Fig.1.33). Several pairs of tonsils are part of a mass of lymphoid tissue encircling the nasal and oral pharynx known as Waldeyer tonsillar tissue, with the palatine tonsils visual with examination and adenoids located above palatine tonsils in the nasopharynx (see Fig. 1.33).

Assessment

Observe clinical manifestations of nasopharyngitis and pharyngitis (see Box 1.7)

In acute infectious pharyngitis, streptococcal infections should be suspected in children older than 2 years old who have pharyngitis without exudate or nasal symptoms.

Tonsillitis (Often Occurs With Pharyngitis)

Tonsils are masses of lymphoid tissue located in the pharyngeal cavity (see Fig. 1.33). Tonsils filter and protect the respiratory and alimentary tract from the invasion by a pathogenic organism and play a role in antibody formation.

Influenza (flu)—Caused by three antigenically distinct orthomyxoviruses: types A and B, which cause epidemic disease, and type C, which is antigenically stable and causes mild disease.

May be subclinical, mild, moderate, or severe

Overt illness

Assessment

- Dry throat and nasal mucosa
- Dry cough
- Tendency toward hoarseness
- Sudden onset of fever and chills
- Flushed face
- Photophobia
- Myalgia
- Hyperesthesia
- Prostration (sometimes)
- Fatigue (sometimes exhaustion)
- Subglottal croup common (especially in infants)

Otitis Media (OM)

OM is the presence of fluid in the middle ear with acute signs and symptoms caused by viruses (e.g., RSV and influenza) and bacteria (e.g., streptococcus pneumoniae, H. influenza, Moraxella catarrhalis). The standard terminology used to define OM is outlined in Box 1.8.

Observe for clinical manifestations of OM that are listed in Box 1.9.

BOX 1.6 Signs and Symptoms Associated With Respiratory Infections in Infants and Small Children

Fever

May be absent in newborn infants

Greatest at ages 6 months to 3 years

- Temperature may reach 39.5°C to 40.5°C (103°F to 105°F), even with mild infections

Often appears as the first sign of infection

Child may be listless and irritable, or somewhat euphoric and more active than normal temporarily; some children talk with unaccustomed rapidity

Tendency to develop high temperatures with infection in certain families

- May precipitate febrile seizures
- Febrile seizures uncommon after 3 or 4 years of age

Meningismus

Meningeal signs without infection of the meninges

Occurs with abrupt onset of fever

Accompanied by:

- Headache
- Pain and stiffness in the back and neck
- Presence of Kernig and Brudzinski signs

Subsides as temperature drops

Anorexia

Common with most childhood illnesses

Frequently the initial evidence of illness

Almost invariably accompanies acute infections in small children

Persists to a greater or lesser degree throughout the febrile stage of illness; often extends into convalescence

Vomiting

Small children vomit readily with illness

A clue to the onset of infection

May precede other signs by several hours

Usually short-lived but may persist during the illness

Diarrhea

Usually mild, transient diarrhea but may become severe

Often accompanies viral respiratory infections

Is a frequent cause of dehydration

Abdominal Pain

Common complaint

Sometimes indistinguishable from the pain of appendicitis

Mesenteric lymphadenitis may be a cause

Muscle spasms from vomiting may be a factor, especially in nervous, tense children

Nasal Blockage

Small nasal passages of infants are easily blocked by mucosal swelling and exudation

Can interfere with respiration and feeding in infants

May contribute to the development of otitis media and sinusitis

Nasal Discharge

Frequent occurrence

May be thin and watery (rhinorrhea) or thick and purulent, depending on the type and/or stage of infection

Associated with itching

May irritate upper lip and skin surrounding the nose

Cough

Common feature

May be evident only during the acute phase

May persist several months after a disease

Respiratory Sounds

Sounds associated with respiratory disease

- Cough
- Hoarseness
- Grunting
- Stridor
- Wheezing

Auscultation

- Wheezing
- Crackles
- Absence of sound

Sore Throat

Frequent complaint of older children

Younger children (unable to describe symptoms) may not complain, even when their throat is highly inflamed. Often the child will refuse to take oral fluids or solids

Infectious Mononucleosis

Infectious mononucleosis is an acute, self-limiting infectious disease primarily caused by EBV and is common among people under 25 years old. Observe for presenting signs and symptoms that may be acute or insidious and vary (see Box 1.10 on clinical manifestations of infectious mononucleosis).

Croup Syndromes

Croup is a general term applied to a symptom complex characterized by hoarseness, a resonant cough described as barking (croupy), varying degrees of inspiratory stridor, and varying degrees of respiratory distress resulting from swelling or obstruction in the region of the larynx and subglottic airway. Croup syndromes are caused by viruses or bacteria and are described according to the affected anatomic area (Table 1.6).

Acute laryngitis—Infection is usually viral; primary clinical manifestation is hoarseness; common illness of older children and adolescents.

Acute laryngotracheobronchitis (LTB)—Viral infection; most common of the croup syndromes; usually occurs in children younger than 5 years, primarily affecting children 6 months to 3 years. The onset is slowly progressive (see Classic manifestations and treatment are listed in Table 1.6)

Acute spasmodic laryngitis (spasmodic croup)—Viral infection with allergic and psychogenic factors in some cases; distinguished from laryngitis and LTB by

BOX 1.7 Clinical Manifestations of Acute Nasopharyngitis and Pharyngitis

Nasopharyngitis

Younger Children

Fever
Irritability, restlessness
Decreased appetite and fluid intake
Sneezing
Nasal mucus (abundant) causing mouth breathing
Vomiting or diarrhea may be present
Decreased activity

Older Children

Dryness and irritation of nose and throat initially
Nasal discharge causing mouth breathing
Chilling sensations
Muscular aches
Cough or sneezing (occasionally)
Physical Assessment Signs
Edema and vasodilation of mucosa

Pharyngitis

Younger Children

Fever
General malaise
Anorexia
Moderate sore throat
Headache

Older Children

Fever (may reach 104°F [40°C])
Headache
Anorexia
Dysphagia
Abdominal pain
Vomiting

Physical Assessment Signs

Younger Children

Mild to moderate hyperemia

Older Children

Mild to bright red, edematous pharynx
Hyperemia of the tonsils and pharynx; may extend to the soft palate and uvula
Often abundant follicular exudate that spreads and coalesces to form pseudomembrane on tonsils
Cervical glands enlarged and tender

characteristic paroxysmal attacks of laryngeal obstruction that occur chiefly at night; usually occurs in children age 1 to 3 years. Onset is sudden, at night (see Table 1.6).

Acute epiglottitis (supraglottitis)—Bacterial (usually *Haemophilus influenzae*) infection; a serious obstructive inflammatory process that requires immediate attention and is a medical emergency; occurs principally in children between 2 and 5 years of age but can occur from

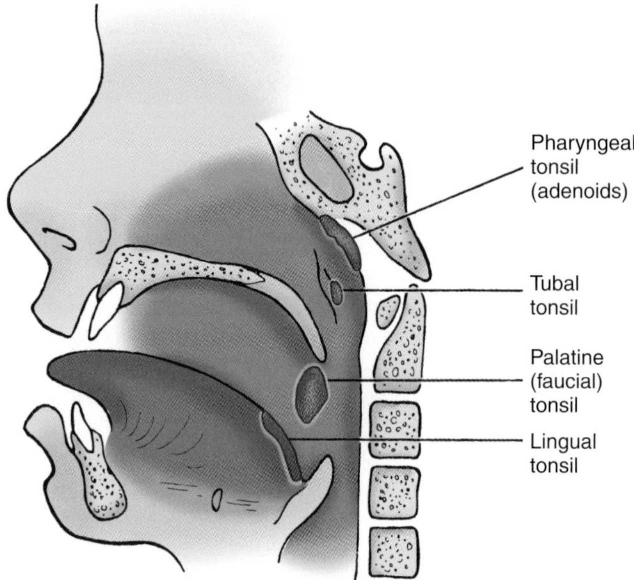

FIG. **1.33** Location of various tonsillar masses. (Added from Essentials 11th ed, Chapter 21, p. 627 Fig 21.3.)

BOX 1.8 Standard Terminology for Otitis Media

Otitis media (OM): An inflammation of the middle ear without reference to etiology or pathogenesis

Acute otitis media (AOM): An inflammation of the middle ear space with a rapid onset of the signs and symptoms of acute infection—namely, fever and otalgia (ear pain)

Otitis media with effusion (OME): Fluid in the middle ear space without symptoms of acute infection

infancy to adulthood; LTB and epiglottitis do not occur together. Onset is abrupt and rapidly progressive. Clinical manifestations and treatment are listed in Table 1.6 in comparison of croup syndromes.

NURSING ALERT

Advise the family to seek medical evaluation of the child or adolescent if:

- Breathing becomes difficult
- Severe abdominal pain develops
- Sore severe throat pain that prevents oral intake
- Respiratory stridor is observed

The child usually goes to bed asymptomatic to awaken complaining of sore throat and pain with swallowing that causes the child to drool. The child will insist on sitting upright, leaning forward (tripod position), with their chin thrust out, mouth open, and tongue protruding.

Throat inspection should be attempted only by experienced personnel when equipment is available to proceed with immediate intubation or tracheostomy.

Acute tracheitis—Bacterial (usually *Staphylococcus aureus*) infection of the mucosa of the upper trachea; is a distinct entity with features of both croup and epiglottitis; may cause

BOX 1.9 Clinical Manifestations of Otitis Media

Acute Otitis Media

Follows an upper respiratory tract infection
Otalgia (earache)
Fever—may or may not be present
Purulent discharge (otorrhea)—may or may not be present

Infants and Very Young Children

Crying, fussiness, restlessness, irritability, especially on lying down
Tendency to rub, hold, or pull affected ear
Rolling head from side to side
Difficulty comforting child
Loss of appetite, refusal to feed

Older Children

Crying or verbalizing feelings of discomfort
Irritability
Lethargy
Loss of appetite

Chronic Otitis Media

- Hearing loss
- Difficulty communicating
- Feeling of fullness, tinnitus, or vertigo may be present

BOX 1.10 Clinical Manifestations of Infectious Mononucleosis

Early Signs

Headache
Epistaxis
Malaise
Fatigue
Chills
Low-grade fever
Loss of appetite
Puffy eyes

Acute Disease

Cardinal Features

Fever
Sore throat
Cervical adenopathy

Common Features

Splenomegaly (may persist for several months)
Palatine petechiae
Macular eruption (especially on trunk)
Exudative pharyngitis or tonsillitis
Hepatic involvement to some degree, often associated with jaundice

TABLE 1.6 Comparison of Croup Syndromes

	Acute Epiglottitis	Acute LTB	Acute Spasmodic Laryngitis	Acute Tracheitis
Age-group affected	2–5 years old but varies	Infant or child younger than 5 years old	1–3 years old	1 month old–6 years old
Etiologic agent	Bacterial	Viral	Viral with allergic component	Viral or bacterial with allergic component
Onset	Rapidly progressive	Slowly progressive	Sudden; at night	Moderately progressive
Major symptoms	Dysphagia Stridor aggravated when supine Drooling High fever Toxic appearance Rapid pulse and respirations	URI Stridor Brassy cough Hoarseness Dyspnea Restlessness Irritability Low-grade fever Nontoxic appearance	URI Croupy cough Stridor Hoarseness Dyspnea Restlessness Symptoms awakening child but disappearing during day Tendency to recur	URI Croupy cough Purulent secretions High fever No response to LTB therapy
Treatment	Airway protection, possible intubation, tracheotomy Humidified oxygen Corticosteroids Fluids Antibiotics Reassurance	Humidified mist if needed Corticosteroids Fluids Reassurance Nebulized epinephrine (possible short-term improvement) Heliox: moderate to severe croup	Cool mist Reassurance	Antibiotics Fluids

LTB, Laryngotracheobronchitis; *URI,* upper respiratory infection.

airway obstruction severe enough to cause respiratory arrest; occurs in children ages 1 month to 6 years. The onset is moderately progressive and believed to be a complication of LTB. Early recognition is essential to prevent life-threatening airway obstruction (see Table 1.6).

Lower Respiratory Tract Infections

Asthma—Exaggerated response of bronchi to infection; most commonly caused by viruses but may be by any variety of upper respiratory infection (URI) pathogens; bronchospasm, exudation, and edema of bronchi; occurs in infancy to adolescence. (See clinical manifestations and treatment listed in Table 1.7 on comparison of conditions affecting the bronchi).

Bronchitis—Inflammation of large airways (trachea and bronchi); usually occurs in association with viral URI, but other agents (e.g., bacteria, fungi, allergic disorders, airborne irritants) can trigger symptoms; seldom occurs as an isolated entity in childhood; affects children in first 4 years of life. Clinical manifestations and treatment are listed in Table 1.7.

Bronchiolitis—Common, acute viral infection usually caused by a respiratory syncytial virus (RSV) with upper respiratory symptoms and lower respiratory infection of bronchioles due to inflammation; usually affects children aged 2 to 12 months; rare after age 2 years. RSV infection is the most frequent cause of hospitalization in children younger than 1-year-old. Clinical manifestations and treatment are listed in Table 1.7.

Pneumonias

Pneumonia, inflammation of the pulmonary parenchyma, is common throughout childhood but occurs more frequently in early childhood. Clinically, pneumonia may occur either as a primary disease or as a complication of another illness. The most useful classification of pneumonia is based on etiology (e.g., viral, bacterial, atypical (mycoplasmal), or aspiration of foreign substances). The clinical manifestations of pneumonia vary depending on the etiological agent, the child's age, the child's systemic reaction to infection, the extent of lesions, and the degree of bronchial and bronchiolar obstruction (see Box 1.11 on General Signs of Pneumonia).

Lobar pneumonia—All or a large segment of one or more pulmonary lobes is involved. When both lungs are affected, it is known as bilateral or double pneumonia.

Bronchopneumonia—Begins in the terminal bronchioles, which become clogged with mucopurulent exudate to form consolidated patches in nearby lobules; also called lobular pneumonia

TABLE 1.7 Comparison of Conditions Affecting the Bronchi

	Asthma[a]	Bronchitis	Bronchiolitis
Description	Exaggerated response of bronchi to a trigger such as URI, animal dander, cold air, exercise Bronchospasm, exudation, and edema of bronchi	Usually occurs in association with URI Seldom an isolated entity	Most common infectious disease of lower airways Maximum obstructive impact at bronchiolar level
Age-group affected	Infancy to adolescence or adulthood	First 4 years of life	Usually children 2–12 months old; rare after 2 years old Peak incidence approximately 6 months old
Etiologic agents	Most often viruses such as RSV in infants but may be any of a variety of URI pathogens	Usually viral Other agents (e.g., bacteria, fungi, allergic disorders, airborne irritants) can trigger symptoms	Viruses, predominantly RSV; also adenoviruses, parainfluenza viruses, human metapneumovirus, and *Mycoplasma pneumoniae*
Predominant characteristics	Wheezing, cough, labored respirations	Persistent dry, hacking cough (worse at night) becoming productive in 2–3 days	Labored respirations, poor feeding, cough, tachypnea, retractions and flaring nares, increased nasal mucus, wheezing, may have fever
Treatment	Inhaled corticosteroids, bronchodilators, leukotriene modifiers, allergen control, control of triggers	Cough suppressants if needed	Supplemental oxygen if saturations ≤90%; bronchodilators (optional) Suction nasopharynx Ensure adequate fluid intake Maintain adequate oxygenation

[a]See Asthma later in the chapter.
RSV, Respiratory syncytial virus; *URI,* upper respiratory infection.

Interstitial pneumonia—The inflammatory process is more or less confined within the alveolar walls (interstitium) and the peribronchial and interlobular tissues.

Pneumonitis is a localized acute inflammation of the lung without the toxemia associated with lobar pneumonia.

The pneumonias are more often classified according to the etiologic agent: viral, atypical (mycoplasma pneumonia), bacterial pneumonia, or pneumonia caused by aspiration of foreign substances. Pneumonia may be caused less often by histoplasmosis, coccidioidomycosis, and other fungi.

Viral pneumonia—Occurs more frequently than bacterial pneumonia; seen in children of all age-groups; often associated with viral URIs. Viruses that cause pneumonia include RSV in infants, parainfluenza, influenza, human metapneumovirus, enterovirus, and adenovirus in older children. The onset may be acute or insidious.

Symptoms variable

Mild—Low-grade fever, slight cough, malaise

Severe—High fever, severe cough, prostration

See other clinical manifestations listed in Box 1.11 on General Signs of Pneumonia.

Atypical pneumonia—Described as community-acquired pneumonia with mycoplasma as the most common etiologic agent in children 5 to 15 years old; occurs principally in fall and winter months; more prevalent in crowded living conditions. Onset may be sudden or insidious.

General systemic symptoms

- Fever
- Chills (older children)
- Headache
- Sore throat

Dry hacking cough: Nonproductive early, then seromucoid sputum, to mucopurulent or blood-streaked

- Fine crepitant crackles over various lung areas

Other clinical manifestations are listed Box 1.11.

Bacterial pneumonia—The most common cause is Streptococcus pneumoniae in both children and adults with other bacterial causes (e.g., *Staphylococcus aureus*, group A streptococcal, chlamydial pneumonias); clinical manifestations differ from other types of pneumonia; individual microorganisms produce a distinct clinical picture. Onset abrupt

- Usually preceded by viral infection
- Toxic, acutely ill appearance
- Fever, usually high
- Malaise
- Rapid, shallow respirations
- Cough
- Chest pain often exaggerated by deep breathing
- Pain may be referred to abdomen
- Chills
- Meningismus

Pulmonary Tuberculosis

Caused by *Mycobacterium tuberculosis;* Tuberculosis (TB) occurs in all ages but is most common in urban, low-income areas and among non-white racial and ethnic groups. The following groups have the greatest rates of latent TB infection: immigrants, international adoptees, refuges or travelers from high-prevalence regions (e.g., Asia, Africa, and Latin America), homeless individuals, inmates in correctional facilities and children with intercurrent infection (especially human immunodeficiency virus [HIV]). Extremely variable and may be asymptomatic or produce a broad range of symptoms (see Box 1.12 listing Clinical Manifestations of Tuberculosis).

Diagnosis is based on information derived from physical examination, history, tuberculin skin testing, radiographic examinations, and culture of the organism (*M. tuberculosis*). The tuberculin skin test is the most important indicator of whether a child has been infected with tubercle bacillus (see Box 1.13 on the recommendation for tuberculin skin test). A positive TB skin test is defined in Box 1.14 with induration and erythema.

BOX 1.11 General Signs of Pneumonia

Fever: Usually high

Respiratory

- Cough: unproductive to productive with whitish sputum
- Tachypnea
- Breath sounds: crackles or rhonchi
- Dullness with percussion
- Chest pain
- Retractions
- Nasal flaring
- Pallor to cyanosis (depends on severity)

Chest radiography: Diffuse or patchy infiltration with peribronchial distribution

Behavior: Irritability, restlessness, lethargic

Gastrointestinal: Anorexia, vomiting, diarrhea, abdominal pain

BOX 1.12 Clinical Manifestations of Tuberculosis

May be asymptomatic or produce a broad range of symptoms:

- Fever
- Malaise
- Anorexia
- Weight loss
- Cough (may or may not be present; progresses slowly over weeks to months)
- Aching pain and tightness in the chest
- Hemoptysis (rare)

With progression:

- Increasing respiratory rate
- Decreased expansion of lung on the affected side
- Diminished breath sounds and crackles
- Dullness to percussion
- Persistent fever
- Generalized symptoms
- Pallor, anemia, weakness, and weight loss

BOX 1.13 Tuberculin Skin Test Recommendations for Infants, Children, and Adolescents

Children for Whom Immediate Tuberculin Skin Test is Indicated

Contact with persons with confirmed or suspected contagious tuberculosis (TB; contact investigation)
Children with radiographic or clinical findings suggesting TB disease
Children immigrating from endemic countries (e.g., Asia, Middle East, Africa, Latin America, countries of the former Soviet Union), including international adoptees
Children with travel histories to endemic countries or significant contact with indigenous persons from such countries

Children Who Should Have Annual Tuberculin Skin Test

Children infected with human immunodeficiency virus (HIV)

Children at Increased Risk for Progression of Infection to Disease

Children with other medical risk factors, including diabetes mellitus, chronic renal failure, malnutrition, and congenital or acquired immunodeficiencies, deserve special consideration. Without recent exposure, these people are not at increased risk of acquiring TB infection. Underlying immune deficiencies associated with these conditions theoretically would enhance the possibility of progression to severe disease. Initial histories of potential exposure to TB should be included for all of these patients. If these histories or local epidemiologic factors suggest a possibility of exposure, immediate and periodic tuberculin skin test (TST) should be considered. An initial TST should be performed before initiation of immunosuppressive therapy, including prolonged steroid administration, for any child with an underlying condition that necessitates immunosuppressive therapy.

From American Academy of Pediatrics, Committee on Infectious Diseases, Kimberlin DW, Brady MT, Jackson MA, Long SS, eds. *Red Book: 2018 Report of the Committee on Infectious Diseases.* 31st ed. Itaca, IL: American Academy of Pediatrics; 2018.

BOX 1.14 Definition of Positive Tuberculin Skin Test Results in Infants, Children, and Adolescents[a]

Induration ≥5 mm

Children in close contact with known or suspected contagious cases of tuberculosis (TB) disease
Children suspected to have TB disease:
Findings on chest radiography consistent with active or previously active TB
Clinical evidence of TB disease[b]
Children receiving immunosuppressive therapy, including immunosuppressive doses of corticosteroids, or who have immunosuppressive conditions, including human immunodeficiency virus (HIV) infection

Induration ≥10 mm

Children at increased risk of disseminated disease:
Children younger than 4 years old
Children with other medical risk conditions, including Hodgkin's disease, lymphoma, diabetes mellitus, chronic renal failure, or malnutrition
Children at increased risk of exposure to TB:
Children born in high-prevalence (TB) regions of the world
Children frequently exposed to adults who are HIV-infected, homeless, users of illicit drugs, residents of nursing homes, incarcerated or institutionalized
Children who travel to high-prevalence (TB) regions of the world

Induration ≥15 mm

Children 4 years old or older without any risk factors

[a]These definitions apply regardless of previous bacillus Calmette-Guérin (BCG) immunization; erythema at the tuberculin skin test (TST) site does not indicate a positive test result. TSTs should be read at 48 to 72 hours after placement.
[b]Evidence by physical examination or laboratory assessment that would include TB in the working differential diagnosis (e.g., meningitis).
From American Academy of Pediatrics, Committee on Infectious Diseases, Kimberlin DW, Brady MT, Jackson MA, Long SS, eds. *Red Book: 2018 Report of the Committee on Infectious Diseases.* 31st ed. Itaca, IL: American Academy of Pediatrics; 2018.

Most children recover from primary TB infection; however, TB infection is a serious disease during the first 2 years of life, during adolescence, and in children who are HIV positive.

Aspiration of Foreign Substances

Inflammation of lung tissue can occur as the result of irritation from foreign material (e.g., vomitus, small objects, oral secretions, inhalation of smoke) and aspiration of food. Foreign body (FB) aspiration can occur at any age but is most common in children 1 to 3 years old.

Foreign body (FB) aspiration—Clinical manifestations and changes produced depend on the degree and location of obstruction and type of FB.

- Choking
- Gagging
- Sternal retractions
- Wheezing
- Cough
- Inability to speak or breathe (larynx)
- Decreased airway entry, dyspnea (bronchi)

Signs of acute distress requiring immediate and quick action

- Becomes cyanotic
- Collapses

FB aspiration may result in life-threatening airway obstruction, especially in infants because of their small airway diameter. It is important to educate parents about the hazards of aspiration in relation to the developmental level of their children and encourage them to teach their children safety.

Aspiration pneumonia—May result from the aspiration of liquids, food, secretions, inert materials, or volatile compounds that enter the lung and cause inflammation and pneumonitis. Aspiration of liquids or food is a particular hazard in children who have difficulty with swallowing; are unable to swallow because of paralysis, weaknesses, debility, congenital anomalies, or absent cough reflex; or are force-fed, especially while crying or breathing rapidly. Irritated mucous membranes may become a site for secondary bacterial infection.

Classic signs and symptoms of aspiration pneumonia include increasing cough or fever, with foul-smelling sputum, deteriorating oxygenation, evidence of infiltrates on chest radiographs, and other signs of lower airway involvement (see Box 1.11 on General Signs of Pneumonia).

Inhalation injury—Results from inhalation of noxious substances are primarily products of incomplete combustion or other noxious gases. Smoke inhalation is a common cause of inhalation injury and results in types of injury: heat (thermal injury to upper airway), chemical (gases generated during material combustion), and systemic injury (gases cause injury by interfering with cellular respiration such as carbon monoxide poisoning).

Heat and chemical clinical manifestations:

- Suspected with a history of flames in a closed space whether burns are present or not
- Sooty material around nose, in sputum
- Singed nasal hairs
- Mucosal burns of nose, lips, mouth, or throat
- Hoarse voice
- Cough
- Inspiratory and expiratory stridor
- Signs of respiratory distress (tachypnea, tachycardia, diminished or abnormal breath sounds)

Systemic injury: Gases that are nontoxic to the airways (e.g., carbon monoxide [CO], hydrogen cyanide) can cause injury and death by interfering with or inhibiting cellular respiration. Clinical manifestations of CO poisoning are secondary to tissue hypoxia and vary according to mild or severe poisoning.

Mild CO poisoning

- Headache
- Visual disturbances
- Irritability
- Nausea

Severe CO poisoning

- Confusion
- Hallucinations
- Ataxia
- Coma
- Pallor
- Cyanosis
- Possibly bright, cherry-red lips and skin (less common)

Assessment of a Child with Common Disorders

The Child with Asthma

Assessment—The child with asthma

Asthma—A complex, chronic inflammatory disorder of the airways characterized by recurring symptoms, airway obstruction, bronchial hyperresponsiveness, and underlying inflammation process (see Fig. 1.34A and B on airway obstruction).

Status asthmaticus is an acute, severe, and prolonged asthma attack in which respiratory distress continues despite vigorous therapeutic measures, especially the administration of sympathomimetics. Status asthmaticus is considered a medical emergency that can result in respiratory failure and death if untreated.

Assessment

Obtain a family history, especially regarding the presence of atopy in family members.

Obtain a health history, including any evidence of atopy (e.g., eczema, rhinitis); evidence of possible precipitating factor(s) or triggers; previous episodes of shortness of

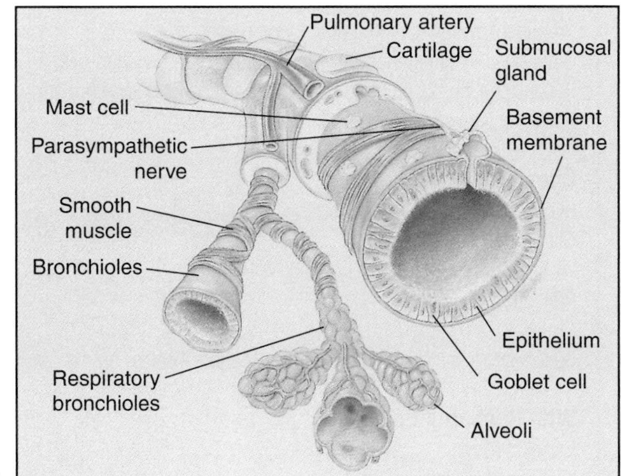

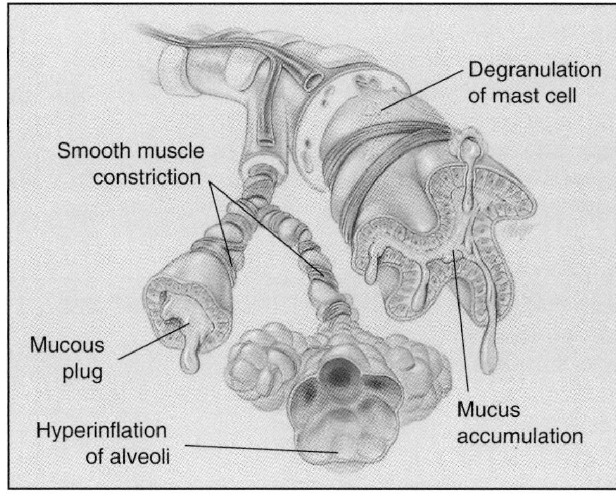

FIG. **1.34** Airway obstruction caused by asthma. (A) Normal lung. (B) Bronchial asthma. Thick mucus, mucosa edema, and smooth muscle spasm causing obstruction of small airways; breathing becomes labored and expiration is difficult. (Modified from Des Jardins, T., & Burton, G. G. [1995]. *Clinical manifestations and assessment of respiratory disease* [3rd ed.]. St Louis: Mosby.)

breath, wheezing, and coughing; and any complaints of prodromal itching at the front of the neck or upper part of the back. Identify the presence of possible triggers or aggravating factors during history taking process (see Box 1.15 on triggers tending to precipitate or aggravate exacerbations).

Observe for clinical manifestations of bronchial asthma (see Box 1.16 on clinical manifestations of asthma).

Assist with diagnostic procedures and tests (e.g., blood gases, electrolytes, pH; oximetry; urine specific gravity; radiography; pulmonary function tests).

The Child with Fluid and Electrolyte Disturbance

Dehydration: is a common body fluid disturbance and occurs whenever the total output of fluid exceeds the total intake, regardless of the underlying cause. Types of dehydration are described according to plasma sodium concentrations since sodium is the primary osmotic force that controls fluid movement between compartments.

Isotonic (isoosmotic, isonatremic)—Electrolyte and water deficits present in approximately balanced proportions which is the primary form of dehydration occurring in children

Hypertonic (hyperosmotic, hypernatremic)—Water loss in excess of electrolyte loss and usually caused by a proportionately larger loss of water or larger intake of electrolytes

Hypotonic (hypoosmotic, hyponatremic)—Electrolyte deficit exceeds water deficit with a greater proportional loss of extracellular fluid, consequently physical signs are more severe with smaller fluid losses than isotonic or hypertonic dehydration

Assessment

Take a detailed health history, especially regarding current health problems (e.g., length of illness, events that may have precipitated symptoms).

Perform a physical assessment.

Observe for clinical manifestations and management of fluid and electrolyte disturbances (see Table 1.8 on disturbances of select fluid and electrolyte balance)

Perform the following specific assessments including the clinical clues to evaluate the extent of dehydration listed in Table 1.9 and clinical manifestations listed in Table 1.10.

Intake and output—Accurate measurements of fluid intake and output are vital to the assessment of dehydration. This includes oral and parenteral intake and losses from urine, stools, vomiting, fistulas, nasogastric suction, sweat, and wound drainage.

BOX 1.15 Triggers Tending to Precipitate or Aggravate Asthma Exacerbations

Allergens
- Outdoor: Trees, shrubs, weeds, grasses, molds, pollens, air pollution, spores
- Indoor: Dust or dust mites, mold, cockroach antigen

Irritants: Tobacco smoke, wood smoke, odors, sprays
Exposure to occupational chemicals
Exercise
Cold air
Changes in weather or temperature
Environmental change: Moving to a new home, starting a new school
Colds and infections
Animals: Cats, dogs, rodents, horses
Medications: Aspirin, nonsteroidal antiinflammatory drugs, antibiotics, beta-blockers
Strong emotions: Fear, anger, laughing, crying
Conditions: Gastroesophageal reflux, tracheoesophageal fistula
Food additives: Sulfite preservatives
Foods: Nuts, milk, or other dairy products
Endocrine factors: Menses, pregnancy, thyroid disease

BOX 1.16 Clinical Manifestations of Asthma

Cough
Hacking, paroxysmal, irritative, and nonproductive
Becomes rattling and productive of frothy, clear, gelatinous sputum

Respiratory-Related Signs
Shortness of breath
Prolonged expiratory phase
Wheezing
May have a malar flush and red ears
Lips deep, dark red color
May progress to cyanosis of nail beds or circumoral cyanosis
Restlessness
Apprehension
Prominent sweating as the attack progresses
Older children sitting upright with shoulders in a hunched-over position, hands on the bed or chair, and arms braced (tripod)
Speaking with short, panting, broken phrases

Chest
Hyperresonance on percussion
Coarse, loud breath sounds
Wheezes throughout the lung fields
Prolonged expiration
Crackles
Generalized inspiratory and expiratory wheezing; increasingly high pitched

With Repeated Episodes
Barrel chest
Elevated shoulders
Use of accessory muscles of respiration
Facial appearance—flattened malar bones, dark circles beneath the eyes, narrow nose, prominent upper teeth

TABLE 1.8 Disturbances of Select Fluid and Electrolyte Balance

Mechanisms and Situations	Manifestations	Management and Nursing Care
Water Depletion		
Failure to absorb or reabsorb water Complete or sudden cessation of intake or prolonged diminished intake: Neglect of intake by self or caregiver—confused, psychotic, unconscious, or helpless Loss from gastrointestinal tract—vomiting, diarrhea, nasogastric suction, fistula Disturbed body fluid chemistry: inappropriate ADH secretion Excessive renal excretion: glycosuria (diabetes) Loss through skin or lungs: Excessive perspiration or evaporation—febrile states, hyperventilation, increased ambient temperature, increased activity (basal metabolic rate) Impaired skin integrity—transudate from injuries Hemorrhage Iatrogenic: Overzealous use of diuretics Improper perioperative fluid replacement Use of radiant warmer or phototherapy	General symptoms dependent to some extent on proportion of electrolytes lost with water Thirst Variable temperature—increased (infection) Dry skin and mucous membranes Poor skin turgor Poor perfusion (decreased pulse, slowed capillary refill time) Weight loss Fatigue Diminished urinary output Irritability and lethargy Tachycardia Tachypnea Altered level of consciousness, disorientation Laboratory findings: High urine specific gravity Increased hematocrit Variable serum electrolytes Variable urine volume Increased blood urea nitrogen Increased serum osmolality	Provide replacement of fluid losses commensurate with volume depletion. Provide maintenance fluids and electrolytes. Determine and correct cause of water depletion. Measure fluid intake and output. Monitor vital signs. Monitor urine specific gravity. Monitor body weight. Monitor serum electrolytes.
Water Excess		
Water intake in excess of output: Excessive oral intake Hypotonic fluid overload Plain water enemas Failure to excrete water in presence of normal intake: Kidney disease Congestive heart failure Malnutrition	Edema: Generalized Pulmonary (moist rales or crackles) Intracutaneous (noted especially in loose areolar tissue) Elevated central venous pressure Hepatomegaly Slow, bounding pulse Weight gain Lethargy Increased spinal fluid pressure Central nervous system manifestations (seizures, coma) Laboratory findings: Low urine specific gravity Decreased serum electrolytes Decreased hematocrit Variable urine volume	Limit fluid intake. Administer diuretics. Monitor vital signs. Monitor neurologic signs as necessary. Determine and treat cause of water excess. Analyze serum electrolytes frequently. Implement seizure precautions.
Sodium Depletion (Hyponatremia)		
Prolonged low-sodium diet Decreased sodium intake Fever Excess sweating Increased water intake without electrolytes Tachypnea (infants) Cystic fibrosis Burns and wounds Vomiting, diarrhea, nasogastric suction, fistulas Adrenal insufficiency Renal disease Diabetic ketoacidosis (DKA) Malnutrition	Associated with water loss: Same as with water loss—dehydration, weakness, dizziness, nausea, abdominal cramps, apprehension Mild—apathy, weakness, nausea, weak pulse Moderate—decreased blood pressure, lethargy Laboratory findings: Sodium concentration <130 mEq/L (may be normal if volume loss) Urine specific gravity depends on water deficit or excess	Determine and treat cause of sodium deficit. Administer IV fluids with appropriate saline concentration. Monitor fluid intake and output.

Continued

TABLE 1.8 Disturbances of Select Fluid and Electrolyte Balance—cont'd

Mechanisms and Situations	Manifestations	Management and Nursing Care
Sodium Excess (Hypernatremia)		
High salt intake—enteral or IV Renal disease Fever Insufficient breast milk intake in neonate (dehydration hypernatremia) High insensible water loss: Increased temperature Increased humidity Hyperventilation Diabetes insipidus Hyperglycemia	Intense thirst Dry, sticky mucous membranes Flushed skin Temperature possibly increased Hoarseness Oliguria Nausea and vomiting Possible progression to disorientation, convulsions, muscle twitching, nuchal rigidity, lethargy at rest, hyperirritability when aroused Laboratory findings: Serum sodium concentration ≤150 mEq/L High plasma volume Alkalosis	Determine and treat cause of sodium excess. Administer IV fluids as prescribed. Measure fluid intake and output. Monitor laboratory data. Monitor neurologic status. Ensure adequate intake of breast milk and provide lactation assistance with new mother-baby pair before hospital discharge.
Potassium Depletion (Hypokalemia)		
Starvation Clinical conditions associated with poor food intake Malabsorption fluid without added potassium Gastrointestinal losses—diarrhea, vomiting, fistulas, nasogastric suction Diuresis Administration of diuretics Administration of corticosteroids Diuretic phase of nephrotic syndrome Healing stage of burns Potassium-losing nephritis Hyperglycemic diuresis (e.g., diabetes mellitus) Familial periodic paralysis IV administration of insulin in DKA Alkalosis	Muscle weakness, cramping, stiffness, paralysis, hyporeflexia Hypotension Cardiac arrhythmias, gallop rhythm Tachycardia or bradycardia Ileus Apathy, drowsiness Irritability Fatigue Laboratory findings: Decreased serum potassium concentration ≥3.5 mEq/L Abnormal ECG—notched or flattened T waves, decreased ST segment, premature ventricular contractions	Determine and treat cause of potassium deficit. Monitor vital signs, including ECG. Administer supplemental potassium. Assess for adequate renal output before administration. For IV replacement, administer potassium slowly. Always monitor ECG for IV bolus potassium replacement. For oral intake, offer high-potassium fluids and foods. Evaluate acid–base status.
Potassium Excess (Hyperkalemia)		
Renal disease Renal failure Adrenal insufficiency (Addison disease) Associated with metabolic acidosis Too-rapid administration of IV potassium chloride Transfusion with old donor blood Severe dehydration Crushing injuries Burns Hemolysis Dehydration Potassium-sparing diuretics Increased intake of potassium (e.g., salt substitutes)	Muscle weakness, flaccid paralysis Twitching Hyperreflexia Bradycardia Ventricular fibrillation and cardiac arrest Oliguria Apnea—respiratory arrest Laboratory findings: High serum potassium concentration ≤5.5 mEq/L Variable urine volume Flat P wave on ECG, peaked T waves, widened QRS complex, increased PR interval	Determine and treat cause of potassium excess. Monitor vital signs, including ECG. Administer exchange resin, if prescribed. Administer IV fluids as prescribed. Administer IV insulin (if ordered) to facilitate movement of potassium into cells. Monitor potassium levels. Evaluate acid-base status.

TABLE 1.8 Disturbances of Select Fluid and Electrolyte Balance—cont'd

Mechanisms and Situations	Manifestations	Management and Nursing Care
Calcium Depletion (Hypocalcemia)		
Inadequate dietary calcium Vitamin D deficiency Rapid transit through gastrointestinal tract Advanced renal insufficiency Administration of diuretics Hypoparathyroidism Alkalosis Calcium trapped in diseased tissues Increased serum protein (albumin) Cow's milk—tetany of the newborn (inappropriate calcium/phosphorus ratio in whole milk for newborn) Exchange transfusion with citrated blood Inadequate parenteral administration in diseased status	Neuromuscular irritability Tingling of nose, ears, fingertips, toes Tetany Laryngospasm Generalized convulsions May be changes in clotting Positive Chvostek and Trousseau signs Hypotension Cardiac arrest Laboratory findings: Decreased serum calcium concentration (8.8–10.8 mEq/L) or increased serum protein levels Prolonged QT interval	Determine and treat cause of calcium deficit. Administer oral calcium supplements as prescribed; administer IV slowly and diluted. Monitor IV site; calcium may cause vascular irritation. Monitor serum calcium, vitamin D, and parathyroid levels. Monitor serum protein levels. Avoid cow's milk in infants younger than 12 months.
Calcium Excess (Hypercalcemia)		
Acidosis Prolonged immobilization Conditions associated with increased bone catabolism Hypoproteinemia Kidney disease Hypervitaminosis D Hyperparathyroidism Hyperthyroidism Excessive IV or oral administration	Constipation Weakness, fatigue Nausea, vomiting Anorexia Dry mouth (thirst) Muscle hypotonicity Bradycardia or cardiac arrest Increased calcium concentration in urine, causing formation of kidney stones Laboratory findings: Increased serum calcium levels or decreased serum protein levels Prolonged QRS complex or PR interval, shortened QT interval	Determine and treat cause of calcium excess. Monitor serum calcium levels. Monitor ECG.

ADH, Antidiuretic hormone; *ECG,* electrocardiogram; *IV,* intravenous.

TABLE 1.9 Evaluating Extent of Dehydration

	LEVEL OF DEHYDRATION		
Clinical Signs	**Mild**	**Moderate**	**Severe**
Weight loss—infants	3%–5%	6%–9%	≤10%
Weight loss—children	3%–4%	6%–8%	10%
Pulse	Normal	Slightly increased	Very increased
Respiratory rate	Normal	Slight tachypnea (rapid)	Hyperpnea (deep and rapid)
Blood pressure	Normal	Normal to orthostatic (>10 mm Hg change)	Orthostatic to shock
Behavior	Normal	Irritable, more thirsty	Hyperirritable to lethargic
Thirst	Slight	Moderate	Intense
Mucous membranes[a]	Normal (moist)	Dry	Parched
Tears	Present	Decreased	Absent, sunken eyes
Anterior fontanel	Normal	Normal to sunken	Sunken
External jugular vein	Visible when supine	Not visible except with supraclavicular pressure	Not visible even with supraclavicular pressure
Skin[a]	Capillary refill >2 s	Slowed capillary refill (2–4 s [decreased turgor])	Very delayed capillary refill (>4 s) and tenting; skin cool, acrocyanotic or mottled
Urine	Decreased	Oliguria	Oliguria or anuria

[a]These signs are less prominent in patients who have hypernatremia.
Data from Jospe N, Forbes G. Fluids and electrolytes—clinical aspects. *Pediatr Rev.* 1996;17(11):395–403; and Steiner MJ, DeWalt DA, Byerly JS. Is this child dehydrated? *J Am Med Assoc.* 2004;291(22):2746–2754.

TABLE 1.10 Clinical Manifestations of Dehydration

Manifestation	Isotonic (Loss of Water and Salt)	Hypotonic (Loss of Salt in Excess of Water)	Hypertonic (Loss of Water in Excess of Salt)
Skin			
• Color	Gray	Gray	Gray
• Temperature	Cold	Cold	Cold or hot
• Turgor	Poor	Very poor	Fair
• Feel	Dry	Clammy	Thickened, doughy
Mucous membranes	Dry	Slightly moist	Parched
Tearing and salivation	Absent	Absent	Absent
Eyeball	Sunken	Sunken	Sunken
Fontanel	Sunken	Sunken	Sunken
Body temperature	Subnormal or elevated	Subnormal or elevated	Subnormal or elevated
Pulse	Rapid	Very rapid	Moderately rapid
Respirations	Rapid	Rapid	Rapid
Behavior	Irritable to lethargic	Lethargic or comatose; convulsions	Marked lethargy with extreme hyperirritability on stimulation

Body weight—Measure regularly and at the same time of day, usually each morning, to detect decreased or increased weight.
Vomitus—Assess for volume, frequency, and type of vomiting
Urine—Assess the frequency, volume, and color of urine.
Sensory alterations—Assess for the presence of thirst.
Fontanel (infants)—Assess sign of sunken appearance with fluid loss
Stools—Assess the frequency, volume, and consistency of stools.
Sweating—Estimate fluid loss from the frequency of clothing and linen change

Assist with diagnostic procedures and tests (e.g., urinalysis, blood chemistry, complete blood count [CBC], blood gases).

The Child with Acute Diarrhea (Gastroenteritis)

Acute diarrhea (gastroenteritis)—A sudden increase in stool frequency and a change in stool consistency, often caused by infectious agents (e.g., bacterial, viral, and parasitic pathogens) or antibiotic therapy or laxative use.

Assessment

Obtain a detailed history of illness including the following:
- Possible ingestion of contaminated food or water
- Possible infection elsewhere (e.g., respiratory or urinary tract infection)

Perform a routine physical assessment.
Observe for manifestations of acute gastroenteritis (e.g., fever, vomiting, frequency and character of stools, urinary output, dietary habits, and recent food intake.
Assess the state of dehydration (see Tables 1.9 and 1.10)
Record fecal output—number, volume, characteristics (watery, blood) and frequency.
Record the presence of associated signs—tenesmus, cramping, vomiting.
Assist with diagnostic procedures (e.g., collect specimens as needed; stools for pH, blood, culture, presence of reducing substances indicating carbohydrate malabsorption or lactase deficiency; urine for pH, specific gravity; CBC, serum electrolytes, creatinine, blood urea nitrogen [BUN]) in the child who has moderate to severe dehydration or who requires hospitalization (see Tables 1.9 and 1.10).
Detect the source of infection (e.g., inquire whether other members of the household have diarrheal symptoms, and refer for treatment as indicated).

The Child with Acute Hepatitis

Hepatitis—An acute or chronic inflammation of the liver that can result from infectious or noninfectious reasons.

Hepatitis of viral origin is caused by at least six types of viruses and the most common types in the United States are hepatitis A, hepatitis B, and hepatitis C (Table 1.11).

- Hepatitis A virus (HAV) is transmitted by the fecal-oral route, contaminated foods, infected feces, or close contact with an infected person.
- Hepatitis B virus (HBV) is found in all body fluids and transmitted parenterally, percutaneously, or transmucosally

TABLE 1.11 Comparison of Clinical Features of Hepatitis Types A, B, and C

Characteristics	Type A	Type B	Type C
Onset	Usually rapid, acute	More insidious	Usually insidious
Fever	Common and early	Less frequent	Less frequent
Anorexia	Common	Mild to moderate	Mild to moderate
Nausea and vomiting	Common	Sometimes present	Mild to moderate
Rash	Rare	Common	Sometimes present
Arthralgia	Rare	Common	Rare
Pruritus	Rare	Sometimes present	Sometimes present
Jaundice	Present (many cases anicteric)	Present	Present

- Hepatitis C virus (HCV) is transmitted parenterally transmitted through exposure to blood or blood products from an HCV-infected person or perinatal transmission virus
- Hepatitis D virus (HDV), occurs in children (rare) already infected with HBV and is transmitted through blood and sexual contact
- Hepatitis E virus (HEV formally known as non-A, non-B hepatitis virus) is transmitted through the fecal-oral route or from contaminated water.
- Hepatitis G virus (HGV) transmitted through blood and blood products

Assessment

Perform a routine physical assessment.

Take a detailed health history, especially regarding the following:

- Contact with persons known to have hepatitis
- Unsafe sanitation practices (e.g., contaminated drinking water)
- Ingestion of certain foods (e.g., raw shellfish taken from polluted water)
- Previous multiple blood transfusions (transmission risk has been significantly reduced due to improvement in donor screening and inactivation procedures for blood and blood products)
- Ingestion of hepatotoxic drugs (e.g., salicylates, sulfonamides, antineoplastic agents, acetaminophen, anticonvulsants)
- Parenteral administration of illicit drugs, or sexual contact with persons who use these drugs

Observe for clinical manifestations of hepatitis including prophylactic treatments (see Table 1.11).

Assist with diagnostic procedures and tests (e.g., serological markers [indicate antibodies or antigens formed in response to the specific virus] for hepatitis A, B, C, liver function tests such as serum aspartate aminotransferase, serum alanine aminotransferase, serum bilirubin, ammonia, albumin) and histologic evidence from liver biopsy.

The Child with Appendicitis

Appendicitis—An inflammation of the vermiform appendix (blind sac at the end of the cecum) is the most common cause of emergency abdominal surgery in childhood. Assessment—The Child with Appendicitis

Assessment

Take a detailed history of illness.

Observe for clinical manifestations of appendicitis as follows:

- Initially, abdominal pain is usually colicky, cramping, and located around the umbilicus
- Pain progresses and becomes constant
- Right lower quadrant abdominal pain (McBurney point)
- Fever
- Rigid abdomen
- Decreased or absent bowel sounds
- Nausea and vomiting (commonly follow the onset of pain)
- Constipation or diarrhea may be present
- Anorexia
- Tachycardia; rapid, shallow breathing
- Pallor
- Lethargy
- Irritability
- Stooped posture

Observe for signs of peritonitis as follows:

- Fever
- Sudden relief from pain (after perforation)
- Subsequent increase in pain, which is usually diffuse and accompanied by rigid guarding of the abdomen
- Progressive abdominal distention
- Tachycardia
- Rapid, shallow breathing
- Pallor
- Chills

- Irritability
- Restlessness

Assist with diagnostic procedures (e.g., laboratory tests such as CBC with rising white blood count with increase bands, rising C-reactive protein, abdominal radiography may be helpful, and CT abdominal scan with 96% accuracy in diagnosing appendicitis).

The Child with Cardiovascular Dysfunction

Cardiac dysfunction—Dysfunction, congenital or acquired, of the heart or the blood vessels

Cardiovascular system—Consists of the heart and blood vessels

Assessment

Assess general appearance, behavior, and function.

- Inspection
  - ***Nutritional state***—Failure to thrive (poor weight gain) or fatigue and/or sweating during feeding is associated with heart disease.
  - ***Color***—Cyanosis is a common feature of congenital heart disease, and pallor is associated with decreased perfusion which may also accompany heart disease.
  - ***Chest deformities***—An enlarged heart sometimes distorts the chest configuration.
  - ***Unusual pulsations***—Visible pulsations of the neck veins are sometimes present.
  - ***Respiratory excursion***—This refers to the ease or difficulty of respiration (e.g., tachypnea, dyspnea, expiratory grunt).
  - ***Clubbing of fingers***—Associated with cyanosis.
  - ***Behavior***—Assuming knee-chest position or squatting is typical of some types of heart disease; exercise intolerance.
- Palpation and percussion
  - ***Chest***—Helps discern heart size and other characteristics (e.g., thrills) associated with heart disease.
  - ***Abdomen***—Hepatomegaly and/or splenomegaly may be evident.
  - ***Peripheral pulses***—Rate, regularity, and amplitude (strength) may reveal discrepancies.

Auscultation

- ***Heart rate and rhythm***—Listen for fast heart rates (tachycardia), slow heart rates (bradycardia), and irregular rhythms.
- ***Character of heart sounds***—Listen for distinct or muffled sounds. murmurs and additional heart sounds.

Assist with diagnostic procedures and tests (e.g., electrocardiography, radiography, echocardiography, blood analysis [blood count, hemoglobin, packed cell volume, blood gases], exercise stress test, cardiac catheterization) (see Table 1.12 on procedures for cardiac diagnosis).

The Child with Congenital Heart Disease

Congenital heart disease—A structural or functional defect of the heart or great vessels present at birth

Assessment

Perform physical assessment with special emphasis on color, pulse (apical, peripheral), respiration, blood pressure, and examination and auscultation of heart and lungs.

Take detailed health history, including evidence of poor weight gain, feeding difficulties, exercise intolerance, unusual posturing, or frequent respiratory tract infections.

Observe the child for manifestations of congenital heart disease. Classification of heart defects correlated with specific defects denotes acyanosis that affects blood flow without oxygen reduction (e.g., increase pulmonary flow, obstruction impedes blood flow) and cyanosis that affects blood flow with oxygen reduction (e.g., increase pulmonary blood flow, mixed blood flow) on comparison of acyanotic-cyanotic and hemodynamic classification systems of congenital heart disease).

Infants

Cyanosis—affects highly vascularized areas; tends to cause a bluish tint to mucous membranes, lips and tongue, conjunctiva, fingers, and toes

Cyanosis, pale gray or pallor may occur during exertion such as crying, feeding, activity; peripheral or central

Abnormal heart rhythms

Dyspnea, especially following physical effort such as feeding, crying, and activity

Fatigue, especially during activity

Delayed growth and development (failure to thrive)

Frequent respiratory tract infections

Feeding difficulties

Hypotonia

Excessive sweating

Syncopal attacks such as paroxysmal hyperpnea, anoxic spells

Older children

Impaired growth

Delicate, frail body build

Abnormal heart rhythms

Fatigue, especially during activity

Effort dyspnea

Orthopnea

Digital clubbing

Squatting for relief of dyspnea

Headache

Epistaxis

Leg fatigue

TABLE 1.12 Procedures for Cardiac Diagnosis

Procedure	Description
Chest radiography (x-ray)	Provides information on heart size and pulmonary blood flow patterns
Electrocardiography (ECG)	Graphic measure of electrical activity of heart
Holter monitor	24-h continuous ECG recording used to assess dysrhythmias
Echocardiography	Use of high-frequency sound waves obtained by a transducer to produce an image of cardiac structures
Transthoracic	Done with transducer on chest
M-mode	One-dimensional graphic view used to estimate ventricular size and function
Two-dimensional	Real-time, cross-sectional views of heart used to identify cardiac structures and cardiac anatomy
Doppler	Shows blood flow patterns and pressure gradients across structures
Fetal	Imaging fetal heart in utero
Transesophageal echocardiography (TEE)	Transducer placed in esophagus behind heart to obtain images of posterior heart structures or in patients with poor images from chest approach
Cardiac catheterization	Imaging study using radiopaque catheters placed in a peripheral blood vessel and advanced into heart to measure pressures and oxygen levels in heart chambers and visualize heart structures and blood flow patterns
Hemodynamics	Measurements of pressures and oxygen saturations in heart chambers
Angiography	Use of contrast material to illuminate heart structures and blood flow patterns
Biopsy	Use of special catheter to remove tiny samples of heart muscle for microscopic evaluation; used in assessing infection, inflammation, or muscle dysfunction disorders; also to evaluate for rejection after heart transplant
Electrophysiology study (EPS)	Special catheters with electrodes inserted to record electrical activity from within the heart; used to diagnose rhythm disturbances
Exercise stress test	Monitoring of heart rate, BP, ECG, and oxygen consumption at rest and during progressive exercise on a treadmill or bicycle
Cardiac MRI	Noninvasive imaging technique; used in evaluation of vascular anatomy outside of the heart (e.g., COA, vascular rings), estimates of ventricular mass and volume

BP, Blood pressure; *COA,* coarctation of the aorta; *MRI,* magnetic resonance imaging.

The Child with Congestive Heart Failure

Assessment—The Child with Congestive Heart Failure

Congestive heart failure—The inability of the heart to pump an adequate amount of blood to the systemic circulation at normal filling pressures to meet the body's metabolic demands.

Assessment

Perform a physical assessment.

Perform a cardiac assessment.

Take a detailed health history, especially regarding previous cardiac problems.

Observe for clinical manifestations of congestive heart failure that vary and are divided into three groups: impaired myocardial function, pulmonary congestion, and systemic venous congestion (see Box 1.17 on clinical manifestations of heart failure)

- Assist with diagnostic procedures and tests (e.g., radiography, electrocardiography, echocardiography).

The Child in Shock (Circulatory Failure)

Shock (circulatory failure)—is a complex clinical syndrome characterized by inadequate tissue perfusion to meet the metabolic demands of the body, resulting in cellular dysfunction and eventual organ failure (Box 1.18).

Stages of Shock:

Compensated shock—Vital organ function is maintained by intrinsic compensatory mechanisms; blood flow is usually normal or increased but generally uneven or maldistributed in the microcirculation.

Decompensated shock—Efficiency of the cardiovascular system gradually diminishes until perfusion in the microcirculation becomes marginal despite compensatory adjustments. The outcomes of circulatory failure that progress beyond the limits of compensation are tissue

BOX 1.17 Clinical Manifestations of Heart Failure

Impaired Myocardial Function
Tachycardia
Sweating (inappropriate)
Decreased urinary output
Fatigue
Weakness
Restlessness
Anorexia
Pale, cool extremities
Weak peripheral pulses
Decreased blood pressure (BP)
Gallop rhythm
Cardiomegaly

Pulmonary Congestion
Tachypnea
Dyspnea
Retractions (infants)
Flaring nares
Exercise intolerance
Orthopnea
Cough, hoarseness
Cyanosis
Wheezing
Grunting

Systemic Venous Congestion
Weight gain
Hepatomegaly
Peripheral edema, especially periorbital
Ascites
Neck vein distention (children)

hypoxia, metabolic acidosis, and eventual dysfunction of all organs.

Irreversible, or terminal, shock—Damage to vital organs such as the heart or brain, is of intensive magnitude that the entire organism will be disrupted regardless of therapeutic intervention; death occurs even if cardiovascular measurements return to normal levels with therapy.

BOX 1.18 Types of Shock

Compensated
Apprehensiveness
Irritability
Unexplained tachycardia
Normal blood pressure (BP)
Narrowing pulse pressure
Thirst
Pallor
Diminished urinary output
Reduced perfusion of extremities

Hypotensive
Confusion and somnolence
Tachypnea
Moderate metabolic acidosis
Oliguria
Cool, pale extremities
Decreased skin turgor
Poor capillary filling

Irreversible
Thready, weak pulse
Hypotension
Periodic breathing or apnea
Anuria
Stupor or coma

Assessment

Maintain vigilance in situations that predispose the patient to shock (e.g., trauma, burns, severe dehydration [vomiting, diarrhea], overwhelming sepsis).

Monitor vital signs, central venous pressure (CVP), capillary refill, intake and output, and cardiac function, initially and continuously.

Observe clinical manifestations of shock in Box 1.19.

Assist with diagnostic procedures and tests (e.g., blood count, blood gases, pH, and sometimes liver function tests, coagulation studies if evidence of bleeding, renal function tests, cultures, electrolytes, electrocardiography).

The Child with Anemia

Anemia—A condition in which the number of red blood cells (RBCs) and/or the hemoglobin concentration is reduced below normal values for age and gender.

Assessment

Perform a physical assessment.

Take a health history, including a detailed dietary history, to identify any deficiencies (e.g., inadequate nutritional intake such as iron deficiency anemia, evidence of pica, the eating of nonfood substances such as clay, ice, or paste).

Observe for clinical manifestations of anemia associated with decreased RBC production, increase RBC loss and increase RBC destruction (see Fig. 1.35 on the classification of anemias).

Assist with diagnostic tests (e.g., complete blood count with differential and reticulocyte count, review peripheral blood smear, iron function test, guaiac fecal occult blood test, vitamin deficiency levels (e.g., B-12 and Folate levels) and may include other tests that focus on coagulation and immune status)

BOX 1.19 Definitions of Systemic Inflammatory Response Syndrome, Infection, and Septic Shock

Systemic inflammatory response syndrome (SIRS): The presence of at least two of the following four criteria, one of which must be abnormal temperature or leukocyte count:

Core temperature of more than 38.5°C (101.3°F) or less than 36°C (96.8°F)

Tachycardia, defined as a mean heart rate more than two standard deviations above normal for age in the absence of external stimulus, chronic drugs, or painful stimuli; or otherwise unexplained persistent elevation over a 0.5- to 4-h period; or, for children younger than 1 year old, bradycardia, defined as a mean heart rate below the 10th percentile for age in the absence of external vagal stimulus, beta-blocker drugs, or CHD; or otherwise unexplained persistent depression over a 0.5-h period

Mean respiratory rate more than two standard deviations above normal for age or mechanical ventilation for an acute process not related to underlying neuromuscular disease or the receipt of general anesthesia

Leukocyte count elevated or depressed for age (not secondary to chemotherapy-induced leukopenia) or more than 10% immature neutrophils

Infection: A suspected or proven (by a positive culture, tissue stain, or PCR test) infection caused by any pathogen; or a clinical syndrome associated with a high probability of infection. Evidence of infection includes positive findings on clinical examination, imaging, or laboratory tests (e.g., white blood cells in a normally sterile body fluid, perforated viscus, chest radiograph consistent with pneumonia, petechial or purpuric rash, or purpura fulminans).

Septic Shock: Severe infection leading to cardiovascular dysfunction (including hypotension, need for treatment with a vasoactive medication, or impaired perfusion) and organ dysfunction in children as severe infection leading to cardiovascular and/or noncardiovascular organ dysfunction.

Adapted from Weiss SL, Peters MJ, Alhazzani W, et al. Surviving sepsis campaign international guidelines for the management of septic shock and sepsis-associated organ dysfunction in children. *Pediatr Crit Care Med.* 2020;21(2); e53–e106; Goldstein B, Giroir B, Randolph A, et al. International pediatric sepsis consensus conference: definitions for sepsis and organ dysfunction in pediatrics. *Pediatr Critical Care Med.* 2005;6(1):2–8.

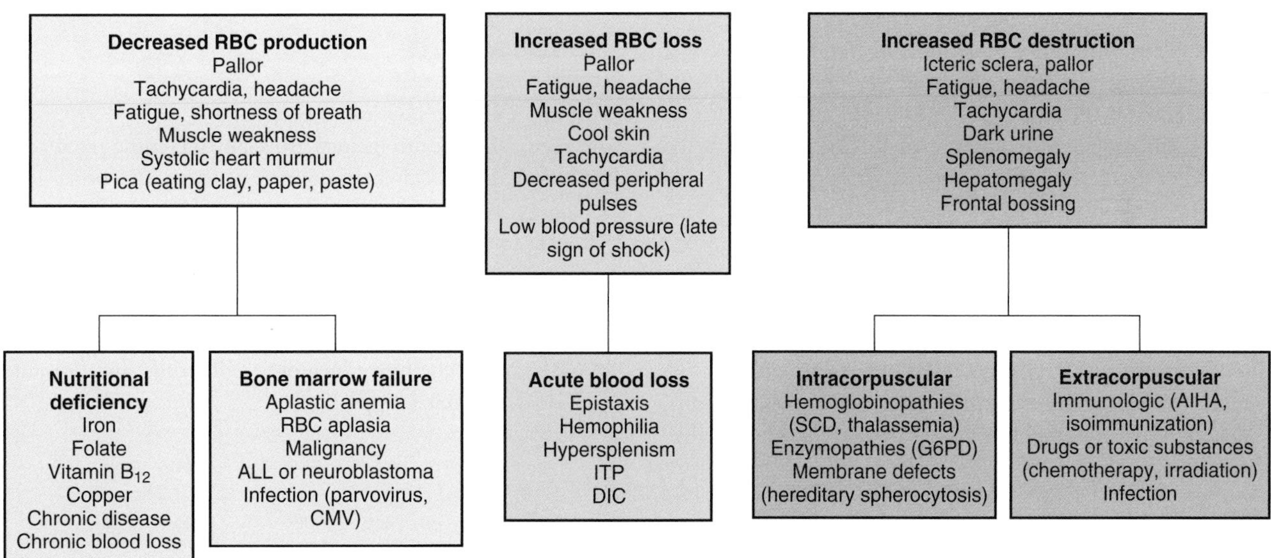

FIG. **1.35** Classifications of anemias. *AIHA,* Autoimmune haemolytic anaemia; *ALL,* acute lymphocytic leukemia; *CMV,* cytomegalovirus; *DIC,* disseminated intravascular coagulopathy; *G6PD,* glucose-6-phosphate dehydrogenase deficiency; *ITP,* immune thrombocytopenia purpura; *RBC,* red blood cell; *SCD,* sickle cell disease. (Added from Essentials 11th ed, Chapter 24, pg 785 Fig 24.1.)

The Child with Renal Failure

Renal failure is the inability of the kidneys to excrete waste material, concentrate urine, and conserve electrolytes

Acute renal injury (ARI)—A condition that results when the kidneys suddenly are unable to regulate the volume and composition of urine appropriately in response to food and fluid intake and needs of the organism.

Assessment

Perform a physical assessment.

Take a detailed health history to reveal symptoms that may be related to glomerulonephritis, obstructive uropathy, or exposure to nephrotoxic chemicals (e.g., ingestion of heavy metals, inhalation of organic solvents or exposure to

BOX 1.20 Clinical Manifestations of Acute Kidney Injury

Clinical Manifestations of Acute Kidney Injury
Specific:
- Oliguria
- Anuria uncommon (except in obstructive disorders)

Nonspecific (may develop):
- Nausea
- Vomiting
- Drowsiness
- Edema
- Hypertension
- Manifestations of underlying disorder or pathologic condition

nephrotoxic drugs such as vancomycin, aminoglycosides, nonsteroidal anti-inflammatory drugs).

Observe for clinical manifestations of acute renal injury. See Box 1.20 on clinical manifestations of acute kidney injury.

Assist with diagnostic tests (e.g., urinalysis, BUN, nonprotein nitrogen, creatinine, serum electrolytes, CBC, blood gases, and specific tests to determine the cause of renal failure).

The Child with Chronic Renal Failure

Chronic renal failure (CRF)— the kidneys are able to maintain the chemical composition of body fluids within normal limits until more than 50% of functional renal capacity is destroyed by disease or injury

The final stage is end-stage renal disease (ESRD), which is irreversible.

Various biochemical substances accumulate in the blood as a result of diminished renal function and produce complications such as the following:

Anemia caused by hematologic dysfunction, including shortened life span of RBCs, impaired RBC production related to decreased production of erythropoietin, prolonged bleeding time, and nutritional anemia

Calcium and phosphorus disturbances resulting in altered bone metabolism, which in turn causes growth arrest or retardation, bone pain, and deformities known as renal osteodystrophy

Growth disturbance, probably caused by such factors as renal osteodystrophy, inadequate nutrition associated with dietary restrictions and loss of appetite, and biochemical abnormalities

Hyperkalemia of dangerous levels

Metabolic acidosis of a sustained nature because of continual hydrogen ion retention and bicarbonate loss

Retention of waste products, especially BUN and creatinine

Water and sodium retention, which contribute to edema and vascular congestion

Assessment

Initial Assessment

Perform a routine physical assessment.

Take a detailed health history, especially including renal dysfunction, eating behavior, frequency of infections, and energy level.

Observe for clinical manifestations of chronic renal failure (see Box 1.21 on clinical manifestations of chronic renal failure).

Assist with diagnostic procedures and tests (e.g., urinalysis, CBC, blood chemistry including glomerular filtration rate [GFR], and renal biopsy).

The Child with Nephrotic Syndrome

Nephrotic syndrome—A clinical state that includes massive proteinuria, hypoalbuminemia, hyperlipidemia, and edema.

Assessment

Perform a physical assessment.

Take a detailed health history, especially relative to recent weight gain or renal dysfunction.

Observe for clinical manifestations of nephrotic syndrome (see Box 1.22 on clinical manifestations of nephrotic syndrome).

Assist with diagnostic procedures and tests (e.g., urinalysis for protein, casts, oval fat bodies, and few RBCs at times; blood analysis for serum protein [total, albumin/globulin ratio, cholesterol]; CBC; serum sodium; renal biopsy).

BOX 1.21 Clinical Manifestations of Chronic Renal Failure

Early signs:
- Loss of normal energy
- Increased fatigue on exertion
- Pallor, subtle (may not be noticed)
- Elevated blood pressure (sometimes)

As the disease progresses:
- Decreased appetite (especially at breakfast)
- Less interest in normal activities
- Increased or decreased urinary output with a compensatory intake of fluid
- Pallor more evident
- Sallow, muddy appearance of skin

Child may complain of:
- Headache
- Muscle cramps
- Nausea

Other signs and symptoms:
- Weight loss
- Facial edema
- Malaise
- Bone or joint pain
- Growth retardation
- Dryness or itching of the skin
- Bruised skin
- Sensory or motor loss (sometimes)
- Amenorrhea (common in adolescent girls)

Uremic syndrome (untreated):
- Gastrointestinal symptoms
- Anorexia
- Nausea and vomiting
- Bleeding tendencies
- Bruises
- Bloody diarrheal stools
- Bleeding from lips and mouth
- Stomatitis
- Intractable itching
- Uremic frost (deposits of urea crystals on skin)
- Unpleasant "uremic" breath odor
- Deep respirations
- Hypertension
- Congestive heart failure
- Pulmonary edema
- Neurologic involvement
- Progressive confusion
- Dulled sensorium
- Coma (ultimately)
- Tremors
- Muscular twitching
- Seizures

BOX 1.22 Clinical Manifestations of Nephrotic Syndrome

Weight gain

Puffiness of face (facial edema):
- Especially around the eyes
- Apparent on arising in the morning
- Subsides during the day

Abdominal swelling (ascites)

Pleural effusion

Labial or scrotal swelling

Edema of intestinal mucosal, possibly causing:
- Diarrhea
- Anorexia
- Poor intestinal absorption

Ankle or leg swelling

Irritability

Easily fatigued

Lethargic

Blood pressure normal or slightly decreased

Susceptibility to infection

Urine alterations:
- Decreased volume
- Frothy

The Child with Cerebral Dysfunction

Cerebral dysfunction—Concerns disorders affecting cerebral structure and function

Assessment

Take a detailed history that provides clues to the etiology of dysfunction.

Family history may offer clues regarding possible genetic disorders with neurologic manifestations

Health history may provide valuable clues regarding the cause of neurologic dysfunction. Information should include Apgar scores, age of developmental milestones, trauma or injury, encounters with animals or insects, ingestion or inhalation of neurotoxic substances or chemicals, acute past illness, and any chronic illnesses such as diabetes mellitus or sickle cell disease)

Perform physical evaluation of infant that includes assessment of:
- Level of alertness
- Size and shape of the head including presence of fontanels

- Motor function including posture, tone, and muscle strength
- Sensory responses
- **Respirations including signs of prolonged apnea, ataxic breathing, paradoxic chest movement** or hyperventilation
- Motility including symmetry in movements and involuntary movements
- Dysmorphic facial features
- Behavioral cues including consolability and habituation
- Deep tendon reflexes
- Cranial nerves

Assess level of consciousness (see Box 1.23 on level of consciousness).

Observe for clinical manifestations of increased intracranial pressure (ICP) in infants and children (see Box 1.24 on clinical manifestation of ICP in infants and children).

Assist with diagnostic procedures and tests (e.g., lumbar puncture, subdural tap, ventricular puncture, electroencephalography, radiography, magnetic resonance imaging [MRI], computed tomography [CT], nuclear brain scan, echoencephalography, positron emission transaxial tomography, real-time ultrasonography, digital subtraction angiography; blood biochemistry [pH, blood gases, ammonia, glucose], electrolytes, clotting studies, complete blood count, liver function tests, blood cultures if fever present, toxicology screen, and blood lead levels if clinically indicated).

BOX 1.23 | Levels of Consciousness

Full consciousness—Awake and alert, orientated to time, place, and person; behavior appropriate for age.
Confusion—Impaired decision making.
Disorientation—Confusion regarding time, place, and/or person; decreased level of consciousness.
Lethargy—Limited spontaneous movement, sluggish speech, drowsiness.
Obtundation—Arousable with stimulation.
Stupor—Remaining in a deep sleep, responsive only to vigorous and repeated stimulation.
Coma—No motor or verbal response to noxious (painful) stimuli.
Persistent vegetative state (PVS)—Permanently lost function of the cerebral cortex. Eyes follow objects only by reflex or when attracted to the direction of loud sounds; all four limbs are spastic but can withdraw from painful stimuli; hands show reflexive grasping and groping; the face can grimace, some food may be swallowed, and the child may groan or cry but utter no words.

Modified from Ball JW, Dains JE, Flynn JA, et al., eds. *Seidel's Guide to Physical Examination.* 9th ed. St. Louis: Elsevier; 2019.

The Child with Seizures

Seizures—is a transient occurrence of signs and/or symptoms due to abnormal excessive and synchronous neuronal activity in the brain[f]

Epilepsy—is defined as two or more unprovoked seizures more than 24 hours apart and can be caused by a variety of pathological processes in the brain.

Assessment

Obtain a detailed health history including prenatal, perinatal, and neonatal events, apnea, colic, and any information regarding previous accidents or serious illnesses or infections.

BOX 1.24 | Clinical Manifestations of Increased Intracranial Pressure in Infants and Children

Infants

Tense, bulging fontanel
Separated cranial sutures
Macewen (cracked-pot) sign
Irritability and restlessness
Drowsiness
Increased sleeping
High-pitched cry
Increased frontooccipital circumference
Distended scalp veins
Poor feeding
Crying when disturbed
Setting-sun sign

Children

Headache
Nausea
Forceful vomiting
Diplopia, blurred vision
Seizures
Indifference, drowsiness
Decline in school performance
Diminished physical activity and motor performance
Increased sleeping
Inability to follow simple commands
Lethargy

Late Signs in Infants and Children

Bradycardia
Decreased motor response to command
Decreased sensory response to painful stimuli
Alterations in pupil size and reactivity
Extension or flexion posturing
Cheyne-Stokes respirations
Papilledema
Decreased consciousness
Coma

Obtain a thorough history of seizure activity including the following:

- Description of the child's behavior during a seizure, especially at the onset
- Age of onset of first seizure
- The time when the seizure occurred—Time of day (e.g., early morning, while awake, or during sleep)
- Any factors that might have precipitated a seizure including fever, infection, head trauma, anxiety, fatigue, sleep deprivation, menstrual cycle, alcohol, activity (e.g., hyperventilation or exposure to strong stimuli such as bright, flashing lights or loud noises)
- Sensory phenomena child experiences
- Duration, progression, and any postictal feelings or behaviors (e.g., confusion, inability to speak, amnesia, headache, and sleep)

Perform a physical and neurologic assessment.

Observe seizure manifestations. Seizures are classified into two major categories with corresponding clinical manifestations: (1) partial seizures that have a local onset and involve a relatively small location in the brain and (2) generalized seizures that involve both hemispheres of the brain from the onset or secondary from partial seizures (see Box 1.25 on classification and clinical manifestations of seizures)

BOX 1.25 | Classification and Clinical Manifestations of Seizures

Classification and Clinical Manifestations of Partial and Generalized Seizures

Partial Seizures

Simple Partial Seizures With Motor Signs

Characterized by the following:
- Localized motor symptoms
- Somatosensory, psychic, and autonomic symptoms
- Abnormal discharges remaining unilateral

Manifestations:
- Aversive seizure (most common motor seizure in children)—Eye or eyes and head turn away from the side of the focus; awareness of movement or loss of consciousness
- Rolandic (Sylvan) seizure—Tonic-clonic movements involving the face, salivation, arrested speech; most common during sleep
- Jacksonian march (rare in children)—Orderly, sequential progression of clonic movements beginning in a foot, hand, or face and moving, or "marching," to adjacent body parts

Simple Partial Seizures With Sensory Signs

Characterized by various sensations, including:
- Numbness, tingling, prickling, paresthesia, or pain originating in one area (e.g., face or extremities) and spreading to other parts of the body
- Visual sensations or formed images
- Motor phenomena such as posturing or hypertonia

Focal Seizures With Impaired Awareness

Observed more often in children from 3 years of age through adolescence

Characterized by the following:
- Period of altered behavior
- Amnesia for event (no recollection of behavior)
- Inability to respond to environment
- Impaired consciousness during event
- Drowsiness or sleep usually following the seizure
- Confusion and amnesia possibly prolonged
- Complex sensory phenomena (aura)—Most frequent sensation is a strange feeling in the pit of the stomach that rises toward the throat and is often accompanied by odd or unpleasant odors or tastes, complex auditory or visual hallucinations, ill-defined feelings of elation or strangeness (e.g., déjà vu, a feeling of familiarity in a strange environment), strong feelings of fear and anxiety, distorted sense of time and self, and in small children emission of a cry or attempt to run for help

Patterns of motor behavior:
- Stereotypic
- Similar with each subsequent seizure
- May suddenly cease activity, appear dazed, stare into space, become confused and apathetic, and become limp or stiff or display some form of posturing
- May be confused
- May perform purposeless, complicated activities in a repetitive manner (automatisms), such as walking, running, kicking, laughing, or speaking incoherently, most often followed by postictal confusion or sleep; may exhibit oropharyngeal activities, such as smacking, chewing, drooling, swallowing, and nausea or abdominal pain followed by stiffness, a fall, and postictal sleep; rarely manifests actions such as rage or temper tantrums; aggressive acts uncommon during a seizure

Generalized Seizures

Tonic-Clonic Seizures (Formerly Known as Grand Mal)

Most common and most dramatic of all seizure manifestations

Occur without warning

Tonic phase lasts approximately 10–20 s

Manifestations:
- Eyes roll upward
- Immediate loss of consciousness
- If standing, falls to floor or ground
- Stiffens in generalized, symmetric tonic contraction of entire body musculature
- Arms usually flexed
- Legs, head, and neck extended
- May utter a peculiar piercing cry
- Apneic, may become cyanotic
- Increased salivation and loss of swallowing reflex

Clonic phase: lasts about 30 s but can vary from only a few seconds to a half-hour or longer

Manifestations:
- Violent jerking movements as the trunk and extremities undergo rhythmic contraction and relaxation
- May foam at the mouth
- May be incontinent of urine and feces

As event ends, movements less intense, occurring at longer intervals, then ceasing entirely

Status epilepticus—Series of seizures at intervals too brief to allow the child to regain consciousness between the time one event ends and the next begins:
- Requires emergency intervention
- Can lead to exhaustion, respiratory failure, and death

BOX 1.25 Classification and Clinical Manifestations of Seizures—cont'd

Postictal state:
Appears to relax
May remain semiconscious and difficult to arouse
May awaken in a few minutes
Remains confused for several hours
Poor coordination
Mild impairment of fine motor movements
May have visual and speech difficulties
May vomit or complain of severe headache
When left alone, usually sleeps for several hours
On awakening is fully conscious
Usually feels tired and complains of sore muscles and headache
No recollection of entire event

Absence Seizures (Formerly Called Petit Mal)
Characterized by the following:
Onset usually between 4 and 12 years of age
More common in girls than in boys
Usually cease at puberty
Brief loss of consciousness
Minimum or no alteration in muscle tone
May go unrecognized because of little change in child's behavior
Abrupt onset; suddenly develops 20 or more attacks daily
Event often mistaken for inattentiveness or daydreaming
Events possibly precipitated by hyperventilation, hypoglycemia, stresses (emotional and physiologic), fatigue, or sleeplessness
Manifestations:
Brief loss of consciousness
Appear without warning or aura
Usually last about 5–10 s
Slight loss of muscle tone may cause child to drop objects
Ability to maintain postural control; seldom falls
Minor movements such as lip smacking, twitching of eyelids or face, or slight hand movements
Not accompanied by incontinence
Amnesia for episode
May need to reorient themselves to previous activity

Atonic and Akinetic Seizures (Also Known as Drop Attacks)
Characterized by the following:
Onset usually between 2 and 5 years of age
Sudden, momentary loss of muscle tone and postural control
Events recurring frequently during the day, particularly in the morning hours and shortly after awakening
Manifestations:
Loss of tone causing the child to fall to the floor violently; unable to break fall by putting out hands; may incur a serious injury to the face, head, or shoulder
Loss of consciousness only momentary

Myoclonic Seizures
May be isolated as benign essential myoclonus
Characterized by the following:
Sudden, brief contractures of a muscle or group of muscles
Occur singly or repetitively
No postictal state
May or may not be symmetric
May or may not include loss of consciousness

Observations During Seizure

General Description
Order of events (before, during, and after)
Duration of seizure
Tonic-clonic—from first signs of event until jerking stops
Absence—from loss of consciousness until consciousness is regained
Focal seizures with impaired awareness—from first sign of unresponsiveness, motor activity, and automatisms until there are signs of responsiveness to the environment

Onset
Time of onset
Significant precipitating events—missed medication dosage, illness, stress, sleep deprivation, menses

Behavior
Change in facial expression
Cry or other sound
Stereotypic or automatous movements
Random activity (wandering)
Position of eyes, head, body, extremities
Unilateral or bilateral posturing of one or more extremities

Movement
Change of position, if any
Site of commencement—hand, thumb, mouth, generalized
Tonic phase—length, parts of body involved
Clonic phase—twitching or jerking movements, parts of body involved, sequence of parts involved, generalized, change in character of movements
Lack of movement or muscle tone of body part or entire body

Face
Color change—pallor, cyanosis, flushing
Perspiration
Mouth—position, deviating to one side, teeth clenched, tongue bitten, frothing at mouth
Lack of expression
Asymmetric expression

Eyes
Position—straight ahead, deviation upward or outward, conjugate, or divergent gaze
Pupils—change in size, equality, reaction to light

Respiratory Effort
Presence and length of apnea

Other
Incontinence

Postictal Observations
Duration of postictal period
State of consciousness
Orientation
Arousability
Motor ability
Any change in motor function
Ability to move all extremities
Paresis or weakness
Speech
Sensations
Complaint of discomfort or pain
Any sensory impairment
Recollection of preseizure sensations or aura

An important nursing responsibility is to observe the seizure episode and accurately document the events (see Box 1.26 on child during a seizure)

Assist with diagnostic procedures and tests (e.g., electroencephalography, skull radiography, echoencephalography, CT brain scan, MRI of brain; CBC and differential (for signs of infection, blood chemistry, serum glucose, BUN, ammonia, calcium, serum amino acids, lactate, and urine organic acids that may indicate metabolic disturbances)

The Child with a Head Injury

Head injury—A pathologic process involving the scalp, skull, meninges, or brain as a result of mechanical force

Concussion—A transient disturbance of brain function, often traumatically induced, that involves a complex pathophysiologic process (Liebig and Congeni, 2016)[g] Sports-related traumatic brain injury, Nelson textbook

Contusion—Petechial hemorrhages or localized bruising along superficial aspects of the brain at the site of impact (coup injury) or a lesion remote from the site of direct trauma (contrecoup injury)

Assessment

Assess **circulation,** airway, and breathing.

Perform neurologic examination focusing on mental status, pupillary responses, motor responses, and assessment of spinal injury (Fig. 1.36 on pediatric coma scale)

Examine scalp and skull for evidence of injury—widely separated sutures, size and tension of fontanels (may indicate intracranial hemorrhage), bruises, lacerations, swelling, depression, drainage, or bleeding from any orifice.

Perform a physical assessment and obtain a history of the event.

Observe for clinical manifestations of head injury (see Box 1.27 on clinical manifestations of acute head injury).

Assist with diagnostic tests (CT scan, MRI, skull x-ray films).

The Child with Acute Bacterial Meningitis

Acute bacterial meningitis—A bacterial infection is an acute inflammation of the meninges and CSF. Suspected bacterial meningitis is a medical emergency that requires immediate recognition and treatment.

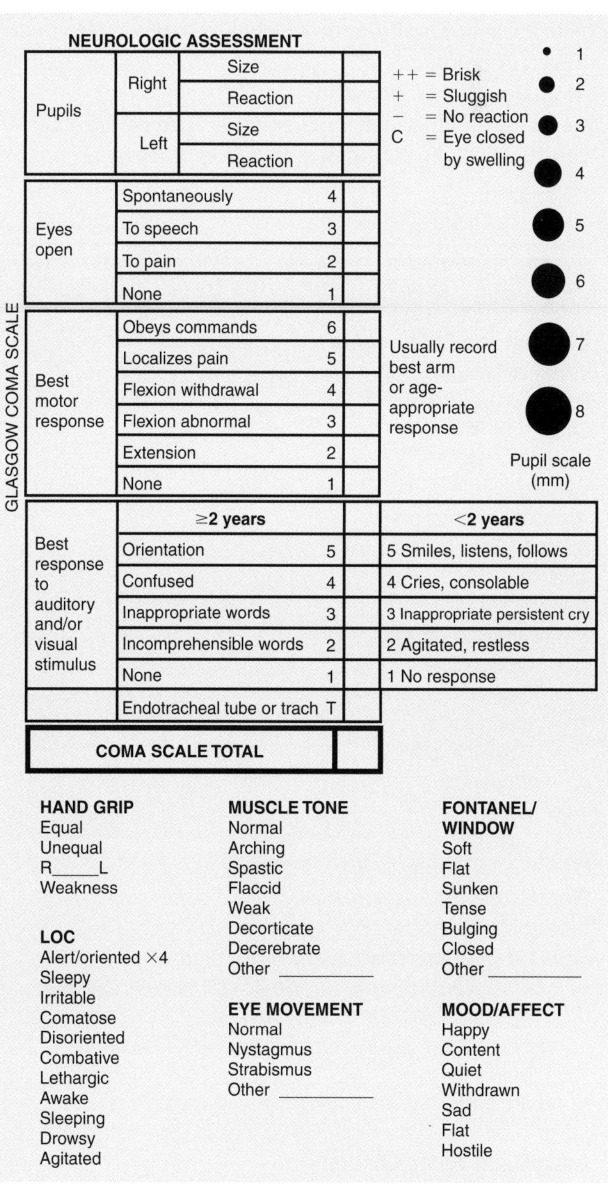

NEUROLOGIC ASSESSMENT

Pupils	Right	Size	
		Reaction	
	Left	Size	
		Reaction	

++ = Brisk
+ = Sluggish
– = No reaction
C = Eye closed by swelling

GLASGOW COMA SCALE

	≥2 years			<2 years
Eyes open	Spontaneously	4		
	To speech	3		
	To pain	2		
	None	1		
Best motor response	Obeys commands	6		Usually record best arm or age-appropriate response
	Localizes pain	5		
	Flexion withdrawal	4		
	Flexion abnormal	3		
	Extension	2		
	None	1		
Best response to auditory and/or visual stimulus	Orientation	5		5 Smiles, listens, follows
	Confused	4		4 Cries, consolable
	Inappropriate words	3		3 Inappropriate persistent cry
	Incomprehensible words	2		2 Agitated, restless
	None	1		1 No response
	Endotracheal tube or trach	T		
COMA SCALE TOTAL				

Pupil scale (mm): 1, 2, 3, 4, 5, 6, 7, 8

HAND GRIP
Equal
Unequal
R____L
Weakness

LOC
Alert/oriented ×4
Sleepy
Irritable
Comatose
Disoriented
Combative
Lethargic
Awake
Sleeping
Drowsy
Agitated

MUSCLE TONE
Normal
Arching
Spastic
Flaccid
Weak
Decorticate
Decerebrate
Other ________

EYE MOVEMENT
Normal
Nystagmus
Strabismus
Other ________

FONTANEL/ WINDOW
Soft
Flat
Sunken
Tense
Bulging
Closed
Other ________

MOOD/AFFECT
Happy
Content
Quiet
Withdrawn
Sad
Flat
Hostile

FIG. **1.36** Pediatric Glasgow Coma Scale.

BOX 1.26 Precautions for the Child During a Seizure

The extent of precautions depends on type, severity, and frequency of seizures. Precautions may include the following:

- Side rails raised when child is sleeping or resting
- Side rails and other hard objects padded
- Waterproof mattress or pad on bed or crib

Appropriate precautions during potentially hazardous activities may include the following:

- Swimming with a companion
- Showers preferred; bathing only with close supervision
- Use of protective helmet and padding during bicycle riding, skateboarding, and skating
- Supervision during use of hazardous machinery or equipment

Have child carry or wear medical identification.

Alert other caregivers to the need for any special precautions.

Child may not drive or operate hazardous machinery or equipment unless seizure free for a designated period (varies by state).

BOX 1.27 Clinical Manifestations of Acute Head Injury

Minor Injury
May or may not lose consciousness
Transient period of confusion
Somnolence
Listlessness
Irritability
Pallor
Vomiting (one or more episodes)

Signs of Progression
- Altered mental status (e.g., difficulty arousing child)
- Mounting agitation
- Development of focal lateral neurologic signs
- Marked changes in vital signs

Severe Injury
Signs of increased intracranial pressure (see Box 27.1)
Bulging fontanel (infant)
Retinal hemorrhages
Extraocular palsies (especially cranial nerve III)
Hemiparesis
Quadriplegia
Elevated temperature
Unsteady gait (older child)
Papilledema (older child)
Retinal hemorrhages

Associated Signs
Scalp trauma
Other injuries (e.g., to extremities)

Assessment

Obtain a detailed health history including previous infection, injury, or exposure.

Perform a physical assessment.

Observe for the clinical manifestations of bacterial meningitis (see Box 1.28 on clinical manifestations of bacterial meningitis).

Assist with diagnostic procedures and tests (e.g., lumbar puncture, spinal fluid pressure, and spinal fluid examination (glucose, protein, gram stain, cultures) and blood cell count.

BOX 1.28 Clinical Manifestations of Bacterial Meningitis

Children and Adolescents
Usually abrupt onset
Fever
Chills
Headache
Vomiting
Alterations in sensorium
Seizures (often the initial sign)
Irritability
Agitation
May develop the following:
- Photophobia
- Delirium
- Hallucinations
- Aggressive behavior
- Drowsiness
- Stupor
- Coma

Nuchal rigidity; may progress to opisthotonos
Positive Kernig and Brudzinski signs
Hyperactivity but variable reflex responses
Signs and symptoms peculiar to individual organisms:
Petechial or purpuric rashes (meningococcal infection), especially when associated with a shock-like state
Joint involvement (meningococcal or *Haemophilus influenzae* infection)
Chronically draining ear (pneumococcal meningitis)

Infants and Young Children
Classic picture (above) rarely seen in children between 3 months and 2 years of age
Fever
Poor feeding
Vomiting
Marked irritability
Frequent seizures (often accompanied by a high-pitched cry)
Bulging fontanel
Nuchal rigidity possible
Brudzinski and Kernig signs are not helpful in diagnosis
Difficult to elicit and evaluate in this age-group
Subdural empyema (*H. influenzae* infection)

Neonates
Specific Signs
Child well at birth but within a few days begins to look and behave poorly
Refuses feedings
Poor sucking ability
Vomiting or diarrhea
Poor tone
Lack of movement
Weak cry
Full, tense, and bulging fontanel may appear late in course of illness
Neck usually supple

Nonspecific Signs That May Be Present
- Hypothermia or fever (depending on the infant's maturity)
- Jaundice
- Irritability
- Drowsiness
- Seizures
- Respiratory irregularities or apnea
- Cyanosis
- Weight loss

The Child with Diabetes Mellitus

Diabetes mellitus (DM)—A chronic disorder of metabolism characterized by hyperglycemia and insulin resistance. DM can be classified into the following categories:

Type 1 (previously called insulin-dependent diabetes mellitus [IDDM])—Characterized by the destruction of the pancreatic beta cells, which produce insulin; this usually leads to absolute insulin deficiency. Type 1 has two forms: Immune-mediated DM results from the autoimmune destruction of beta cells and Idiopathic type 1 which is rare and has no known cause.

Type 2 (previously called non–insulin-dependent diabetes mellitus [NIDDM])—Usually arises because of insulin resistance, in which the body fails to use insulin properly, combined with relative (not absolute) insulin deficiency (see Table 1.13 on characteristics of type 1 and 2)

Assessment

Perform a physical assessment.

Obtain a detailed health history including a family history of diabetes, weight loss, frequency of drinking and voiding, increased appetite, diminished activity level, behavior changes, and other clinical manifestations of type 1 diabetes mellitus including the 3 cardinal signs of diabetes (polyphagia, polyuria, and polydipsia). See Box 1.29 on clinical manifestations of type 1 DM

Daily monitoring of blood glucose levels is an essential aspect of appropriate DM management. Plasma blood glucose and hemoglobin A1c goal ranges are listed in Table 1.14. Even with close monitoring of blood glucose levels, a child may frequently experience symptoms of hypoglycemia (see Table 1.15 for a comparison of hypoglycemia and hyperglycemia).

Perform or assist with diagnostic procedures and tests (e.g., fasting blood glucose, serum insulin levels, urine for ketones and glucose, blood glucose, hemoglobin A1c, serum islet cell antibody level).

The Child with a Fracture

Fracture—A break in the continuity of a bone caused when the resistance of the bone against the stress being exerted yields to a stress or force

Comminuted fracture—Small fragments of bone are broken from the fractured shaft and lie in surrounding tissue (rare in children).

Complete fracture—Fracture fragments are separated.

Complicated fracture—Bone fragments cause damage to other organs or tissues (e.g., lung, liver, bladder).

Incomplete fracture—Fracture fragments remain attached.

Open or compound fracture—Fracture has an open wound through which the bone protrudes.

Simple or closed fracture—Fracture does not produce a break in the skin.

Most frequent fractures in children (see Box 1.30 and Fig. 1.37 on types of fractures in children)

Assessment

Obtain a detailed history including the event, previous injury, and experience with health personnel.

Observe for clinical manifestations of fracture (see Box 1.31 on clinical manifestations of fracture).

Assist with diagnostic procedures and tests (e.g., radiographic films).

Assessment of the Extremity in a Cast or Traction

—four major categories of cast used for fractures: upper extremity to immobilize the wrist or elbow, lower extremity to immobilize ankle or knee, spinal and cervical to immobilize the spine and spica casts to immobilize the hip and knee.

Compartment syndrome is a serious complication that results from the compression of nerves, blood vessels, and muscles inside a closed space. The six Ps of ischemia from vascular, soft tissue, nerve, or bone injury should be included in an assessment of any injury (see Box 1.32 on compartment syndrome evaluation)

The Child Who is Maltreated

Child maltreatment—A broad term that includes intentional physical abuse or neglect, emotional abuse or neglect, and sexual abuse of children, usually by an adult

Emotional abuse or psychological maltreatment—The deliberate attempt to destroy or significantly impair a child's self-esteem or competence

Emotional neglect—Failure to meet the child's needs for affection, attention, and emotional nurturance

Physical abuse—The deliberate infliction of physical injury on a child

Physical neglect—The deprivation of necessities, such as food, clothing, shelter, supervision, medical care, and education

TABLE 1.13 Characteristics of Type 1 and Type 2 Diabetes Mellitus

Characteristic	Type 1	Type 2
Age at onset	<20 years	Increasingly occurring in younger children
Type of onset	Abrupt	Gradual
Sex ratio	Affects males slightly more than females	Females outnumber males
Percentage of diabetic population	5%–8%	85%–90%
Heredity:		
Family history	Sometimes	Frequently
Human leukocyte antigen	Associations	No association
Twin concordance	25%–50%	90%–100%
Ethnic distribution	Primarily whites	Increased incidence in American Indians, Hispanics, African Americans
Presenting symptoms	Three Ps common—polyuria, polydipsia, polyphagia	May be related to long-term complications
Nutritional status	Underweight	Overweight
Insulin (natural):		
Pancreatic content	Usually none	>50% normal
Serum insulin	Low to absent	High or low
Primary resistance	Minimum	Marked
Islet cell antibodies	80%–85%	<5%
Therapy:		
Insulin	Always	20%–30% of patients
Oral agents	Ineffective	Often effective
Diet only	Ineffective	Often effective
Chronic complications	>80%	Variable
Ketoacidosis	Common	Infrequent

BOX 1.29 Clinical Manifestations of Type 1 Diabetes Mellitus

Clinical Manifestations of Type 1 Diabetes Mellitus
- Polyphagia
- Polyuria
- Polydipsia
- Weight loss
- Enuresis or nocturia
- Irritability; "not himself" or "not herself"
- Shortened attention span
- Lowered frustration tolerance
- Dry skin
- Blurred vision
- Poor wound healing
- Fatigue
- Flushed skin
- Headache
- Frequent infections
- Hyperglycemia
  - Elevated blood glucose levels
  - Glucosuria
- Diabetic ketosis
  - Ketones and glucose in urine
  - Dehydration in some cases
- Diabetic ketoacidosis (DKA)
  - Dehydration
  - Electrolyte imbalance
  - Acidosis
  - Deep, rapid breathing (Kussmaul respirations)

TABLE 1.14 Plasma Blood Glucose and Hemoglobin A1c Goals for Type 1 Diabetes Mellitus by Age-Group

Age	Value[a] Before Meals (mg/dL)	Value[a] at Bedtime/ Overnight (mg/dL)	Hemoglobin A1c (%)	Implications
Toddlers and preschoolers (<6 years)	100–180	110–200	≤8.5% (but ≥7.5%)	High risk and vulnerability to hypoglycemia
School age (6–12 years)	90–180	100–180	<8%	Risks of hypoglycemia and relatively low risk of complications before puberty
Adolescents (>12 years) and young adults	90–130	90–150	<7.5%	Risk of hypoglycemia Developmental and psychologic issues

[a]Plasma blood glucose goal range.

Modified from American Diabetes Association; Standards of Medical Care in Diabetes. *Diabetes Care* 1 January 2005; 28 (suppl_1): s4–s36. https://doi.org/10.2337/diacare.28.suppl_1.S4.

TABLE 1.15 Comparison of Manifestations of Hypoglycemia and Hyperglycemia

Variable	Hypoglycemia	Hyperglycemia
Onset	Rapid (minutes)	Gradual (days)
Mood	Labile, irritable, nervous, weepy	Lethargic
Mental status	Difficulty concentrating, speaking, focusing, coordinating Nightmares	Dulled sensorium Confusion
Inward feeling	Shaky feeling	Thirst
	Hunger	Weakness
	Headache	Nausea and vomiting
	Dizziness	Abdominal pain
Skin	Pallor Sweating	Flushed Signs of dehydration
Mucous membranes	Normal	Dry, crusty
Respirations	Shallow, normal	Deep, rapid (Kussmaul)
Pulse	Tachycardia, palpitations	Less rapid, weak
Breath odor	Normal	Fruity, acetone
Neurologic	Tremors	Diminished reflexes Paresthesia
Ominous signs	Late: Hyperreflexia, dilated pupils, seizure Shock, coma	Acidosis, coma
Blood:		
Glucose	Low: <60 mg/dL	High: ≥200 mg/dL
Ketones	Negative	High, large
Osmolarity	Normal	High
pH	Normal	Low (≤7.25)
Hematocrit	Normal	High
Bicarbonate	Normal	<20 mEq/L
Urine:		
Output	Normal	Polyuria (early) to oliguria (late)
Glucose	Negative	Enuresis, nocturia
Ketones	Negative or trace	High
Visual	Diplopia	Blurred vision

Continued

BOX 1.30 Types of Fractures in Children

Plastic deformation: Occurs when the bone is bent but not broken. A child's flexible bone can be bent 45 degrees or more before breaking. However, if bent, the bone will straighten slowly but not completely, producing some deformity but without the angulation seen when the bone breaks. Bends occur most commonly in the ulna and fibula, often in association with fractures of the radius and tibia.

Buckle, or **torus, fracture:** Produced by compression of the porous bone; appears as a raised or bulging projection at the fracture site. These fractures occur in the most porous portion of the bone near the metaphysis (the portion of the bone shaft adjacent to the epiphysis) and are more common in young children.

Greenstick fracture: Occurs when a bone is angulated beyond the limits of bending. The compressed side bends, and the tension side fails, causing an incomplete fracture similar to the break observed when a green stick is broken.

Complete fracture: Divides the bone fragments. These fragments often remain attached by a **periosteal hinge**, which can aid or hinder reduction.

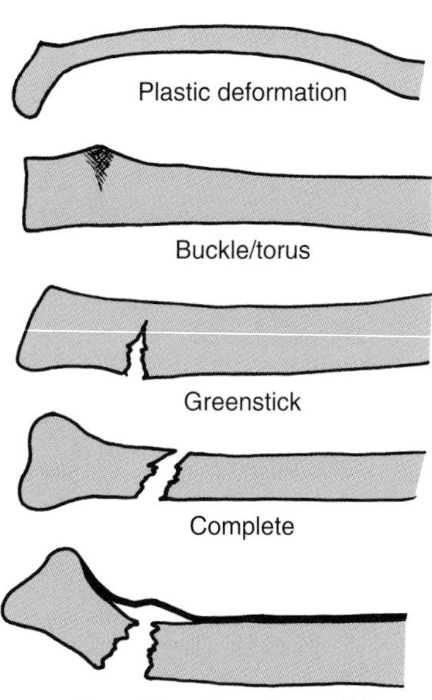

FIG. **1.37** Types of fractures in children. (Added from Essentials 11th ed, Chapter 29, pg 975 Fig. 29.2.)

Munchausen syndrome by proxy or medical abuse or factitious disorder—A rare but serious form of child abuse in which the caregivers deliberately exaggerate or fabricate histories and symptoms or induce symptoms

BOX 1.31 Clinical Manifestations of a Fracture

Signs of injury:
- Generalized swelling
- Pain or tenderness
- Deformity
- Diminished functional use of affected limb or digit

May also demonstrate:
- Bruising
- Severe muscular rigidity
- Crepitus (grating sensation at fracture site)

BOX 1.32 Compartment Syndrome Evaluation

Assess the extent of injury—"the 6 Ps":

- **Pain:** Severe pain that is not relieved by analgesics or elevation of the limb, movement that increases pain
- **Pulselessness:** Inability to palpate a pulse distal to the fracture or compartment
- **Pallor:** Pale-appearing skin, poor perfusion, capillary refill greater than 3 s
- **Paresthesia:** Tingling or burning sensations
- **Paralysis:** Inability to move extremity or digits
- **Pressure:** Involved limb or digits may feel tense and warm; skin is tight, shiny; pressure within the compartment is elevated

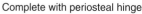

Sexual abuse—is one of the most devastating types of child maltreatment. Defined by the US Department of Health and Human services (2012) as employment, use, persuasion, inducement, enticement, or coercion of any child to engage in, or assist any other person to engage in, sexually explicit conduct or any stimulation of such conduct; or rape, molestation, prostitution, or other forms of sexual exploitation of children; or incest with children.

Assessment

Perform an assessment with special attention to clinical manifestations of potential child maltreatment (see Box 1.33 on clinical manifestations of potential child maltreatment).

All evidence collected must adhere to strict guidelines (see nursing care guidelines).

BOX 1.33 Clinical Manifestations of Potential Child Maltreatment

Clinical Manifestations of Potential Child Maltreatment

Physical Neglect

Suggestive Physical Findings

Growth failures
Signs of malnutrition, such as thin extremities, abdominal distention, lack of subcutaneous fat
Poor personal hygiene
Unclean or inappropriate dress
Evidence of poor health care, such as delayed immunization, untreated infections, frequent colds
Frequent injuries from lack of supervision

Suggestive Behaviors

Dull and inactive affect; excessively passive or sleepy
Self-stimulatory behaviors, such as finger-sucking or rocking
Begging or stealing food
Absenteeism from school
Substance abuse
Vandalism or shoplifting

Emotional Abuse and Neglect

Suggestive Physical Findings

Growth failure (failure to thrive)
Eating or feeding disorder
Enuresis
Sleep disorder

Suggestive Behaviors

Self-stimulatory behaviors, such as biting, rocking, or sucking
During infancy, lack of social smile and stranger anxiety
Withdrawal from environment and people
Unusual fearfulness
Antisocial behavior, such as destructiveness, stealing, cruelty to animals or people
Extremes of behavior, such as overly compliant and passive or aggressive and demanding
Lags in emotional and intellectual development, especially language
Suicide attempts

Physical Abuse

Suggestive Physical Findings

Bruises and welts (may be in various stages of healing)
- On face, lips, mouth, back, buttocks, thighs, or areas of torso
- Regular patterns descriptive of object used, such as belt buckle, hand, wire hanger, chain, wooden spoon, squeeze or pinch marks
- May be present in various stages of healing

Burns
- On soles, palms, back, or buttocks
- Patterns descriptive of object used, such as round cigar or cigarette burns; sharply demarcated areas from immersion in scalding water; rope burns on wrists or ankles from being bound; burns in the shape of an iron, radiator, or electric stove burner
- Absence of "splash" marks and presence of symmetric burns
- Stun gun injury: Lesions circular, fairly uniform (≤0.5 cm), and paired about 5 cm apart

Fractures and dislocations
- Skull, nose, or facial structures
- Injury denoting type of abuse, such as spiral fracture or dislocation from twisting of an extremity or whiplash from shaking the child
- Multiple new or old fractures in various stages of healing

Lacerations and abrasions
- On backs of arms, legs, torso, face, or external genitalia
- Unusual symptoms, such as abdominal swelling, pain, and vomiting from punching
- Descriptive marks, such as from human bites or pulling out of hair

Chemical
- Unexplained repeated poisoning, especially drug overdose
- Unexplained sudden illness, such as hypoglycemia from insulin administration

Suggestive Behaviors

Wary of physical contact with adults
Apparent fear of parents or going home
Lying very still while surveying the environment
Inappropriate reaction to injury, such as failure to cry from pain
Lack of reaction to frightening events
Apprehensive when hearing other children cry
Indiscriminate friendliness and displays of affection
Superficial relationships
Acting-out behavior, such as aggression, to seek attention
Withdrawal behavior

Sexual Abuse

Suggestive Physical Findings

Bruises, bleeding, lacerations, or irritation of external genitalia, anus, mouth, or throat
Torn, stained, or bloody underclothing
Pain on urination or pain, swelling, and itching of genital area
Penile discharge
Sexually transmitted disease, nonspecific vaginitis
Difficulty in walking or sitting
Unusual odor in the genital area
Recurrent urinary tract infections
Presence of sperm
Pregnancy in young adolescent

Suggestive Behaviors

Sudden emergence of sexually related problems, including excessive or public masturbation, age-inappropriate sexual play, promiscuity, or overtly seductive behavior
Withdrawn behavior, excessive daydreaming
Preoccupation with fantasies, especially in play
Poor relationships with peers
Sudden changes, such as anxiety, loss or gain of weight, clinging behavior
In incestuous relationships, excessive anger at mother for not protecting daughter
Regressive behavior, such as bedwetting or thumb sucking
Sudden onset of phobias or fears, particularly fears of the dark, men, strangers, or particular settings or situations (e.g., undue fear of leaving the house or staying at the daycare center or the babysitter's house)
Running away from home
Substance abuse, particularly of alcohol or mood-elevating drugs
Profound and rapid personality changes, especially extreme depression, hostility, and aggression (often accompanied by social withdrawal)
Rapidly declining school performance
Suicidal attempts or ideation

GUIDELINES

Nursing Care

Recording assessment data in suspected abuse:

History of Injury:

- Date, time, and place of occurrence
- Sequence of events with recorded times.
- Time-lapse between the occurrence of injury and initiation of treatment
- Interview with the child when appropriate, including verbal quotations and information from drawings or other play activities.
- Interview parents, witnesses, and other significant persons, including their verbal quotations.

Description of parent-child interactions (e.g., verbal interactions, eye contact, touching, parental concern).

Names, ages, and conditions of other children in the home (if possible).

Physical examination:

Location, size, shape, and color of bruises, approximate location, size and shape on drawing of body outline

Distinguishing characteristics of bruise

Symmetry or asymmetry of injury; presence of other injuries

Degree of pain, any bone tenderness

Evidence of past injuries, general state of health, hygiene

Development level of child; screening test (see Developmental Assessment)

All states and provinces in North America have laws for mandatory reporting of child maltreatment. Suspected child abuse is reported to local authorities (telephone numbers usually listed under child abuse or call child abuse hotline: 800-422-4453).

Assist with diagnostic procedures and tests that relate directly to the type of potential maltreatment (e.g., radiology, collection of specimens for examination).

The Child with Burns

Burns—The destruction of body surface area caused by extreme heat sources but may also result from exposure to cold, chemicals, electricity, or radiation

Burn severity criteria

Minor burns—Partial-thickness burns of less than 10% of body surface area (BSA)

Moderate burns—Partial-thickness burns of 10% to 20% of BSA (age-related; see Major, or critical, burns)

Major, or critical, burns

Burns complicated by respiratory tract injury

Partial-thickness burns of 20% or more of BSA

Burns of face, hands, feet, or genitalia, even if they appear to be partial thickness

All full-thickness burns

Any child younger than 2 years of age, unless the burn is very small and very superficial (20% or more of BSA considered critical in a child younger than 2 years of age)

Electric burns that penetrate

Deep chemical burns

Respiratory tract damage

Burns complicated by fractures or soft tissue injury

Burns complicated by concurrent illness, such as obesity, diabetes, epilepsy, or cardiac or renal disease

Assessment

Obtain a history of burn injury including general health and child's age, time of injury, nature of the burning agent, duration of contact, location of wounds, whether the injury occurred in an enclosed area, presence of respiratory involvement, and any associated injury (e.g., irritated or injured eyes, nasopharynx for erythema or edema, bruises, fractures, internal injuries) or condition.

Perform physical assessment (e.g., level of consciousness [LOC], vital signs, weight status, pain),

Assess for estimated distribution of burn injury based on the percentage of BSA involved (see Fig. 1.37). The extent and depth of the burn, the causative agent, the body area involved, the patient's age, concomitant injuries, and illness determine the severity of the injury.

Observe for depth of burn injury with associated clinical manifestations (Figs. 1.38 and 1.39) on the estimation of burn distribution, classification of burn depth, and clinical manifestations in children. A burn is a three-dimensional wound that is assessed in relation to the depth of injury described as superficial (epidural injury only), partial-thickness (epidermal and varying degrees of the dermal layer) full-thickness (entire epidermis and dermis and subcutaneous tissue that may extend to underlying structures [e.g., muscle, fascia, and bone]). Because the skin of infants is so thin, they are likely to sustain deeper injuries compared to older children.

Assist with diagnostic procedures and tests depends on the causative agent, depth, and extent of injury and complications (e.g., blood count, urinalysis, wound cultures).

The Child with Attention Deficit Hyperactivity Disorder

Attention deficit hyperactivity disorder (ADHD)—An illness consisting of developmentally inappropriate degrees of inattention, impulsivity, and hyperactivity.

Assessment

Perform a comprehensive age-appropriate physical assessment including vision and hearing screening, and a detailed neurologic examination.

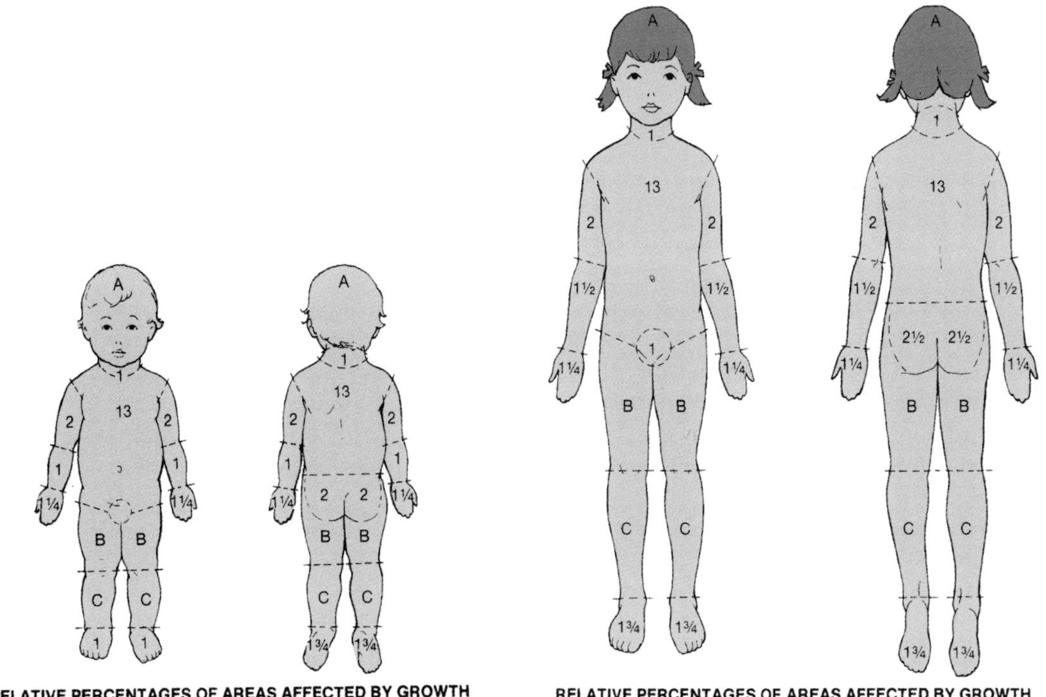

RELATIVE PERCENTAGES OF AREAS AFFECTED BY GROWTH

AREA	BIRTH	AGE 1 YR	AGE 5 YR
A = ½ of head	9½	8½	6½
B = ½ of one thigh	2¾	3¼	4
C = ½ of one leg	2½	2½	2¾

A

RELATIVE PERCENTAGES OF AREAS AFFECTED BY GROWTH

AREA	AGE 10 YR	AGE 15 YR	ADULT
A = ½ of head	5½	4½	3½
B = ½ of one thigh	4½	4½	4¾
C = ½ of one leg	3	3¼	3½

B

FIG. **1.38** Estimation of distribution of burns in children. (A) Children from birth to age 5 years. (B) Older children.

Skin layers	Burn type	Degree	Wound Appearance	Wound Sensation	Course of Healing
Epidermis Sweat duct Capillary	Partial-Thickness Burn	1st Degree	Epidermis remains intact and without blisters Erythema; skin blanches with pressure	Painful	Discomfort lasts 48–72 h. Desquamation occurs in 3–7 days.
Sebaceous gland Nerve endings **Dermis** Hair follicle	Partial-Thickness Burn	2nd Degree	Wet, shiny, weeping surface Blisters Wound blanches with pressure	Painful Very sensitive to touch, air currents	Superficial partial-thickness burn heals in <21 days. Deep partial-thickness burn requires >21 days for healing. Healing rates vary with burn depth and presence or absence of infection.
Sweat gland Fat Blood vessels	Full-Thickness Burn	3rd Degree	Color variable (i.e., deep red, white, black, brown) Surface dry Thrombosed vessels visible No blanching	Insensate (↓ pinprick sensation)	Autografting is required for healing.
Bone	Full-Thickness Burn	4th Degree	Color variable Charring visible in deepest areas Extremity movement limited	Insensate	Amputation of extremities is likely. Autografting is required for healing.

FIG. **1.39** Classification of burn depth according to depth of injury. (From Black, J. M. [2009]. *Medicalsurgical nursing: Clinical management for positive outcomes.* Philadelphia: Saunders.)

Perform a developmental assessment.

Obtain a detailed family and behavioral history including the following:

- History of excessive fussiness and irritability as an infant and toddler
- History of destructive or aggressive behavior as a small child
- History of disciplinary problems in early childhood
- Some evidence suggests that one parent may have had similar problems as a child; therefore, a history of the parents' childhoods is imperative.
- Note if other children in the family have been diagnosed with ADHD or have behaviors consistent with ADHD.
- Inquire about family daily routines, including mealtimes and time set aside for schoolwork and play time (to determine if the environment is a potential cause for distractions related to learning).

Observe for clinical manifestations associated with the ADHD three subtypes.

Inattentive type: six or more symptoms of inattention (e.g., distracted easily, trouble concentrating on a task, poor organizational skills, processing information slowly, difficulty following directions, losing items needed to complete a task, and other symptoms) but fewer than six symptoms of hyperactivity-impulsivity that persisted for at least 6 months to a degree that is inconsistent with developmental level and negatively impacts directly on social and academic/occupational activities.[h]

Hyperactive-impulsive type: six or more symptoms of hyperactivity-impulsivity (e.g., squirming and fidgeting, talking constantly, impatient, interrupting, difficulty sitting still, difficulty engaging in quiet activities, and other symptoms) but fewer than six symptoms of inattention that persisted at least 6 months to a degree that is inconsistent with developmental level and negatively impacts directly on social and academic/occupational activities.[h]

Combined type: six or more symptoms of inattention and six or more symptoms of hyperactivity-impulsivity that have persisted for at least 6 months to a degree that is inconsistent with developmental level and negatively impacts directly on social and academic/occupational activities.[h] Most children and adolescents with ADHD have the combined type. For older children and adults (age 17 or older) at least five symptoms are required for a diagnosis of each subtype.

Assist with diagnostic tests (e.g., electroencephalogram [EEG], blood lead levels, and thyroid levels to rule out potential organic causes, lead poisoning; neurologic evaluation; hearing and vision screening, psychometric testing). The Diagnostic and Statistical Manual of Mental Disorders (DSM-5) is used across United States to diagnose children and adults with ADHD, as it includes diagnostic evaluation of behavior.

The Child with Poisoning

Assessment—The Child with Toxic Ingestion, Inhalation, or Absorption of injurious agents

Poisoning—The condition or physical state produced when a substance is applied to body surfaces, ingested, injected, inhaled, or absorbed and subsequently causes structural damage or disturbance of function

Assessment

Perform a physical assessment including vital signs, mental status (e.g., state of consciousness, neurological signs), respiratory and circulatory signs and symptoms.

Obtain a detailed history regarding what, when, and how much of a toxic substance has entered the body and if possible obtain evidence of ingestion, inhalation, or absorption of toxic substances (e.g., pills, containers, plants).

Observe for clinical manifestations characteristic of specific poison and treatment (see Box 1.34 on selected poisonings in children).

Assist with diagnostic tests (e.g., blood levels of toxins with each toxic ingestion, inhalation, and absorption diagnosed individually).

The Child with Lead Poisoning

Lead poisoning (plumbism)—Acute or chronic ingestion or inhalation of lead-containing substances, resulting in physical and mental dysfunction

Assessment

Perform a physical assessment.

Obtain a history of possible sources of lead in the child's environment (see Box 1.35 sources of lead). Lead does cross the placenta and can be harmful to the unborn child, therefore it is important to assess the pregnant mother for any lead exposure (pica or any of the listed sources of lead).

Observe for clinical manifestations of lead poisoning (see Fig. 1.40 on the main effects of lead on body systems).

Assist with diagnostic procedures and tests (e.g., the blood-lead level is the gold-standard for assessing the risk of harm,[i] erythrocyte-protoporphyrin level, bone

[h] Substance Abuse and Mental Health Services Administrational DSM-5 changes: Implications for child's serious emotional disturbance [Internet] (2016). Rockville (MD).

[i] Markowitz M. Lead poisoning: an update. *Pediatr Rev.* 2021;42(6):302–315.

BOX 1.34 Selected Poisonings in Children

Corrosives (Strong Acids or Alkalis)

Drain, toilet, and oven cleaners
Electric dishwasher detergent (liquid because of its higher pH, is more hazardous than granular)
Mildew remover
Batteries
Clinitest tablets
Denture cleaners
Bleach

Clinical Manifestations

Severe burning pain in the mouth, throat, and stomach
White, swollen mucous membranes; edema of the lips, tongue, and pharynx (respiratory obstruction)
Coughing, hemoptysis
Drooling and inability to clear secretions
Signs of shock
Anxiety and agitation

Comments

Household bleach is a frequently ingested corrosive but rarely causes serious damage.
Liquid corrosives are easily ingested and cause more damage than granular or solid preparations. Liquids may also be aspirated, causing upper airway injury.
Solid products tend to stick to and burn tissues, causing localized damage.

Treatment

Inducing emesis is contraindicated (vomiting redamages the mucosa).
Contact the PCC immediately. If the PCC or medical advice and treatment are not immediately available, it may be appropriate to dilute corrosive with water or milk (usually ≤120 mL [4 oz]).
Do not neutralize. Neutralization can cause an exothermic reaction (which produces heat and causes increased symptoms or produces a thermal burn in addition to a chemical burn).
Maintain patent airway as needed.
Administer analgesics.
Give oral fluids when tolerated.
Esophageal stricture may require repeated dilations or surgery.

Hydrocarbons

Gasoline
Kerosene
Lamp oil
Mineral seal oil (found in furniture polish)
Lighter fluid
Turpentine
Paint thinner and remover (some types)

Clinical Manifestations

Gagging, choking, and coughing
Burning throat and stomach
Nausea
Vomiting
Alterations in sensorium, such as lethargy
Weakness
Respiratory symptoms of pulmonary involvement
- Tachypnea
- Cyanosis
- Retractions
- Grunting

Comments

Immediate danger is aspiration (even small amounts can cause bronchitis and chemical pneumonia).
Gasoline, kerosene, lighter fluid, mineral seal oil, and turpentine cause severe pneumonia.

Treatment

Inducing emesis is generally contraindicated.
Gastric decontamination and emptying are questionable even when the hydrocarbon contains a heavy metal or pesticide; if gastric lavage must be performed, a cuffed endotracheal tube should be in place before lavage because of a high risk of aspiration.
Symptomatic treatment of chemical pneumonia includes high humidity, oxygen, hydration, and acetaminophen.

Acetaminophen

Clinical Manifestations

Occurs in four stages post ingestion:
0–24 h
- Nausea
- Vomiting
- Sweating
- Pallor

24–72 h
- Patient improves
- May have right upper quadrant abdominal pain

72–96 h
- Pain in right upper quadrant
- Jaundice
- Vomiting
- Confusion
- Stupor
- Coagulation abnormalities
- Sometimes renal failure, pancreatitis

More than 5 days
- Resolution of hepatoxicity or progress to multiple organ failure
- May be fatal

Comments

This is the most common accidental drug poisoning in children.
Toxicity occurs from acute ingestion. Toxic dose is 150 mg/kg or greater in children.

Treatment

Antidote *N*-acetylcysteine (Mucomyst) is equally effective given intravenously or orally. When given orally may first be diluted in fruit juice or soda because of the antidote's offensive odor. An antiemetic may be given if vomiting occurs.
Given as 1 loading dose followed by 17 additional doses in different dosages. IV administration is given as a continuous infusion.

Aspirin (Acetylsalicylic Acid)

Clinical Manifestations

Acute poisoning (early symptoms):
- Nausea

Continued

BOX 1.34 Selected Poisonings in Children—cont'd

Hyperventilation
Vomiting
Tinnitus
Acute poisoning (later symptoms):
Hyperactivity
Fever
Confusion
Seizures
Renal failure
Respiratory failure
Chronic poisoning:
Same as listed above but with subtle onset and nonspecific symptoms (often mistaken for viral illness)
Bleeding tendencies

Comments

May be caused by acute ingestion (severe toxicity occurs with 300–500 mg/kg).
May be caused by chronic ingestion (i.e., >100 mg/kg/day for ≥2 days); can be more serious than acute ingestion.
Time to peak serum salicylate level can vary with enteric aspirin or the presence of concretions (bezoars).

Treatment

Hospitalization is necessary for severe toxicity.
Activated charcoal is given as soon as possible (unless contraindicated by altered mental status). If bowel sounds are present, may be repeated every 4 h until charcoal appears in the stool.
Lavage will not remove concretions of ASA.
Sodium bicarbonate transfusions are used to correct metabolic acidosis, and urinary alkalinization may be effective in enhancing elimination; hypokalemia may interfere with achieving urinary alkalinization.
Be aware of the risk of fluid overload and pulmonary edema.
Use external cooling for hyperpyrexia.
Administer anticonvulsants if seizures are present.
Provide oxygen and ventilation for respiratory depression.
Administer vitamin K for bleeding.
In severe cases, hemodialysis (not peritoneal dialysis) is used.

Iron

Mineral supplements or vitamins containing iron

Clinical Manifestations

Occurs in five stages (may have a significant variation in symptoms and their progression):
Within 6 h (if the child does not develop gastrointestinal symptoms in 6 h, toxicity is unlikely)
Vomiting
Hematemesis
Diarrhea
Hematochezia (bloody stools)
Abdominal pain
Severe toxicity may have tachypnea, tachycardia, hypotension, coma
Latency period—up to 24 h of apparent improvement
12–24 h
Metabolic acidosis
Fever
Hyperglycemia
Bleeding
Seizures
Shock
Death (may occur)
2–5 days
Jaundice
Liver failure
Hypoglycemia
Coma
2–5 weeks
Pyloric stenosis or duodenal obstruction may occur secondary to scarring.

Comments

Factors related to the frequency of iron poisoning include:
Widespread availability
Packaging of large quantities in individual containers
Lack of parental awareness of iron toxicity
Resemblance of iron tablets to candy (e.g., M&Ms)
Toxic dose is based on the amount of elemental iron ingested. Common preparations include ferrous sulfate (20% elemental iron), ferrous gluconate (12%), and ferrous fumarate (33%). Ingestions of 20 to 60 mg/kg are considered mildly to moderately toxic, and >60 mg/kg is severely toxic and may be fatal.

Treatment

Hospitalization is required when more than mild gastroenteritis is present.
Use whole bowel irrigation if radiopaque tablets are visible on abdominal x-ray; may need to be given via nasogastric tube.
Emesis empties the stomach more effectively than lavage.
Activated charcoal does not absorb iron.
Chelation therapy with deferoxamine should be used in severe intoxication (may turn urine red to orange).
If IV deferoxamine is given too rapidly, hypotension, facial flushing, rash, urticaria, tachycardia, and shock may occur; stop the infusion, maintain the IV line with normal saline, and notify the practitioner immediately.

Plants

Clinical Manifestations

Depends on the type of plant ingested.
May cause local irritation of the oropharynx and the entire gastrointestinal tract.
May cause respiratory, renal, and central nervous system symptoms.
Topical contact with plants can cause dermatitis.

Comments

Plants are some of the most frequently ingested substances.
They rarely cause serious problems, although some plant ingestions can be fatal.
Plants can also cause choking and allergic reactions.

Treatment

Wash from skin or eyes.
Provide supportive care as needed.

BOX 1.35 | Sources of Lead

Lead-based paint in deteriorating condition
Lead solder
Lead crystal
Battery casings
Lead fishing sinkers
Lead curtain weights
Lead bullets
Some of these may contain lead:
- Ceramic ware
- Water
- Pottery
- Pewter
- Dyes
- Industrial factories
- Vinyl miniblinds
- Playground equipment
- Collectible toys
- Some imported toys or children's metal jewelry
- Artists' paints
- Pool cue chalk

Occupations and hobbies involving lead:
- Battery and aircraft manufacturing
- Lead smelting
- Brass foundry work
- Radiator repair
- Construction work
- Furniture refinishing
- Bridge repair work
- Painting contracting
- Mining
- Ceramics work
- Stained-glass making
- Jewelry making

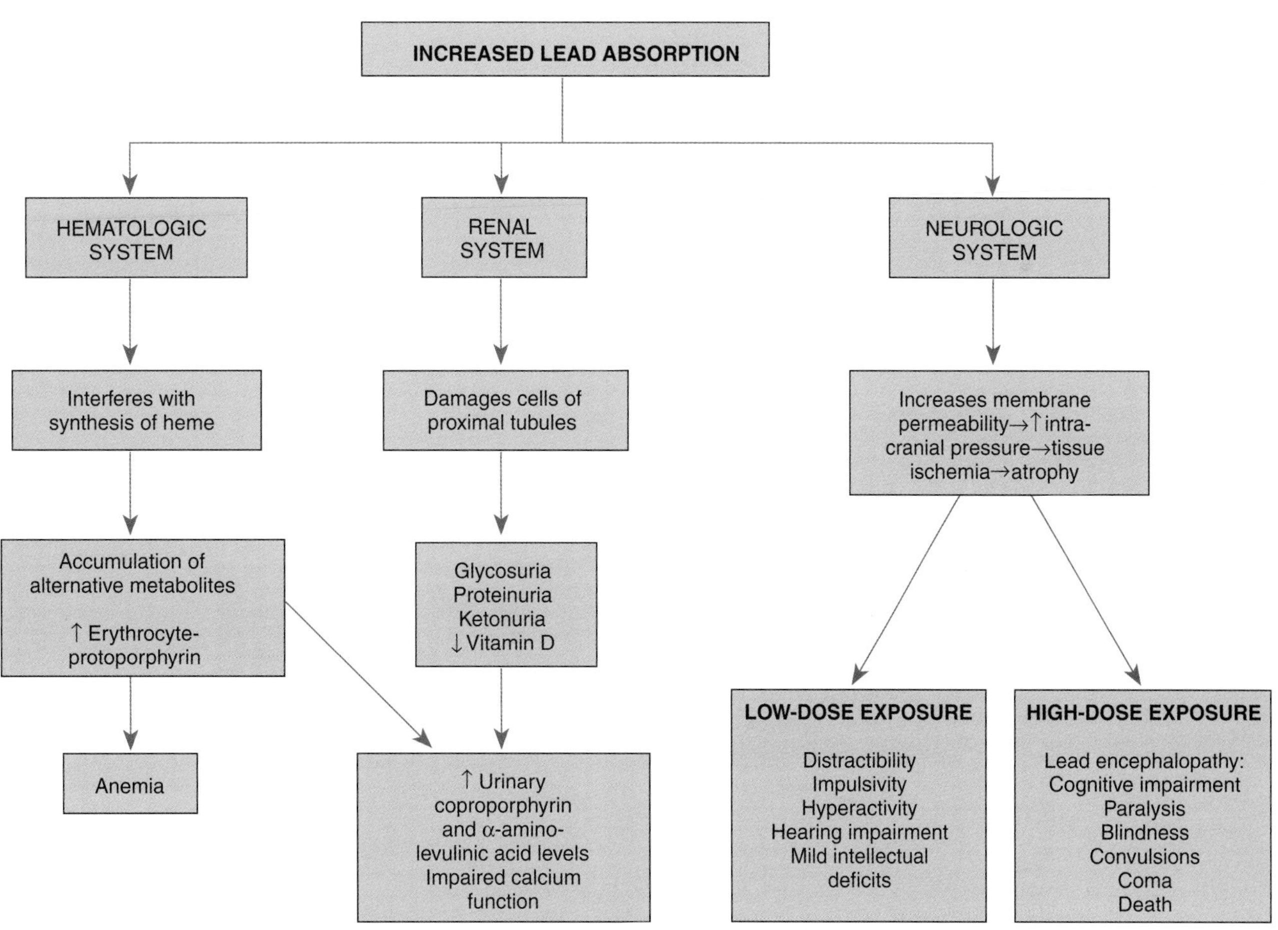

FIG. **1.40** Main effects of lead on body systems. (Added from Essentials 11th ed, Chapter 13. p. 386, Fig. 13.7.)

radiography, urinalysis and CBC and differential, and lead mobilization test). Newer laboratory methods, such as inductively coupled plasma mass spectrometry enable the measurement of nomograms/deciliter amounts of lead in plasma.[i]

The Child with a Communicable Disease

Communicable disease—An illness caused by a specific infectious agent or its toxic products through a direct or indirect mode of transmission of that agent from a reservoir

Assessment and recognition of communicable diseases—a child with a communicable disease

Obtain detailed history including recent exposure to known communicable disease, the occurrence of initial symptoms, immunization history

Perform physical exam—nurse must be familiar with the infectious agent and recognize the communicable disease immediately and institute appropriate preventive and supportive interventions (see Figs. 1.41–1.45 of communicable diseases)

Observe the clinical manifestations of the communicable disease and institution of treatment (see Table 1.16 on communicable diseases of childhood describes the more common communicable diseases of childhood, clinical manifestations, therapeutic management, and nursing care management).

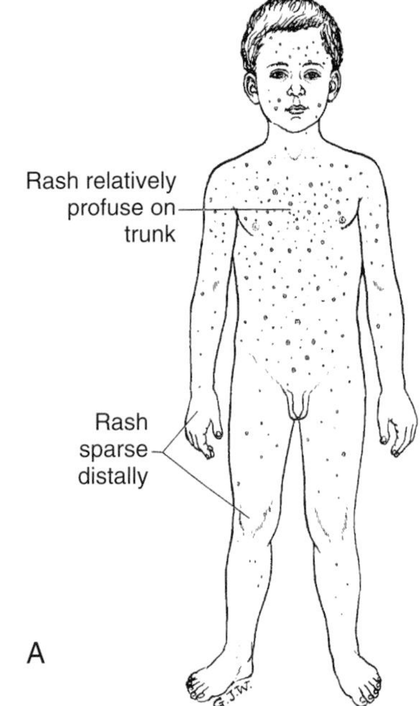

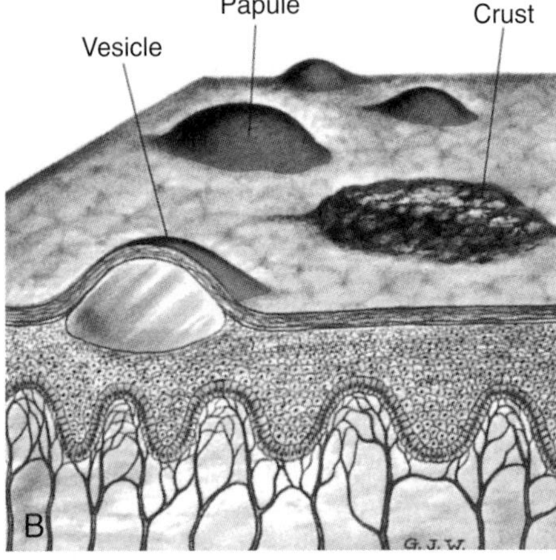

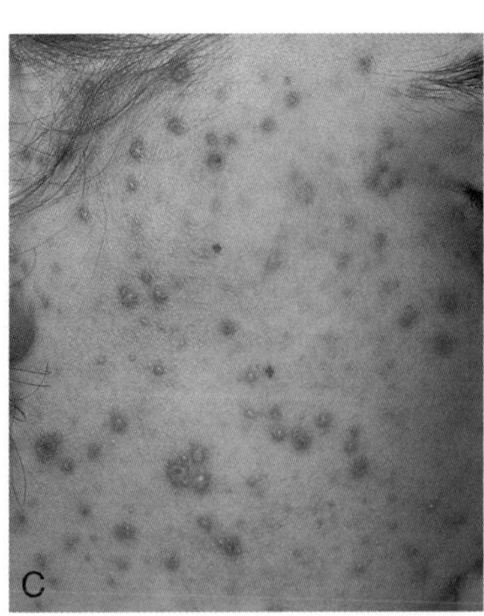

FIG. **1.41** Chickenpox (varicella). (A) Progression of disease. (B) Simultaneous stages of lesions. (C) Clinical view. (C, From Habif TP. Clinical Dermatology: A Color Guide to Diagnosis and Therapy. 6th ed. St. Louis, MO: Mosby; 2016.)

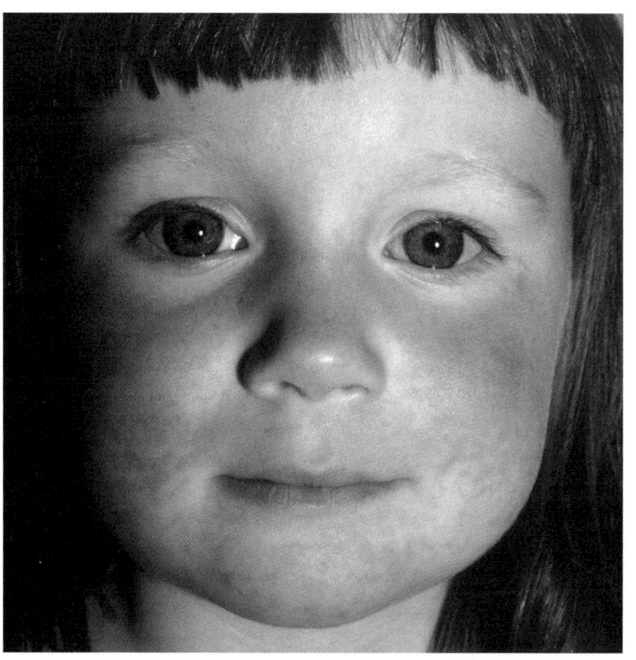

FIG. **1.42** Erythema infectiosum (fifth disease). (From Habif TP. Clinical Dermatology: A Color Guide to Diagnosis and Therapy. [6th ed.]. St. Louis, MO: Mosby; 2016.)

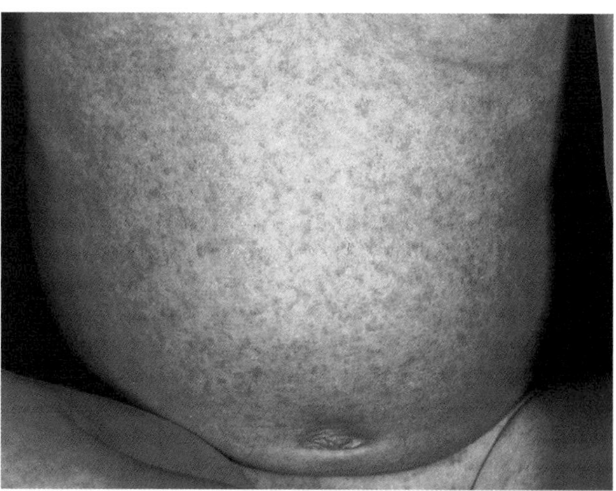

FIG. **1.43** Exanthem subitum (roseola infantum). (From Habif TP. Clinical Dermatology: A Color Guide to Diagnosis and Therapy. [6th ed.]. St. Louis, MO: Mosby; 2016.)

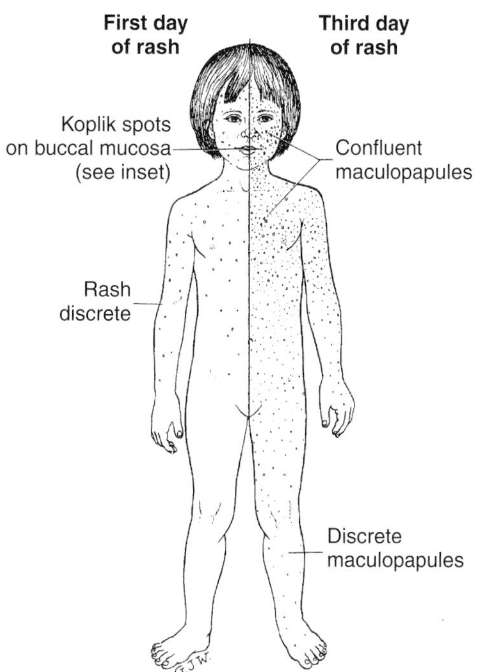

FIG. **1.44** Measles (rubeola). Progression of disease.

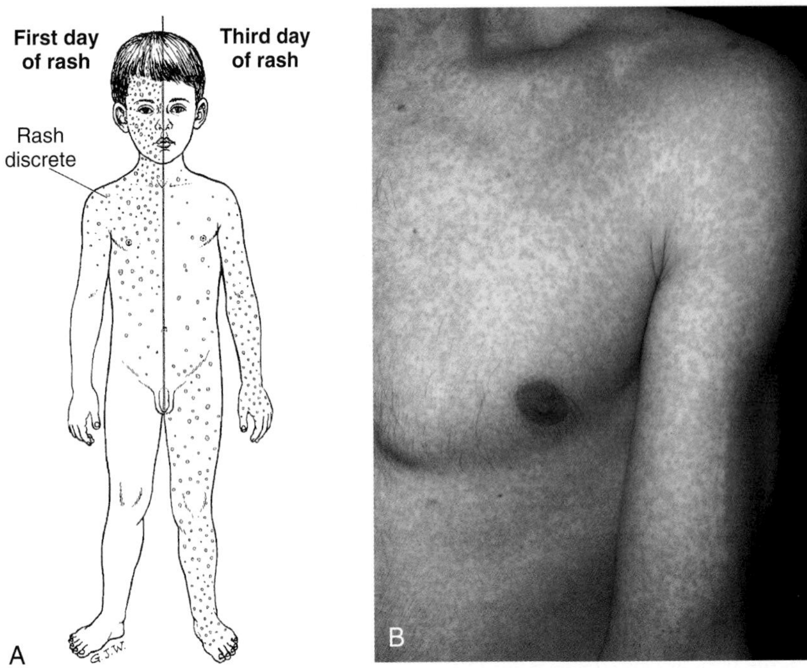

FIG. **1.45** (A) Rubella (German measles). (B) Progression of rash.

Family Assessment

Obtain detailed history. Family assessment involves both the structure and function and is an important component of the history-taking process

Family structure—The composition of the family (who usually lives in the home) consists of individuals, each with a socially recognize status and position, who interact with one another on a regular, recurring basis in socially sanctioned ways

Family function—refers to the interaction of family members, especially the quality of those relationships and interactions.

In its broadest sense, "family" refers to all those individuals who are significant to the nuclear unit, including relatives, friends, and social groups (e.g., the school and church). The nurse elicits information on family structure and function by interviewing family members regarding family characteristics, activities, and cultural and religious traditions that provide insight into family dynamics and relationships.

Initiating a Comprehensive Family Assessment

See Box 1.36 for a family assessment interview.

Nutritional Assessment

A nutritional assessment is an essential component of a nutritional assessment. Its purpose is to evaluate the child's nutritional status—the condition of health as it relates to the state of balance between nutrient intake and nutrient expenditure or need. A thorough nutritional assessment includes information about dietary intake, clinical assessment of nutritional status, anthropometric measures, sociodemographic data, and biochemical status.

Dietary History

Information about dietary intake usually begins with a dietary history and may be coupled with a detailed account of actual food intake using a daily food diary. The nurse should analyze the daily food diary for variety and amounts of foods as suggested in MyPlate.gov (see Fig. 1.46 on MyPlate) which describes the five food groups forming the foundation for a healthy diet. It is important for nurses to focus on preventive strategies, such as referring parents and parents-to-be to MyPlate Kids'Place,

TABLE 1.16 Communicable Diseases of Childhood

Disease	Clinical Manifestations	Therapeutic Management and Complications	Nursing Care Management
Chickenpox (Varicella) (Fig. 1.41)			
Agents—Varicella-zoster virus (VZV) **Source**—Primary secretions of respiratory tract of infected persons; to a lesser degree, skin lesions (scabs not infectious) **Transmissions**—Direct contact, droplet (airborne) spread, and contaminated objects **Incubation period**—2–3 weeks, usually 14–16 days **Period of communicability**—Probably 1 day before eruption of lesions (prodromal period) to 6 days after first crop of vesicles when crusts have formed	**Prodromal stage**—Slight fever, malaise, and anorexia for first 24 h; rash highly pruritic; begins as macule, rapidly progresses to papule and then vesicle (surrounded by erythematous base; becomes umbilicated and cloudy; breaks easily and forms crusts); all three stages (papule, vesicle, crust) present in varying degrees at one time **Distribution**—Centripetal, spreading to face and proximal extremities but sparse on distal limbs and less on areas not exposed to heat (i.e., from clothing or sun) **Constitutional signs and symptoms**—Elevated temperature from lymphadenopathy, irritability from pruritus	**Specific**—Antiviral agent acyclovir (Zovirax); varicella-zoster immune globulin or intravenous immunoglobulin (IVIG) after exposure in high-risk children **Supportive**—Diphenhydramine hydrochloride or antihistamines to relieve itching; skin care to prevent secondary bacterial infection **Complications**—Secondary bacterial infections (abscesses, cellulitis, necrotizing fasciitis, pneumonia, sepsis) Encephalitis Varicella pneumonia (rare in healthy children) Hemorrhagic varicella (tiny hemorrhages in vesicles and numerous petechiae in skin) Chronic or transient thrombocytopenia **Preventive**—Childhood immunization	Maintain Standard, Airborne, and Contact Precautions if hospitalized until all lesions are crusted; for immunized child with mild breakthrough varicella, isolate until no new lesions are seen. Keep child in home away from susceptible individuals until vesicles have dried (usually 1 wk after onset of disease) and isolate high-risk children from infected children. Administer skin care: give bath and change clothes and linens daily; administer topical calamine lotion; keep child's fingernails short and clean; apply mittens if child scratches. Keep child cool (may decrease number of lesions). Lessen pruritus; keep child occupied. Remove loose crusts that rub and irritate skin. Teach child to apply pressure to pruritic area rather than scratching it. Avoid use of aspirin (possible association with Reye syndrome).
Diphtheria			
Agent—*Corynebacterium diphtheriae* **Source**—Discharges from mucous membranes of nose and nasopharynx, skin, and other lesions of infected person **Transmission**—Direct contact with infected person, a carrier, or contaminated articles **Incubation period**—Usually 2–5 days, possibly longer **Period of communicability**—Variable; until virulent bacilli are no longer present (identified by three negative cultures); usually 2 weeks but as long as 4 weeks	Vary according to anatomic location of pseudomembrane **Nasal**—Resembles common cold, serosanguineous mucopurulent nasal discharge without constitutional symptoms; may have frank epistaxis **Tonsillar-pharyngeal**—Malaise; anorexia; sore throat; low-grade fever; pulse increased above expected for temperature within 24 h; smooth, adherent, white or gray membrane; lymphadenitis possibly pronounced ("bull's neck"); in severe cases, toxemia, septic shock, and death within 6–10 days **Laryngeal**—Fever, hoarseness, cough, with or without previous signs listed; potential airway obstruction; apprehensive; dyspneic retractions; cyanosis	Equine antitoxin (usually intravenously); preceded by skin or conjunctival test to rule out sensitivity to horse serum Antibiotics (penicillin G procaine or erythromycin) in addition to equine antitoxin Complete bed rest (prevention of myocarditis) Tracheostomy for airway obstruction Treatment of infected contacts and carriers **Complications**—Toxic cardiomyopathy (week 2–3) Toxic neuropathy **Preventive**—Childhood immunization	Follow Standard and Droplet Precautions until two cultures are negative for *C. diphtheriae;* use Contact Precautions with cutaneous manifestations. Administer antibiotics in timely manner. Participate in sensitivity testing; have epinephrine available. Administer complete care to maintain bed rest. Use suctioning as needed. Observe respiration for signs of obstruction. Administer humidified oxygen as prescribed.

Continued

TABLE 1.16 Communicable Diseases of Childhood—cont'd

Disease	Clinical Manifestations	Therapeutic Management and Complications	Nursing Care Management
Erythema Infectiosum (Fifth Disease) (Fig. 1.42)			
Agent—Human parvovirus B19 **Source**—Infected persons, mainly school-age children **Transmission**—Respiratory secretions and blood, blood products **Incubation period**—4 to 14 days; may be as long as 21 days **Period of communicability**—Uncertain but before onset of symptoms in children with aplastic crisis	Rash appears in three stages: **I**—Erythema on face, chiefly on cheeks ("slapped face" appearance); disappears by 1–4 days **II**—About 1 day after rash appears on face, maculopapular red spots appear, symmetrically distributed on upper and lower extremities; rash progresses from proximal to distal surfaces and may last ≥1 week **III**—Rash subsides but reappears if skin is irritated or traumatized (sun, heat, cold, friction) In children with aplastic crisis, rash usually absent and prodromal illness includes fever, myalgia, lethargy, nausea, vomiting, and abdominal pain Child with sickle cell disease may have concurrent vasoocclusive crisis	**Symptomatic and supportive**—Antipyretics, analgesics, antiinflammatory drugs Possible blood transfusion for transient aplastic anemia **Complications**—Self-limited arthritis and arthralgia (arthritis may become chronic); more common in adult women May result in serious complications (anemia, hydrops) or fetal death if mother infected during pregnancy (primarily second trimester) Aplastic crisis in children with hemolytic disease or immunodeficiency Myocarditis (rare)	Isolation of child is not necessary, except hospitalized child (immunosuppressed or with aplastic crises) suspected of parvovirus infection is placed on Droplet Precautions and Standard Precautions. Pregnant women need not be excluded from workplace where parvovirus infection is present; they should not care for patients with aplastic crises. Explain low risk of fetal death to those in contact with affected children; assist with routine fetal ultrasound for detection of fetal hydrops.
Exanthem Subitum (Roseola Infantum) (Fig. 1.43)			
Agent—Human herpesvirus 6 (HHV-6; rarely HHV-7) **Source**—Possibly acquired from saliva of healthy adult person; entry via nasal, buccal, or conjunctival mucosa **Transmission**—Year round; no reported contact with infected individual in most cases (virtually limited to children <3 years but peak age is 6–15 months) **Incubation period**—Usually 5–15 days **Period of communicability**—Unknown	Persistent high fever >39.5°C (103°F) for 3–7 days in child who appears well Precipitous drop in fever to normal with appearance of rash Bulging fontanel **Rash**—Discrete rose-pink macules or maculopapules appearing first on trunk, then spreading to neck, face, and extremities; nonpruritic; fades on pressure; lasts 1–2 days **Associated signs and symptoms**—Cervical and postauricular lymphadenopathy, inflamed pharynx, cough, coryza	Nonspecific Antipyretics to control fever **Complications**—Recurrent febrile seizures (possibly from latent infection of central nervous system that is reactivated by fever) Encephalitis Hepatitis (rare)	**Use Standard Precautions.** Teach parents measures for lowering temperature (antipyretic drugs); ensure adequate parental understanding of specific antipyretic dosage to prevent accidental overdose. If child is prone to seizures, discuss appropriate precautions and possibility of recurrent febrile seizures.

TABLE 1.16 Communicable Diseases of Childhood—cont'd

Disease	Clinical Manifestations	Therapeutic Management and Complications	Nursing Care Management
Mumps			
Agent—Paramyxovirus **Source**—Saliva of infected persons **Transmission**—Direct contact with or droplet spread from an infected person **Incubation period**—14 to 21 days **Period of communicability**—Most communicable immediately before and after swelling begins	**Prodromal stage**—Fever, headache, malaise, and anorexia for 24 h, followed by "earache" that is aggravated by chewing **Parotitis**—By third day, parotid gland(s) (either unilateral or bilateral) enlarges and reaches maximum size in 1–3 days; accompanied by pain and tenderness; other exocrine glands (submandibular) may also be swollen	**Preventive**—Childhood immunization **Symptomatic and supportive**—Analgesics for pain and antipyretics for fever Intravenous fluid if needed for child who refuses to drink or vomits because of meningoencephalitis **Complications**—Sensorineural deafness Postinfectious encephalitis Myocarditis Arthritis Hepatitis Epididymo-orchitis Oophoritis Pancreatitis Sterility (extremely rare in adult men) Meningitis	Maintain isolation during period of communicability; institute Droplet and Contact Precautions during hospitalization. Encourage rest and decreased activity during prodromal phase until swelling subsides. Give analgesics for pain; if child is unwilling to swallow pills or tablets medication, use elixir form. Encourage fluids and soft, bland foods; avoid foods requiring chewing. Apply hot or cold compresses to neck, whichever is more comforting. To relieve orchitis, provide hot or cold packs for analgesia and scrotal elevation.
Measles (Rubeola) (Fig. 1.44)			
Agent—Virus **Source**—Respiratory tract secretions, blood, and urine of infected person **Transmission**—Usually by direct contact with droplets of infected person; primarily in the winter **Incubation period**—10 to 20 days **Period of communicability**—From 4 days before to 5 days after rash appears but mainly during prodromal (catarrhal) stage	**Prodromal (catarrhal) stage**—Fever and malaise, followed in 24 h by coryza, cough, conjunctivitis, Koplik spots (small, irregular red spots with a minute, bluish-white center first seen on buccal mucosa opposite molars 2 days before rash); symptoms gradually increasing in severity until second day after rash appears, when they begin to subside **Rash**—Appears 3–4 days after onset of prodromal stage; begins as erythematous maculopapular eruption on face and gradually spreads downward; more severe in earlier sites (appears confluent) and less intense in later sites (appears discrete); after 3–4 days assumes brownish appearance, and fine desquamation occurs over area of extensive involvement **Constitutional signs and symptoms**—Anorexia, abdominal pain, malaise, generalized lymphadenopathy	**Preventive**—Childhood immunization **Supportive**—Bed rest during febrile period; antipyretics Antibiotics to prevent secondary bacterial infection in high-risk children **Complications**—Otitis media Pneumonia (bacterial) Obstructive laryngitis and laryngotracheitis Encephalitis (rare but has high mortality) **Treatment**—Administer vitamin A (World Health Organization recommendation) for children with acute illness: 200,000 IU for children ≥12 months old; 100,000 IU for children 6–11 months old; 50,000 IU for infants <6 months old (Kimberlin et al., 2018	Maintain isolation until fifth day of rash; if child is hospitalized, institute Airborne Precautions. Encourage rest during prodromal stage; provide quiet activity. **Fever**—Instruct parents to administer antipyretics; avoid chilling; if child is prone to seizures, institute appropriate precautions. **Eye care**—Dim lights if photophobia present; clean eyelids with warm saline solution to remove secretions or crusts; keep child from rubbing eyes. **Coryza, cough**—Use cool-mist vaporizer; protect skin around nares with layer of petrolatum; encourage fluids and soft, bland foods. **Skin care**—Keep skin clean; use tepid baths as necessary.

Continued

TABLE 1.16 Communicable Diseases of Childhood—cont'd

Disease	Clinical Manifestations	Therapeutic Management and Complications	Nursing Care Management
Pertussis (Whooping Cough)			
Agent—*Bordetella pertussis* **Source**—Discharge from respiratory tract of infected persons **Transmission**—Direct contact or droplet spread from infected person; indirect contact with freshly contaminated articles **Incubation period**—6 to 20 days; usually 7–10 days **Period of communicability**—Greatest during catarrhal stage before onset of paroxysms	**Catarrhal stage**—Begins with symptoms of upper respiratory tract infection, such as coryza, sneezing, lacrimation, cough, and low-grade fever; symptoms continue for 1–2 weeks, when dry, hacking cough becomes more severe **Paroxysmal stage**—Cough most common at night, consists of short, rapid coughs followed by sudden inspiration associated with a high-pitched crowing sound or "whoop"; during paroxysms, cheeks become flushed or cyanotic, eyes bulge, and tongue protrudes; paroxysm may continue until thick mucus plug is dislodged; vomiting frequently follows attack; stage generally lasts 4–6 weeks, followed by convalescent stage Infants <6 months old may not have characteristic whoop cough but have difficulty maintaining adequate oxygenation with amount of secretions, frequent vomiting of mucus and formula or breast milk Pertussis may occur in adolescents and adults with varying manifestations; cough and whoop may be absent, but as many as 50% of adolescents may have a cough for up to 10 weeks (Kimberlin et al., 2018) Additional symptoms in adolescents include difficulty breathing and posttussive vomiting (*see also* the Pertussis section earlier in the chapter for discussion of pertussis immunization schedule.)	**Preventive**—Immunization; current belief is that childhood immunizations for pertussis do not confer lifelong immunity to adolescents and adults, so a pertussis booster is recommended for adolescents (see the Pertussis section earlier in the chapter) Antimicrobial therapy (e.g., erythromycin, clarithromycin, azithromycin) **Supportive**—Hospitalization sometimes required for infants, children who are dehydrated, or those who have complications Increased oxygen intake and humidity Adequate fluids Intensive care and mechanical ventilation if needed for infants <6 months old **Complications**—Pneumonia (usual cause of death in younger children) Atelectasis Otitis media Seizures Hemorrhage (scleral, conjunctival, epistaxis; pulmonary hemorrhage in neonate) Weight loss and dehydration Hernias (umbilical and inguinal) Prolapsed rectum Complications reported among adolescents include syncope, sleep disturbance, rib fractures, incontinence, and pneumonia (Kimberlin et al., 2018)	Maintain isolation during catarrhal stage; if child is hospitalized, institute Standard and Droplet Precautions. Obtain nasopharyngeal culture for diagnosis. Encourage oral fluids; offer small amount of fluids frequently. Ensure adequate oxygenation during paroxysms; position infant on side to decrease chance of aspiration with vomiting. Provide humidified oxygen; suction as needed to prevent choking on secretions. Observe for signs of airway obstruction (e.g., increased restlessness, apprehension, retractions, cyanosis). Encourage compliance with antibiotic therapy for household contacts. Encourage adolescents to obtain pertussis booster (Tdap) (see Pertussis section earlier in the chapter). Use Standard and Droplet Precautions in health care workers exposed to children with persistent cough and high suspicion of pertussis.

TABLE 1.16 Communicable Diseases of Childhood—cont'd

Disease	Clinical Manifestations	Therapeutic Management and Complications	Nursing Care Management
Poliomyelitis			
Agent—Enteroviruses, three types: type 1, most frequent cause of paralysis, both epidemic and endemic; type 2, least frequently associated with paralysis; type 3, second most frequently associated with paralysis **Source**—Feces and oropharyngeal secretions of infected persons, especially young children **Transmission**—Direct contact with persons with apparent or inapparent active infection; spread via fecal-oral and pharyngeal-oropharyngeal routes; vaccine-acquired paralytic polio may occur as a result of the live oral polio vaccination (no longer available in the United States) **Incubation period**—Usually 7–14 days, with range of 5–35 days **Period of communicability**—Not exactly known; virus present in throat and feces shortly after infection and persists for about 1 week in throat and 4–6 weeks in feces	May be manifested in three different forms: **Abortive or inapparent**—Fever, uneasiness, sore throat, headache, anorexia, vomiting, abdominal pain; lasts a few hours to a few days **Nonparalytic**—Same manifestations as abortive but more severe, with pain and stiffness in neck, back, and legs **Paralytic**—Initial course similar to nonparalytic type, followed by recovery and then signs of central nervous system paralysis	**Preventive**—Childhood immunization **Supportive**—Complete bed rest during acute phase Mechanical or assisted ventilation in case of respiratory paralysis Physical therapy for muscles after acute stage **Complications**—Permanent paralysis Respiratory arrest Hypertension Kidney stones from demineralization of bone during prolonged immobility	**Institute Contact Precautions**. Administer mild sedatives as necessary to relieve anxiety and promote rest. Participate in physical therapy procedures (use of moist hot packs and range-of-motion exercises). Position child to maintain body alignment and prevent contractures or skin breakdown; use footboard or appropriate orthoses to prevent foot drop; use pressure mattress for prolonged immobility. Encourage child to perform activities of daily living to capability; promote early ambulation with assistive devices; administer analgesics for maximum comfort during physical activity; give high-protein diet and bowel management for prolonged immobility. Observe for respiratory paralysis (e.g., difficulty talking, ineffective cough, inability to hold breath, shallow and rapid respirations); report such signs and symptoms to practitioner.

Continued

ASSESSMENT 1

TABLE 1.16 Communicable Diseases of Childhood—cont'd

Disease	Clinical Manifestations	Therapeutic Management and Complications	Nursing Care Management
Rubella (German Measles) (Fig. 1.45)			
Agent—Rubella virus **Source**—Primarily nasopharyngeal secretions of person with apparent or inapparent infection; virus also present in blood, stool, and urine **Incubation period**—14 to 21 days **Period of communicability**—7 days before to about 5 days after appearance of rash **Constitutional signs and symptoms**—Occasionally low-grade fever, headache, malaise, and lymphadenopathy	**Prodromal stage**—Absent in children, present in adults and adolescents; consists of low-grade fever, headache, malaise, anorexia, mild conjunctivitis, coryza, sore throat, cough, and lymphadenopathy; lasts 1–5 days, subsides 1 day after appearance of rash **Rash**—First appears on face and rapidly spreads downward to neck, arms, trunk, and legs; by end of first day, body is covered with discrete, pinkish-red maculopapular exanthema; disappears in same order as it began and is usually gone by third day	**Preventive**—Childhood immunization No treatment necessary other than antipyretics for low-grade fever and analgesics for discomfort **Complications**—Rare (arthritis, encephalitis, or purpura); most benign of all childhood communicable diseases; greatest danger is teratogenic effect on fetus	Institute Droplet Precautions. Reassure parents of benign nature of illness in affected child. Use comfort measures as necessary. Avoid contact with pregnant women. Monitor rubella titer in pregnant adolescent.
Scarlet Fever			
Agent—Group A beta-hemolytic streptococci **Source**—Usually from nasopharyngeal secretions of infected persons and carriers **Transmission**—Direct contact with infected person or droplet spread; indirectly by contact with contaminated articles or ingestion of contaminated milk or other food **Incubation period**—2 to 5 days, with range of 1–7 days **Period of communicability**—During incubation period and clinical illness, approximately 10 days; during first 2 weeks of carrier phase, although may persist for months	**Prodromal stage**—Abrupt high fever, pulse increased out of proportion to fever, vomiting, headache, chills, malaise, abdominal pain, halitosis **Enanthema**—Tonsils enlarged, edematous, reddened, and covered with patches of exudates; in severe cases appearance resembles membrane seen in diphtheria; pharynx is edematous and beefy red; during first 1–2 days tongue is coated and papillae become red and swollen (white strawberry tongue); by fourth or fifth day white coat sloughs off, leaving prominent papillae (red strawberry tongue); palate is covered with erythematous punctate lesions **Exanthema**—Rash appears within 12 h after prodromal signs; red pinhead-sized punctate lesions rapidly become generalized but are absent on face, which becomes flushed with striking circumoral pallor; rash more intense in folds of joints; by end of first week desquamation begins (fine, sandpaper-like on torso; sheetlike sloughing on palms and soles), which may be complete by 3 weeks or longer	Full course of penicillin (or erythromycin in penicillin-sensitive children) or oral cephalosporin Antibiotic therapy for newly diagnosed carriers (nose or throat cultures positive for streptococci) **Supportive**—Rest during febrile phase, analgesics for sore throat; antipruritics for rash if bothersome **Complications**—Peritonsillar and retropharyngeal abscess Sinusitis Otitis media Acute glomerulonephritis Acute rheumatic fever Polyarthritis (uncommon)	Institute Standard and Droplet Precautions until 24 h after initiation of treatment. Ensure compliance with oral antibiotic therapy; intramuscular benzathine penicillin G [Bicillin] may be given. Encourage rest during febrile phase; provide quiet activity during convalescent period. Relieve discomfort of sore throat with analgesics, gargles, lozenges, antiseptic throat sprays, and inhalation of cool mist. Encourage fluids during febrile phase; avoid irritating liquids (e.g., citrus juices) or rough foods (e.g., chips); when child can eat, begin with soft diet. Advise parents to consult practitioner if fever persists after beginning therapy. Discuss procedures for preventing spread of infection—discard toothbrush; avoid sharing drinking and eating utensils.

Tdap, Tetanus, diphtheria toxoids, and acellular pertussis vaccine.

BOX 1.36 Family Assessment Interview

General Guidelines

Schedule the interview with the family at a time that is most convenient for all parties; include as many family members as possible; clearly state the purpose of the interview.

Begin the interview by asking each person's name and their relationships to one another.

Restate the purpose of the interview and the objective.

Keep the initial conversation general to put members at ease and to learn the "big picture" of the family.

Identify major concerns and reflect these back to the family to be certain that all parties receive the same message.

Terminate the interview with a summary of what was discussed and a plan for additional sessions, if needed.

Structural Assessment Areas

Family Composition

Immediate members of the household (names, ages, and relationships)

Significant extended family members

Previous marriages, separations, death of spouses, or divorces

Home and Community Environment

Type of dwelling, number of rooms, occupants

Sleeping arrangements

Number of floors, accessibility of stairs and elevators

Adequacy of utilities

Safety features (fire escape, smoke and carbon monoxide detectors, guardrails on windows, use of car restraint)

Environmental hazards (e.g., chipped paint, poor sanitation, pollution, heavy street traffic)

Availability and location of health care facilities, schools, play areas

Relationship with neighbors

Recent crises or changes in home

Child's reaction and adjustment to recent stresses

Occupation and Education of Family Members

Types of employment

Work schedules

Work satisfaction

Exposure to environmental or industrial hazards

Sources of income and adequacy

Effect of illness on financial status

Highest degree or grade level attained

Cultural and Religious Traditions

Religious beliefs and practices

Cultural and ethnic beliefs and practices

Language spoken in home

Assessment questions include the following:

- Does the family identify with a religious or ethnic group? Are both parents from that group?
- How is religious or ethnic background part of family life?
- What special religious or cultural traditions are practiced in the home (e.g., food choices and preparation)?
- Where were family members born, and how long have they lived in this country?
- What language does the family speak most frequently?
- Do they speak and understand English?
- What do they believe causes health or illness?
- What religious or ethnic beliefs influence the family's perception of illness and its treatment?
- What methods are used to prevent or treat illness?
- How does the family know when a health problem needs medical attention?
- Who does the family contact when a member is ill?
- Does the family rely on cultural or religious healers or remedies? If so, ask them to describe the type of healer or remedy.
- Who does the family go to for support (clergy, medical healer, relatives)?
- Does the family experience discrimination because of their race, beliefs, or practices? Ask them to describe.

Functional Assessment Areas

Family Interactions and Roles

Interactions refer to ways in which family members relate to each other. The chief concern is the amount of intimacy and closeness among the members, especially spouses.

Roles refer to behaviors of people as they assume a different status or position.

Observations include the following:

- Family members' responses to each other (cordial, hostile, cool, loving, patient, short tempered)
- Obvious roles of leadership versus submission
- Support and attention shown to various members

Assessment questions include the following:

- What activities does the family perform together?
- Who do family members talk to when something is bothering them?
- What are family members' household chores?
- Who usually oversees what is happening with the children, such as at school or health care?
- How easy or difficult is it for the family to change or accept new responsibilities for household tasks?

Power, Decision Making, and Problem Solving

Power refers to an individual member's control over others in the family; it is manifested through family decision making and problem solving.

The chief concern is the clarity of boundaries of power between parents and children.

One method of assessment involves offering a hypothetical conflict or problem, such as a child failing school, and asking the family how they would handle this situation.

Assessment questions include the following:

- Who usually makes the decisions in the family?
- If one parent makes a decision, can the child appeal to the other parent to change it?
- What input do children have in making decisions or discussing rules?
- Who makes and enforces the rules?
- What happens when a rule is broken?

Communication

Communication is concerned with clarity and directness of communication patterns.

Further assessment includes periodically asking family members if they understood what was just said and to repeat the message.

Observations include the following:

- Who speaks to whom

Continued

BOX 1.36 Family Assessment Interview—cont'd

- If one person speaks for another or interrupts
- If members appear uninterested when certain individuals speak
- If there is agreement between verbal and nonverbal messages

Assessment questions include the following:

- How often do family members wait until others are through talking before "having their say?"
- Do parents or older siblings tend to lecture and preach?
- Do parents tend to "talk down" to the children?

Expression of Feelings and Individuality

Expressions are concerned with personal space and freedom to grow, with limits and structure needed for guidance.

Observing patterns of communication offers clues to how freely feelings are expressed.

Assessment questions include the following:

- Is it okay for family members to get angry or sad?
- Who gets angry most of the time? What do they do?
- If someone is upset, how do other family members try to comfort this person?
- Who comforts specific family members?
- When someone wants to do something, such as try out for a new sport or get a job, what is the family's response (offer assistance, discouragement, or no advice)?

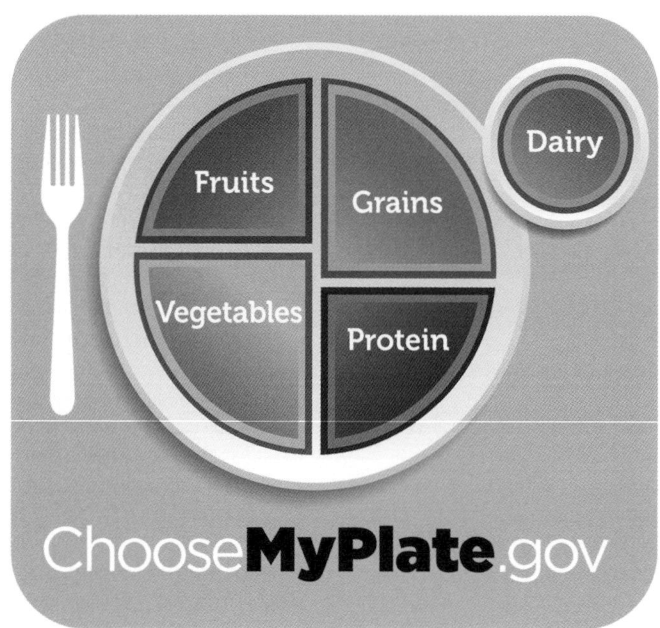

FIG. **1.46** MyPlate advocates building a healthy plate by making half of one's plate fruits and vegetables and the other half grains and lean protein. Avoiding oversized portions, making half of grains whole grains and drinking fat-free or low-fat (1%) milk are among the recommendations for a healthy diet. Logo of Choosemyplate.gov with a plate divided into four parts labeled as fruits, grains, vegetables, and protein and a glass labeled as dairy. (From US Department of Agriculture, Center for Nutrition Policy and Promotion. [2015]. MyPlate.http://www.ChooseMyPlate.gov. Adapted from Essentials 11th ed. Chapter 4, p. 71, Fig 4.4.)

which provide resources to help families build healthy meals and encourage physical activity among their children with the aim of decreasing the incidence of childhood obesity

Observe clinical manifestations of nutritional assessment that is correlated with possible nutritional deficiency or excess (see Table 1.17 on Nutrition-Focused Clinical Findings)

Assist with diagnostic procedures and tests: A number of biochemical tests are available for studying nutritional status. Common laboratory procedures related to nutritional status include measurement of CBCD, transferrin, albumin or pre-albumin, creatinine, and nitrogen and at times fasting serum glucose, lipids, and liver function tests are included.

Sleep Assessment

A sleep history is usually taken during the general health history. However, when sleep problems are identified, a more detailed history of sleep and awake patterns is needed for planning appropriate interventions. Sleep problems tend to be common in young children. The following information includes a summary of a comprehensive sleep history.

TABLE 1.17 Nutrition-Focused Clinical Findings

Normal Findings	Abnormal Findings	Possible Nutrient Deficiencies
Physical Growth		
Normal weight gain and linear growth for age and gender	Weight loss, poor weight gain, linear growth failure	Protein, fat, calories, zinc, iodine, sodium, other essential nutrients
Normal skeletal development without obvious deformity	Kyphosis, genu varum (bowing of extremities) or genu valgum (knock knees), rickets, history of nontraumatic fractures	Calcium, vitamin D, phosphorus
Skin		
Smooth, slightly dry to touch, elastic and firm, absence of lesions, uniform color appropriate to genetic background	Dry, rough, scaly	Vitamin A, essential fatty acids
	Dermatitis	Essential fatty acids, zinc, niacin, riboflavin, tryptophan
	Petechiae	Riboflavin, vitamin C
	Delayed wound healing	Vitamin C, zinc
	Scaly dermatitis on exposed surfaces	Riboflavin, vitamin C, zinc, niacin, tryptophan
	Wrinkled, flabby	Niacin
	Crusted lesions around orifices, especially nares	Protein, calories, zinc
	Poor turgor	Water, sodium
	Depigmentation	Protein, calories
	Pallor (anemia)	Iron, folic acid; vitamins B12, C, and E (in premature infants); pyridoxine
Hair		
Lustrous, silky smooth, strong, elastic, distributed symmetrically	Stringy, friable, dull, dry, thin	Protein, calories, zinc, biotin, essential fatty acids
	Alopecia	Protein, calories, zinc, biotin, essential fatty acids, selenium
	Depigmentation	Protein, calories, copper
	Raised areas around hair follicles	Vitamin C
Nails		
Symmetric and smooth	Transverse lines	Protein
	Flaky	Magnesium
	Poorly blanched	Vitamins A and D
	Brittle nails, spooning	Iron
Eyes		
Clear, bright, moist	Dull, dry with Bitot spots (buildup of keratin superficially in the conjunctiva)	Vitamin A
Good night vision	Night blindness	Vitamin A
Conjunctiva—pink, glossy, tolerates light exposure	Burning, itching, photophobia	Riboflavin
Mouth		
Lips—smooth, moist, darker color than skin, absence of lesions	Fissures and inflammation at corners	Riboflavin
	Dry, swollen	Vitamins B6 and B12, iron, folate, riboflavin, niacin
Gums—firm, pink, stippled	Spongy, friable, inflamed, bluish red or black, bleed easily	Vitamin C
Mucous membranes—bright pink, smooth, moist	Stomatitis	Niacin
	Dry mucous membranes	Water, zinc
Tongue—moist pink with slightly rough texture, no lesions, normal taste sensation	Glossitis (swollen, inflamed, smooth, and dark red)	Niacin, riboflavin, folate, vitamins B6 and B12, iron
	Diminished taste sensation	Zinc
Teeth—uniform white color, smooth, intact; normal eruption begins at 4–12 months	Defective enamel	Vitamins A, C, and D; calcium; phosphorus
	Caries	Fluoride, vitamin D
	Delayed dentition	Malnutrition

Adapted from Green Corkins K, Teague EE. Pediatric nutrition assessment: anthropometrics to zinc. *Nutr Clin Prac.* 2017;32(1), 40–51; National Institutes of Health, Office of Dietary Supplements. (n.d.). Vitamin and mineral fact sheets. Retrieved from https://ods.od.nih.gov/factsheets/list-VitaminsMinerals/

Assessment of Sleep Problems During Infancy and Early Childhood

History of a sleep problem in young children include:
Parents and/or child's description of sleep problems.
Inquire about the onset, duration, character, and frequency of sleep problem.
Circumstances surrounding onset (e.g., the birth of a sibling, start of toilet training, death of significant other, move from crib to bed)
Circumstances that aggravate the problem (e.g., overtiredness, family conflict, disrupted routine [visitors])
Remedies used to correct the problem, and results of interventions
Clinical description of typical infant and early childhood sleep problem with associated management (see Table 1.18 on selected disturbances during infancy and early childhood)

TABLE 1.18 Selected Sleep Disturbances During Infancy and Early Childhood

Disorder and Description	Management
Nighttime Feeding	
Child has a prolonged need for middle-of-night bottle-feeding or breastfeeding. Child goes to sleep at breast or with bottle. Awakenings are frequent (may be hourly). Child returns to sleep after feeding; other comfort measures (e.g., rocking or holding) are usually ineffective.	Increase daytime feeding intervals to >4 h (may need to be done gradually). Offer last feeding as late as possible at night; may need to gradually reduce amount of formula or length of breastfeeding. Offer no bottles in bed. Put to bed awake. When child is crying, check at progressively longer intervals each night; reassure child but do not hold, rock, take to parent's bed, or give bottle or pacifier.
Developmental Night Crying	
Child ages 6–12 months with undisturbed nighttime sleep now awakens abruptly; may be accompanied by nightmares.	Reassure parents that this phase is temporary. Enter room immediately to check on child but keep reassurances brief. Avoid feeding, rocking, taking to parent's bed, or any other routine that may initiate trained night crying.
Refusal to Go to Sleep	
Child resists bedtime and comes out of room repeatedly. Nighttime sleep may be continuous, but frequent awakenings and refusal to return to sleep may occur and become a problem if parent allows child to deviate from usual sleep pattern.	Evaluate whether hour of sleep is too early (child may resist sleep if not tired). Assist parents in establishing consistent before-bedtime routine and enforcing consistent limits regarding child's bedtime behavior. If child persists in leaving bedroom, close door for progressively longer periods. Use reward system with child to provide motivation.
Trained Night Crying (Inappropriate Sleep Associations)	
Child typically falls asleep in place other than own bed (e.g., rocking chair, parent's bed) and is brought to own bed while asleep; on awakening, cries until usual routine is instituted (e.g., rocking).	Put child in own bed when awake. If possible, arrange sleeping area separate from other family members. When child is crying, check at progressively longer intervals each night; reassure child but do not resume usual routine.
Nighttime Fears	
Child resists going to bed or wakes during the night because of fears. Child seeks parent's physical presence and falls asleep easily with parent nearby, unless fear is overwhelming.	Evaluate whether hour of sleep is too early (child may fantasize when nothing to do but think in dark room). Calmly reassure frightened child; keeping night-light on may be helpful. Use reward system with child to provide motivation to deal with fears. Avoid patterns that can lead to additional problems (e.g., sleeping with child, taking child to parent's room). If child's fear is overwhelming, consider desensitization (e.g., progressively spending longer time alone; consult professional help for protracted fears). Distinguish between nightmares and sleep terrors (confused partial arousals).

Modified from Ferber R. Behavioral "insomnia" in the child. *Psychiatr Clin North Am.* 10(4):641–653.

Growth Measurements

General Trends in Physical Growth During Childhood

Age	Weight[a]	Height[a]
Infants		
Birth to 6 months	Weekly gain: 140–200 g (5–7 ounces) Birth weight doubles by end of first 4–7 months[b]	Monthly gain: 2.5 cm (1 inch)
6–12 months	Weight gain: 85–140 g (3–5 ounces) Birth weight triples by end of first year[b]	Monthly gain: 1.25 cm (0.5 inch) Birth length increases by approximately 50% by end of first year
Toddlers	Birth weight quadruples by age 2½ years	Height at age 2 years is approximately 50% of eventual adult height Gain during second year: about 12 cm (4.7 inches) Gain during third year: about 6–8 cm (2.4–3.2 inches)
Preschoolers	Yearly gain: 2–3 kg (4.5–6.5 pounds)	Birth length doubles by age 4 years Yearly gain: 5–7.5 cm (2–3 inches)
School-age children	Yearly gain: 2–3 kg (4.5–6.5 pounds)	Yearly gain after age 7 years: 5 cm (2 inches) Birth length triples by about age 13 years
Pubertal Growth Spurt		
Females (10–14 years)	Weight gain: 7–25 kg (15.5–55 pounds) Mean: 17.5 kg (38.5 pounds)	Height gain: 5–25 cm (2–10 inches); approximately 95% of mature height achieved by onset of menarche or skeletal age of 13 years Mean: 20.5 cm (8 inches)
Males (11–16 years)	Weight gain: 7–30 kg (15.5–66 pounds) Mean: 23.7 kg (52.2 pounds)	Height gain: 10–30 cm (4–12 inches); approximately 95% of mature height achieved by skeletal age of 15 years Mean: 27.5 cm (11 inches)

[a]Yearly height and weight gains for each age group represent averaged estimates from a variety of sources.
[b]Jung E, Czajka-Narins DM. Birth weight doubling and tripling times: an updated look at the effects of birth weight, sex, race, and type of feeding. *Am J Clin Nutr*. 1985;42:182–189, has shown the mean doubling time for birth weight to be 4.7 months and mean tripling time to be 14.7 months.

Sequence of Tooth Eruption and Shedding

See Fig. 1.47.

Growth Charts

The Centers for Disease Control and Prevention recommends that the World Health Organization growth standards be used to monitor growth for infants and children between the ages of 0 and 2 years old. Because breastfeeding is the recommended standard for infant feeding, the World Health Organization growth charts are used; they reflect growth patterns among children who were predominately breastfed for at least 4 months and are still breastfeeding at 12 months old. The Centers for Disease Control and Prevention growth charts (www.cdc.gov/growthcharts) are used for children 2 years old and older.

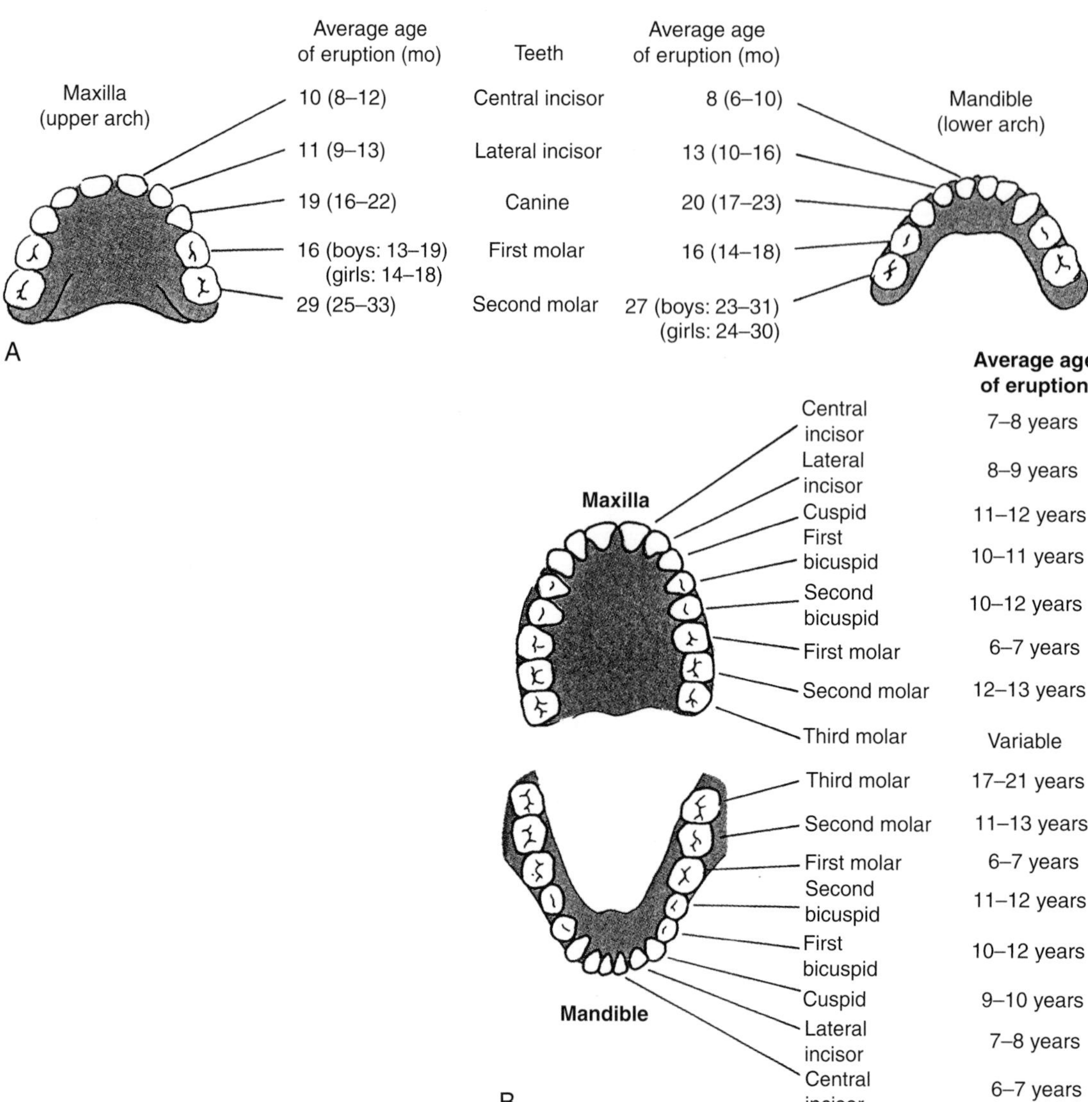

FIG. **1.47** (A) Sequence of eruption of primary teeth. Range represents ± standard deviation, or 67% of subjects studied. (B) Sequence of eruption of secondary teeth. (Data from Dean JA, McDonald RE, Avery DR. McDonald and Avery's Dentistry for the Child and Adolescent. 9th ed. St. Louis: Mosby; 2011.)

Body Mass Index Formula

English Formula

BMI = (Weight in pounds ÷ Height in inches) ÷ Height in inches × 703

Fractions and ounces must be entered as decimal values.[j]

Example: A 33-pound, 4-ounce child is 37⅝ inches tall.

BMI = (33.25 pounds ÷ 37.625 * inches) ÷ 37.625 inches×703 = 16.5

Fraction	Ounces	Decimal	Fraction	Ounces	Decimal
⅛	2	0.125	⅝	10	0.625
¼	4	0.25	¾	12	0.75
⅜	6	0.375	⅞	14	0.875
½	8	0.5			

Metric Formula

BMI = (Weight in kilograms ÷ Height in meters) ÷ Height in meters

or

BMI = (Weight in kilograms ÷ Height in cm) ÷ Height in cm × 10,000

Example: A 16.9-kg child is 105.2 cm tall.

BMI = (16.9 ÷ 105.2cm) ÷ 105.2cm × 10,000 = 15.3

Sexual Maturation

The Tanner stages[k] were developed by Dr. J.M. Tanner and colleagues. Tanner stages describe the stages of pubertal growth and are numbered from stage 1 (immature) to stage 5 (mature) for both males and females. In females, the Tanner stages describe pubertal development based on breast size and the shape and distribution of pubic hair. In males, the Tanner stages describe pubertal development based on the size and shape of the penis and scrotum and the shape and distribution of pubic hair.[l] The usual sequence of appearance of maturational changes is presented in Box 1.37 on maturational changes.

[k] Kuczmarski RJ, Ogden CL, Grummer-Strawn LM, et al. *CDC Growth Charts: United States. Advance Data From Vital and Health Statistics, No 314.* Hyattsville, MD: NCHS; June 8, 2000.

[l] Tanner JM. *Growth of Adolescents.* Oxford: Blackwell Scientific Publications; 1962.

Sexual Maturation in Males

The first pubescent changes in boys are testicular enlargement accompanied by thinning, reddening, and increased looseness of the scrotum (Fig. 1.48). These events usually occur between 9½ and 14 years.

Sexual Maturation in Females

In most girls, the initial indication of puberty is the appearance of breast buds, an event known as thelarche which occurs between 8 and 13 years old (Fig. 1.49). This is followed in approximately 2 to 6 months by growth of pubic hair on the mons pubis, known as adrenarche (Fig. 1.50).

Assessment of Development

The use of a developmental screening test is an essential component of developmental assessment as it quickly and reliably identifies children whose developmental level is below normal for their age and who require further investigation. In the past, the most widely used developmental screening test for young children was the Denver Developmental Screening Test II (DDST II) which was rerevised from the DDST-R. The American Academy of Neurology and the Child Neurology Society state that research has found that the DDST II is insensitive and lacks specificity, and neither the American Academy of Neurology nor the Child Neurology Society recommends the use of the Denver II for primary care developmental screening.

There are several parent-report developmental screening tools that are reliable and valid. One of the most common high-quality screening tool is the Ages and Stages Questionnaires (ASQ) which include 19 age-specific surveys that ask parents or other caregivers about developmental skills common in daily life for children 1 month to 5½ years old (see Box 1.38). Children whose development appears to fall significantly below the results of other children their age are flagged for further evaluation. The ASQ is a universal 10 to 15 minutes screening tool that can be used in pediatric clinics to identify children at risk for developmental delays. Also, a comprehensive list of child developmental assessment tools has been developed by the National Early Childhood Technical Assistance Center as part of its cooperative agreement with the US Office of Special Education Programs.[m]

[m] Early Childhood Technical Assistance Center (2020). Screening tools for children birth to age five years with potential for remote administration. Obtained February 2022 from https://ectacenter.org/topics/earlyid/remote asp.; Ringwalt S. *Developmental Screening and Assessment Instruments With an Emphasis on Social and Emotional Development for Young Children Ages Birth Through Five.* Chapel Hill: The University of North Carolina, FPG Child Development Institute, National Early Childhood Technical Assistance Center; 2008.

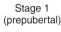

BOX 1.37 Usual Sequence of Maturational Changes

Girls

Breast changes
Rapid increase in height and weight
Growth of pubic hair
Appearance of axillary hair
Menstruation (usually begins 2 years after first signs)
Abrupt deceleration of linear growth

Boys

Enlargement of testicles
Growth of pubic hair, axillary hair, hair on upper lip, hair on face and elsewhere on body (facial hair usually appears about 2 years after appearance of pubic hair)
Rapid increase in height
Changes in the larynx and consequently the voice (usually take place along with growth of the penis)
Nocturnal emissions
Abrupt deceleration of linear growth

Stage 1 (prepubertal)

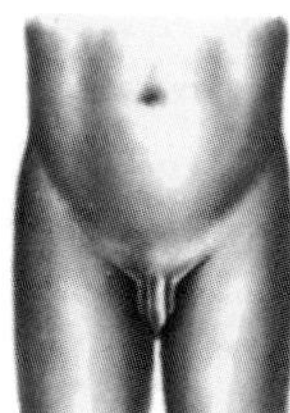

No pubic hair; essentially the same as during childhood; no distinction between hair on pubis and over the abdomen

Stage 2 (pubertal)

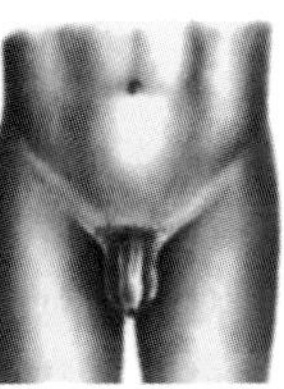

Initial enlargement of scrotum and testes; reddening and textural changes of scrotal skin; sparse growth of long, straight, downy, and slightly pigmented hair at base of penis

Stage 3

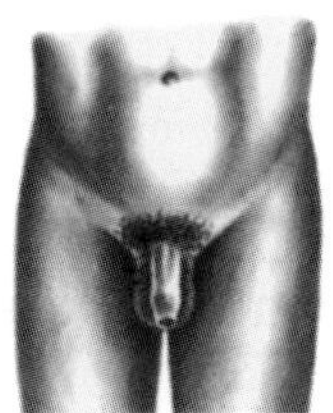

Initial enlargement of penis, mainly in length; testes and scrotum further enlarged; hair darker, coarser, and curly and spread sparsely over entire pubis

Stage 4

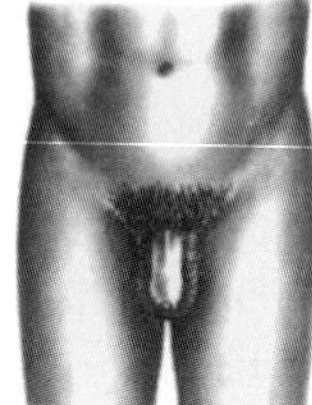

Increased size of penis with growth in diameter and development of glans; glans larger and broader; scrotum darker; pubic hair more abundant with curling but restricted to pubic area

Stage 5

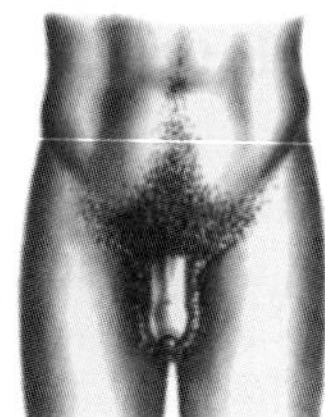

Testes, scrotum, and penis adult in size and shape; hair adult in quantity and type with spread to inner surface of thighs

FIG. **1.48** Developmental stages of secondary sex characteristics and genital development in boys. (Modified from Marshall WA, Tanner JM. Variations in the pattern of pubertal changes in boys, Arch Dis Child. 1970;45[239]:13–23; Tanner JM. Growth at Adolescence. Springfield, Ill: CC Thomas; 1995.)

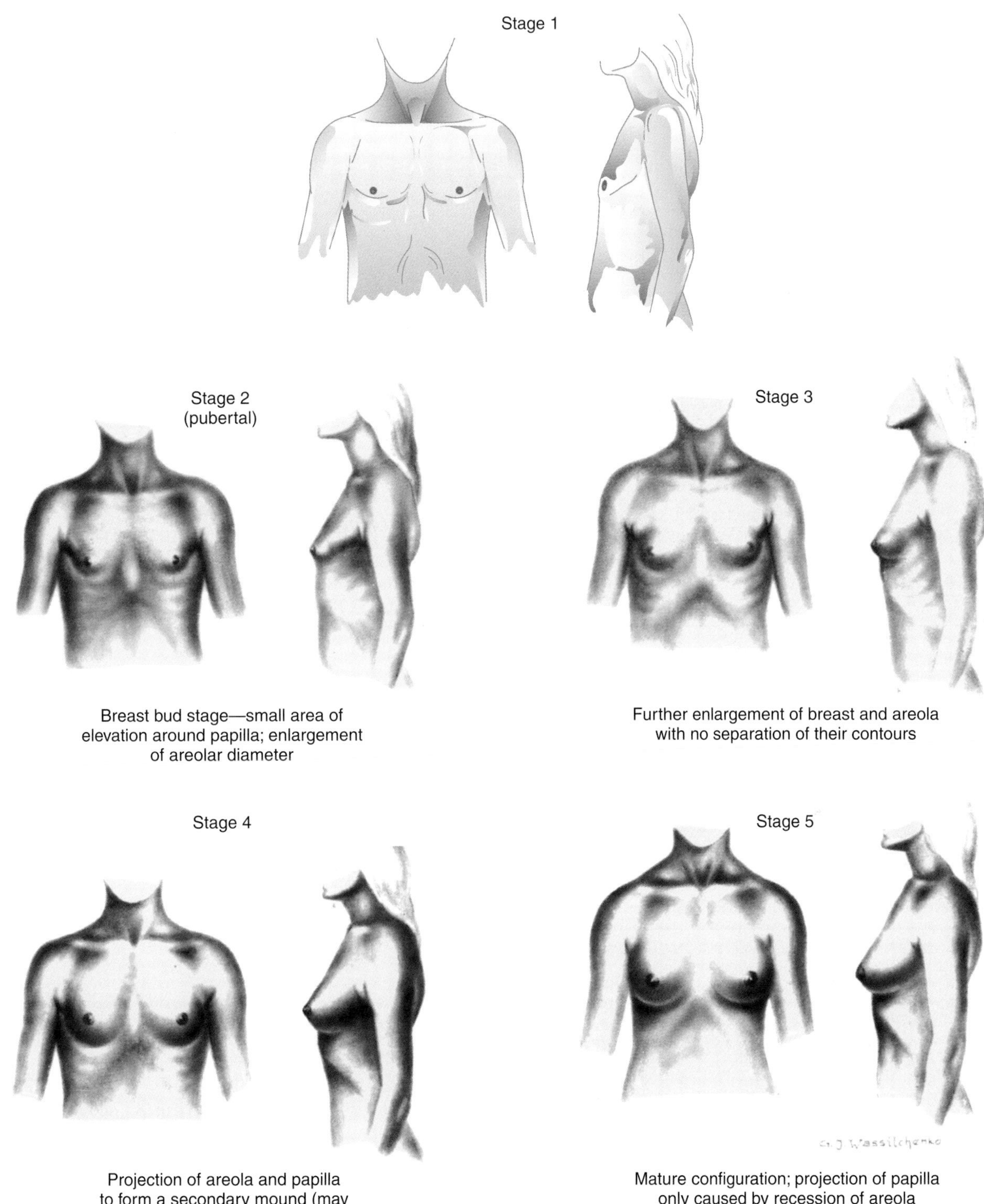

Stage 1
Stage 2
(pubertal)
Stage 3
Breast bud stage—small area of elevation around papilla; enlargement of areolar diameter
Further enlargement of breast and areola with no separation of their contours
Stage 4
Stage 5
Projection of areola and papilla to form a secondary mound (may not occur in all girls)
Mature configuration; projection of papilla only caused by recession of areola into general contour

FIG. **1.49** Development of the breast in girls. Stage 1 (prepubertal-elevation of papilla only) is not shown. (Modified from Marshall WA, Tanner JM. Variations in pattern of pubertal changes in girls, Arch Dis Child. 1969;44[235]:291–303; Tanner JM. Growth at Adolescence. Springfield, IL: CC Thomas; 1995.)

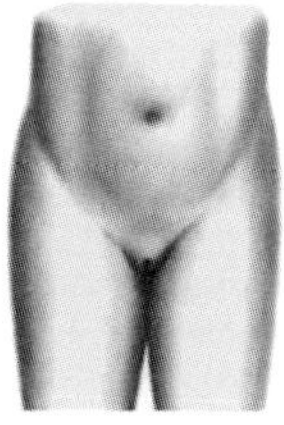

Stage 1
(prepubertal)
No pubic hair; essentially the same as during childhood; no distinction between hair on pubis and over the abdomen

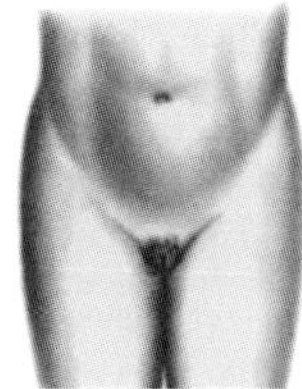

Stage 2
Sparse growth of long, straight, downy, and slightly pigmented hair extending along labia; between stages 2 and 3 begins to appear on pubis

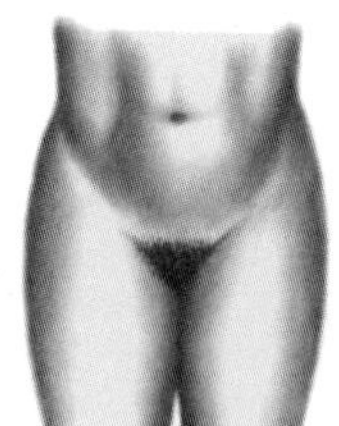

Stage 3
Hair darker, coarser, and curly and spread sparsely over entire pubis in the typical female triangle

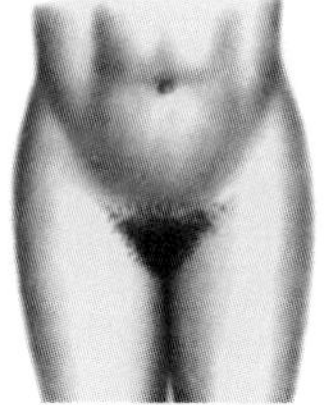

Stage 4
Pubic hair denser, curled, and adult in distribution but less abundant and restricted to the pubic area

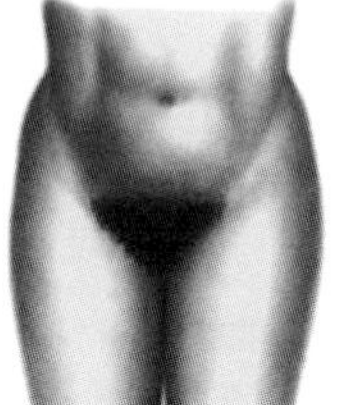

Stage 5
Hair adult in quantity, type, and pattern with spread to inner aspect of thighs

FIG. **1.50** Growth of pubic hair in girls. (Modified from Marshall WA, Tanner JM. Variations in the pattern of pubertal changes in girls, Arch Dis Child. 1969;44[235]:291–303; Tanner JM. Growth at Adolescence. Springfield, Ill: CC Thomas; 1955.)

BOX 1.38 Ages and Stages Questionnaires[a]

Type of screening: Developmental (ASQ-3) and social-emotional (ASQ:SE)
Age range: 1–66 months old for ASQ-3, 3–66 months old for ASQ:SE
Number of questionnaires: 21 for ASQ-3, 8 for ASQ:SE
Number of items: About 30 per questionnaire
Online components: Data management and questionnaire completion
Reading level of items: fourth to sixth grade
Who completes it: Parents
Time to complete: 10–15 min
Who scores it: Professionals
Time to score: 2–3 min
Languages: English and Spanish (for other languages, visit https://agesandstages.com)

[a]Information on the Ages & Stages Questionnaires (ASQ) can be found at https://agesandstages.com.

Assessment of Language and Speech

Assessment: Language and speech characteristics development relate to neurologic competence and cognitive development and are environmentally stimulated with the rate of development varying from child to child (e.g., bilingual children, a child attending preschool). The most critical period for speech development occurs during the pre-school years, with progression to the use of structurally complete sentences, grammatical usage, and intelligibility by end of 5 years of age (see major developmental characteristics of Language and Speech).

Major Developmental Characteristics of Language and Speech

Age (year)	Normal Language Development	Normal Speech Development	Intelligibility
1	Says two or three words with meaning	Omits most final and some initial consonants	Usually no more than 25% intelligible to unfamiliar listener
	Imitates sounds of animals	Substitutes consonants *m, w, p, b, k, g, n, t, d,* and *h* for more difficult sounds	Height of unintelligible jargon at age 18 months

Major Developmental Characteristics of Language and Speech—cont'd

Age (year)	Normal Language Development	Normal Speech Development	Intelligibility
2	Uses two- or three-word phrases Has vocabulary of about 300 words Uses "I," "me," and "you"	Uses above consonants with vowels, but inconsistently and with much substitution Omission of final consonants Articulation lags behind vocabulary	At age 2 years, 50% intelligible in context
3	Says four- or five-word sentences Has vocabulary of about 900 words Uses "who," "what," and "where" in asking questions Uses plurals, pronouns, and prepositions	Masters *b, t, d, k,* and *g*; sounds *r* and *l* may still be unclear; omits or substitutes *w* Repetitions and hesitations common	At age 3 years, 75% intelligible
4–5	Has vocabulary of 1500–2100 words Able to use most grammatical forms correctly, such as past tense of verb with "yesterday" Uses complete sentences with nouns, verbs, prepositions, adjectives, adverbs, and conjunctions	Masters *f* and *v*; may still distort *r, l, s, z, sh, ch, y,* and *th* Little or no omission of initial or final consonants	Speech is 100% intelligible, although some sounds are still imperfect
5–6	Has vocabulary of 3000 words Comprehends "if," "because," and "why"	Masters *r, l,* and *th;* may still distort *s, z, sh, ch,* and *j* (usually mastered by age 7½–8 years)	

Assessment of Communication Impairment

Key questions for language disorders

1. How old was your child when he or she spoke his or her first words?
2. How old was your child when he or she began to put words into sentences?
3. Does your child have difficulty learning new vocabulary words?
4. Does your child omit words from sentences (i.e., do sentences sound telegraphic?) or use short or incomplete sentences?
5. Does your child have trouble with grammar, such as using the verbs is, am, are, was, and were?
6. Can your child follow two or three directions given at once?
7. Do you have to repeat directions or questions?
8. Does your child respond appropriately to questions?
9. Does your child ask questions beginning with who, what, where, and why?
10. Does it seem that your child has made little or no progress in speech and language in the last 6 to 12 months?

Key questions for speech impairment

1. Does your child ever stammer or repeat sounds or words?
2. Does your child seem anxious or frustrated when trying to express an idea?
3. Have you noted certain behaviors, such as blinking, jerking the head, or attempting to rephrase thoughts with different words when your child stammers?
4. What do you do when any of these occurs?
5. Does your child omit sounds from words?
6. Does it seem like your child uses *t, d, k,* or *g* in place of most other consonants when speaking?
7. Does your child omit sounds from words or replace the correct consonant with another one (e.g., "rabbit" with "wabbit")?
8. Do you have any difficulty understanding your child's speech?
9. Has anyone else ever remarked about having difficulty understanding your child?
10. Has there been any recent change in the sound of your child's voice?

Clues for Detecting Communication Impairment

Language Disability

Assigning meaning to words
- First words not uttered before the second birthday
  - Vocabulary size is reduced for age or fails to show a steady increase
  - Difficulty in describing characteristics of objects, although may be able to name them
  - Infrequent use of modifier words (adjectives, adverbs)
- Excessive use of jargon past age 18 months

Organizing words into sentences
- First sentences not uttered before the third birthday
  - Short and incomplete sentences
  - Tendency to omit words (articles, prepositions)
  - Misuse of the "be," "do," and "can" verb forms
  - Difficulty understanding and producing questions
- Plateaus at an early developmental level; uses easy speech patterns

Altering word forms
- Omission of endings for plurals and tenses
  - Inappropriate use of plurals and tense endings
- Inaccurate use of possessive words

Speech Impairment

Dysfluency (stuttering)
- Noticeable repetition of sounds, words, or phrases after age 4 years
- Obvious frustration when attempting to communicate
- Demonstration of struggling behavior while talking (head jerks, blinks, retrials, circumlocution)
- Embarrassment about their own speech

Articulation deficiency
- Intelligibility of conversational speech absent by age 3 years
- Omission of consonants at beginning of words by age 3 years and at end of words by age 4 years
- Persisting articulation faults after age 7 years
- Omission of a sound where one should occur
- Distortion of a sound
- Substitution of an incorrect sound for a correct one

Voice disorders
- Deviations in pitch (too high or too low, especially for age and gender); monotone
- Deviations in loudness
- Deviations in quality (hypernasality, hyponasality)

Guidelines for Referral Regarding Communication Impairment

Regardless of age, refer child with signs that suggest hearing impairment for further evaluation

2 years of age
- Failure to speak any meaningful words spontaneously
- Consistent use of gestures rather than vocalizations
- Difficulty in following verbal directions
- Failure to respond consistently to sound

3 years of age
- Speech is largely unintelligible
- Failure to use sentences of three or more words
- Frequent omission of initial consonants
- Use of vowels rather than consonants

5 years of age
- Stutters or has any other type of dysfluency
- Sentence structure noticeably impaired
- Substitutes easily produced sounds for more difficult ones
- Omits word endings (e.g., plurals, tenses of verbs)

School age
- Poor voice quality (monotonous, loud, or barely audible)
- Vocal pitch inappropriate for age and gender
- Any distortions, omissions, or substitutions of sounds after age 7 years
- Connected speech characterized by the use of unusual confusions or reversals

Assessment of Vision

Major Developmental Characteristics of Vision

Birth
- Visual acuity 20/100 to 20/400[n]
- Pupillary and corneal (blink) reflexes present
- Able to fixate on moving object in a range of 45 degrees when held 20 to 25 cm (8 to 10 inches) away
- Cannot integrate head and eye movements well (doll's eye reflex—eyes lag behind if head is rotated to one side)

4 weeks of age
- Can follow in a range of 90 degrees
- Can watch parent intently as he or she speaks to an infant
- Tear glands begin to function
- Visual acuity is hyperoptic because of less spherical eyeball than in adult

6 to 12 weeks of age
- Has peripheral vision to 180 degrees
- Binocular vision begins at age 6 weeks, is well established by age 4 months

- Convergence on near objects begins by age 6 weeks, is well developed by age 3 months
- Doll's eye reflex disappears

12 to 20 weeks of age

- Recognizes feeding bottle
- Able to fixate on a 1.25-cm (0.5-inch) block
- Looks at hand while sitting or lying on back
- Able to accommodate to near objects

20 to 28 weeks of age

- Adjusts posture to see an object
- Able to rescue a dropped toy
- Develops color preference for yellow and red
- Able to discriminate among simple geometric forms
- Prefers more complex visual stimuli
- Develops hand-eye coordination

28 to 44 weeks of age

- Can fixate on very small objects
- Depth perception begins to develop.
- Lack of binocular vision indicates strabismus.

44 to 52 weeks of age

- Visual acuity 20/40 to 20/60
- Visual loss may develop if strabismus is present.
- Can follow rapidly moving objects[o]

Visual Impairment

Visual impairment encompasses both partial visual impairment and severe permanent impairment and is a common problem during childhood that is usually identified through vision screening. The most common type of visual impairment in children is refractive errors. In addition to these eye disorders, other visual problems can be the result of infection and trauma (see Emergency Treatment box)

Special Tests of Visual Acuity and Eye Examination Guidelines

Table 1.19 provides a list of visual screening tests for children and guidelines for referral. The current recommendation by the American Academy of Ophthalmology is for LEA symbols as one of the preferred optotypes for testing preliterate children.[p] Listed below is a detailed procedure to administer both the Snellen (widely used visual test) and the LEA Symbols screening test.

[p] Loh AR, Chiang MF. Pediatric vision screening. *Pediatr Rev.* 2018;39(5):225–234.

TABLE 1.19 Eye Examination Guidelines[a]

Function	Recommended Tests	Referral Criteria	Comments
3–5 Years Old			
Distance visual acuity	Snellen letters Snellen numbers Tumbling E HOTV Picture test: • Allen figures • LEA symbols	1. Less than four of six correct on 20-foot (6-m) line with either eye tested at 10 feet (3 m) monocularly (i.e., <10/20 or 20/40) *or* 2. Two-line difference between eyes, even within passing range (i.e., 10/12.5 and 10/20 or 20/25 and 20/40)	1. Tests are listed in decreasing order of cognitive difficulty; highest test that child is capable of performing should be used; in general, tumbling E or HOTV test should be used for children 3–5 years old and Snellen letters or numbers for children 6 years old and older. 2. Testing distance of 10 feet (3 m) is recommended for all visual acuity tests. 3. Line of figures is preferred over single figures. 4. Nontested eye should be covered by occluder held by examiner or by adhesive occluder patch applied to eye; examiner must ensure that it is not possible to peek with nontested eye.

Continued

TABLE 1.19 Eye Examination Guidelines[a]—cont'd

Function	Recommended Tests	Referral Criteria	Comments
Ocular alignment	Cross cover test at 10 feet (3 m) Random dot E stereo test at 18 inches (40 cm) Simultaneous red reflex test (Bruckner test)	Any eye movement Less than four of six correct Any asymmetry of pupil color, size, brightness	Child must be fixing on a target while cross cover test is performed. Use direct ophthalmoscope to view both red reflexes simultaneously in a darkened room from 2 to 3 feet (0.6–0.9 m) away; detects asymmetric refractive errors as well.
Ocular media clarity (cataracts, tumors, and so on)	Red reflex	White pupil, dark spots, absent reflex	Use direct ophthalmoscope in a darkened room. View eyes separately at 12–18 inches (30–45 cm); white reflex indicates possible retinoblastoma.
6 Years Old and Older			
Distance visual acuity	Snellen letters Snellen numbers Tumbling E HOTV Picture test: • Allen figures • LEA symbols	1. Less than four of six correct on 15-foot (4.5-m) line with either eye tested at 10 feet (3 m) monocularly (i.e., <10/15 or 20/30)*or* 2. Two-line difference between eyes, even within the passing range (i.e., 10/10 and 10/15 or 20/20 and 20/30)	1. Tests are listed in decreasing order of cognitive difficulty; highest test that child is capable of performing should be used; in general, tumbling E or HOTV test should be used for children 3–5 years old and Snellen letters or numbers for children 6 years old and older. 2. Testing distance of 10 feet (3 m) is recommended for all visual acuity tests. 3. Line of figures is preferred over single figures. 4. Nontested eye should be covered by occluder held by examiner or by adhesive occluder patch applied to eye; examiner must ensure that it is not possible to peek with nontested eye.
Ocular alignment	Cross cover test at 10 feet (3 m) Random dot E stereo test at 18 inches (40 cm) Simultaneous red reflex test (Bruckner test)	Any eye movement Less than four of six correct Any asymmetry of pupil color, size, brightness	Child must be fixing on target while cross cover test is performed. Use direct ophthalmoscope to view both red reflexes simultaneously in a darkened room from 2 to 3 feet (0.6–0.9 m) away; detects asymmetric refractive errors as well.
Ocular media clarity (e.g., cataracts, tumors)	Red reflex	White pupil, dark spots, absent reflex	Use direct ophthalmoscope in a darkened room. View eyes separately at 12–18 inches (30–45 cm); white reflex indicates possible retinoblastoma.

[a]Assessing visual acuity (vision screening) is one of the most sensitive techniques for detection of eye abnormalities in children. The American Academy of Pediatrics Section on Ophthalmology, in cooperation with American Association for Pediatric Ophthalmology and Strabismus and American Academy of Ophthalmology, has developed these guidelines to be used by physicians, nurses, educational institutions, public health departments, and other professionals who perform vision evaluation services.
From American Academy of Pediatrics, Committee on Practice and Ambulatory Medicine, Section on Ophthalmology. Eye examination in infants, children, and young adults by pediatricians. *Pediatrics.* 2003;111(4):902–907.

Snellen Screening

The Snellen Screening (Fig. 1.51A and B) is the most widely used technique in clinical practice for measuring visual acuity.[q]

Preparation

1. Hang the Snellen chart (see Fig. 1.51) on a light-colored wall so that the 20- to 30-foot lines are at eye level when children 6 to 12 years old are tested in the standing position.

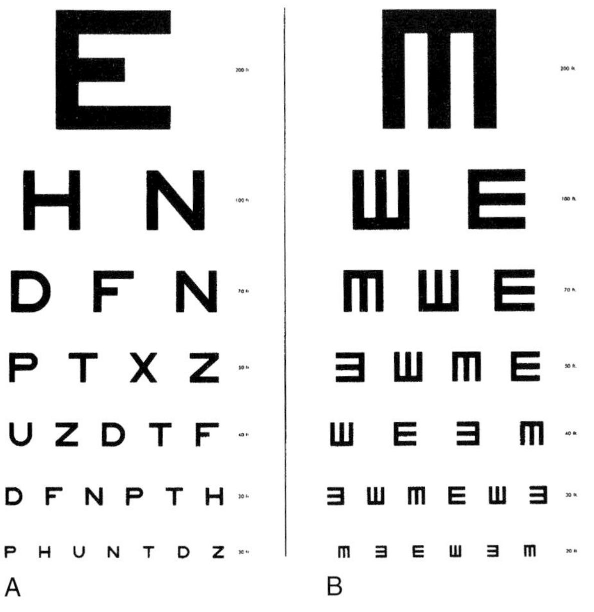

FIG. **1.51** A Snellen chart. (A) Letter (alphabet) chart. (B) Symbol E chart.

2. Secure the chart to the wall with double-stick tape on the back side of all four corners. If the chart must be reversed for use of the letter or E chart, secure it at the top and bottom with tacks. Make sure that the chart does not swing when in place.
3. The illumination intensity on the chart should be 10- to 30-foot candles, without any glare from windows or light fixtures. The illumination should be checked with a light meter.
4. Mark an exact 20-foot distance from the chart. Mark the floor with a piece of tape or "footprints" positioned so that the heels touch the 20-foot line.[r]

[r]Modified from recommendations of *Prevent Blindness America: Guide to testing distance visual acuity,* Schaumburg, Ill, 1995, Prevent Blindness America. Azzam D, Ronquillo Y. Snellen Chart. In: *StatPearls* [Internet]. Treasure Island (FL): StatPearls Publishing; 2022 January (Updated 2021), Available from: https://www.ncbi.nlm.nih.gov/books/NBK558961/; A Tsui E, Patel P. Calculated decisions: visual acuity testing (Snellen Chart). *Emerg Med Pract.* 2020;22(4):CD1–CD2.

Procedure

1. Place the child at the 20-foot mark, with the heel edging the line if the child is standing, or with the back of the chair placed at the marker if the child is seated.
2. If the E chart is used, accustom the child to identifying which direction the legs of the E are pointing. Use a demonstration E card for this purpose.
3. Teach the child to use the occluder to cover one eye. Instruct the child to keep both eyes open during the test. Provide a clean cover card for each child, and discard after use.
4. If the child wears glasses, test only with glasses on.
5. Test both eyes together, then the right eye, then the left eye.
6. Begin with the 40- or 30-foot line, and proceed with test to include the 20-foot line.
7. With a child suspected to have low vision, begin with the 20-foot line and proceed until the child can no longer correctly read three out of four or four out of six symbols on a line.
8. Use covers on the Snellen chart to expose only one symbol or one line at a time. When screening kindergarten-age or older children, expose one line, but a pointer may be used to point to one symbol at a time.

Recording and Referral

1. Record the last line the child read correctly (three out of four or four out of six symbols).
2. Record visual acuity as a fraction. The numerator represents the distance from the chart, and the denominator represents the last line read correctly. For example, 20/30 means that the child read the 30-foot line at a 20-foot distance.
3. Observe the child's eyes during testing, and record any evidence of squinting, head tilting, thrusting the head forward, excessive blinking, tearing, or redness.
4. Make referrals after a second screening has been made on children with visual concerns.

LEA Symbols Screening

LEA Symbols Chart (Fig. 1.52)—designed for visual acuity screening in young children to eliminate the problems of language barriers. Research-supported LEA symbols tests are better for visual acuity assessment as compared with Snellen E charts for visual acuity measurements on preschool children[s]

[s]Vivekanand U, Gonsalves SS. Is LEA symbol better compared to Snellen Chart for visual acuity assessment in preschool children?. *Rom J Ophtalmol.* 2019;63(1):35–37.

Preparation

1. Measure the exact 10-foot distance from the chart for preschool children
2. Set up LEA Symbol Chart at the correct height (the correct height where the child's eyes will focus on the chart while sitting or standing)

Procedure

1. Show all the symbols on a card to the child and practice by naming the symbols before using the chart
2. Position the child at the correct distance from the chart

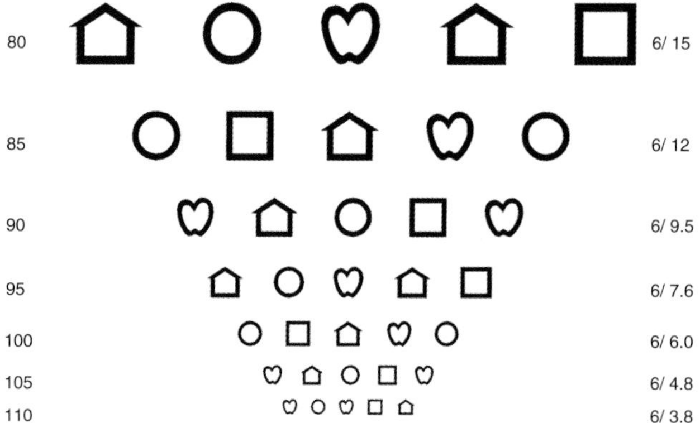

FIG. **1.52** LEA Symbols Chart consist of lines of four different symbols, arranged in combinations of five symbols per line.

3. Test binocular vision first
4. Point to one of the smaller symbols and ask the child to name the symbol or match the correct symbol on the card in front of them
5. Move down the chart until the child is unable to correctly identify four out of five symbols on that line
6. Visual acuity is recorded as the last line on which four of the five symbols are identified correctly across the line.
7. Proceed to test each eye separately using the same progression as with binocular vision testing
8. Test the right eye first (occluding the left eye using a different smaller lower triangle line which eliminates the risk of memorizing.
9. To pass, the child must be able to at least correctly identify four of five symbols on the line
10. Repeat the procedure to test the left eye, covering the right eye.
11. Observe the eyes during testing and record concerns (e.g., squinting, head tilting, tearing, excessive blinking).
12. Visual acuity is recorded as a Snellen notation (found in the right margin of the Lea Symbols Chart)
13. Make a referral after a second screening has been made on children with visual concerns.

Assessment of Hearing

Major Developmental Characteristics of Hearing

Major Developmental Clinical Manifestations listed from birth to 48 months:

Birth; American Academy of Pediatrics, Joint Committee on Infant Hearing (2007) recommends universal hearing screening of all newborns before discharge from the birthing hospital.

- Responds to loud noise with startle reflex
- Responds to the sound of human voice more readily than to any other sound
- Becomes quiet with low-pitched sounds, such as lullaby, metronome, or heartbeat

2 to 3 months of age

- Turns head to the side when sound is made at the level of ear

3 to 4 months of age

- Locates sound by turning head to the side and looking in the same direction

4 to 6 months of age

- Can localize sounds made below the ear, which is followed by localization of sound made above the ear; will turn head to the side and then look up or down
- Begins to imitate sounds

6 to 8 months of age

- Locates sounds by turning head in a curving arc
- Responds to own name

8 to 10 months of age

- Localizes sounds by turning head diagonally and directly toward the sound

10 to 12 months of age

- Knows several words and their meanings, such as "no" and the names of family members
- Learns to control and adjust own response to sound, such as listening for the sound to occur again

18 months of age

- Begins to discriminate between harshly dissimilar sounds, such as the sounds of a doorbell and a train

24 months of age

- Refines gross discriminative skills

36 months of age

- Begins to distinguish more subtle differences in speech sounds, such as between "e" and "er"

48 months of age

- Begins to distinguish between similar sounds such as *f* and *th* or between *f* and *s*
- Listening becomes considerably refined
- Able to be tested with an audiometer

Assessment of Child for Hearing Impairment

Obtain detailed history of hearing impairment regarding any family members with childhood hearing impairment, anatomic malformations of the head or neck, low birth weight, severe perinatal asphyxia, perinatal infection (e.g., cytomegalovirus, rubella, herpes, syphilis, toxoplasmosis, bacterial meningitis), maternal prenatal substance abuse, chronic ear infections, cerebral palsy, Down syndrome, prolonged neonatal oxygen supplements, administration of ototoxic drugs, exposure to loud environmental noises and loud noises combined toxic substances (e.g., smoking or second-hand smoking) that produce a synergistic effect on hearing causing hearing loss.

Observe for Clinical Manifestations of Hearing Impairment

See Box 1.39 on Clinical Manifestations of Hearing Impairment.

The nurse must operate under a high index of suspicion for those children who may have conditions associated with hearing loss (see detailed history) or whose parents are concerned about hearing loss and who have developed behaviors that indicate auditory impairment. Several types of hearing tests are available and recommended for screening infants and children (see Table 1.20 on auditory tests for infants and children).

Hearing impairment is expressed in terms of a decibel (dB). Hearing impairment can be classified according to the hearing threshold level (the measurement of an individual's hearing threshold by means of an audiometer) and the degree of symptom severity as it affects speech (see Table 1.21 on Classification of Hearing Impairment Based on Symptom Severity).

BOX 1.39 Clinical Manifestations of Hearing Impairment

Lack of startle or blink reflex to a loud sound
Failure to be awakened by loud environmental noises
Failure to localize a source of sound by 6 months old
Absence of babble or voice inflections by 7 months old
General indifference to sound
Lack of response to the spoken word; failure to follow verbal directions
Response to loud noises as opposed to the voice

Children

Use of gestures rather than verbalization to express desires, especially after 15 months old
Failure to develop intelligible speech by 24 months old
Monotone and unintelligible speech; lessened laughter
Vocal play, head banging, or foot stamping for vibratory sensation
Yelling or screeching to express pleasure, needs, or annoyance
Asking to have statements repeated or answering them incorrectly
Greater response to facial expression and gestures than to verbal explanation
Avoidance of social interaction; prefer to play alone
Inquiring, sometimes confused facial expression
Suspicious alertness alternating with cooperation
Frequent stubbornness because of lack of comprehension
Irritability at not making themselves understood
Shy, timid, and withdrawn behavior
Frequent appearance of being "in a world of their own" or markedly inattentive

TABLE 1.20 Auditory Tests for Infants and Children

Age	Auditory Test	Type of Measurement	Procedure
Newborns	Auditory brainstem response (ABR)	Electrophysiologic measurement of activity in auditory nerve and brainstem pathways	Placement of electrodes on child's head detects auditory stimuli presented though earphones one ear at a time.
Infants	Behavioral audiometry	Used to observe behavior in response to certain sounds heard through speakers or earphones	The child's responses to the sounds heard are observed.
Toddlers	Play audiometry	Uses an audiometer to transmit sounds at different volumes and pitches	The toddler is asked to do something with a toy (e.g., touch a toy, move a toy) every time the sound is heard.

Continued

TABLE 1.20 Auditory Tests for Infants and Children—cont'd

Age	Auditory Test	Type of Measurement	Procedure
Children and adolescents	Pure tone audiometry	Uses an audiometer that produces sounds at different volumes and pitches in the child's ears	The child is asked to respond in some way when the tone is heard in the earphone.
	Tympanometry (also called *impedance* or *admittance*)	Determines how the middle ear is functioning and detects any changes in pressure in the middle ear	A soft plastic tip is placed over the ear canal, and the tympanometer measures tympanic membrane movement when the pressure changes.
All ages	Evoked optoacoustic emissions (EOAE)	Physiologic test specifically measuring cochlear (outer hair cell) response to presentation of stimulus	Small probe containing sensitive microphone is placed in ear canal for stimulus delivery and response detection.

TABLE 1.21 Classification of Hearing Impairment Based on Symptom Severity

Hearing Level (dB)	Effect
Slight: 16–25	Has difficulty hearing faint or distant speech Usually is unaware of hearing difficulty Likely to achieve in school but may have problems No speech defects
Mild to moderate: 26–55	May have speech difficulties Understands face-to-face conversational speech at 0.9–1.5 m (3–5 feet)
Moderately severe: 56–70	Unable to understand conversational speech unless loud Considerable difficulty with group or classroom discussion Requires special speech training
Severe: 71–90	May hear a loud voice if nearby May be able to identify loud environmental noises Can distinguish vowels but not most consonants Requires speech training
Profound: 91	May hear only loud sounds Requires extensive speech training

dB, Decibels.

Summary of Growth and Development

This summary of growth and development offers a broad overview of the significant physical, psychosocial, and mental achievements during childhood. It begins with a comparison of cognitive and personality development throughout the life span according to different theorists. Following are summaries of the specific developmental milestones associated with each major age group of children.

Personality, Moral, and Cognitive Development

Stage and Age	Psychosexual Stages (Freud)	Psychosocial Stages (Erikson)	Cognitive Stages (Piaget)	Moral Judgment Stages (Kohlberg)
I Infancy (Birth-1 year)	Oral sensory	Trust vs. mistrust	Sensorimotor (birth to 18 months)	
II Toddlerhood (1–3 years)	Anal-urethral	Autonomy vs. shame and doubt	Preoperational thought, preconceptual phase (transductive reasoning; e.g., specific to specific) (2–4 years)	Preconventional (premoral) level Punishment and obedience orientation
III Early Childhood (3–6 years)	Phallic locomotion	Initiative vs. guilt	Preoperational thought, intuitive phase (transductive reasoning) (4–7 years)	Preconventional (premoral) level Naïve instrumental orientation
IV Middle Childhood (6–12 years)	Latency	Industry vs. inferiority	Concrete operations (inductive reasoning and beginning logic)	Conventional level Good-boy, nice-girl orientation Law-and-order orientation
V Adolescence (13–18 years)	Genitality	Identity and repudiation vs. identity confusion	Formal operations (deductive and abstract reasoning)	Postconventional or principled level Social-contract orientation Universal ethical principle orientation (no longer included in revised theory)
VI Early Adulthood		Intimacy and solidarity vs. isolation		
VII Young and Middle Adulthood		Generativity vs. self-absorption		
VIII Later Adulthood		Ego integrity vs. despair		

Growth and Development During Infancy

Physical	Gross Motor	Fine Motor
1 Month		
Weight gain of 150–210 g (5–7 ounces) weekly for first 6 months Height gain of 2.5 cm (1 inch) monthly for first 6 months Head circumference increases by 2 cm (0.75 inch) monthly for first 3 months Primitive reflexes present and strong Doll's eye reflex and dance reflex fading Obligatory nose breathing (most infants)	Assumes flexed position with pelvis high but knees not under abdomen when prone (at birth, knees flexed under abdomen)[a] Can turn head from side to side when prone; lifts head momentarily from bed[a] Has marked head lag, especially when pulled from lying to sitting position Holds head momentarily parallel and in midline when suspended in prone position Assumes asymmetric tonic neck reflex position when supine When infant is held in standing position, body limp at knees and hips In sitting position back is uniformly rounded, head control is absent	Hands predominantly closed Grasp reflex strong Hand clenches on contact with rattle
2 Months		
Posterior fontanel closed Crawling reflex disappears	Assumes less flexed position when prone—hips flat, legs extended, arms flexed, head to side[a] Less head lag when pulled to sitting position Can maintain head in same plane as rest of body when held in ventral suspension When infant is prone, can lift head almost 45 degrees off table When infant is held in sitting position, head is held up but bends forward Assumes symmetric tonic neck position intermittently	Hands frequently open Grasp reflex fading
3 Months		
Primitive reflexes fading	Able to hold head more erect when sitting but still bobs forward Has only slight head lag when pulled to sitting position Assumes symmetric body positioning Able to raise head and shoulders from prone position to a 45- to 90-degree angle from table; bears weight on forearms When infant is held in standing position, able to bear slight fraction of weight on legs Regards own hand	Actively holds rattle but will not reach for it[a] Grasp reflex absent Hands kept loosely open Clutches own hand; pulls at blankets and clothes

Sensory	Vocalization	Socialization and Cognition
Able to fixate on moving object in range of 45 degrees when held at a distance of 20–25 cm (8–10 inches) Visual acuity approaches 20/100[b] Follows light to midline Quiets when hears a voice	Cries to express displeasure Makes small, throaty sounds Makes comfort sounds during feeding	Is in sensorimotor phase—stage I, use of reflexes (birth-1 month), and stage II, primary circular reactions (1–4 months) Watches parent's face intently as she or he talks to infant
Binocular fixation and convergence to near objects beginning When infant is supine, follows dangling toy from side to point beyond midline Visually searches to locate sounds Turns head to side when sound is made at level of ear	Vocalizes, distinct from crying[a] Crying becomes differentiated Coos Vocalizes to familiar voice	Demonstrates social smile in response to various stimuli[a]
Follows object to periphery (180 degrees) Locates sound by turning head to side and looking in same direction[a] Begins to have ability to coordinate stimuli from various sense organs	Squeals to show pleasure[a] Coos, babbles, chuckles Vocalizes when smiling "Talks" a great deal when spoken to Less crying during periods of wakefulness	Displays considerable interest in surroundings Ceases crying when parent enters room Can recognize familiar faces and objects, such as feeding bottle Shows awareness of strange situations

Continued

Growth and Development During Infancy—cont'd

Physical	Gross Motor	Fine Motor
4 Months		
Drooling begins Moro, tonic neck, and rooting reflexes have disappeared[a]	Has almost no head lag when pulled to sitting position[a] Balances head well in sitting position[a] Back less rounded, curved only in lumbar area Able to sit erect if propped up Able to raise head and chest off surface to angle of 90 degrees Assumes predominant symmetric position Rolls from back to side[a]	Inspects and plays with hands; pulls clothing or blanket over face in play[a] Tries to reach object with hand but overshoots Grasps object with both hands Plays with rattle placed in hand, shakes it, but cannot pick it up if dropped Can carry objects to mouth
5 Months		
Beginning signs of tooth eruption Birth weight doubles	No head lag when pulled to sitting position When infant is sitting, able to hold head erect and steady Able to sit for longer periods when back is well supported Back straight When infant is prone, assumes symmetric positioning with arms extended Can turn over from abdomen to back[a] When infant is supine, puts feet to mouth	Able to grasp objects voluntarily[a] Uses palmar grasp, bidextrous approach Plays with toes Takes objects directly to mouth Holds one cube while regarding a second one
6 Months		
Growth rate may begin to decline Weight gain of 90–150 g (3–5 ounces) weekly for next 6 months Height gain of 1.25 cm (0.5 inch) monthly for next 6 months Teething may begin with eruption of two lower central incisors[a] Chewing and biting occur[a]	When infant is prone, can lift chest and upper abdomen off table, bearing weight on hands When infant is about to be pulled to a sitting position, lifts head Sits in highchair with back straight Rolls from back to abdomen When infant is held in standing position, bears almost all of weight Hand regard absent	Resecures a dropped object Drops one cube when another is given Grasps and manipulates small objects Holds bottle Grasps feet and pulls to mouth
7 Months		
Eruption of lower central incisors	When infant is supine, spontaneously lifts head off table Sits, leaning forward on hands[a] When infant is prone, bears weight on one hand Sits erect momentarily Bears full weight on feet When infant is held in standing position, bounces actively	Transfers objects from one hand to the other[a] Has unidextrous approach and grasp Holds two cubes more than momentarily Bangs cube on table Rakes at a small object

Sensory	Vocalization	Socialization and Cognition
Able to accommodate to near objects Binocular vision fairly well established Can focus on a 1.25-cm (½-inch) block Beginning eye-hand coordination	Makes consonant sounds *n, k, g, p,* and *b* Laughs aloud[a] Vocalization changes according to mood	Is in stage III, secondary circular reactions Demands attention by fussing; becomes bored if left alone Enjoys social interaction with people Anticipates feeding when sees bottle or mother if breast-feeding Shows excitement with whole body, squeals, breathes heavily Shows interest in strange stimuli Begins to show memory
Visually pursues a dropped object Is able to sustain visual inspection of an object Can localize sounds made below the ear	Squeals Makes vowel cooing sounds interspersed with consonant sounds (e.g., ah-goo)	Smiles at mirror image Pats bottle or breast with both hands More enthusiastically playful but may have rapid mood swings Is able to discriminate strangers from family Vocalizes displeasure when object is taken away Discovers parts of body
Adjusts posture to see an object Prefers more complex visual stimuli Can localize sounds made above the ear Will turn head to the side, then look up or down	Begins to imitate sounds[a] Babbling resembles one-syllable utterances—*ma, mu, da, di, hi*[a] Vocalizes to toys, mirror image Takes pleasure in hearing own sounds (self-reinforcement)	Recognizes parents; begins to fear strangers Holds arms out to be picked up Has definite likes and dislikes Begins to imitate (cough, protrusion of tongue) Excites on hearing footsteps Briefly searches for a dropped object (object permanence beginning)[a] Frequent mood swings—From crying to laughing with little or no provocation
Can fixate on very small objects[a] Responds to own name Localizes sound by turning head in an arc Beginning awareness of depth and space Has taste preferences	Produces vowel sounds and chained syllables—*baba, dada, kaka*[a] Vocalizes four distinct vowel sounds "Talks" when others are talking	Increasing fear of strangers; shows signs of fretfulness when parent disappears[a] Imitates simple acts and noises Tries to attract attention by coughing or snorting Plays peek-a-boo Demonstrates dislike of food by keeping lips closed Exhibits oral aggressiveness in biting and mouthing Demonstrates expectation in response to repetition of stimuli

Continued

Growth and Development During Infancy—cont'd

Physical	Gross Motor	Fine Motor
8 Months		
Begins to show regular patterns in bladder and bowel elimination Parachute reflex appears	Sits steadily unsupported[a] Readily bears weight on legs when supported; may stand holding on to furniture Adjusts posture to reach an object	Has beginning pincer grasp using index, fourth, and fifth fingers against lower part of thumb Releases objects at will Rings bell purposely Retains two cubes while regarding third cube Secures an object by pulling on a string Reaches persistently for toys out of reach
9 Months		
Eruption of upper central incisors may begin	Creeps on hands and knees Sits steadily on floor for prolonged time (10 min) Recovers balance when leans forward but cannot do so when leaning sideways Pulls self to standing position and stands holding on to furniture[a]	Uses thumb and index finger in crude pincer grasp[a] Preference for use of dominant hand now evident Grasps third cube Compares two cubes by bringing them together
10 Months		
Labyrinth-righting reflex is strongest—when infant is in prone or supine position; is able to raise head	Can change from prone to sitting position Stands while holding on to furniture, sits by falling down Recovers balance easily while sitting While child is standing, lifts one foot to take a step	Crude release of an object beginning Grasps bell by handle
11 Months		
Eruption of lower lateral incisors may begin	When child is sitting, pivots to reach toward back to pick up an object Cruises or walks holding on to furniture or with both hands held[a]	Explores objects more thoroughly (e.g., clapper inside bell) Has neat pincer grasp Drops object deliberately for it to be picked up Puts one object after another into a container (sequential play) Able to manipulate an object to remove it from tight-fitting enclosure

Sensory	Vocalization	Socialization and Cognition
	Makes consonant sounds *t*, *d*, and *w* Listens selectively to familiar words Utterances signal emphasis and emotion Combines syllables, such as *dada*, but does not ascribe meaning to them	Increasing anxiety over loss of parent, particularly mother, and fear of strangers Responds to word "no" Dislikes dressing, diaper change
Localizes sounds by turning head diagonally and directly toward sound Depth perception increasing	Responds to simple verbal commands Comprehends "no-no"	Parent (usually mother) is increasingly important for own sake Shows increasing interest in pleasing parent Begins to show fears of going to bed and being left alone Puts arms in front of face to avoid having it washed
	Says "dada," "mama" with meaning Comprehends "bye-bye" May say one word (e.g., "hi," "bye," "no")	Inhibits behavior to verbal command of "no-no" or own name Imitates facial expressions; waves bye-bye Extends toy to another person but will not release it Develops object permanence[a] Repeats actions that attract attention and cause laughter Pulls clothes of another to attract attention Plays interactive games such as pat-a-cake Reacts to adult anger; cries when scolded Demonstrates independence in dressing, feeding, locomotive skills, and testing of parents Looks at and follows pictures in a book
	Imitates definite speech sounds	Experiences joy and satisfaction when a task is mastered Reacts to restrictions with frustration Rolls ball to another on request Anticipates body gestures when a familiar nursery rhyme or story is being told (e.g., holds toes and feet in response to "This little piggy went to market") Plays games such as up-down, so big, or peek-a-boo Shakes head for "no"

Continued

Growth and Development During Infancy—cont'd

Physical	Gross Motor	Fine Motor
12 Months		
Birth weight tripled[a] Birth length increased by 50%[a] Head and chest circumference equal (head circumference 46 cm [18 inches]) Has six to eight deciduous teeth Anterior fontanel almost closed Landau reflex fading Babinski reflex disappears Lumbar curve develops; lordosis evident during walking	Walks with one hand held[a] Cruises well May attempt to stand alone momentarily; may attempt first step alone[a] Can sit down from standing position without help	Releases cube in cup Attempts to build two-block tower but fails Tries to insert a pellet into a narrow-necked bottle but fails Can turn pages in a book, many at a time

[a]Milestones that represent essential integrative aspects of development that lay the foundation for the achievement of more advanced skills.
[b]Degree of visual acuity varies according to vision measurement procedure used.

Sensory	Vocalization	Socialization and Cognition
Discriminates simple geometric forms (e.g., circle) Amblyopia may develop with lack of binocularity Can follow rapidly moving object Controls and adjusts response to sound; listens for sound to recur	Says three to five words besides "dada," "mama"[a] Comprehends meaning of several words (comprehension always precedes verbalization) Recognizes objects by name Imitates animal sounds Understands simple verbal commands (e.g., "Give it to me," "Show me your eyes")	Shows emotions such as jealousy, affection (may give hug or kiss on request), anger, fear Enjoys familiar surroundings and explores away from parent Is fearful In strange situation; clings to parent May develop habit of security blanket or favorite toy Has increasing determination to practice locomotion skills Searches for an object even if it has not been hidden, but searches only where object was last seen [a]

Growth and Development During Toddler Years

Physical	Gross Motor	Fine Motor
15 Months		
Steady growth in height and weight Head circumference 48 cm (19 inches) Weight 11 kg (24 pounds) Height 78.7 cm (31 inches)	Walks without help (usually since age 13 months) Creeps up stairs Kneels without support Cannot walk around corners or stop suddenly without losing balance without support Assumes standing position without support Cannot throw ball without falling	Constantly casting objects to floor Builds tower of two cubes Holds two cubes in one hand Releases a pellet into a narrow-necked bottle Scribbles spontaneously Uses cup well, but often rotates spoon before it reaches mouth
18 Months		
Physiologic anorexia from decreased growth needs Anterior fontanel closed Physiologically able to control sphincters	Runs clumsily, falls often Walks upstairs with one hand held Pulls and pushes toys Jumps in place with both feet Seats self on chair Throws ball overhand without falling	Builds tower of three or four cubes Release, prehension, and reach well developed Turns pages in a book two or three at a time In drawing, makes stroke imitatively Manages spoon without rotation
24 Months		
Head circumference 49–50 cm (19.5–20 inches) Chest circumference exceeds head circumference. Lateral diameter of chest exceeds anteroposterior diameter. Usual weight gain of 1.8–2.7 kg (4–6 pounds) Usual gain in height of 10–12.5 cm (4–5 inches) Adult height approximately double height at 2 years May have demonstrated readiness for beginning daytime control of bowel and bladder Primary dentition of 16 teeth	Goes up and down stairs alone with 2 feet on each step Runs fairly well, with wide stance Picks up object without falling Kicks ball forward without overbalancing	Builds tower of six or seven cubes Aligns two or more cubes like a train Turns pages of book one at a time In drawing, imitates vertical and circular strokes Turns doorknob, unscrews lid
30 Months		
Birth weight quadrupled Primary dentition (20 teeth) completed May have daytime bowel and bladder control	Jumps with both feet Jumps from chair or step Stands on one foot momentarily Takes a few steps on tiptoe	Builds tower of eight cubes Adds chimney to train of cubes Good hand-finger coordination; holds crayon with fingers rather than fist In drawing, imitates vertical and horizontal strokes, makes two or more strokes for cross; draws circles

Sensory	Vocalization	Socialization
Able to Identify geometric forms; places round object into appropriate hole Binocular vision well developed Displays an intense and prolonged interest in pictures	Uses expressive jargon Says four to six words, including names Asks for objects by pointing Understands simple commands May headshake to gesture "no" Uses "no" even while agreeing to the request. Uses common gestures, such as putting cup to mouth when empty.	Tolerates some separation from parent Less likely to fear strangers Beginning to imitate parents, such as cleaning house (sweeping, dusting), folding clothes, mowing lawn May discard bottle Kisses and hugs parents, may kiss pictures in a book Expressive of emotions, has temper tantrums
	Says 10 or more words Points to a common object, such as shoe or ball, and to two or three body parts Forms word combinations Forms gestures-word combinations (points while naming) Forms gesture-gesture combinations	Great imitator (domestic mimicry) Takes off gloves, socks, and shoes and unzips Temper tantrums may be more evident Beginning awareness of ownership ("my toy") May develop dependence on transitional objects, such as security blanket
Accommodation well developed In geometric discrimination, able to insert square block into oblong space	Has vocabulary of approximately 300 words Uses two- to three-word phrases Uses pronouns "I," "me," "you" Understands directional commands Gives first name; refers to self by name Verbalizes need for toileting, food, or drink Talks incessantly Able to remember and imitate arbitrary sequences of manual actions and gestures	Stage of parallel play Has sustained attention span Temper tantrums decreasing Pulls people to show them something Increased independence from mother Dresses self in simple clothing Develops visual recognition and verbal self-reference ("me big") Develops awareness that feelings and desires of others may be different and begins to explore implications and consequences
	Gives first and last names Refers to self by appropriate pronoun Uses plurals Names one color	Separates more easily from parent In play, helps put things away, can carry breakable objects, pushes with good steering Begins to note gender differences; knows own gender May attend to toilet needs without help, except for wiping Emotions expand to include pride, shame, guilt, embarrassment

Growth and Development During Preschool Years

Physical	Gross Motor	Fine Motor	Language
3 Years			
Usual weight gain of 1.8–2.7 kg (4–6 pounds) Average weight of 14.6 kg (32 pounds) Usual gain in height of 7.5 cm (3inches) per year Average height of 95 cm (3 feet, 1-½ inches) May have achieved nighttime control of bowel and bladder	Rides tricycle Jumps off bottom step Stands on one foot for a few seconds Goes up stairs using alternate feet, may still come down using both feet on step Broad jumps May try to dance, but balance may not be adequate	Builds tower of 9 or 10 cubes Builds bridge with three cubes Adeptly places small pellets in narrow-necked bottle In drawing, copies a circle, imitates a cross, names what has been drawn, cannot draw stick figure but may make circle with facial features	Has vocabulary of about 900 words Uses primarily "telegraphic" speech Uses complete sentences of three or four words Talks incessantly regardless of whether anyone is paying attention Repeats sentence of six syllables Asks many questions
4 Years			
Growth rate is similar to previous year Average weight of 16.5 kg (36.5 pounds) Average height of 103 cm (3 feet 4½ inches) Length at birth is doubled Maximum potential for development of amblyopia	Skips and hops on one foot Catches ball reliably Throws ball overhand Walks down stairs using alternate footing	Uses scissors successfully to cut out picture following outline Can lace shoes but may not be able to tie bow In drawing, copies a square, traces a cross and diamond, adds three parts to stick figure	Has vocabulary of 1500 words or more Uses sentences of four or five words Questioning is at peak Tells exaggerated stories Knows simple songs May be mildly profane if associates with older children Obeys prepositional phrases, such as "under," "on top of," "beside," "in back of," or "in front of" Names one or more colors Comprehends analogies, such as, "If ice is cold, fire is_________"

Socialization	Cognition	Family Relationships
Dresses self almost completely if helped with back buttons and told which shoe is right or left Pulls on shoes Has increased attention span Feeds self completely Can prepare simple meals, such as cold cereal and milk Can help set table; can dry dishes without breaking any May have fears, especially of dark and of going to bed Knows own gender and gender of others Play is parallel and associative; begins to learn simple games but often follows own rules; begins to share	Is in preconceptual phase Is egocentric in thought and behavior Has beginning understanding of time; uses many time-oriented expressions; talks about past and future as much as about present; pretends to tell time Has improved concept of space as demonstrated in understanding of prepositions and ability to follow directional command Has beginning ability to view concepts from another perspective	Attempts to please parents and conform to their expectations Is less jealous of younger sibling; may be opportune time for birth of additional sibling Is aware of family relationships and gender-role functions Boys tend to identify more with father or other male figure Has increased ability to separate easily and comfortably from parents for short periods
Very independent Tends to be selfish and impatient Aggressive physically as well as verbally Takes pride in accomplishments Has mood swings Shows off dramatically, enjoys entertaining others Tells family tales to others with no restraint Still has many fears Play is associative: Imaginary playmates are common Uses dramatic, imaginative, and imitative devices Sexual exploration and curiosity demonstrated through play, such as being "doctor" or "nurse"	Is in phase of intuitive thought Causality is still related to proximity of events Understands time better, especially in terms of sequence of daily events Unable to conserve matter Judges everything according to one dimension, such as height, width, or order Immediate perceptual clues dominate judgment Is beginning to develop less egocentrism and more social awareness May count correctly but has poor mathematic concept of numbers Obeys because parents have set limits, not because of understanding of right and wrong	Rebels if parents expect too much, such as impeccable table manners Takes aggression and frustration out on parents or siblings Dos and don'ts become important May have rivalry with older or younger siblings; may resent older sibling's privileges and younger sibling's invasion of privacy and possessions May "run away" from home Identifies strongly with parent of opposite gender Is able to run simple errands outside the home

Continued

Growth and Development During Preschool Years—cont'd

Physical	Gross Motor	Fine Motor	Language
5 Years			
Average weight of 18.5 kg (41 pounds) Average height of 110 cm (3 feet, 7½ inches) Eruption of permanent dentition may begin Handedness is established (about 90% are right handed)	Skips and hops on alternate feet Throws and catches ball well Jumps rope Skates with good balance Walks backward with heel to toe. Jumps from Jumps from the height of 12 inches and lands on toes Balances on alternate feet with eyes closed	Ties shoelaces Uses scissors, simple tools, or pencil very well In drawing, copies a diamond and triangle; adds seven to nine parts to stick figure; prints a few letters, numbers, or words, such as first name	Has vocabulary of about 2100 words Uses sentences of six to eight words, with all parts of speech Names coins (e.g., nickel, dime) Names four or more colors Describes drawing or comment and enumeration Knows names of days of week, months, and other time-associated words Knows composition of articles, such as, "A shoe is made of ____" Can follow three commands in succession

Socialization	Cognition	Family Relationships
Less rebellious and quarrelsome than at age 4 years More settled and eager to get down to business Not as open and accessible in thoughts and behavior as in earlier years Independent but trustworthy; not foolhardy; more responsible Has fewer fears; relies on outer authority to control world Eager to do things right and to please; tries to "live by the rules" Has better manners Cares for self totally, occasionally needs supervision in dress or hygiene Not ready for concentrated close work or small print because of slight farsightedness and still unrefined eye-hand coordination Play is associative; tries to follow rules but may cheat to avoid losing	Begins to question what parents think by comparing them with age-mates and other adults May note prejudice and bias in outside world Is more able to view another's perspective but tolerates differences rather than understanding them May begin to show understanding of conservation of numbers through counting objects regardless of arrangement Uses time-oriented words with increased understanding Cautious about factual information regarding world	Gets along well with parents May seek out parent more often than at age 4 years for reassurance and security, especially when entering school Begins to question parents' thinking and principles Strongly identifies with parent of same gender, especially boys with their fathers Enjoys activities such as sports, cooking, shopping with parent of same gender

Growth and Development During School-Age Years

Physical and Motor	Mental	Adaptive	Personal-Social
6 Years			
Height and weight gain continues slowly Weight: 16–23.3 kg (35.5–58 pounds); height: 106.7–123.5 cm (42–49 inches) Central mandibular incisors erupt Loses first tooth Gradual increase in dexterity Active age; constant activity Often returns to finger feeding More aware of hand as a tool Likes to draw, print, and color Vision reaches maturity	Develops concept of numbers Counts 13 pennies Knows whether it is morning or afternoon Defines common objects such as fork and chair in terms of their use Obeys triple commands in succession Knows right and left hands Says which is pretty and which is ugly of a series of drawings of faces Describes the objects in a picture rather than simply enumerating them Attends first grade	At table, uses knife to spread butter or jam on bread At play, cuts, folds, and pastes paper toys, sews crudely if needle is threaded Takes bath without supervision; performs bedtime activities alone Reads from memory; enjoys oral spelling game Likes table games, checkers, simple card games Giggles a lot Sometimes steals money or attractive items Has difficulty owning up to misdeeds Tries out own abilities	Can share and cooperate better Has great need for children of own age Will cheat to win Often engages in rough play Often jealous of younger brother or sister Does what adults are seen doing May have occasional temper tantrums Is a boaster Is more independent, probably influence of school Has own way of doing things Increases socialization
7 Years			
Begins to grow at least 5 cm (2 inches) a year Weight: 17.7–30 kg (39–66 pounds); height: 111.8–129.5 cm (44–51 inches) Maxillary central incisors and lateral mandibular incisors erupt Jaw begins to expand to accommodate permanent teeth More cautious in approaches to new performances Repeats performances to master them Jaw begins to expand to accommodate permanent teeth	Notes that certain parts are missing from pictures Can copy a diamond Repeats three numbers backward Develops concept of time; reads ordinary clock or watch correctly to nearest quarter hour; uses clock for practical purposes Attends second grade More mechanical in reading; often does not stop at the end of a sentence, skips words such as "it," "the," and "he"	Uses table knife for cutting meat; may need help with tough or difficult pieces Brushes and combs hair acceptably without help May steal Likes to help and have a choice Is less resistant and stubborn	Is becoming a real member of the family group Takes part in group play Boys prefer playing with boys; girls prefer playing with girls Spends a lot of time alone; does not require a lot of companionship
8–9 Years			
Continues to grow at least 5 cm (2 inches) a year Weight: 19.6–39.6 kg (43–87 pounds); height: 116.8–141.8 cm (46–56 inches) Lateral incisors (maxillary) and mandibular cuspids erupt Movement fluid, often graceful and poised Always on the go; jumps, chases, skips	Gives similarities and differences between two things from memory Counts backward from 20 to 1; understands concept of reversibility Repeats days of the week and months in order; knows the date Describes common objects in detail, not merely their use	Makes use of common tools such as hammer, saw, or screwdriver Uses household and sewing utensils Helps with routine household tasks such as dusting, sweeping Assumes responsibility for share of household chores Looks after all of own needs at table	Is easy to get along with at home Likes the reward system Dramatizes Is more sociable Is better behaved Is interested in boy-girl relationships but will not admit it Goes about home and community freely, alone, or with friends

Growth and Development During School-Age Years—cont'd

Physical and Motor	Mental	Adaptive	Personal-Social
Increased smoothness and speed in fine motor control; uses cursive writing Dresses self completely Likely to overdo; hard to quiet down after recess More limber; bones grow faster than ligaments	Gives similarities and differences between 2 things from memory Count backward from 20 to 1; understands concept of reversibility Repeats days of the week and months in order; knows the date Describes common objects in detail; not merely their use Makes change out of a quarter Attends third and fourth grades Reads more; may plan to wake up early just to read Reads classic books but also enjoys comics More aware of time; can be relied on to get to school on time Can grasp concepts of parts and whole (fractions) Understands concepts of space, cause and effect, nesting (puzzles), and conservation (permanence of mass and volume) Classifies objects by more than one quality; has collections Produces simple paintings or drawings	Makes use of common tools such as hammer, saw, screwdriver Uses household and sewing utensils Assumes responsibility for share of household chores Looks after all of own needs at table Buys useful articles; exercises some choice in making purchases Runs useful errands Likes pictorial magazines Likes school; wants to answer all the questions Is afraid of failing a grade; is ashamed of bad grades Is more critical of self Takes music and sport lessons	Is easy to get along with at home Likes the reward system Dramatizes Is more sociable Is better behaved Is interested in boy-girl relationships but will not admit it Goes about home and community freely, alone or with friends Likes to compete and play games Shows preference in friends and groups Plays mostly with groups of own gender but is beginning to mix Develops modesty Compares self with others Enjoys organizations, clubs, and group sports
10–12 Years			
Boys: Slow growth in height and rapid weight gain; may become obese in this period Girls: Pubescent changes may begin to appear; body lines soften and round out Weight: 24.3–58 kg (54–128 pounds); height: 127–162.5 cm (50–64 inches) Remainder of teeth will erupt and tend toward full development (except wisdom teeth)	Writes brief stories Attends fifth to seventh grades Writes occasional short letters to friends or relatives on own initiative Uses telephone for practical purposes Responds to magazine, radio, or other advertising Reads for practical information or own enjoyment—Stories or library books of adventure or romance, or animal stories	Makes useful tools or does easy repair work Cooks or sews in small way Raises pets Washes and dries own hair; is responsible for a thorough job of cleaning hair but may need reminding to do so Is sometimes left alone at home for an hour or so Is successful in looking after own needs or those of other children left in his or her care	Loves friends; talks about them constantly Chooses friends more selectively; may have a best friend Enjoys conversation Develops beginning interest in opposite gender Is more diplomatic Likes family; family really has meaning Likes mother and wants to please her in many ways Demonstrates affection Likes father, who is adored and idolized Respects parents

Growth and Development During Adolescence

Early Adolescence (11–14 Years)	Middle Adolescence (14–17 Years)	Late Adolescence (17–20 Years)
Growth		
Rapidly accelerating growth Reaches peak velocity Secondary sex characteristics appear	Growth decelerating in girls Stature reaches 95% of adult height Secondary sex characteristics well advanced	Physically mature Structure and reproductive growth almost complete
Cognition		
Explores newfound ability for limited abstract thought Clumsy groping for new values and energies Comparison of "normality" with peers of same gender	Developing capacity for abstract thinking Enjoys intellectual powers, often in idealistic terms Concern with philosophic, political, and social problems	Established abstract thought Can perceive and act on long-range operations Able to view problems comprehensively Intellectual and functional identity established
Identity		
Preoccupied with rapid bodily changes Trying out of various roles Measurement of attractiveness by acceptance or rejection of peers Conformity to group norms Decline in self-esteem	Modifies bodily image Self-centered; increased narcissism Tendency toward inner experience and self-discovery Has a rich fantasy life Idealistic Able to perceive future implications of current behavior and decisions; variable application	Bodily image and gender role definition nearly secured Mature sexual identity Phase of consolidation of identity Increase in self-esteem Comfortable with physical growth Social roles defined and articulated
Relationships With Parents		
Defining independence-dependence boundaries Strong desire to remain dependent on parents while trying to detach No major conflicts over parental control	Major conflicts over independence and control Low point in parent-child relationship Greatest push for emancipation; disengagement Final and irreversible emotional detachment from parents; mourning	Emotional and physical separation from parents completed Independence from family with less conflict Emancipation nearly secured
Relationships With Peers		
Seeks peer affiliations to counter instability generated by rapid change Upsurge of close idealized friendships with members of the same gender Struggle for mastery takes place within peer group	Strong need for identity to affirm self-image Behavioral standards set by peer group Acceptance by peers extremely important—Fear of rejection Exploration of ability to attract the opposite gender	Peer group recedes in importance in favor of individual friendship. Testing of romantic relationships against possibility of permanent alliance Relationships characterized by giving and sharing
Sexuality		
Self-exploration and evaluation Limited dating, usually group Limited intimacy	Multiple plural relationships Internal identification of heterosexuality, homosexual, or bisexual attractions Exploration of "self-appeal" Feeling of "being in love" Tentative establishment of relationships	Forms stable relationships and attachment to another Growing capacity for mutuality and reciprocity Dating as a romantic pair May publicly identify as LGBT (lesbian, gay, bisexual, transgender) Intimacy involves commitment rather than exploration and romanticism.

Growth and Development During Adolescence—cont'd

Early Adolescence (11–14 Years)	Middle Adolescence (14–17 Years)	Late Adolescence (17–20 Years)
Psychologic Health		
Wide mood swings Intense daydreaming Anger outwardly expressed with moodiness, temper outbursts, and verbal insults and name calling	Tendency toward inner experiences; more introspective Tendency to withdraw when upset or feelings are hurt Vacillation of emotions in time and range Feelings of inadequacy common; difficulty in asking for help	More constancy of emotion Anger more apt to be concealed

ATRAUMATIC CARE

Reducing Distress From Otoscopy in Young Children

Make examining the ear a game by explaining that you are looking for a "big elephant" in the ear. This kind of fairy tale is an absorbing distraction and usually elicits cooperation. After the ear has been examined, clarify that "looking for elephants" was only pretending and thank the child for letting you look in his or her ear. Another great distraction technique is asking the child to put a finger on the opposite ear to keep the light from getting out.

ATRAUMATIC CARE

Encouraging Deep Breaths

Ask the child to "blow out" the light on an otoscope or pocket flashlight; discreetly turn off the light on the last try so that the child feels successful.

Place a cotton ball in the child's palm; ask the child to blow the ball into the air and have the parent catch it.

Place a small tissue on the top of a pencil and ask the child to blow the tissue off.

Have the child blow a pinwheel or a party horn.

ATRAUMATIC CARE

Encouraging Opening the Mouth for Examination

Perform the examination in front of a mirror.

Let the child first examine someone else's mouth, such as the parent, the nurse, or a puppet; then examine the child's mouth.

Instruct the child to tilt the head back slightly, breathe deeply through the mouth, and hold the breath; this action lowers the tongue to the floor of the mouth without using a tongue blade.

EMERGENCY TREATMENT

Eye Injuries

Foreign Object

Examine the eye for the presence of a foreign body (evert upper eyelid to examine the upper eye).

Remove a freely movable object with a pointed corner of gauze pad lightly moistened with water.

Do not irrigate the eye or attempt to remove a penetrating object (see Penetrating Injuries).

Caution child against rubbing the eye.

Chemical Burns

Irrigate the eye copiously with tap water for 15–20 min.

Evert the upper eyelid to flush thoroughly.

Hold the child's head with the eye under a tap of running lukewarm water.

Take the child to an emergency department.

Have the child rest with eyes closed.

Keep room darkened.

Ultraviolet Burns

If the skin is burned, patch both eyes (make certain eyelids are completely closed); secure dressing with Kling bandages wrapped around the head rather than with tape.

Have the child rest with eyes closed.

Refer to an ophthalmologist.

Hematoma ("Black Eye")

Use a flashlight to check for gross hyphema (hemorrhage into anterior chamber; visible fluid meniscus across iris; more easily seen in light-colored than in brown eyes).

Apply ice for the first 24 h to reduce swelling if no hyphema is present.

Refer to an ophthalmologist immediately if hyphema is present.

Have the child rest with eyes closed.

Penetrating Injuries

Take the child to an emergency department.

Never remove an object that has penetrated the eye.

Follow strict aseptic technique in examining the eye.

Observe for:

- Aqueous or vitreous leaks (fluid leaking from point of penetration)
- Hyphema
- Shape and equality of pupils, reaction to light, prolapsed iris (not perfectly circular)

Apply a Fox shield if available (not a regular eye patch) and apply the patch over the unaffected eye to prevent bilateral movement.

Maintain bed rest with the child in a 30-degree Fowler position.

Caution child against rubbing the eye.

Refer to an ophthalmologist.

Health Promotion

Symbol ▶ indicates material that may be photocopied and distributed to families.

Preventive Pediatric Health Care

The American Academy of Pediatrics (AAP) Bright Futures provides an evidence-based guideline for pediatric preventive health care from infancy through adolescence. Table 2.1 describes essential components of the health care visit at each developmental stage.

Nutrition

Dietary Reference Intakes

The National Academy of Medicine (formally known as Institute of Medicine [IOM]) developed guidelines for nutritional intake that encompass the Recommended Dietary Allowances (RDAs) yet extended the scope to include additional parameters related to nutritional intake. The dietary reference intakes (DRIs) are a set of evidenced-based nutrient reference values that are used to assess and plan dietary intake applicable to healthy individuals. The DRIs are composed of the following categories (Table 2.2):

Estimated average requirements (EARs): Estimated to meet the nutrient requirement of half of healthy individuals for a specific age and gender group.

Recommended Dietary Allowance (RDA): Sufficient to meet the nutrient requirement of nearly all healthy individuals for a specific age and gender group.

Tolerable upper-limit level (UL): Highest nutrient intake level likely to pose no risk of adverse effects.

Adequate intakes (AIs): Based on estimates of nutrient intake by healthy individuals.

The US Department of Agriculture has an online interactive DRI tool for health care professionals to calculate daily nutrient recommendations based on age, gender, height, weight, and activity level, although it is important to note that individual requirements may vary (tool available at https://www.nal.usda.gov/human-nutrition-and-food-safety/dri-calculator).

An additional dietary resource is MyPlate, which is a colorful plate showing the five main food groups (fruits, grains, vegetables, protein, and dairy) for the intended purpose of involving children and their families in making appropriate food choices (see Fig. 1.46 in Unit 1). The MyPlate online interactive feature allows the individual to select (click on) a specific food group and see choices for foods in that group. Appropriate serving sizes are suggested, and vegetarian substitutions are also provided. MyPlate resources include the newly designed website MyPlate.gov (https://www.myplate.gov) based on the Dietary Guidelines for Americans, 2020–2025.[a]

Dietary Guidelines

The American Heart Association dietary guidelines (Table 2.2) may also be used to encourage healthy dietary intakes designed to decrease obesity and cardiovascular risk factors and subsequent cardiovascular disease, which is now known to occur in young children as well as adults. For more information on healthy dietary habits and child nutrition, visit the American Heart Association website, available at https://www.heart.org/nutrition-basics/di.

The Dietary Guidelines for Americans, 2020–2025 ninth edition was issued jointly by the US Departments of Agriculture and of Health and Human Services in December 2020 (Table 2.3). It is the first to provide recommendations by life stage, from birth to older adulthood, and is grounded in the current body of scientific evidence on diet and health outcomes with aims to promote health and prevent chronic diseases.[a]

Fluoride Supplementation

The widespread decline in dental caries in many developed countries, including the United States, has been largely attributed to use of fluoride.[b] Fluoride has three main actions: promotes enamel remineralization, reduces enamel demineralization, and inhibits bacterial metabolism and acid production. The US Preventive Services

[b] Clark MB, Keels MA, Slayton RL, et al. Fluoride use in caries prevention in the primary care setting. *Pediatrics.* 2020;146(6):e2020034637.

[a] Snetselaar LG, de Jesus JM, DeSilva DM, Stoody EE. Dietary Guidelines for Americans, 2020–2025: understanding the scientific process, guidelines, and key recommendations. *Nutr Today.* 2021;56(6):287–295.

TABLE 2.1 Recommendations for Preventive Health Care, American Association of Pediatrics Bright Futures

	INFANCY								EARLY CHILDHOOD						
AGE	**Prenatal**	**Newborn**	**3-5 d**	**By 1 mo**	**2 mo**	**4 mo**	**6 mo**	**9 mo**	**12 mo**	**15 mo**	**18 mo**	**24 mo**	**30 mo**	**3 y**	**4 y**
HISTORY Initial/Interval	●	●	●	●	●	●	●	●	●	●	●	●	●	●	●
MEASUREMENTS															
Length/Height and Weight		●	●	●	●	●	●	●	●	●	●	●	●	●	●
Head Circumference		●	●	●	●	●	●	●	●	●	●	●			
Weight for Length		●	●	●	●	●	●	●	●	●	●				
Body Mass Index												●	●	●	●
Blood Pressure		★	★	★	★	★	★	★	★	★	★	★	★	●	●
SENSORY SCREENING															
Vision		★	★	★	★	★	★	★	★	★	★	★	★	●	●
Hearing		●	● →	→	→	★	★	★	★	★	★	★	★	★	●
DEVELOPMENTAL/BEHAVIORAL HEALTH															
Developmental Screening								●			●		●		
Autism Spectrum Disorder Screening											●	●			
Developmental Surveillance		●	●	●	●	●	●		●	●		●		●	●
Psychosocial/Behavioral Assessment		●	●	●	●	●	●	●	●	●	●	●	●	●	●
Tobacco, Alcohol, or Drug Use Assessment															
Depression Screening															
Maternal Depression Screening				●	●	●	●								
PHYSICAL EXAMINATION		●	●	●	●	●	●	●	●	●	●	●	●	●	●
PROCEDURES															
Newborn Blood		●	● →	→	→										
Newborn Bilirubin		●													
Critical Congenital Heart Defect		●													
Immunization		●	●	●	●	●	●	●	●	●	●	●	●	●	●
Anemia						★			●	★	★	★	★	★	★
Lead							★	★	● ★		★	● ★		★	★
Tuberculosis				★			★		★			★		★	★
Dyslipidemia												★			★
Sexually Transmitted Infections															
HIV															
Cervical Dysplasia															
ORAL HEALTH							●	●	★		★	★	★	★	★
Fluoride Varnish							←	—	—	—	●	—	—	—	—
Fluoride Supplementation							★	★	★		★	★	★	★	★
ANTICIPATORY GUIDANCE	●	●	●	●	●	●	●	●	●	●	●	●	●	●	●

KEY: ● = to be performed ★ = risk assessment to be performed with appropriate action to follow, if positive

←—●—→ = range during which a service may be provided

	MIDDLE CHILDHOOD						ADOLESCENCE							
AGE	5 y	6 y	7 y	8 y	9 y	10 y	11 y	12 y	13 y	14 y	15 y	16 y	17 y	18 y
HISTORY Initial/Interval	●	●	●	●	●	●	●	●	●	●	●	●	●	●
MEASUREMENTS														
Length/Height and Weight	●	●	●	●	●	●	●	●	●	●	●	●	●	●
Head Circumference														
Weight for Length														
Body Mass Index	●	●	●	●	●	●	●	●	●	●	●	●	●	●
Blood Pressure	●	●	●	●	●	●	●	●	●	●	●	●	●	●
SENSORY SCREENING														
Vision	●	●	★	●	★	●	★	●	★	★	●	★	★	★
Hearing	●	●	★	●	★	●	←	—	●	→	←	●	→	
DEVELOPMENTAL/BEHAVIORAL HEALTH														
Developmental Screening														
Autism Spectrum Disorder Screening														
Developmental Surveillance	●	●	●	●	●	●	●	●	●	●	●	●	●	●
Psychosocial/Behavioral Assessment	●	●	●	●	●	●	●	●	●	●	●	●	●	●
Tobacco, Alcohol, or Drug Use Assessment							★	★	★	★	★	★	★	★
Depression Screening								●	●	●	●	●	●	●
Maternal Depression Screening														
PHYSICAL EXAMINATION	●	●	●	●	●	●	●	●	●	●	●	●	●	●
PROCEDURES														
Newborn Blood														
Newborn Bilirubin														
Critical Congenital Heart Defect														
Immunization	●	●	●	●	●	●	●	●	●	●	●	●	●	●
Anemia	★	★	★	★	★	★	★	★	★	★	★	★	★	★
Lead	★	★												
Tuberculosis	★	★	★	★	★	★	★	★	★	★	★	★	★	★
Dyslipidemia		★		★	←	●	→	★	★	★	★	★		
Sexually Transmitted Infections							★	★	★	★	★	★	★	★
HIV							★	★	★	★	←	—	●	→
Cervical Dysplasia														
ORAL HEALTH	★	★												
Fluoride Varnish	►													
Fluoride Supplementation	★	★	★	★	★	★	★	★	★	★	★	★		
ANTICIPATORY GUIDANCE	●	●	●	●	●	●	●	●	●	●	●	●	●	●

BFNC 2019.PSMAR
3-351/0319

Courtesy of American Academy of Pediatrics.

TABLE 2.2 Dietary Reference Intakes[a]

DRI Populations and Life Stage Groups	Recommended Dietary Allowance (RDA)	Estimated Average Requirements (EARs)	Adequate Intake (AI)	Tolerable Upper Intake Level (UL)
• Pregnancy and lactation • Birth to 6 months • 7–12 months • 1–3 years • 4–8 years • 9–13 years • 14–18 years • 19–30 years • 31–50 years • 51–70 years • >70 years	Average daily dietary intake level sufficient to meet the nutrient requirement of most healthy individuals in a given life stage or gender group. May be used to evaluate nutrient intake of a given population (e.g., vegetarian).	Daily nutrient intake value estimated to meet the requirement of half the healthy persons in a given life stage or gender group (used to assess dietary adequacy and is the basis for RDAs).	Recommended intake value based on observed or experimentally determined approximations of nutrient intake by a group of healthy persons, which are assumed to be adequate when an RDA cannot be determined. In healthy breastfed infants (0–6 months), AI is the mean intake.[b]	Highest level of daily nutrient intake likely to pose no risk of adverse effects for most individuals in the general population. Risk increases as intake above the UL increases. May be used to set limits on nutrient supplementation, especially for vitamins and minerals that could be harmful.
Clinical Applications				
Potassium undetermined intake. b 400 mg/day[b] undetermined				
Sodium undetermined db. 110 mg/day[b] undetermined				
Infant 0–6 months (both sexes)				
Folate				
• Pregnant 19–30-year-old women	600 mcg/day	520 mcg/day	400 mcg/day[c]	1000 mcg/day
Iron				
• 4–8-year-old boys	10 mg/day	4.1 mg/day	10 mg/day	40 mg/day
Vitamin C				
• 16-year-old girls	65 mg/day	56 mg/day	65 mg/day	1800 mg/day

[a]Portions adapted from Dietary Reference Intakes (DRIs). *Food and Nutrition Board, Institute of Medicine, National Academy of Sciences*; 2004. Available at www.nap.edu; and Dietary Reference Intakes (DRI). *The essential guide to Nutrient Requirements Council Foundation, Institute of Medicine, National Academy of Sciences*; 2006. Available at www.nap.edu.
[b]National Academies of Sciences, Engineering, and Medicine. *Dietary Reference Intakes for Sodium and Potassium.* Washington, DC: The National Academies Press; 2019. Available at https://doi.org/10.17226/25353.
[c]Women of childbearing age and with expectation of becoming pregnant should consume 400 mcg/day from supplements or fortified foods, or both, in addition to intake of folate from a varied diet.
DRIs, Dietary reference intakes.
See also Unit 1 for select DRI values.

Task Force (USPSTF) concluded that there is a moderate benefit of preventing future dental caries with oral fluoride supplementation at recommended doses in children 6 months or older whose water supply is deficient in fluoride (see Community Focus on Fluoride Supplementation). In addition, it should be noted that deficient fluoride may be present in well water, and most purchased bottled water has suboptimal concentrations of fluoride unless fluoride was added and listed by the manufacturer. Fluoride supplementation is not required in children for the first 6 months because of the risk of dental fluorosis. USPSTF (2021) recommends that primary care clinicians prescribe oral fluoride supplementation starting at age 6 months for children whose water supply is deficient in fluoride.[c]

[c]US Preventive Services Task Force. Screening and interventions to prevent dental caries in children younger than 5 years: US Preventive Services Task Force Recommendation Statement. *JAMA.* 2021;326(21):2172–2178.

TABLE 2.3 Daily Estimated Calories and Recommended Servings for Grains, Fruits, Vegetables, and Dairy Products by Age and Gender

	1 Year	2–3 Years	4–8 Years	9–13 Years	14–18 Years
Kilocalories[a]					
Female	900 kcal	1000 kcal	1200 kcal	1600 kcal	1800 kcal
Male	900 kcal	1000 kcal	1400 kcal	1800 kcal	2200 kcal
Fat (% of total kcal)	30%–40%	30%–35%	25%–35%	25%–35%	25%–35%
Milk or dairy[b]	2 cups[c]	2 cups	2 cups	3 cups	3 cups
Lean Meat or Beans					
Female	1½ oz	2 oz	3 oz	5 oz	5 oz
Male	1½ oz	2 oz	4 oz	5 oz	6 oz
Fruits[d]					
Female	1 cup	1 cup	1½ cups	1½ cups	1½ cups
Male	1 cup	1 cup	1½ cups	1½ cups	2 cups
Vegetables[d]					
Female	¾ cup	1 cup	1 cup	2 cups	2½ cups
Male	¾ cup	1 cup	1½ cups	2½ cups	3 cups
Grains[e]					
Female	2 oz	3 oz	4 oz	5 oz	6 oz
Male	2 oz	3 oz	5 oz	6 oz	7 oz

[a]For children age 2 years and older. Nutrient and energy contributions from each group are calculated according to the nutrient-dense forms of food in each group (e.g., lean meats and fat-free milk).
[b]Milk listed is fat-free except for children younger than age 2 years. If 1%, 2%, or whole-fat milk is substituted, this will use, for each cup, 19, 39, or 63 kcal, respectively, of discretionary calories and add 2.6, 5.1, or 9 g, respectively, of fat, of which 1.3, 2.6, or 4.6 g, respectively, are saturated fat.
[c]For 1-year-old children, calculations are based on 2%-fat milk. If 2 cups of whole milk are substituted, 48 kcal of discretionary calories will be used. The American Academy of Pediatrics recommends that low-fat or reduced-fat milk not be started before age 2 years.
[d]Serving sizes are ¼ cup for age 1 year, ⅓ cup for ages 2 to 3 years, and ½ cup for age 4 years and older. A variety of vegetables should be selected from each subgroup over the week.
[e]Half of all grains should be whole grains.
Estimates are based on sedentary lifestyle. Increased physical activity requires additional calories by 0 to 200 kcal/day for moderately active children and 200 to 400 kcal/day for very physically active children.
Data from American Heart Association Editorial Staff and Reviewed by Science and Medicine Advisers. *Dietary recommendations for healthy children*; 2018. Available at https//www.heart.org>eat smart>nutrition-basics>di…; U.S. Department of Agriculture, U.S. Department of Health and Human Services. *Dietary Guidelines for Americans, 2020–2025.* 9th ed. December 2020. Available at DietaryGuidelined.gov.

Commercially Prepared Formulas

Commercially prepared formulas are altered from cow's milk by removing butterfat, decreasing the protein content, and adding vegetable oil and carbohydrate. The standard cow's milk–based formulas, regardless of the commercial brand, have essentially the same compositions of vitamins, minerals, protein, carbohydrates, and essential amino acids with minor variations, such as the source of carbohydrate, nucleotides to enhance immune function; and long-chain polyunsaturated fatty acids (LCPUFAs). Docosahexaenoic acid (DHA)- and arachidonic acid (AA)-containing formulas have shown improved brain function and visual acuity compared with formulas without DHA and AA. The US Food and Drug Administration regulates the manufacture of infant formula in the United States to ensure product safety. There are four main categories of commercially prepared infant formulas: (1) cow's milk–based formula, available in 20 kcal/fl oz as liquid (ready to feed), powder (requires reconstitution with water), or a concentrated liquid (requires dilution with water); (2) soy-based formulas, available commercially in ready-to-feed 20 kcal/fl oz or powder and concentrated liquid forms, commonly used for children who are lactose or cow's milk

COMMUNITY FOCUS

Fluoride Supplementation[a]

Age	FLUORIDE CONCENTRATION IN LOCAL WATER SUPPLY (PPM)		
	<0.3	0.3–0.6	>0.6
Birth to 6 months	0	0	0
6 months to 3 years	0.25[b]	0	0
3–6 years	0.50	0.25	0
6 years to at least 16 years	1	0.50	0

[a]Must know fluoride concentration in patient's drinking water before prescribing fluoride supplements.
[b]All values are milligrams of fluoride supplement per day.

From American Academy of Pediatric Dentistry. Fluoride therapy. In: *The Reference Manual of Pediatric Dentistry.* Chicago, IL: The American Academy of Pediatric Dentistry; 2021:302–305. From www.aapd.org/media/Policies_Guidelines/G_FluorideTherapy.pdf.

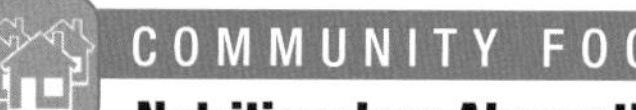

COMMUNITY FOCUS

Nutrition: Iron Absorption

To ensure that children receive an adequate supply of iron from foods, consider the following factors that may *increase* or *decrease* iron absorption:

Increase

Acidity (low pH)—Administer iron between meals (gastric hydrochloric acid)
Ascorbic acid (vitamin C)—Administer iron with citrus juice, fruit, or multivitamin preparation
Vitamin A
Tissue need
Meat, fish, poultry
Cooking in cast iron pots

Decrease

Alkalinity (high pH)—Avoid antacid preparations.
Phosphates—Milk is unfavorable vehicle for iron administration.
Phytates—Found in cereals
Calcium (e.g., dairy products, calcium supplement)
Oxalates—Found in fruits and vegetables (e.g., plums, strawberries, currants, green beans, spinach, rhubarb, sweet potatoes, and tomatoes)
Tannins—Found in tea, coffee
Tissue (cellular) saturation
Malabsorptive disorders
Disturbances that cause diarrhea or steatorrhea
Infection

protein intolerant; (3) casein- or whey-hydrolysate formulas, commercially available in ready-to-feed and powder forms and used primarily for children who cannot tolerate or digest cow's milk- or soy-based formulas; and (4) amino acid formulas available in powder form and designed for infants who are extremely sensitive to cow milk–based, soy-based, and partially hydrolyzed casein- and whey-based formulas.

A variety of formulas are manufactured for infants and children with special needs. A formula company representative provides books that describe the purpose and content of each formula for the medical provider and the parent or caregiver. The Child Care Food Program (2017) provides an approved infant formula list that is available: https://childrensnutritionofflorida.org/provider-resources/. The infant formula list is not inclusive because new formulas are continually being developed. The selection of the commercial prepared formula is based on a variety of factors (e.g., heath professional advice, availability, parent's preference and experience, infant's medical condition). The AAP (2020) review on the selection of infant formula is available at: https://publications.aap.org/pediatricsinreview/article-abstract/32/5/179/32831/Infant-Formulas?redirectedFrom=fulltext.

Proper Preparation, Handling, and Storage of Breast Milk (Human Milk) and Infant Formula (Instructions)

Prior to expressing breast milk or preparing formula, the individual must wash hands thoroughly with soap and warm water. If expressing human milk, ensure pump parts are thoroughly cleaned before use. If preparing formula, wash all equipment used to prepare the formula (including the cans of formula) with soap and water. Sterilizing bottles, caps, and nipples or other associated items may be done in a dishwasher or commercial home sterilizer or boiling water after each use and according to manufacture instructions.

It is essential to follow the manufacturer's instructions for preparing the formula to ensure the infant receives adequate calories and fluid for growth. Powdered and concentrated formula are prepared using boiled water, including bottled water, and then the formula is bottled and refrigerated, if not used immediately. Do not use a microwave to warm human milk or infant formula. Warm safely, if desired, by placing the sealed container of human milk or infant formula in a bowl of warm water or under warm running water.

Refrigerate freshly expressed human milk within 4 hours for up to 4 days. Previously frozen and thawed human milk should be used within 24 hours. Thawed human milk should never be refrozen. Any human milk or formula remaining in the bottle after feeding should be discarded because it is an excellent media for bacterial growth. Opened cans of ready-to-feed or concentrated formula are covered and refrigerated immediately until the next feeding. Parents should be cautioned not to alter the reconstitution or dilution of the infant formula except under the specific directions of the primary practitioner.

More information on storing and handling human milk is available at https://www.cdc.gov/breastfeeding/recommendations/index.htm. More information on storing and preparing powdered infant formula is available at cdc.gov/nutrition/downloads/prepare-store-powered-infant-formula-508.pdf. Additional information on how to clean, sanitize, and store infant feeding items is available at https://www.cdc.gov/hygiene/childcare/clean-sanitize.html.

Guidelines for Feeding During the First Year

Birth to 6 Months (Breast- or Bottle-Feeding)

Breast-Feeding

Breast milk is the most desirable complete diet for infants during the first 6 months after birth.[d] The AAP recommends breast-feeding until the infant is 1 year old or older with the gradual introduction of nutritionally adequate solid foods, especially iron-rich foods.[d] Breastfeeding is switched to whole cow's milk after 12 months of age or even later depending on the parents' preference.

In exclusively breastfed infants 4 months and older, an iron supplement of 1 mg/kg/day is recommended until iron-rich complementary foods are introduced. A supplement of oral vitamin D (400 International units/day) is also recommended.

Formula

Iron-fortified commercial formula is a complete food for infants during the first 6 months after birth, if breast-feeding is unavailable.[d] The AAP recommends iron-fortified formula be used for infants who are not breastfed or who are partially breastfed, from birth to 12 months of age with the gradual introduction of nutritionally adequate solid foods at approximately 4 to 6 months of age.[d] After 12 months of age, the commercial formula is switched whole cow's milk.

Formula-fed infants require fluoride supplements (0.25 mg) after age 6 months when the concentration of fluoride in the local water supply is less than 0.3 parts per million (ppm).

Evaporated milk formula requires supplements of vitamin C, iron, and fluoride (in accordance with the fluoride content of the local water supply) after age 6 months.

4 to 12 Months (Solid Foods)

Solids may be added by age 4 to 6 months.

First foods are strained, pureed, or finely mashed.

Finger foods such as teething crackers and raw fruit or vegetables can be introduced by age 6 to 7 months.

Chopped/cut table food or commercially prepared junior foods can be started by age 9 to 12 months.

With the exception of iron-rich cereal initially, the order of introducing foods is variable; a recommended sequence is strained fruit, followed by vegetables, then meat. However, some clinicians prefer to add vegetables before fruit.

Introduce one food at a time, usually at intervals of 4 to 7 days, to identify food allergies.

Introduce solid foods when the infant is hungry.

Begin spoon feeding by pushing food to back of tongue because infants' natural tendency is to thrust the tongue forward.

Use a small spoon with a straight handle; begin with 1 or 2 tsp. of food; gradually increase to 2 to 3 Tbsp. per feeding.

As the quantity of solids increases, decrease the quantity of formula to prevent overfeeding. Limit formula to approximately 960 mL (32 ounces) daily.

Juice should not be introduced into the diet of infant before 12 months of age unless clinically indicated, and intake of juice should be limited, at most, to 120 mL (4 ounces) daily to toddlers 1 through 3 years of age as recommended by the AAP.[d]

Never introduce foods by mixing them with the formula in the bottle.

Cereal—Start at 4 to 6 Months Old

Introduce commercially prepared, iron-fortified infant cereals, and administer daily until age 18 months.

Rice cereal is usually introduced first because of its low allergenic potential.

Parents may discontinue supplemental iron once iron-fortified cereal is given.

[d] Heyman MB, Abrams SA, Section on Gastroenterology, Hepatology, and Nutrition; Committee on Nutrition. Fruit juice in infants, children, and adolescents: current recommendations. *Pediatrics.* 2017;139(6):e20170967; Snetselaar LG, de Jesus JM, DeSilva DM, Stoody EE. Dietary guidelines for Americans, 2020–2025: understanding the scientific process, guidelines, and key recommendations. *Nutr Today.* 2021;56(6):287–295.

Fruits and Vegetables—Start at 6 to 8 Months Old

Apple sauce, bananas, and pears are usually well tolerated.

Avoid fruits and vegetables marketed in cans that are not specifically designed for infants, because of variable and sometimes high content and addition of salt, sugar, and/or preservatives.

Offer fruit juice only from a cup, not a bottle, to reduce the development of early childhood caries. Limit fruit juice to no more than 4 ounces per day with the introduction of fruit juice after 12 months of age.

Meat, Fish, and Poultry

Avoid fatty meats.

Prepare meats by baking, broiling, steaming, or poaching.

Include organ meats such as liver, which has a high iron, vitamin A, and vitamin B complex content.

If soup is given, be sure all ingredients are familiar to child's diet.

Avoid commercial meat and vegetable combinations because their protein content is low.

Eggs and Cheese

Serve egg yolk hard boiled and mashed, soft cooked, or poached.

Introduce egg white in small quantities (1 teaspoon) after the first year of age to detect an allergy.

Use cheese as a substitute for meat and as a finger food.

Developmental Milestones Associated With Feeding

Age (Months)	Development
Birth	Has sucking, rooting, and swallowing reflexes Feels hunger and indicates desire for food by crying; expresses satiety by falling asleep
1	Has strong extrusion reflex
3–4	Extrusion reflex fading Begins to develop hand-eye coordination
4–5	Can approximate lips to the rim of a cup
5–6	Can use fingers to feed self a cracker
6–7	Chews and bites May hold own bottle but may prefer for bottle to be held
7–9	Refuses food by keeping lips closed; has taste preferences Holds a spoon and plays with it during feeding May drink from a straw Drinks from a cup with assistance
9–12	Picks up small morsels of food (finger foods) and feeds self Holds own bottle and drinks from it Drinks from a cup without assistance but spills some Uses spoon with much spilling
12–18	Drools less Drinks well from a cup but may drop it when finished Holds cup with both hands Begins to use a spoon but turns it before reaching mouth
24	Uses straw Chews food with mouth closed and shifts food in mouth Distinguishes between finger foods and spoon foods Holds small cup in one hand; replaces cup without dropping Uses spoon correctly but with some spilling
36	Spills small amount from spoon Begins to use fork; holds it in fist Uses adult pattern of chewing, which involves rotary action of jaw
48	Rarely spills when using spoon Serves self-finger foods Eats with fork; held with fingers
54	Uses fork in preference to spoon
72	Spreads with knife

HEALTH PROMOTION 2

Immunizations

Keeping Current on Vaccine Recommendations

In the United States, two organizations, the Committee on Infectious Diseases of the American Academy of Pediatrics and the Advisory Committee on Immunization Practices (ACIP) of the Centers for Disease Control and Prevention, govern the recommendations for immunization policies and procedures. It is much easier to keep current if you know where to look for the official recommendations of the AAP and the Centers for Disease Control and Prevention's ACIP. The primary sources are publications and the Internet. You can also contact each organization at the following addresses to request information:

American Academy of Pediatrics
345 Park Boulevard
Itasca, IL 60143
Phone: 800/433-9016
Fax: 847/434-8000
Website: www.aap.org

Centers for Disease Control and Prevention
1600 Clifton Road
Atlanta, GA 30333
Phone: 404-639-3311
Information: 800-232-4636
Website: www.cdc.gov

Vaccine and immunization information: www.cdc.gov/vaccines

The AAP's *Report of the Committee on Infectious Diseases,* known as the *Red Book,* is an authoritative source of information on vaccines and other important pediatric infectious diseases. The Red Book (2021) recommends timely immunization of infants, children, adolescents, and adults, with ongoing immunization efforts to be maintained and strengthened.[e]

Because of constant changes in the pharmaceutical industry, trade names of single and combination vaccines in this section may differ from those currently available. The reader is encouraged to access the vaccine page of the Center for Biologics Evaluation and Research of the US Food and Drug Administration for the latest licensed vaccine trade names: http://www.fda.gov/BiologicsBloodVaccines/Vaccines/ApprovedProducts/ucm093833.htm.

[e] Report of the Committee on Infectious Diseases. Active and passive immunization. In: Kimberlin DW, Barnett ED, Lynfield R, Sawyer MH, eds. *Red Book 2021–2014: Report of the Committee on Infectious Diseases.* 32nd ed. Itasca, IL: American Academy of Pediatrics; 2021.

VACCINES APPROVED FOR IMMUNIZATION AND DISTRIBUTED IN THE UNITED STATES AND THEIR ROUTES OF ADMINISTRATION[A]

Vaccine	Type	Route of Administration
Anthrax	Inactivated[b]	IM or SC
BCG	Live bacteria	Percutaneous using multiple puncture device
Cholera	Live attenuated bacteria	Oral
COVID-19	mRNA, protein subunit, viral vector	IM
Dengue[c]	Live attenuated chimeric viruses	SC
Diphtheria-tetanus (DT, Td)	Toxoids	IM
DTaP	Toxoids and inactivated bacterial components	IM
DTaP, hepatitis B, and IPV	Toxoids and inactivated bacterial components, recombinant viral antigen, inactivated virus	IM
DTaP-IPV	Toxoids and inactivated bacterial components, inactivated virus	IM
DTaP, hepatitis B, Hib (*Haemophilus influenzae* type b), and IPV	Toxoids and inactivated bacterial components, recombinant viral antigen, polysaccharide-protein conjugate, inactivated virus	IM
Hepatitis A (HepA)	Inactivated virus	IM
Hepatitis B (HepB)	Recombinant viral antigen	IM
Hepatitis A-hepatitis B	Inactivated virus and recombinant viral antigens	IM
Hib (*Haemophilus influenzae* type b) conjugate (tetanus toxoid)	Bacterial polysaccharide-protein conjugate	IM
Hib conjugate (meningococcal protein conjugate)	Bacterial polysaccharide-protein conjugate	IM
Human papillomavirus (9vHPV)	Recombinant viral antigens	IM
Influenza (IIV)	Inactivated viral components	IM
Influenza (IIV)	Inactivated viral components	ID[d]
Influenza (LAIV)	Live attenuated viruses	Intranasal
Japanese encephalitis	Inactivated virus	IM
Meningococcal ACWY conjugate (MCV4 or MenACWY)	Bacterial polysaccharide-protein conjugate	IM

VACCINES APPROVED FOR IMMUNIZATION AND DISTRIBUTED IN THE UNITED STATES AND THEIR ROUTES OF ADMINISTRATION[A]—cont'd

Vaccine	Type	Route of Administration
Meningococcal serogroup B (MenB)	Bacterial recombinant protein	IM
MMR	Live attenuated viruses	SC
MMRV	Live attenuated viruses	SC
Pneumococcal polysaccharide (PPSV23)	Bacterial polysaccharide	IM or SC
Pneumococcal conjugate (PCV13)	Bacterial polysaccharide-protein conjugate	IM
Poliovirus (IPV)	Inactivated viruses	SC or IM
Rabies	Inactivated virus	IM
Rotavirus (RV1 and RV5)	Live attenuated virus	Oral
Tdap	Toxoids and inactivated bacterial components	IM
Tetanus	Toxoid	IM
Typhoid	Bacterial capsular polysaccharide	IM
Typhoid	Live attenuated bacteria	Oral
Varicella (VAR)	Live attenuated virus	SC
Yellow Fever	Live attenuated virus	SC
Zoster (HZ/su)	Recombinant viral antigens	IM

[a]Other vaccines approved in the United States but not distributed include adenovirus (types 4, 7), anthrax, smallpox, H5N1 influenza vaccines, influenza A (H1N1) monovalent 2009 vaccine, JE-virus vaccine (JE-VAX), pneumococcal conjugate vaccine (PCV7), HepB-Hib (Comvax), and bivalent HPV vaccine (Cervarix). The US Food and Drug Administration maintains a website listing currently approved vaccines in the United States (www.fda.gov/vaccines-blood-biologics/vaccines/vaccines-licensed-use-united-states). The American Academy of Pediatrics maintains a website (http://aapredbook.aappublications.org/news/vaccstatus.dtl) showing status of licensure and recommendations for newer vaccines.

[b]https://pediatrics.aappublications.org/content/133/5/e1411. Anthrax vaccine is not approved for use in children. Federal/state authorities would oversee emergency use under an investigational new drug application for children, should the need arise.

[c]Dengue vaccine is indicated only for individuals 9 through 16 years of age with laboratory confirmed prior dengue infection and living in areas with endemic infection.

[d]Intradermal influenza vaccine is recommended only for people 18 through 64 years of age.

BCG, Bacille Calmette-Guérin; *DT,* diphtheria and tetanus toxoids (for children younger than 7 years of age); *DTaP,* diphtheria and tetanus toxoids and acellular pertussis, adsorbed; *Hib, Haemophilus influenzae* type b; *HPV,* human papillomavirus; *ID,* intradermal; *IM,* intramuscular; *IPV,* inactivated poliovirus; *MMR,* live measles, mumps, rubella; *MMRV,* live measles, mumps, rubella, varicella (monovalent measles, mumps, and rubella components are not being produced in the United States); *PRP-T,* polyribosylribitol phosphate-tetanus toxoid; *SC,* subcutaneous; *Td,* diphtheria and tetanus toxoids (for children 7 years of age or older and adults); *Tdap,* tetanus toxoid, reduced diphtheria toxoid, and acellular pertussis.

Modified from American Academy of Pediatrics. Active and passive immunization. In Kimberlin DW, Barnett E, Lynfield R, Sawyer M, eds. *Red Book 2021–2024: Report of the Committee on Infectious Diseases.* 32nd ed. Itasca, IL: The Academy of Pediatrics; 2021.

Vaccine Hesitancy and Vaccine Refusal (Parents and Caregivers)

There is a growing issue of parental vaccine hesitancy or refusal that is identified as a top 10 threat to global health by the World Health Organization (WHO) (2019).[f] The WHO Strategic Advisory Group of Experts' Immunization Report on Vaccine Hesitancy described vaccine hesitancy as delay in acceptance or refusal of vaccines despite availability of vaccine services.[f] Vaccine hesitancy includes a broad spectrum of attitudes, beliefs, and behaviors regarding vaccine refusal and intentional vaccine delay.[g]

[f]Bianco A, Mascaro V, Zucco R, Pavia M. Parent perspectives on childhood vaccination: how to deal with vaccine hesitancy and refusal? *Vaccine.* 2019;37(7):984–990; Ryan J, Malinga T. Interventions for vaccine hesitancy. *Curr Opin Immunol.* 2021;71:89–91; Spencer JP, Trondsen Pawlowski RH, Thomas S. Vaccine adverse events: separating myth from reality. *Am Fam Physician.* 2017;95(12):786–794.

[g]World Health Organization (WHO). *Ten threats to global health in 2019*; 2019. Available at https://www.who.int/news-room/spotlight/ten-threats-to-global-health-in-2019.

Mass-media (e.g., social media, intranet, independent news outlets) represent a source used by parents to seek vaccine information that may contribute to vaccine hesitancy and refusal by providing inaccurate and incomplete information (e.g., misconceptions about vaccines, safety).[g]

Health care providers should inquire regarding the reasons why children are undervaccinated or unvaccinated and provide the parent or caregiver with reliable evidence-based vaccine information. It is imperative the health care provider improve parental trust in vaccinations not only by providing accurate vaccine information but emphasizing the important benefits of vaccination weighted against the unvaccinated risk. Additional research is needed to identify the most effective communication strategies to reduce vaccine hesitancy and vaccine refusal.

Since massive amounts of online vaccine misinformation have been identified in several studies, there are multiple credible information sources available on immunizations that are provided for clinicians and parents to correct false and misleading statements.[h] The Centers for Disease Control and Prevention offers a valuable online personalized resource tool for parents and clinicians. The vaccine assessment tool applies from birth to 18 years old; it asks a few pertinent questions, then lists vaccines the child may need based on the answers to the questions. Clinicians can use this tool for children to serve as a reminder for parents. Nurses should note that the personalized tool is based on the current immunization schedule and may need to be adjusted with the yearly updates from the AAP and the ACIP. The tool is available at www2a.cdc.gov.

A publication of the Centers for Disease Control and Prevention, *Morbidity and Mortality Weekly Report (MMWR),* contains comprehensive reviews of the literature and important background data regarding vaccine efficacy and side effects. An electronic copy of the vaccine data is available from the centers' website at www.cdc.gov.

Vaccine information statements (VISs) are available by calling your state or local health department. A wide variety of immunization information and resources for the public and health professionals can also be downloaded from the Immunization Action Coalition's website at www.immunize.org/vis or Centers for Disease Control and Prevention's website at www.cdc.gov. Some translations are available. Another resource to keep up to date on vaccines that are licensed and commercially available is the US Food and Drug Administration's Center for Biologics Evaluation and Research report for each year, which is available at www.fda.gov/BiologicsBloodVaccines/Vaccines/default.htm.

[h] Garrett R, Young SD. Online misinformation and vaccine hesitancy. *Transl Behav Med.* 2021;11(12):2194–2199.

Possible Side Effects of Recommended Childhood Immunizations and Nursing Responsibilities

Immunization	Reaction	Nursing Responsibilities
COVID-19	Well tolerated, mild side effects soreness and redness at injection site, fever, chills, tiredness, headache for 24-48 h usually after second dose	Advise parents of possible mild side effects. see general comments to parents.[a]
Hepatitis B virus	Well tolerated, few side effects Soreness at the injection site or fever. Vaccine prepared from yeast cultures	Explain to parents the reason for this immunization. Consider that cost for three injections may be a factor. If child has a yeast hypersensitivity, then consult with allergist prior to giving hepatitis B vaccine.
Diphtheria, tetanus, acellular pertussis (DTaP) or DTP Tetanus, diphtheria, acellular pertussis (Tdap)	Fever usually within 24–48 h Soreness, redness, and swelling at injection site Drowsiness, fretfulness, anorexia, vomiting, loss of consciousness, convulsions, persistent inconsolable crying episodes for 3 h or more, generalized or focal neurologic signs, rarely a fever (>40.5°C [105°F]), or systemic allergic reaction may occur. Reactions may have delayed onset and last several days, but gradually disappear. Reactions to DTap tend to be more severe if they occurred with previous vaccination Pain, erythema, or swelling at the injection site, mild fever, headache, fatigue, nausea, vomiting, diarrhea, or stomachache. Highly purified acellular vaccine is recommended because is associated with fewer local and systemic side effects.	Nursing responsibilities include explanation to parent's reason for DTaP or DTP and Tdap immunizations. Instruction regarding DTaP/DTP, Tdap on possible side effects and recommendation for prophylactic use of acetaminophen every 4–6 h × 3 doses. Advise parents to notify practitioner immediately of any unusual side effects, such as fever (temperature at or above 40.5°C [105°F]) within 48 h after vaccination; collapse or shock-like state within 48 h. after receiving dose of DTaP/DPT; seizures within 3 days of receiving dose of DTaP/DPT; Guillain-Barré syndrome within 6 weeks after receiving dose; or persistent, inconsolable crying lasting ≥3 h within 48 h after receiving dose of DTaP/DPT. Before administering next dose of DTaP/DPT/Td or Tdap inquire about any previous reactions, especially those listed above.
Haemophilus influenzae type b	Mild local reactions (erythema, pain, swelling) at injection site and fever	Advise parents of possible mild side effects. See general comment to parents.[a]
Poliovirus (IPV)	Mild local reaction (soreness, pain, erythema) at injection site Rare reactions possible Trace amounts of neomycin, streptomycin, and polymyxin B may be present in IPV	Advise parents of safety of IPV (i.e., no vaccine-associated polio paralysis with inactivated virus). Inquire regarding any documented anaphylactic reactions to neomycin. If so, then avoid the vaccine. See general comment to parents.[a]

Immunization	Reaction	Nursing Responsibilities
Measles, Mumps, Rubella (MMR)	Soreness, erythema at injection site. Anorexia, malaise, rash, and fever, lymphadenopathy, mild rash, or temporary joint stiffness and pain Rarely febrile seizures or temporary thrombocytopenia occur. Life-threatening in people with serious immune problems.	Advise parents of more common side effects, and recommend use of antipyretics (acetaminophen) for fever. If persistent fever with other obvious signs of illness occurs, have parents notify physician immediately. Advise parent's joint swelling and pain side effect; assure them that these symptoms will disappear. See general comment to parents.[a]
Varicella	Pain, tenderness, or redness at injection site Mild, vaccine-associated maculopapular or varicelliform rash at injection site or elsewhere	Advise parents of possible side effects. If necessary, recommend use of acetaminophen for pain. See general comment to parents.[a]
Hepatitis A	Soreness, redness at the injection site. Fever, headache, tiredness, or loss of appetite	Explain to parents and teens rationale for immunization. Encourage parents in high-risk areas to immunize children, especially teens and preteens.
Pneumococcal (PCV13 and PPSV23)	Soreness, erythema, swelling at the injection site. Fever, chills, fussiness, headache, decreased appetite, drowsiness, interrupted sleep, diarrhea, vomiting, and hives. Young children may be at increased risk for febrile seizure if PCV is given with inactivated influenza vaccine May develop muscle aches with PPV	Explain to parents benefits and rationale for vaccination in children younger than age 2 years and older than age 2 years if in high-risk category.
Meningococcal ACWY (serogroups A, C, W, Y)	Pain and erythema at injection site, fever, headache, fatigue, malaise, chills, anorexia, vomiting, diarrhea, rash	Explain to parents the benefits and rationale for immunization, especially in adolescents and in small children at higher risk for meningococcal disease.
Meningococcal B (serotype B	Soreness, erythema or swelling at injection site. Fever, chills, fatigue, headache, nausea, diarrhea, or muscle and joint pain	
Influenza	Inactivated vaccine (IIV)—Fever and local reactions (soreness, erythema, pain), fever, muscle aches, headache. Small risk of Guillain-Barre syndrome. Young children who obtain inactivated influenza vaccine along with pneumococcal vaccine may have slight increased risk of a febrile seizure Live-attenuated influenza vaccine (LAIV)—Fever, rhinitis, nasal congestion, runny nose, wheezing, headache, vomiting, muscle aches, cough, sore throat Same reactions may occur with H1N1 vaccines NOTE: Children with severe anaphylactic reaction to chicken or egg protein should not receive the inactivated influenza egg-based vaccine.	Explain to parents and adolescents rationale for vaccine; explain that the vaccine will not give the child a case of influenza. Influenza vaccine contains small amounts of egg protein. If a child has a severe allergy to egg, then consult an allergist to determine the best course of action
Human papillomavirus	Localized pain, swelling and erythema, fever or headache Syncope in adolescents	Explain to parents the benefit and rationale for immunization and necessity of completing vaccination series. Observe for 15 min after vaccine administration Vaccines should not be given to pregnant female, but may be given to lactating female HPV4 contains baker's yeast.[b]

(Continued)

Immunization	Reaction	Nursing Responsibilities
Rotavirus (RV1 [Rotarix] and RV5 [RotaTeq])	Irritability or temporary diarrhea, vomiting, runny nose and sore throat, ear infection, wheezing and coughing. RV1 oral applicator contains latex—avoid use in children with latex sensitivity. Children with known immunocompetence should be carefully evaluated for risk and benefits before administration of rotavirus vaccine. Slight risk of intussusception usually within a week after dose given. Multiple vaccines are in development to avoid cases of intussusception[c]	Explain to parent's rationale for immunization. Assess for latex exposure and allergy, presence of acute moderate-to-severe gastroenteritis at time of administration; preterm infants should receive age-appropriate dose of rotavirus vaccine prior to discharge from NICU or nursery.

[a]General comment to parents regarding each immunization: Benefit of being protected by immunization is believed to greatly outweigh risk from the disease.
[b]Adapted from Centers for Disease Control and Prevention (2022). Kroger A, Bahta L, Hunter P. (2022). General best practice guidelines for immunization. In: *Best Practices Guidance of the Advisory Committee on Immunization Practices (ACIP). Vaccine Recommendations and Guidelines of the ACIP*. Assessed from https://www.cdc.gov/vaccines/hcp/acip-recs/general-recs/.
[c]Cárcamo-Calvo R, Muñoz C, Buesa J, et al. The rotavirus vaccine landscape, an update. *Pathogens*. 2021;10(5):520. https://doi.org/10.3390/pathogens10050520
DTaP, Diphtheria-tetanus–acellular pertussis; *DTP,* diphtheria-tetanus-pertussis; *MMR,* measles-mumps-rubella vaccine; *Td,* Tetanus-diphtheria; *PCV13,* Pneumococcal Conjugate Vaccine; *PPSV23,* Pneumococcal Polysaccharide); *IIV,* inactivated influenza vaccine. Combination vaccines are available (see immunization schedule); *NICU,* neonatal intensive care unit; *Tdap,* tetanus toxoid, reduced diphtheria toxoid, and acellular pertussis (booster).
Modified from The Academy and Centers for Disease Control and Prevention. General recommendations on immunizations: recommendations of the Advisory Committee on Immunization Practices (ACIP). *MMWR Recommendations Rep*. 2011;60(2):1–61. Accessed on March 18, 2022 at http://www.cdc.gov/mmwr/pdf/rr/rr6002.pdf.

Safety and Injury Prevention

A home safety checklist can be presented to parents to increase their awareness of danger areas in the home and assist in implementing safety devices and practices before injury occurs.

Child Safety Home Checklist

Safety: Fire, Electrical, Burns

- Guards in front of or around any heating appliance, fireplace, or furnace (including floor furnace)[i]
- Electrical wires hidden or out of reach[i]
- No frayed or broken wires; no overloaded sockets
- Plastic guards or caps over electrical outlets; furniture in front of outlets[i]
- Hanging tablecloths out of reach, away from open fires[i]
- Smoke detectors tested and operating properly
- Matches and other lighters (e.g., butane) stored out of child's reach[i]
- Small stoves, heaters, and other hot objects (cigarettes, candles, coffee pots, slow cookers) placed where they cannot be tipped over or reached by children
- Hot water heater set at 48.9°C or lower
- Pot handles turned toward back of stove or toward center of table
- No loose clothing worn near stove
- No cooking or eating hot foods or liquids with child standing nearby or sitting in lap
- All small appliances, such as iron, turned off, disconnected, and placed out of reach when not in use
- Cool, not hot, mist vaporizer used
- Fire extinguisher available on each floor and checked periodically
- Electrical fuse box and gas shutoff accessible
- Family escape plan in case of fire practiced periodically; fire escape ladder available on upper-level floors
- Telephone number of fire or rescue squad and address of home with nearest cross street posted near phone

[i]Safety measures are specific for homes with young children. All safety measures should be implemented in homes where children reside and in homes they visit frequently, such as those of grandparents or babysitters.

Safety: Suffocation and Aspiration

- Small objects stored out of reach[i]
- Toys inspected for small, removable parts or long strings[i]
- Hanging crib toys and mobiles placed out of reach
- Plastic bags stored away from young child's reach; large plastic garment bags discarded after tying in knots[i]
- Mattress or pillow should not be covered with plastic or in such a way that is accessible to child[i]
- Crib designed according to federal regulations (crib slats <2.375 inches [6 cm] apart) with snug-fitting mattress[j]
- Crib positioned away from other furniture or windows[i]
- Portable play yard sides up and locked at all times while in use[i]
- Accordion-style gates not used[i]
- Bathroom doors kept closed, and toilet seats down[i]
- Faucets turned off firmly[i]
- Pool fenced with locked gate
- Proper safety equipment at poolside
- Electric garage door openers stored safely and garage door adjusted to rise when door strikes object
- Doors of ovens, trunks, dishwashers, refrigerators, and front-loading clothes washers and dryers kept closed[i]
- Unused appliance, such as refrigerators securely closed with lock or doors removed[i]
- Food served in small, noncylindric pieces[i]
- Toy chests without lids or with lids that securely lock in open position[i]
- Buckets and wading pools kept empty when not in use[i]
- Clothesline above head level
- At least one member of household trained in basic life support (cardiopulmonary resuscitation [CPR]) including first aid for infant choking and the Heimlich maneuver

Safety: Poisoning

- Toxic substances, including batteries, placed out of reach, preferably in locked cabinet
- Toxic plants hung or placed out of reach[i]
- Telephone number of local poison control center (800-222-1222) and home address with nearest cross street posted near phone
- Excess quantities of cleaning fluid, paints, pesticides, drugs, and other toxic substances not stored in home
- Used containers of poisonous substances discarded where child cannot obtain access
- Medicines clearly labeled in childproof containers and stored out of reach
- Household cleaners, disinfectants, and insecticides kept in their original containers, separate from food and out of reach
- Smoking only allowed in outside areas away from children and children play areas

Safety: Falls

- Nonskid mats, strips, or surfaces in tubs and showers
- Exits, halls, and passageways in rooms kept clear of toys, furniture, boxes, and other items that could be obstructive
- Stairs and halls well lit, with switches at both top and bottom
- Sturdy handrails for all steps and stairways
- Nothing stored on stairways
- Treads, risers, and carpeting in good repair
- Glass doors and walls marked with decals
- Safety glass used in doors, windows, and walls
- Gates on top and bottom of staircases and elevated areas, such as porch or fire escape[i]
- Guardrails on upstairs windows with locks that limit height of window opening and access to areas such as fire escape[i]
- Crib's side rails raised to full height; mattress lowered as child grows.[i]
- Restraints used in high chairs or other baby furniture, and wheeled walkers not used[i]
- Scatter rugs secured in place or used with nonskid backing
- Walks, patios, and driveways in good repair

Safety: Bodily Injury

- Knives and power tools stored safely and unloaded firearms stored safely in locked cabinet
- Furniture anchored so child cannot pull down on top of self when climbing or pulling to stand
- Garden tools returned to storage racks after use
- Pets properly restrained when appropriate and immunized for rabies
- Swings, slides, and other outdoor play equipment kept in safe condition
- Yard free of broken glass, nail-studded boards, and other litter
- Cement birdbaths placed where young child cannot tip them over[i]

[j] Federal regulations are available from the U.S. Consumer Product Safety Commission, 800-638-2772; http://(www.cpsc.gov).

Injury Prevention During Infancy

Injuries are a major cause of death during infancy, especially in children 6 to 12 months of age.

Constant vigilance, awareness, and supervision are essential as children gain increased locomotor and manipulative skills that are coupled with an insatiable curiosity about the environment.

Safety Promotion and Injury Prevention During Infancy

Birth to 4 Months Old

Major Developmental Accomplishments

Exhibits involuntary reflexes (e.g., crawling reflex may propel infant forward or backward; startle reflex may cause the body to jerk)

May roll over
Has increasing eye-hand coordination and voluntary grasp reflex

Injury Prevention

Aspiration

Aspiration is not as great a danger to this age group, but parents should begin practicing safeguarding early (see 4 to 7 Months Old).
Never shake baby powder directly on infant; place powder in hand and then on infant's skin; store container closed and out of the infant's reach.
Hold infant for feeding; do not prop bottle.
Know emergency procedures for choking.
Use pacifier with one-piece construction and loop handle.

Burns

Install smoke detectors in home.
Do not use microwave oven to warm formula; always check temperature of liquid before feeding.
Check bathwater.
Do not pour hot liquids when infant is close by, such as sitting on lap.
Beware of cigarette ashes that may fall on infant.
Do not leave infant in sun for more than a few minutes; keep exposed areas covered.
Wash flame-retardant clothes according to label directions.
Use cool-mist vaporizers.
Do not leave child in parked car.
Check surface heat of car restraint before placing child in seat.

Suffocation and drowning

Keep all plastic bags stored out of infant's reach; discard large plastic garment bags after tying in a knot.
Do not cover mattress with plastic.
Use firm mattress and loose blankets with no pillows.
Make certain crib design follows federal regulations and mattress fits snugly—crib slats 2.375 inches (6 cm) apart.[k]
Position crib away from other furniture and away from radiators.
Do not tie pacifier on a string around infant's neck.
Remove bibs at bedtime.
Never leave infant alone in bath.
Do not leave infant younger than 12 months old alone on adult or youth mattress or beanbag-type seats.

Motor vehicles

Transport infant in federally approved, rear-facing car seat, preferably in back seat.
Do not place infant on seat (of car) or in lap.
Do not place child in a carriage or stroller behind a parked car.
Do not place infant or child in front passenger seat with an air bag.
Do not leave infant unattended in car.

Falls

Use crib with fixed, raised rails.
Never leave infant alone on a raised, unguarded surface.
When in doubt as to where to place child, use floor.
Restrain child in infant seat, and never leave child unattended while the seat is resting on a raised surface.
Avoid using a high chair until child can sit well with support.

Accidental poisoning. Poisoning is not as great a danger to this age group, but parents should begin practicing safeguards early (see 4 to 7 Months Old).

Bodily damage

Keep sharp or jagged objects, such as knives and broken glass, out of child's reach.
Keep diaper pins closed and away from infant.

Four to 7 Months Old

Major Developmental Accomplishments

Rolls over
Sits momentarily
Grasps and manipulates small objects
Resecures a dropped object
Has well-developed eye-hand coordination
Can focus on and locate small objects
Has prominent mouthing (oral fixation)
Can push up on hands and knees
Crawls backward

Injury Prevention

Aspiration

Keep buttons, beads, syringe caps, and other small objects out of infant's reach.
Keep floor free of any small objects.
Do not feed infant hard candy, nuts, food with pits or seeds, or whole or circular pieces of hot dog.
Exercise caution when giving teething biscuits because large chunks may be broken off and aspirated.
Do not feed infant while he or she is lying down.
Inspect toys for removable parts.
Keep baby powder, if used, out of reach.
Avoid storing cleaning fluid, paints, pesticides, and other toxic substances within infant's reach.
Know telephone number of local poison control center (800-222-1222) (usually listed in front of telephone directory).

Suffocation

Keep all latex balloons out of reach.
Remove all crib toys that are strung across crib or play yard when child begins to push up on hands or knees or is 5 months old.

Burns

Keep water faucets out of reach.
Place hot objects (cigarettes, candles, incense) on high surface out of child's reach.
Limit exposure to sun; apply sunscreen.

---

[k]Information on many items such as cribs or walkers is available from US Consumer Product Safety Commission, 800-638-2772; http://www.cpsc.gov/.

Falls

Restrain in a high chair.
Keep crib rails raised to full height.

Motor vehicles See Birth to 4 Months Old.

Accidental poisoning

Make certain that paint for furniture or toys does not contain lead.
Place toxic substances on a high shelf or in a locked cabinet.
Hang plants or place on high surface rather than on floor.
Know telephone number of local poison control center (800-222-1222) (usually listed in front of telephone directory).

Bodily damage

Give toys that are smooth and rounded, preferably made of wood or plastic.
Avoid long, pointed objects as toys.
Avoid toys that are excessively loud.
Keep sharp objects out of infant's reach.

Eight to 12 Months Old

Major Developmental Accomplishments

Crawls or creeps
Stands holding on to furniture
Stands alone
Cruises around furniture
Walks
Climbs
Pulls on objects
Throws objects
Picks up small objects; has pincer grasp
Explores by putting objects in mouth
Dislikes being restrained
Explores away from parent
Increasingly understands simple commands and phrases

Injury Prevention

Aspiration

Keep small objects off floor, off furniture, and out of reach of children.
Take care when feeding solid table food to give very small pieces.
Do not use beanbag toys or allow child to play with dried beans.
See also 4 to 7 Months Old.

Bodily damage See 4 to 7 Months Old.

Avoid placing televisions or other large objects on top of furniture, which may be overturned when infant pulls self to standing position.

Falls

Avoid walkers, especially near stairs.[k]
Ensure that furniture is sturdy enough for child to pull self to standing position and cruise.
Fence stairways at top and bottom if child has access to either end.[k]
Dress infant in safe shoes and clothing (soles that do not "catch" on floor, tied shoelaces, pant legs that do not touch floor)

Suffocation and drowning

Keep doors of ovens, dishwashers, refrigerators, coolers, and front-loading clothes washers and dryers closed at all times.
If storing an unused large appliance, such as a refrigerator, remove the door.
Supervise contact with inflated balloons; immediately discard popped balloons and keep uninflated balloons out of reach.
Fence swimming pools and other bodies of standing water, such as decorative fountains; lock gate to swimming pools so that only adult can access.
Always supervise when near any source of water, such as cleaning buckets, drainage areas, toilets.
Keep bathroom doors closed.
Eliminate unnecessary pools of water.
Keep one hand on child at all times when in tub.

Accidental poisoning

Administer medications as a drug, not as a candy.
Do not administer medications unless prescribed by a practitioner.
Return medications and poisons to safe storage area immediately after use; replace caps properly if a child-protector cap is used.
Have poison control center number (800-222-1222) on telephone and refrigerator.

Burns

Place guards in front of or around any heating appliance, fireplace, or furnace.
Keep electrical wires hidden or out of reach.
Place plastic guards over electrical outlets; place furniture in front of outlets.
Keep hanging tablecloths out of reach (child may pull down hot liquids or heavy or sharp objects).

Injury Prevention During Early Childhood

Early childhood (ages 1 to 5 years) encompasses the unrestricted freedom of locomotion combined with an unawareness of danger within the environment that is associated with injuries. Specific categories of injuries and appropriate prevention are best understood by associating them with the major growth and developmental achievements of this age bracket on injury prevention during early childhood.

Developmental Abilities Related to Risk of Injury	Injury Prevention
Motor Vehicles	
Walks, runs, and climbs Able to open doors and gates Can ride tricycle Can throw ball and other objects	Use federally approved car restraint per manufacturer's recommendations for weight and height. Supervise child while playing outside. Do not allow child to play on curb or behind a parked car. Do not permit child to play in pile of leaves, snow, or large cardboard container in trafficked area. Supervise tricycle riding; have child wear helmet. Limit playing in driveways with parked cars or provide physical barriers limiting access. Lock fences and doors if not directly supervising children. Teach child to obey pedestrian safety rules: • Obey traffic regulations; cross only at crosswalks and only when traffic signal indicates it is safe. • Stand back a step from the curb until it is time to cross. • Look left, right, and left again, and check for turning cars before crossing street. • Use sidewalks; when there is no sidewalk, walk on the left, facing traffic. • Wear light colors at night, and attach fluorescent material to clothing.
Drowning	
Able to explore if left unsupervised Has great curiosity Helpless in water; unaware of its danger; depth of water has no significance	Supervise closely when near any source of water, including buckets. Never, under any circumstance, leave unsupervised in bathtub. Keep bathroom doors closed and lid down on toilet. Have fence around swimming pool and lock gate.[k]
Burns	
Able to reach heights by climbing, stretching, and standing on toes Pulls objects Explores any holes or opening Can open drawers and closets Unaware of potential sources of heat or fire Plays with mechanical objects	Turn pot handles toward back of stove. Place electric appliances, such as coffee maker and popcorn machine, toward back of counter. Place guardrails in front of radiators, fireplaces, and other heating elements. Store matches and cigarette lighters in locked or inaccessible area; discard carefully. Place burning candles, incense, hot foods, and cigarettes out of reach. Do not let tablecloth hang within child's reach. Do not let electric cord from iron or other appliance hang within child's reach. Cover electrical outlets with protective plastic caps. Keep electrical wires hidden or out of reach. Do not allow child to play with electrical appliance, wires, or lighters. Stress danger of open flames; teach what "hot" means. Always check bathwater temperature; adjust water heater temperature to 49°C (120°F) or lower; do not allow children to play with faucets. Apply a sunscreen when child is exposed to sunlight (all year round).

Developmental Abilities Related to Risk of Injury	Injury Prevention
Accidental Poisoning	
Explores by putting objects in mouth Can open drawers, closets, and most containers Climbs Cannot read labels Does not know safe dose or amount	Place all potentially toxic agents, including cosmetics, personal care items, cleaning products, pesticides, and medications, out of reach or in a locked cabinet. Caution against eating nonedible items, such as plants. Replace medications or poisons immediately in locked cabinet; replace child-guard caps promptly. Administer medications as a drug, not as a candy. Do not store large surplus of toxic agents. Promptly discard empty poison containers; never reuse to store a food item or other poison. Teach child not to play in trash containers. Never remove labels from containers of toxic substances. Know number of nearest poison control center: 800-222-1222.
Falls	
Able to open doors and some windows Goes up and down stairs Depth perception unrefined	Use window guards; do not rely on screens to stop falls. Place gates at top and bottom of stairs. Keep doors locked, or use childproof doorknob covers at entry to stairs, high porch, or other elevated area, including laundry chute. Ensure safe and effective barriers on porches, balconies, decks. Remove unsecured or scatter rugs. Apply nonskid decals in bathtub or shower. Keep crib rails fully raised and mattress at lowest level. Place carpeting under crib and in bathroom. Keep large toys and bumper pads out of crib or play yard (child can use these as "stairs" to climb out) and then move to youth bed when child is able to climb out of crib. Avoid using mobile walker, especially near stairs. Dress in safe clothing (soles that do not "catch" on floor, tied shoelaces, pant legs that do not touch floor). Keep child restrained in vehicle; never leave unattended in vehicle or shopping cart. Never leave child unattended in high chair. Supervise at playgrounds; select play areas with soft ground cover and safe equipment.
Choking and Suffocation	
Puts things in mouth May swallow hard or inedible pieces of food	Avoid large, round chunks of meat, such as whole hot dogs (slice lengthwise into short pieces). Avoid fruit with pits, fish with bones, hard candy, chewing gum, nuts, popcorn, grapes, and marshmallows. Choose large, sturdy toys without sharp edges or small removable parts. Discard old refrigerators, ovens, and so on, and remove the door. Install smoke and carbon monoxide alarms; change batteries every 6 months. Develop a fire escape plan for the entire family, and have drills. Keep automatic garage door transmitter in an inaccessible place. Select safe toy boxes or chests without heavy, hinged lids. Keep venetian blind cords out of child's reach. Remove drawstrings from clothing; shorten essential drawstrings to 15.24 cm (6 inches) or less. Avoid contact with round, hollow, semirigid plastic items such as half of a plastic ball.

Developmental Abilities Related to Risk of Injury	Injury Prevention
Bodily Injury	
Still clumsy in many skills Easily distracted from tasks Unaware of potential danger from strangers or other people	Avoid giving sharp or pointed objects (e.g., knives, scissors, toothpicks), especially when walking or running. Do not allow lollipops or similar objects in mouth when walking or running. Teach safety precautions (e.g., to carry knife or scissors with pointed end away from face). Store all dangerous tools, garden equipment, and firearms in locked cabinet. Be alert to danger of unsupervised animals and household pets. Use safety glass on large glassed areas, such as sliding glass doors. Teach child name, address, and phone number and to ask for help from appropriate people (cashier, security guard, police officer) if lost; have identification on child (sewn in clothes, inside shoe). Teach stranger safety: • Avoid personalized clothing in public places. • Never go with a stranger. • Tell parents if anyone makes child feel uncomfortable in any way. • Always listen to child's concerns regarding others' behavior. • Teach child to say "no" when confronted with uncomfortable situations

Injury Prevention During School-Age Years

School-age children have developed refined muscular coordination and control and can apply their cognitive capacities to their behavior; however, their injuries usually depend on environmental dangers, adult protection, and child's behavior patterns. The section Family-Centered Care provides safety guidelines for bicycle, skateboard, inline skate, and scooter guidance during the school years.

Developmental Abilities Related to Risk of Injury	Injury Prevention
Motor Vehicle Accidents	
Is increasingly involved in activities away from home Is excited by speed and motion Is easily distracted by environment Can be reasoned with	Educate child on proper use of seat belts while a passenger in a vehicle. Maintain discipline while the child is a passenger in a vehicle (e.g., ensure that children keep arms inside, do not lean against doors, and do not interfere with driver). Remind parents and children that no one should ride in the bed of a pickup truck. Emphasize safe pedestrian behavior. Insist on child wearing safety apparel (e.g., helmet) when applicable, such as while riding bicycle, motorcycle, moped, or all-terrain vehicle (ATV) (see Family-Centered Care).
Drowning	
Is apt to overdo May work hard to perfect a skill Has cautious, but not fearful, gross motor actions Likes swimming	Teach child to swim. Teach basic rules of water safety. Select safe and supervised places to swim. Check sufficient water depth for diving. Caution child to swim with a companion. Ensure that child uses an approved flotation device in water or boat. Advocate for legislation requiring fencing around pools. Learn cardiopulmonary resuscitation.

Developmental Abilities Related to Risk of Injury	Injury Prevention
Burns	
Has increasing independence Is adventurous Enjoys trying new things	Make certain home has smoke detectors. Set water heaters to 48.9°C (120°F) to avoid scald burns. Instruct child on behavior in areas involving contact with potential burn hazards (e.g., gasoline, matches, bonfires or barbecues, lighter fluid, firecrackers, cigarette lighters, cooking utensils, chemistry sets). Instruct child to avoid climbing or flying kite around high-tension wires. Instruct child in proper behavior in the event of fire (e.g., fire drills at home and school). Teach child safe cooking (use low heat; avoid any frying; be careful of steam burns, scalds, or exploding foods, especially from microwaving).
Poisoning	
Adheres to group rules May be easily influenced by peers Has strong allegiance to friends	Educate child on hazards of taking nonprescription drugs and chemicals, including aspirin and alcohol. Teach child to say "no" if offered illegal or dangerous drugs or alcohol. Keep potentially dangerous products in properly labeled receptacles, preferably out of reach.
Bodily Damage	
Has increased physical skills Needs strenuous physical activity Is interested in acquiring new skills and perfecting attained skills Is daring and adventurous, especially with peers Frequently plays in hazardous places Confidence often exceeds physical capacity Desires group loyalty and has strong need for friends' approval Delights in physical activity Attempts hazardous feats Accompanies friends to potentially hazardous facilities Is likely to overdo Growth in height exceeds muscular growth and coordination	Help provide facilities for supervised activities. Encourage playing in safe places. Keep firearms safely locked up except under adult supervision. Teach proper care of, use of, and respect for potentially dangerous devices (e.g., power tools, firecrackers). Teach children not to tease or surprise dogs, invade their territory, take dogs' toys, or interfere with dogs' feeding. Stress use of eye, ear, or mouth protection when using potentially hazardous objects or devices or when engaging in potentially hazardous sports. Do not permit use of trampolines except as part of supervised training. Teach safety regarding use of corrective devices (glasses); if child wears contact lenses, monitor duration of wear to prevent corneal damage. Stress careful selection, use, and maintenance of sports and recreation equipment, such as skateboards and inline skates (see Family-Centered Care). Emphasize proper conditioning, safe practices, and use of safety equipment for sports or recreational activities. Caution against engaging in hazardous sports, such as those involving trampolines. Use safety glass and decals on large glassed areas, such as sliding glass doors. Use window guards to prevent falls. Teach name, address, and phone number, and emphasize that child should ask for help from appropriate people (e.g., cashier, security guard, police) if lost; have identification on child (e.g., sewn in clothes, inside shoe).

Developmental Abilities Related to Risk of Injury	Injury Prevention
	Teach safety and stranger safety: • Avoid personalized clothing in public places. • Never go with a stranger. • Have child tell parents if anyone makes child feel uncomfortable in any way. • Teach child to say "no" when confronted by uncomfortable situations. • Always listen to child's concerns regarding others' behavior.

Family-Centered Care

Bicycle Safety

- Always wear a properly fitted bicycle helmet that is approved by the US Consumer Product Safety Commission; replace a damaged or outgrown helmet.
- Ride bicycles with traffic and away from parked cars.
- Ride single file.
- Walk bicycles through busy intersections only at crosswalks.
- Give hand signals well in advance of turning or stopping.
- Keep as close to the curb as practical.
- Watch for drain grates, potholes, soft shoulders, loose dirt, and gravel.
- Keep both hands on handlebars except when signaling.
- Never ride double on a bicycle.
- Do not carry packages that interfere with vision or control; do not drag objects behind a bike.
- Watch for and yield to pedestrians.
- Watch for cars backing up or pulling out of driveways; be especially careful at intersections.
- Look left, right, and then left before turning into traffic or roadway.
- Never hitch a ride on a truck or other vehicle.
- Learn rules of the road and respect for traffic officers.
- Obey all local ordinances.
- Wear shoes that fit securely while riding.
- Wear light colors at night and attach fluorescent material to clothing and bicycle.
- Equip the bicycle with proper lights and reflectors.
- Be certain the bicycle is the correct size for rider.
- Equip the bicycle with proper lights and reflectors.
- Children riding as passengers must wear appropriate-size helmets and sit in specially designed protective seats.

Data from Brudvik C. Injuries caused by small wheel devices. *Prev Sci.* 2006;7:313–320; and American Academy of Pediatrics, Committee on Injury and Poison Prevention. In-line skating injuries in children and adolescents. *Pediatrics.* 2009;123(5):1421–1422.

Skateboard, Inline Skate, and Scooter Safety

- Children younger than 5 years old should not use skateboards or inline skates because they are not developmentally prepared to protect themselves from injury. Children ages 6 to 10 years should use these only with close adult supervision.
- The age when children are ready to use inline skates safely is not known because of differences in the ability to acquire the skills needed to participate in the sport. Novice skaters should learn indoors on a flat, smooth surface. Children who ride skateboards, inline skates, or scooters should wear helmets and other protective equipment, especially on their knees, wrists, and elbows, to prevent injury.
- Skateboards, inline skates, and scooters should never be used near traffic or in streets. Their use should be prohibited on streets and highways. Activities that bring skateboards together (e.g., "catching a ride") are especially dangerous.
- Some types of use, such as riding homemade ramps on hard surfaces, may be particularly hazardous.

Injury Prevention During Adolescence

Injuries account for substantial morbidity among adolescents. Their propensity for risk-taking behavior plus feelings of indestructibility make adolescents especially prone to injuries. The leading causes of injury-related morbidity among adolescents include vehicular crashes, firearms, drowning, poisoning, burns, and falls. Unintentional vehicle injuries and death are highest injury among teens that are often associated with texting, talking on phone, lack of experience, driving too fast,

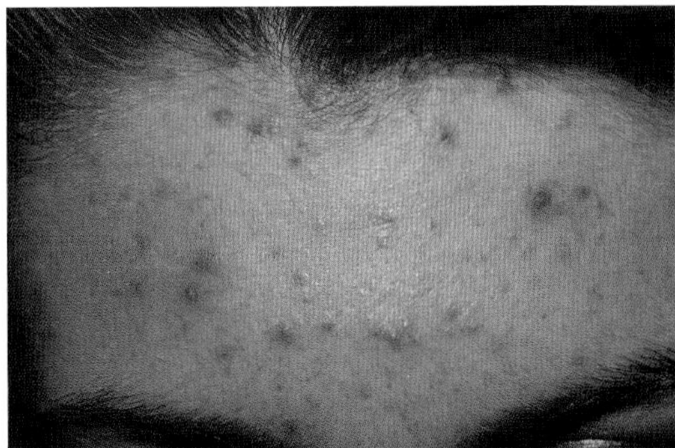

FIG. **1** Acne vulgaris. (From Weston WL. *Color Textbook of Pediatric Dermatology*. 4th ed. Philadelphia: Mosby; 2007.)

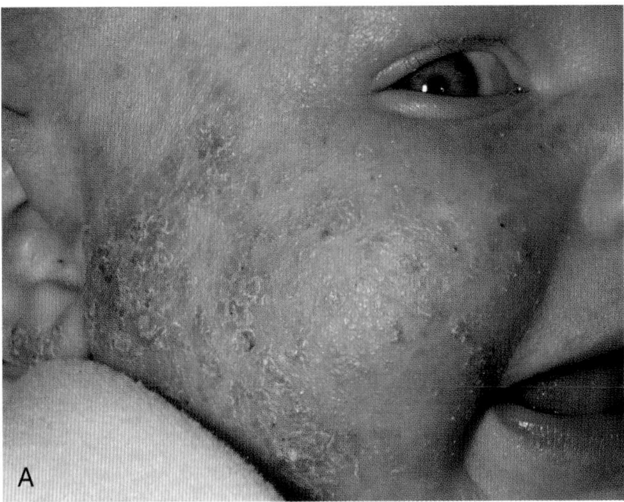

FIG. **2A** Atopic dermatitis. (From Habif T. *Clinical Dermatology: A Color Guide to Diagnosis and Therapy*. 5th ed. Philadelphia: Mosby; 2010.)

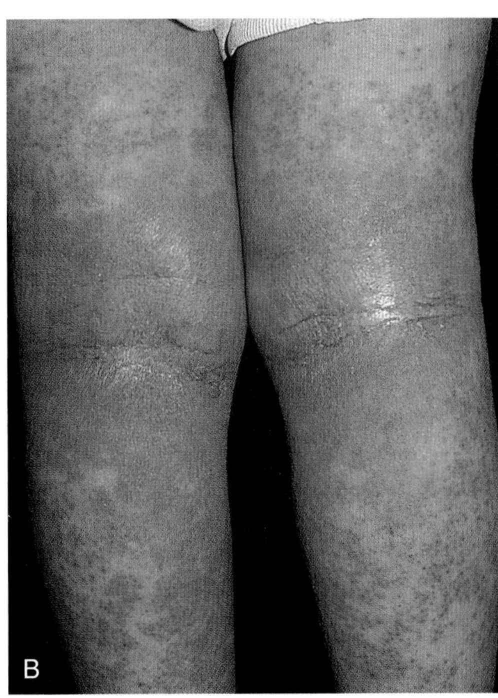

FIG. **2B** Atopic dermatitis. (From White GM, Cox NH. *Diseases of the Skin: A Color Atlas and Text*. 2nd ed. Edinburgh: Mosby; 2006.)

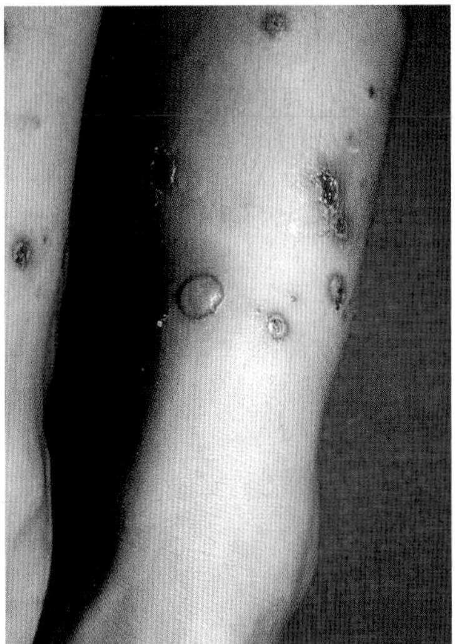

FIG. **3** Bullous Impetigo. (From James WD, Berger TG, Elston DM. *Andrews' Diseases of the Skin: Clinical Dermatology*. 10th ed. Edinburgh: Saunders; 2006.)

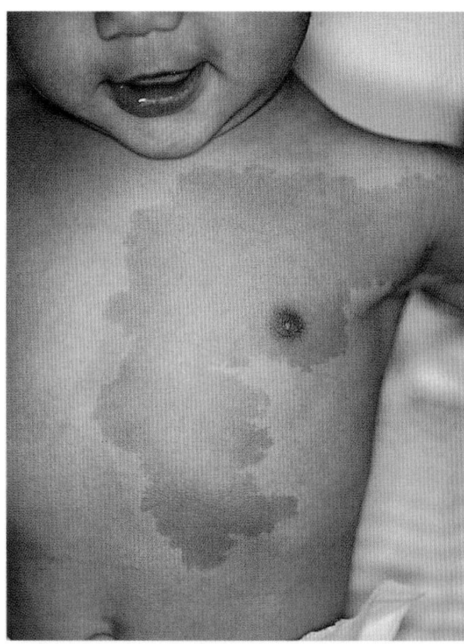

FIG. **4** Café-au-lait spots. (From Eichenfield LF, Frieden IJ, Esterly NB. *Neonatal Dermatology*. 2nd ed. Philadelphia: Saunders; 2008.)

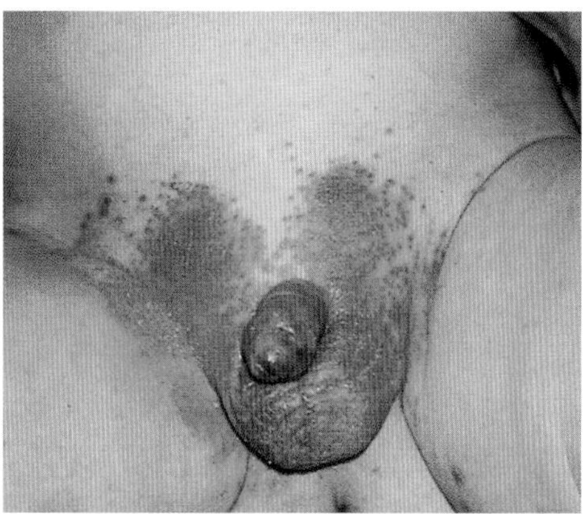

FIG. **5** Candidiasis. (From Feigin RD, Cherry D, eds. *Textbook of Pediatric Infectious Diseases*. 6th ed. Philadelphia: Saunders; 2009.)

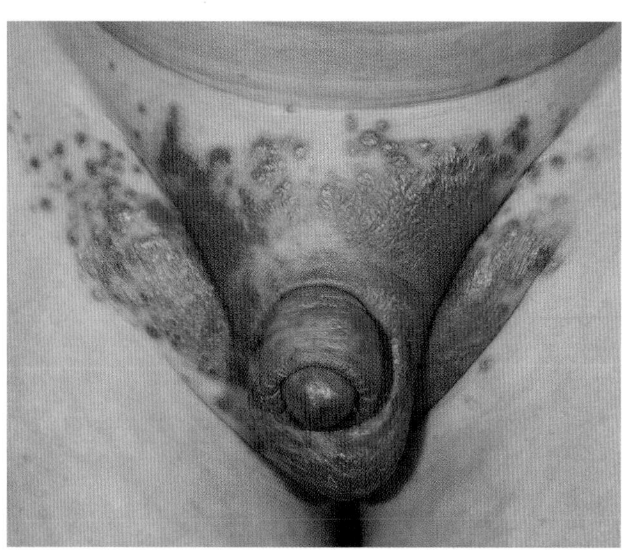

FIG. **6** Diaper dermatitis. (From Habif T. *Clinical Dermatology: A Color Guide to Diagnosis and Therapy*. 5th ed. Philadelphia: Mosby; 2010.)

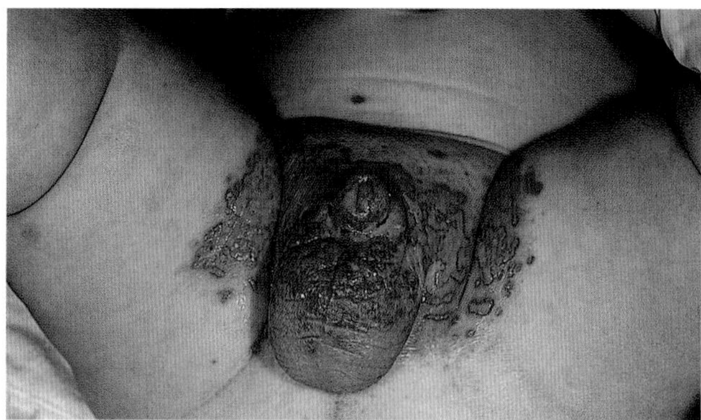

FIG. **7** Herpes simplex. (From Callen JP, Greer KE, Paller AS, Swinyer LJ. *Color Atlas of Dermatology*. 2nd ed. Philadelphia; Saunders; 2000.)

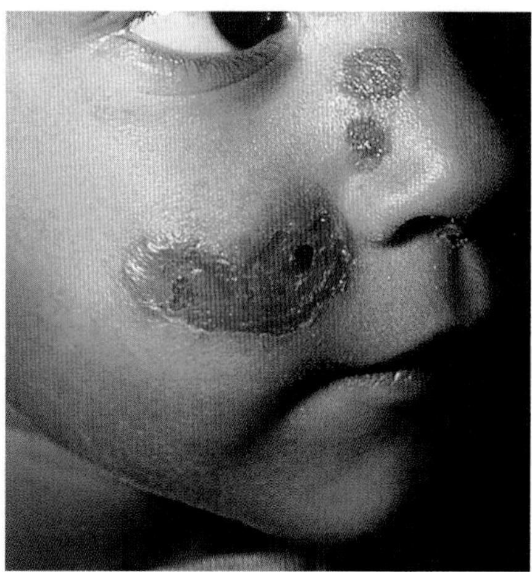

FIG. **8** Impetigo. (From James WD, Berger TG, Elston DM. *Andrews' Diseases of the Skin: Clinical Dermatology*. 10th ed. Edinburgh: Saunders; 2006.)

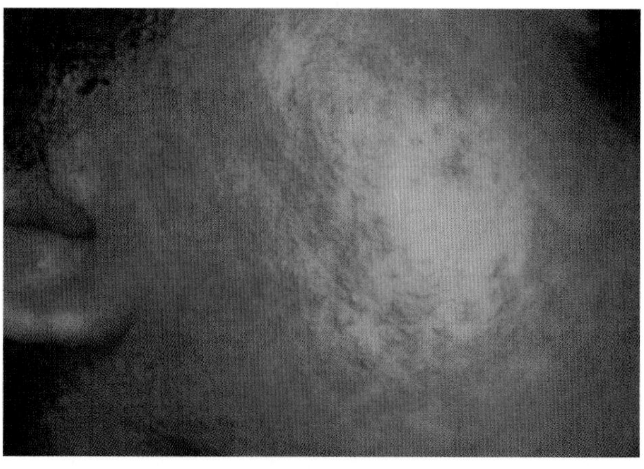

Measles Rash

FIG. **9** Measles. (From Feigin RD, Cherry D, eds. *Textbook of Pediatric Infectious Diseases*. 6th ed. Philadelphia: Saunders; 2009.)

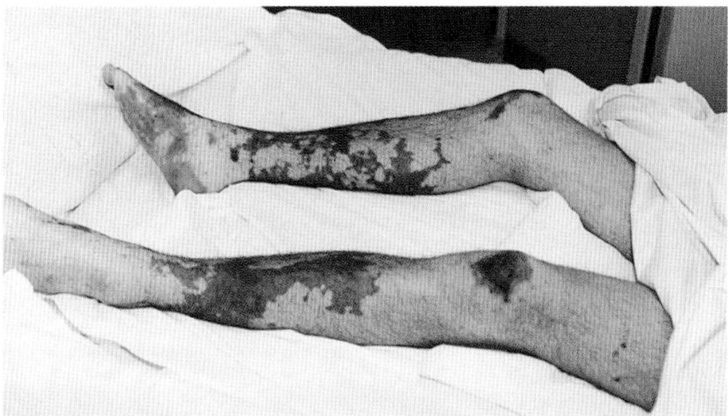

FIG. **10** Meningococcemia. (From Hockenberry MJ, Wilson D. *Wong's Nursing Care of Infants and Children*. 9th ed. St Louis: Mosby; 2010.)

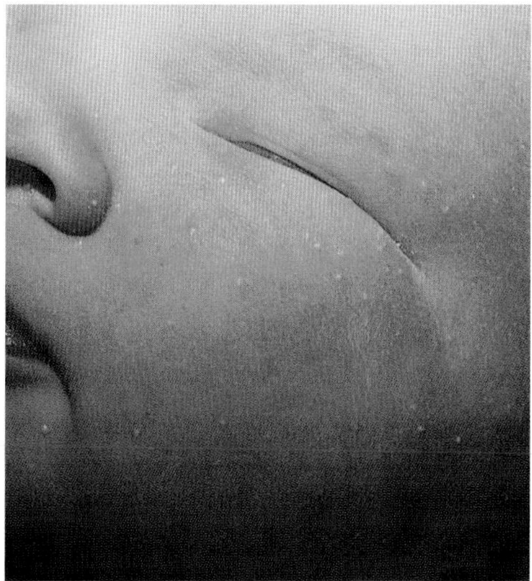

FIG. **11** Milia. (From White GM, Cox NH. *Diseases of the Skin: A Color Atlas and Text*. 2nd ed. Edinburgh: Mosby; 2006.)

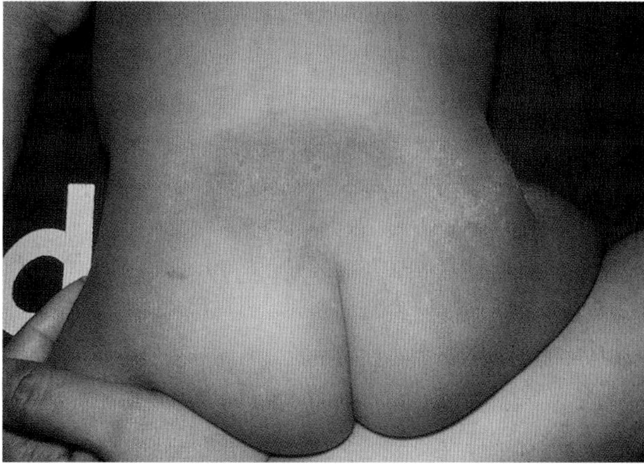

FIG. **12** Mongolian spot. (From Swartz MH. *Textbook of Physical Diagnosis: History and Examination*. 6th ed. Philadelphia: Saunders; 2009.)

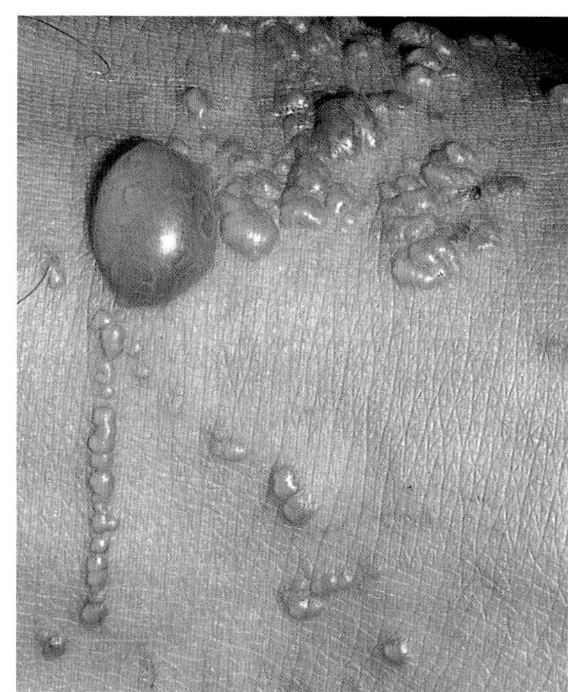

FIG. **13** Poison ivy. (From Habif T. *Clinical Dermatology: A Color Guide to Diagnosis and Therapy.* 5th ed. Philadelphia: Mosby; 2010.)

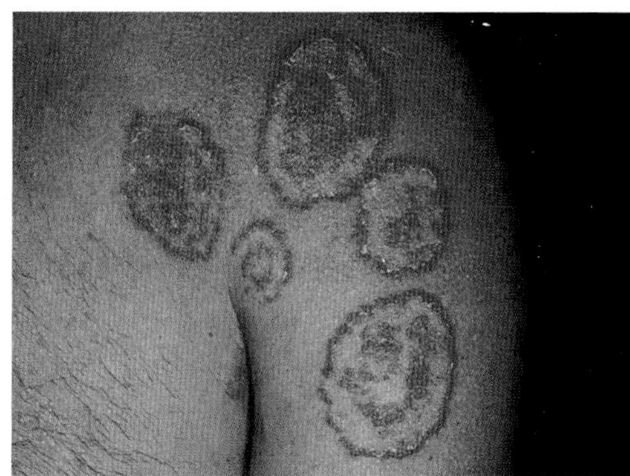

FIG. **14** Ringworm. (From Callen JP, Greer KE, Paller AS, Swinyer LJ. *Color Atlas of Dermatology*. 2nd ed. Philadelphia: Saunders; 2000.)

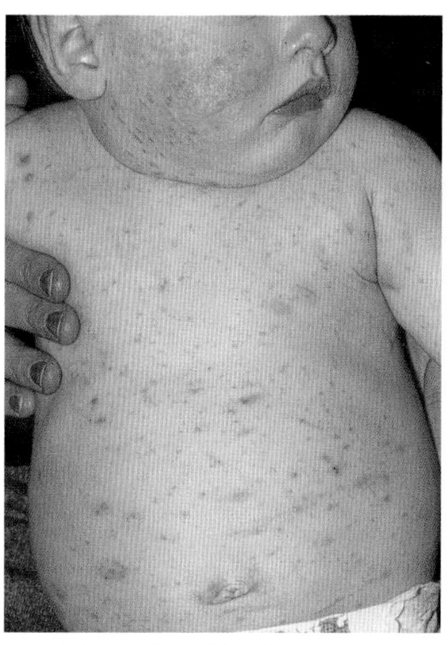

FIG. **15** Scabies. (From White GM, Cox NH. *Diseases of the Skin: A Color Atlas and Text*. 2nd ed. Edinburgh: Mosby; 2006.)

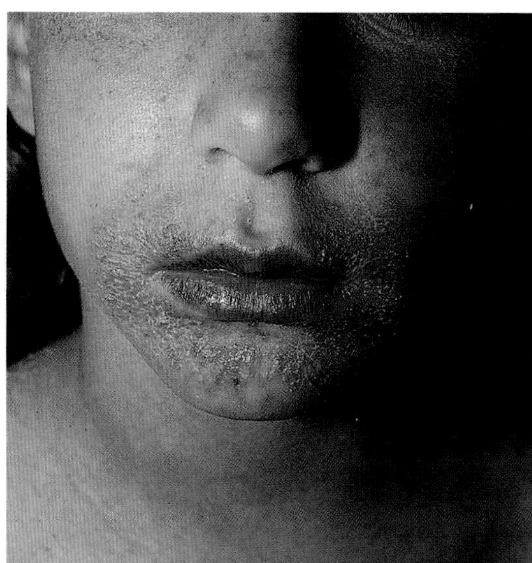

FIG. **16** Scalded skin syndrome. (From Callen JP, Greer KE, Paller AS, Swinyer LJ. *Color Atlas of Dermatology*. 2nd ed. Philadelphia: Saunders; 2000.)

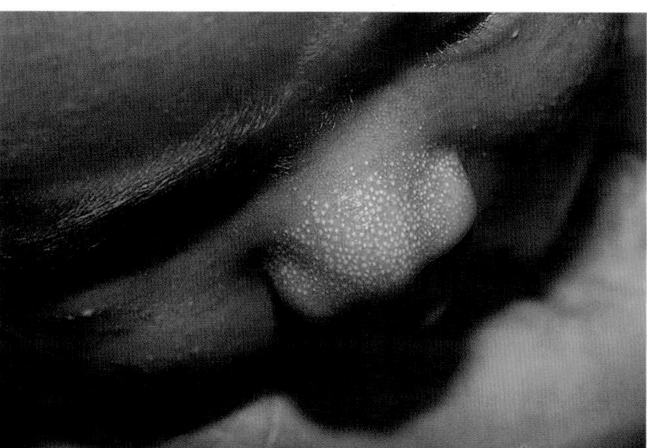

FIG. **17** Sebaceous gland hyperplasia. (From White GM, Cox NH. *Diseases of the Skin: A Color Atlas and Text*. 2nd ed. Edinburgh: Mosby; 2006.)

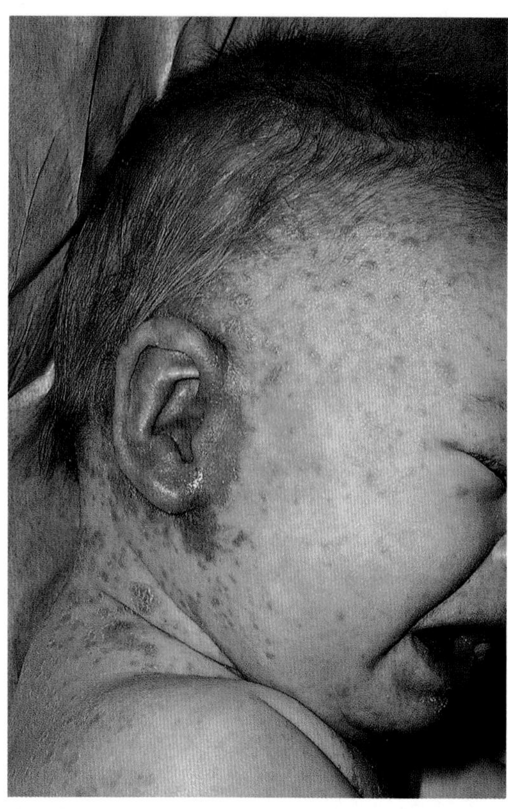

FIG. **18** Seborrheic dermatitis. (From Habif T. *Clinical Dermatology: A Color Guide to Diagnosis and Therapy*. 5th ed. Philadelphia: Mosby; 2010.)

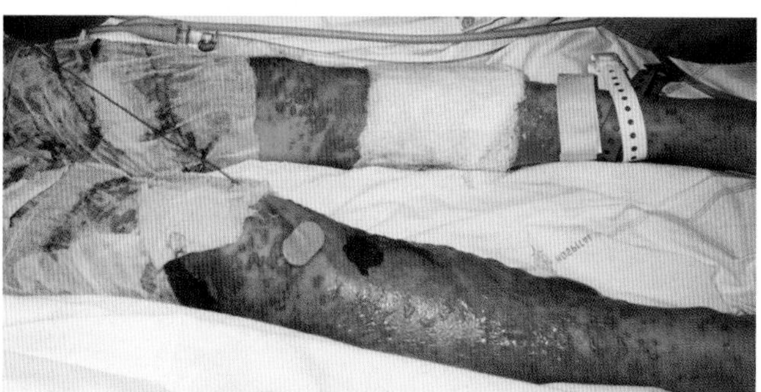

FIG. **19** Stevens–Johnson syndrome. (From Hockenberry MJ, Wilson D. *Wong's Nursing Care of Infants and Children*. 9th ed. St Louis: Mosby; 2010.)

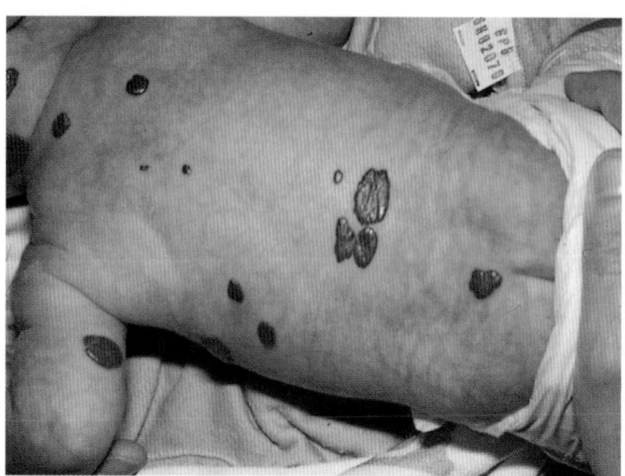

FIG. **20** Strawberry hemangioma. (From Zitelli BJ, Davis HW. *Atlas of Pediatric Physical Diagnosis*. 5th ed. St Louis: Mosby; 2007.)

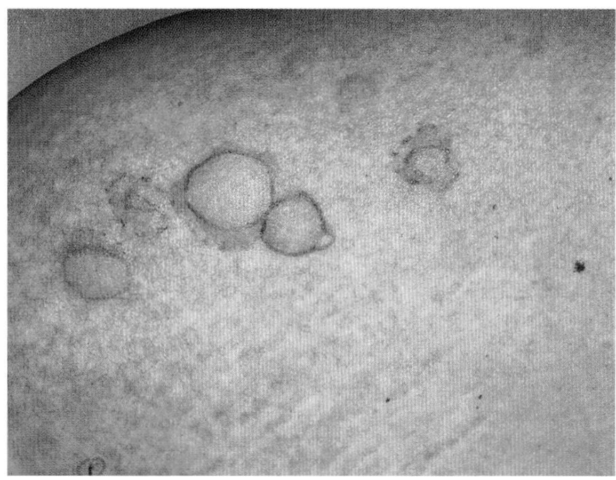

FIG. **21** Urticaria. (From White GM, Cox NH. *Diseases of the Skin: A Color Atlas and Text*. 2nd ed. Edinburgh: Mosby; 2006.)

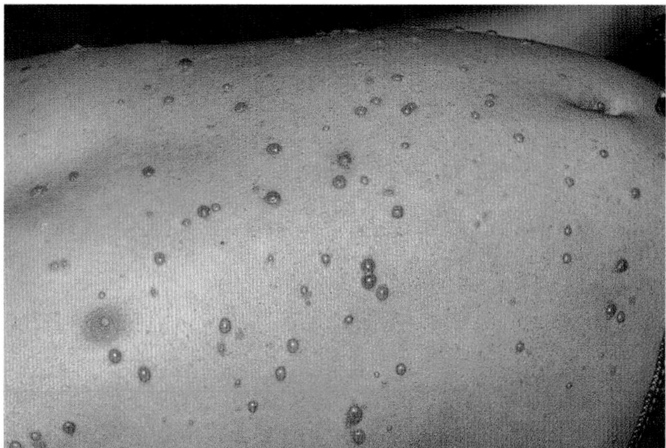

FIG. **22** Varicella zoster. (From White GM, Cox NH. *Diseases of the Skin: A Color Atlas and Text*. 2nd ed. Edinburgh: Mosby; 2006.)

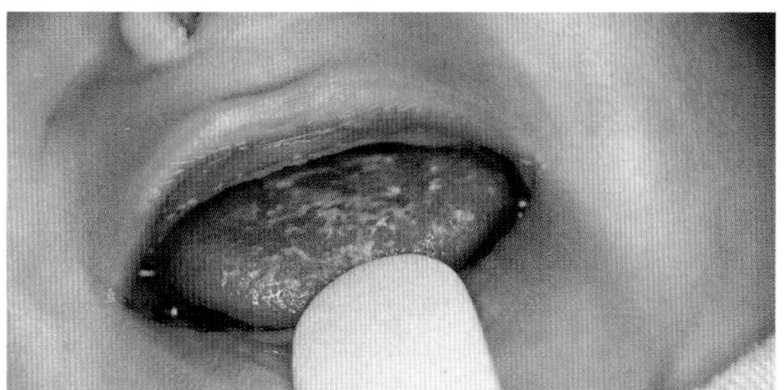

FIG. **23** White patches on the tongue in an infant with thrush. (Reprinted with permission from Morelli JG, Torres-Zegarra C. *Pediatric Dermatology*. 3rd ed. St Louis: Elsevier; 2021.)

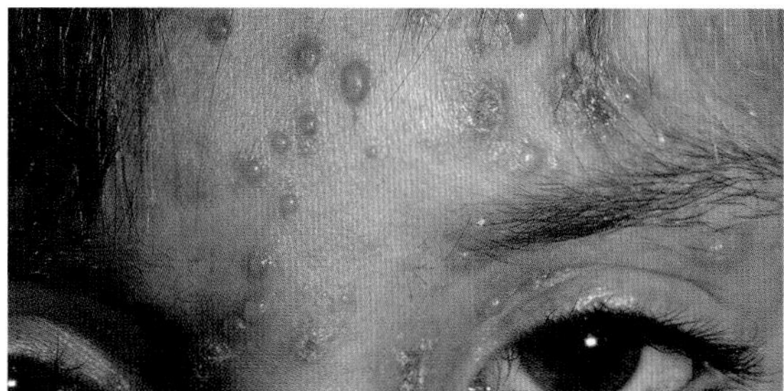

FIG. **24** Varicella. Multiple discrete vesicles and crusted lesion on a child's face. (Reprinted with permission from Morelli JG, Torres-Zegarra C. *Pediatric Dermatology*. 3rd ed. St Louis: Elsevier; 2021.)

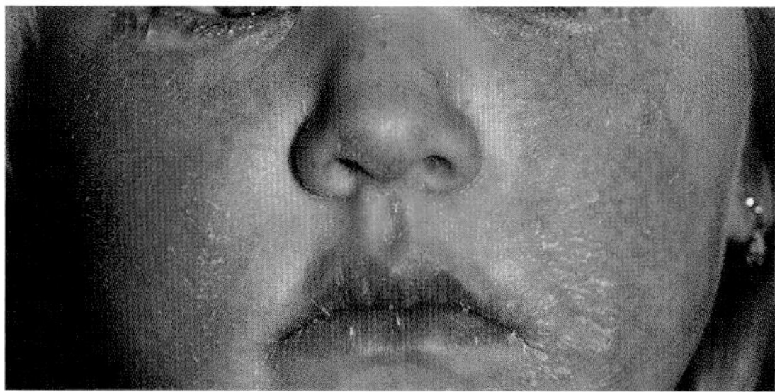

FIG. **25** Child with Staphylococcus scaled skin syndrome. Painful red cheeks with initial perioral crusting. (Reprinted with permission from Morelli JG, Torres-Zegarra C. *Pediatric Dermatology*. 3rd ed. St Louis: Elsevier; 2021.)

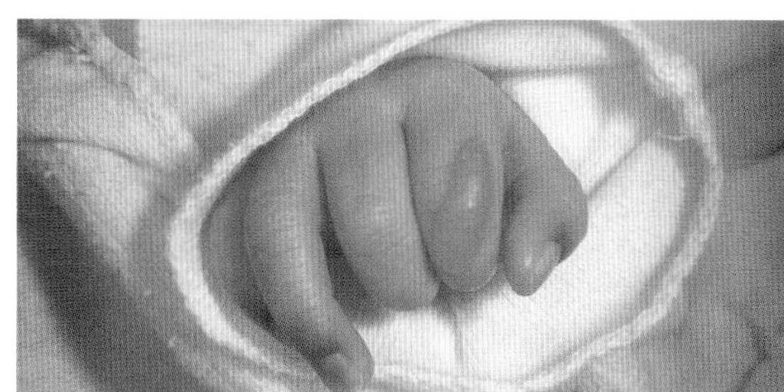

FIG. **26** Sucking blister. Oral noninflammatory blister on a finger of a newborn. (Reprinted with permission from Morelli JG, Torres-Zegarra C. *Pediatric Dermatology*. 3rd ed. St Louis: Elsevier; 2021.)

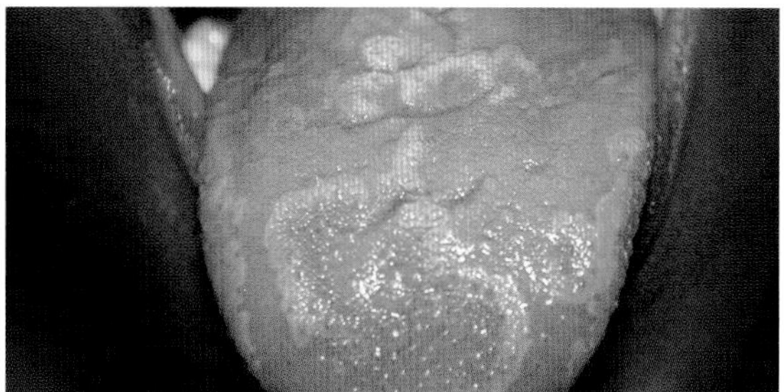

FIG. **27** Geographic tongue. Raised gray borders delineate smooth, pink areas of a child's tongue. (Reprinted with permission from Morelli JG, Torres-Zegarra C. *Pediatric Dermatology*. 3rd ed. St Louis: Elsevier; 2021.)

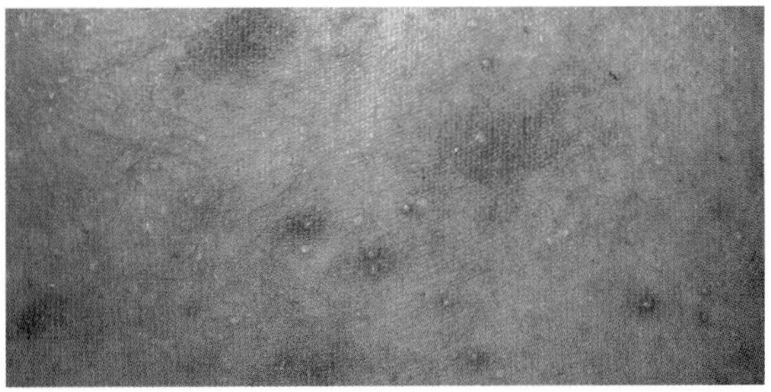

FIG. **28** Erythema toxicum. Red macules, papules, and pustules in a newborn. (Reprinted with permission from Morelli JG, Torres-Zegarra C. *Pediatric Dermatology*. 3rd ed. St Louis: Elsevier; 2021.)

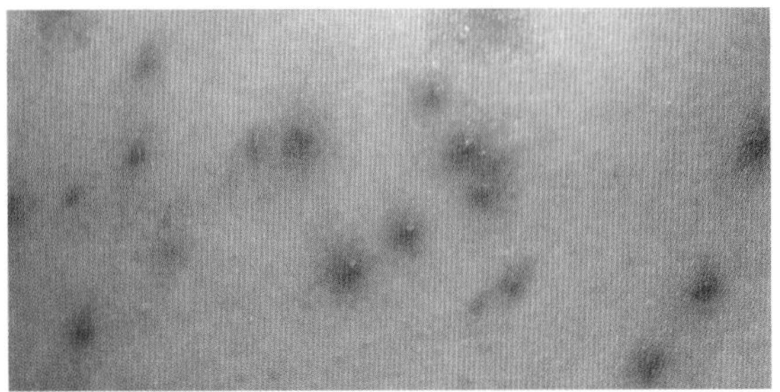

FIG. **29** Staphylococcal superficial folliculitis. Multiple pustules on a red base. (Reprinted with permission from Morelli JG, Torres-Zegarra C. *Pediatric Dermatology*. 3rd ed. St Louis: Elsevier; 2021.)

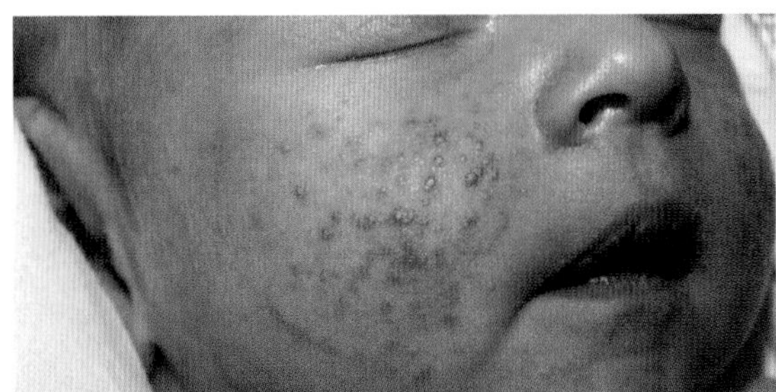

FIG. **30** Neonatal acne. Papules and pustules on a cheek of a 3-week-old infant. (Reprinted with permission from Morelli JG, Torres-Zegarra C. *Pediatric Dermatology*. 3rd ed. St Louis: Elsevier; 2021.)

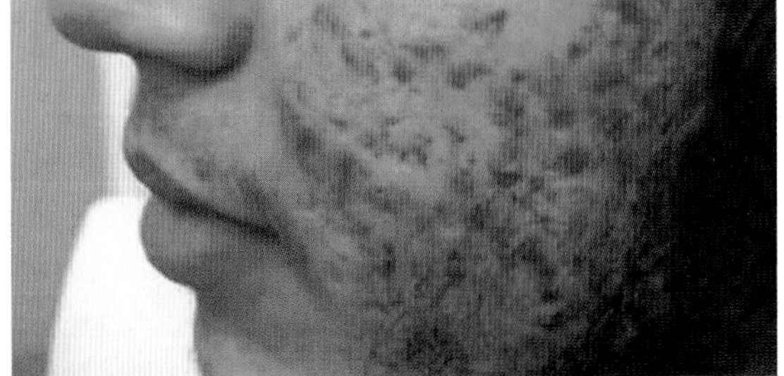

FIG. **31** Acne scarring following nodulocystic acne. Reprinted with permission from Morelli JG, Torres-Zegarra C. *Pediatric Dermatology*. 3rd ed. St Louis: Elsevier; 2021.

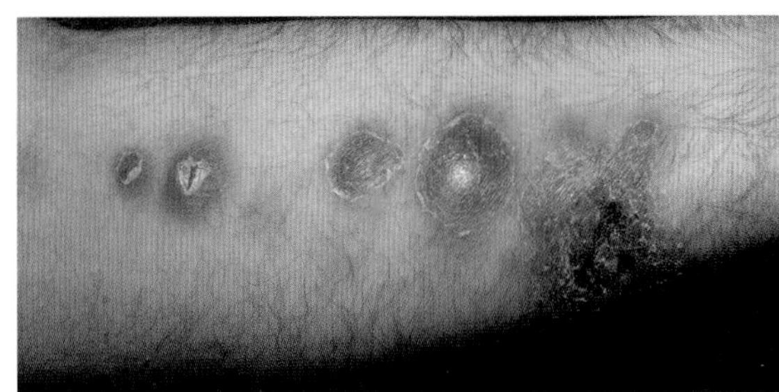

FIG. **32** Staphylococcal furunculosis. Multiple tender red nodules on a teen's arm. (Reprinted with permission from Morelli JG, Torres-Zegarra C. *Pediatric Dermatology*. 3rd ed. St Louis: Elsevier; 2021.)

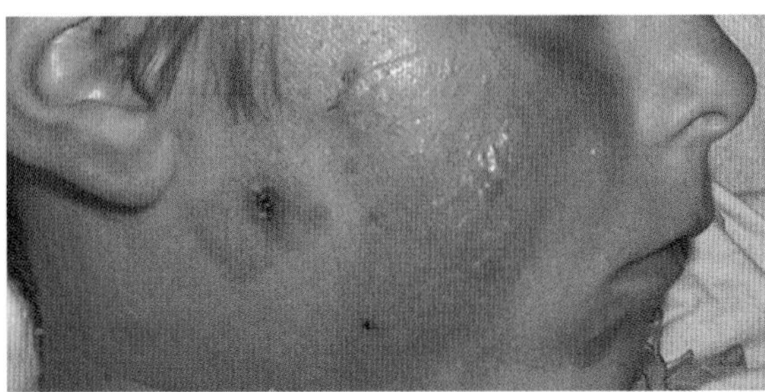

FIG. **33** Cellulitis of the cheek of a child with red-tender skin following a puncture wound. (Reprinted with permission from Morelli JG, Torres-Zegarra C. *Pediatric Dermatology*. 3rd ed. St Louis: Elsevier; 2021.)

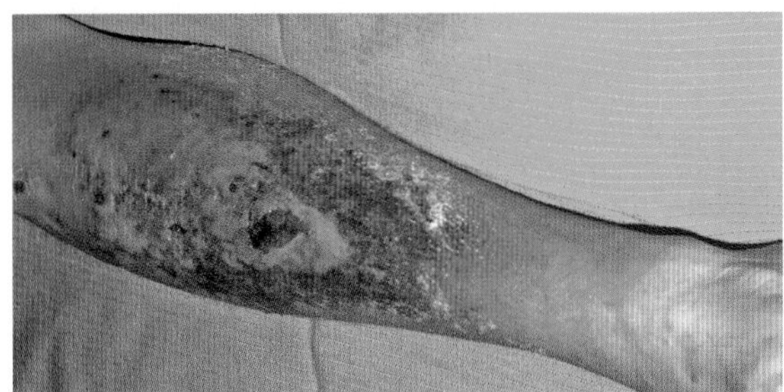

FIG. **34** Necrotizing fasciitis. Painful, red, swollen leg with black necrotic areas. (Reprinted with permission from Morelli JG, Torres-Zegarra C. *Pediatric Dermatology*. 3rd ed. St Louis: Elsevier; 2021.)

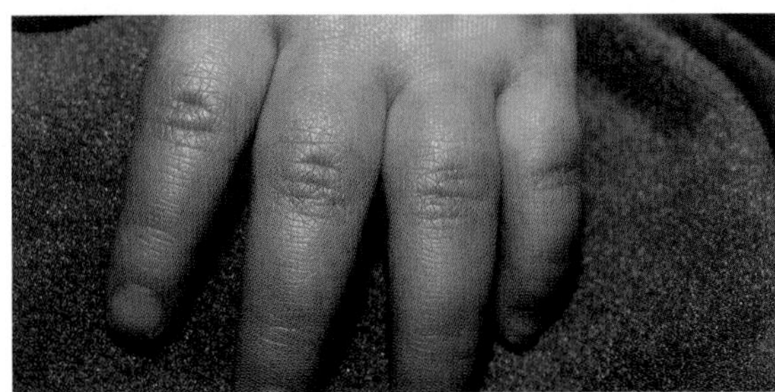

FIG. **35** Diffuse swelling and redness of the fingers in Kawaski disease. (Reprinted with permission from Morelli JG, Torres-Zegarra C. *Pediatric Dermatology*. 3rd ed. St Louis: Elsevier; 2021.)

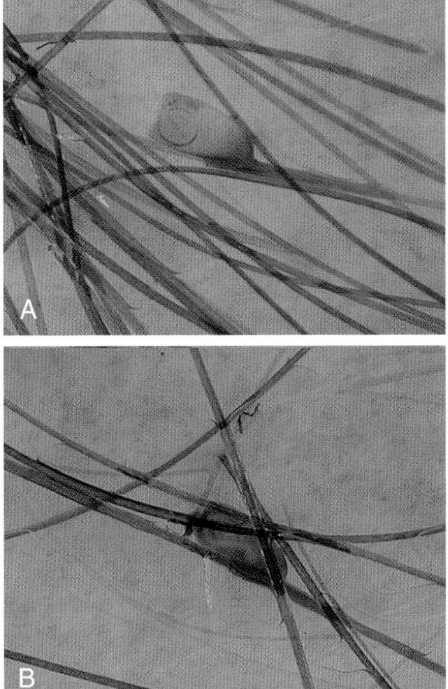

FIG. **36** (A) Empty nit case. (B) Viable nits. (A) Close-up of tiny insects that live in hairs. (B) Close-up of tiny insects that within 1/4 inch of the scalp on strands of hair. (From Di Stefani A, Hofmann-Wellenhof R, Zalaudek I. Dermoscopy for diagnosis and treatment monitoring of pediculosis capitis. *J Am Acad Dermatol.* 2006;54[5]:909–911.)

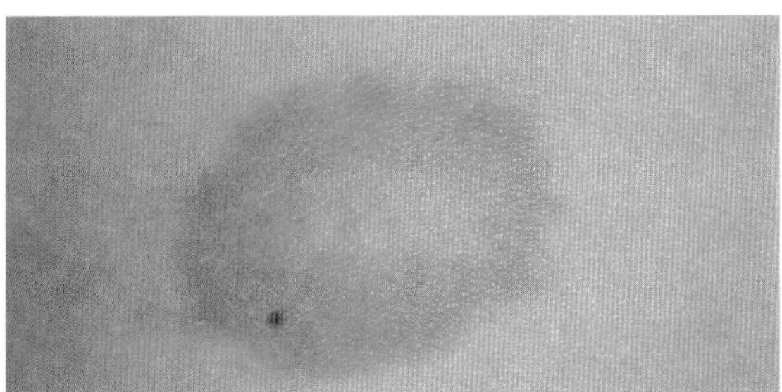

FIG. **37** Papular urticaria. Giant red flare following an insect bite. (Reprinted with permission from Morelli JG, Torres-Zegarra C. *Pediatric Dermatology*. 3rd ed. St Louis: Elsevier; 2021.)

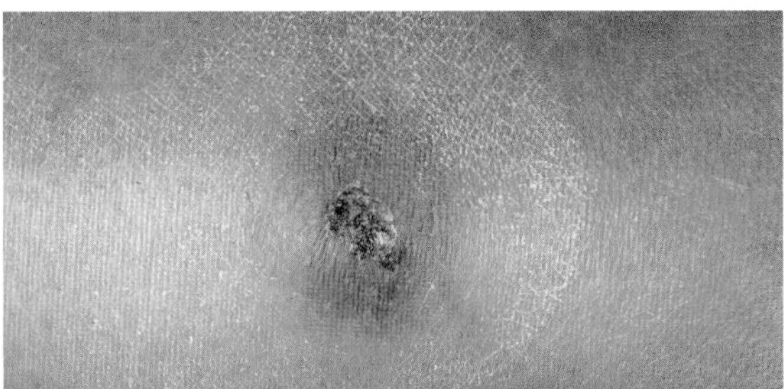

FIG. **38** Venomous spider bite. Central necrosis and indurated red border in brown recluse spider bite. (Reprinted with permission from Morelli JG, Torres-Zegarra C. *Pediatric Dermatology*. 3rd ed. St Louis: Elsevier; 2021.)

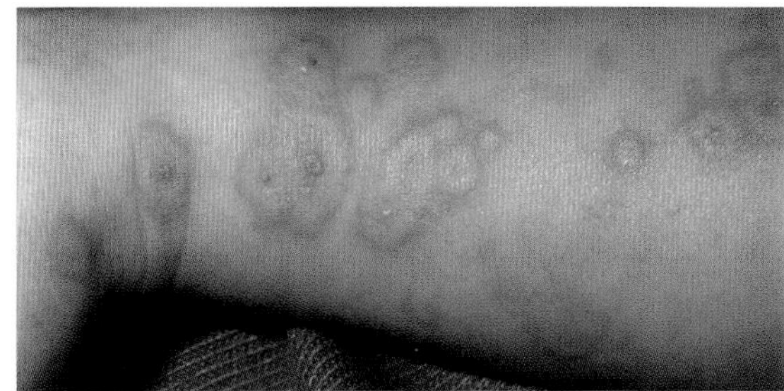

FIG. **39** Papules. Early target lesions with a central dusk and an outer edematous zone. (Reprinted with permission from Morelli JG, Torres-Zegarra C. *Pediatric Dermatology*. 3rd ed. St Louis: Elsevier; 2021.)

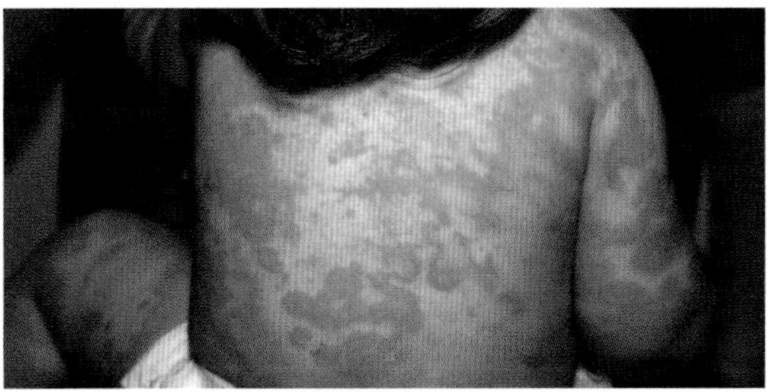

FIG. **40** Urticarial drug eruption with partially clearing areas due to cefaclor. (Reprinted with permission from Morelli JG, Torres-Zegarra C. *Pediatric Dermatology*. 3rd ed. St Louis: Elsevier; 2021.)

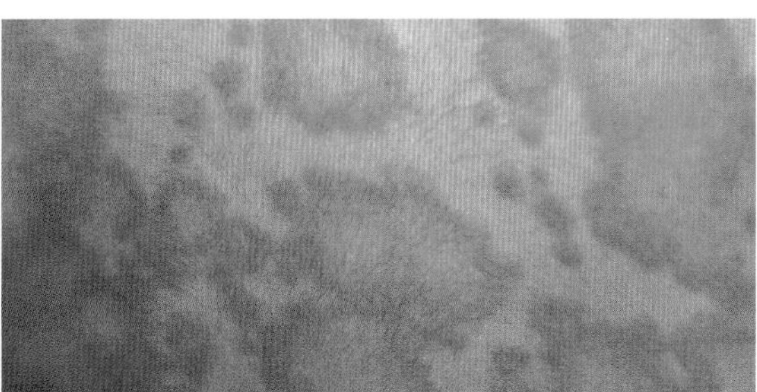

FIG. **41** Multiple shapes of urticarial lesions in a child. (Reprinted with permission from Morelli JG, Torres-Zegarra C. *Pediatric Dermatology*. 3rd ed. St Louis: Elsevier; 2021.)

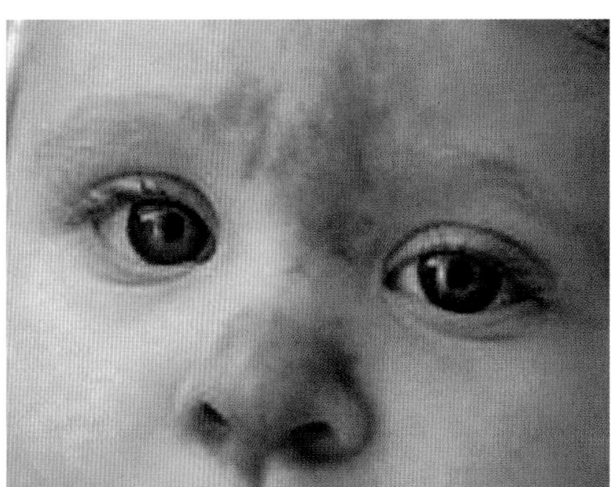

FIG. **42** Extensive nevus simplex in an infant. When the nose is involved regression is unlikely. (Reprinted with permission from Morelli JG, Torres-Zegarra C. *Pediatric Dermatology*. 3rd ed. St Louis: Elsevier; 2021.)

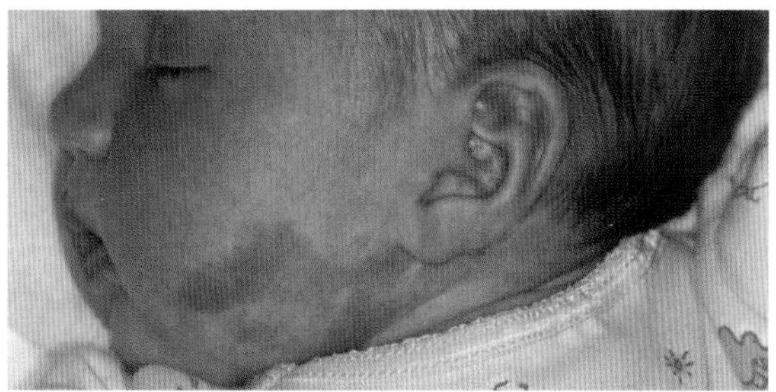

FIG. **43** Port-wine stain (capillary malformation) on the cheek of a newborn. (Reprinted with permission from Morelli JG, Torres-Zegarra C. *Pediatric Dermatology*. 3rd ed. St Louis: Elsevier; 2021.)

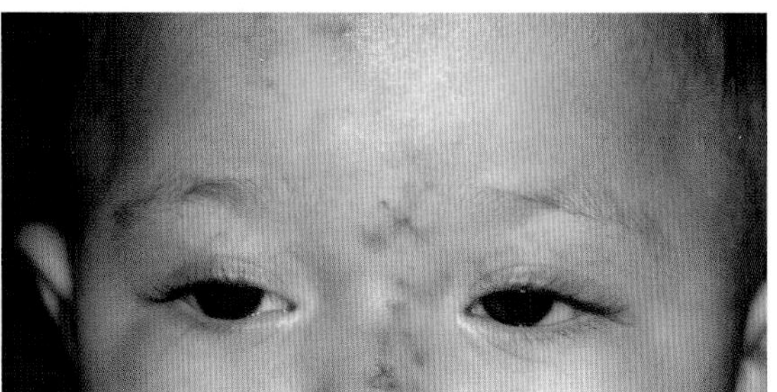

FIG. **44** Prominent dilated veins in a child with venous malformation. (Reprinted with permission from Morelli JG, Torres-Zegarra C. *Pediatric Dermatology*. 3rd ed. St Louis: Elsevier; 2021.)

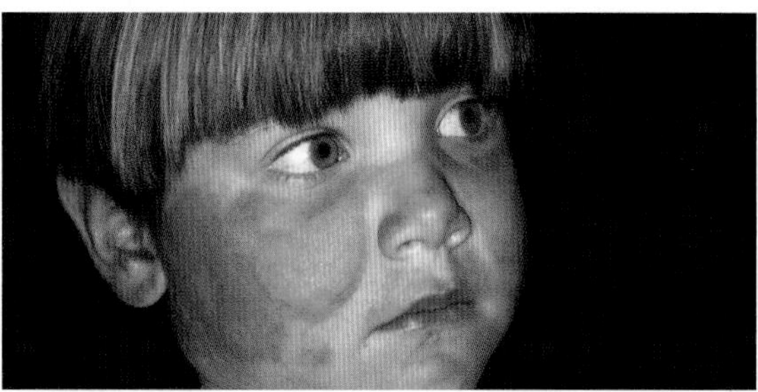

FIG. **45** Butterfly rash of childhood acute systemic lupus erythematosus (SLE). (Reprinted with permission from Morelli JG, Torres-Zegarra C. *Pediatric Dermatology*. 3rd ed. St Louis: Elsevier; 2021.)

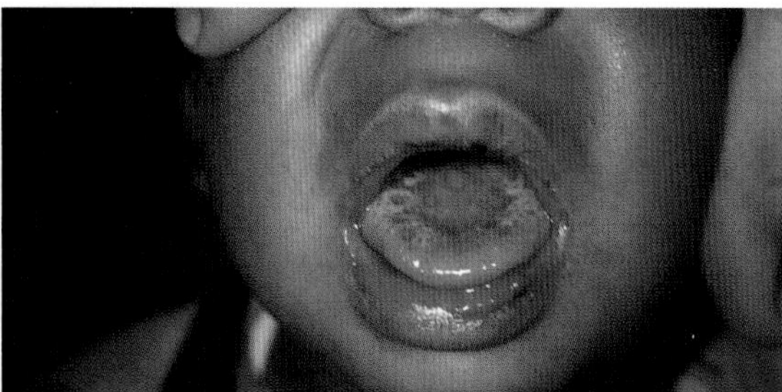

FIG. **46** Primary herpes gingivostomatitis. Perioral and lip vesicles in a 10-month-old infant. (Reprinted with permission from Morelli JG, Torres-Zegarra C. *Pediatric Dermatology*. 3rd ed. St Louis: Elsevier; 2021.)

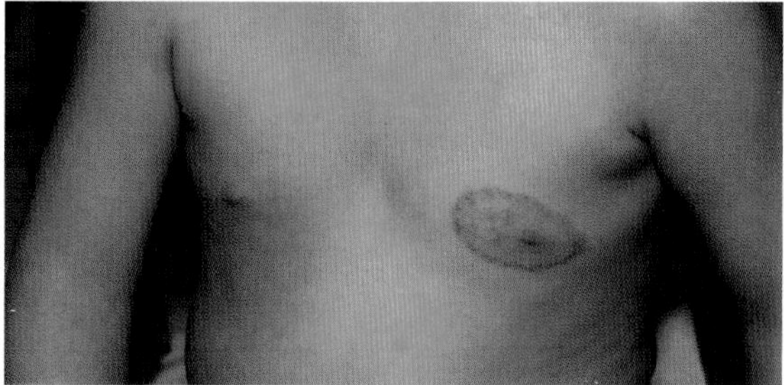

FIG. **47** Red scaly plaque with partial clearing in the center on a boy with tinea corporis. (Reprinted with permission from Morelli JG, Torres-Zegarra C. *Pediatric Dermatology*. 3rd ed. St Louis: Elsevier; 2021.)

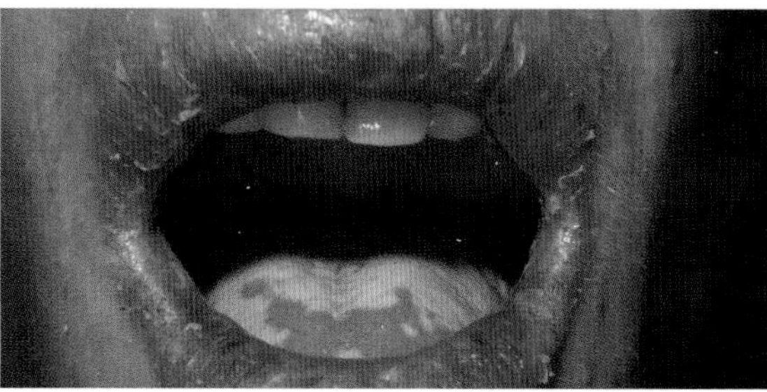

FIG. **48** Mucocutaneous candidiasis in immune deficiency showing white-coated tongue and dry, fissured lips. (Reprinted with permission from Morelli JG, Torres-Zegarra C. *Pediatric Dermatology*. 3rd ed. St Louis: Elsevier; 2021.)

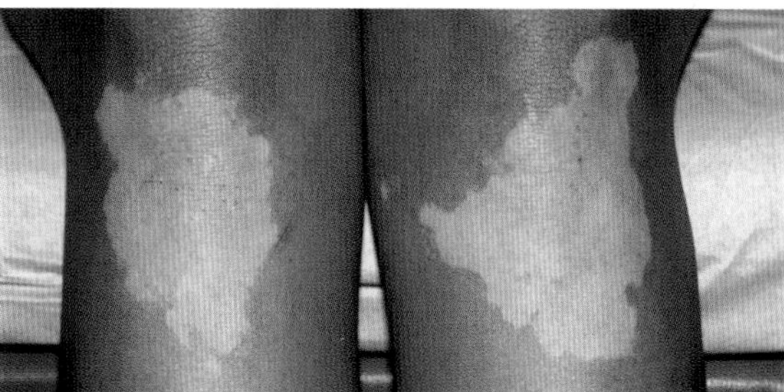

FIG. **49** Symmetric acral vitiligo. (Reprinted with permission from Morelli JG, Torres-Zegarra C. *Pediatric Dermatology*. 3rd ed. St Louis: Elsevier; 2021.)

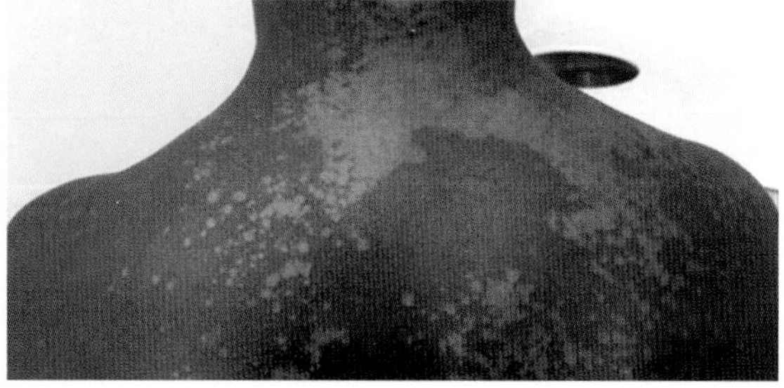

FIG. **50** Hypopigmented macules of tinea versicolor on the back of a teenager. (Reprinted with permission from Morelli JG, Torres-Zegarra C. *Pediatric Dermatology*. 3rd ed. St Louis: Elsevier; 2021.)

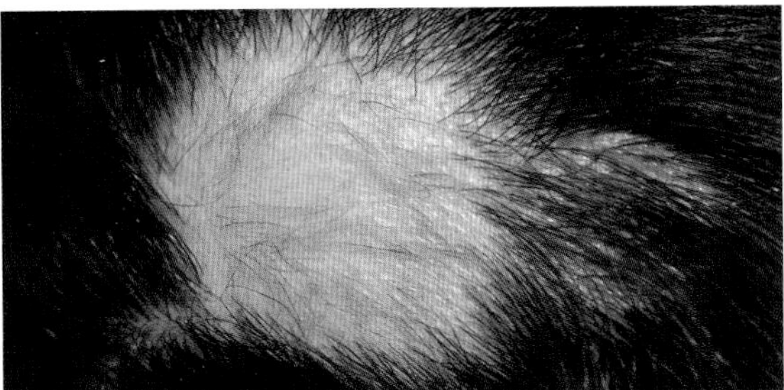

FIG. **51** Round patch of complete hair loss without scalp change in a child with alopecia areata. (Reprinted with permission from Morelli JG, Torres-Zegarra C. *Pediatric Dermatology*. 3rd ed. St Louis: Elsevier; 2021.)

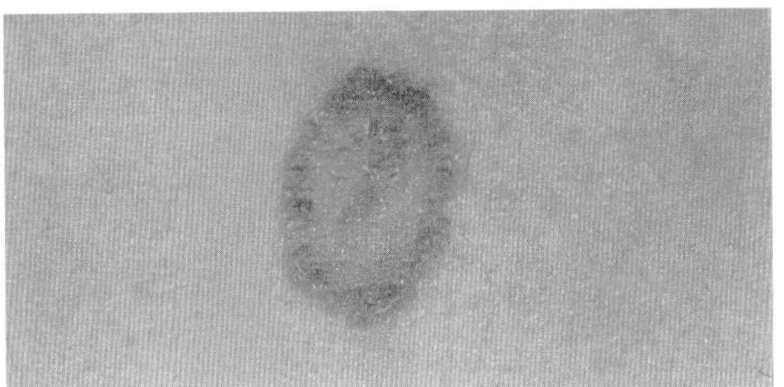

FIG. **52** Tinea corporis. Scaly red border on an annular lesion. (Reprinted with permission from Morelli JG, Torres-Zegarra C. *Pediatric Dermatology*. 3rd ed. St Louis: Elsevier; 2021.)

First intention (clean incision)

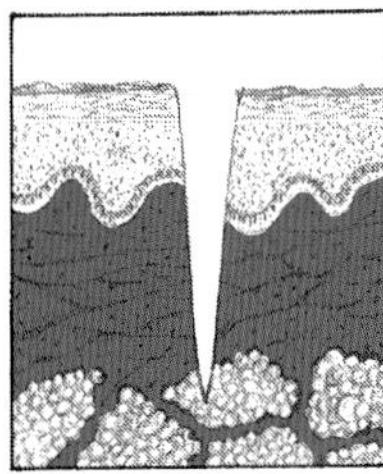

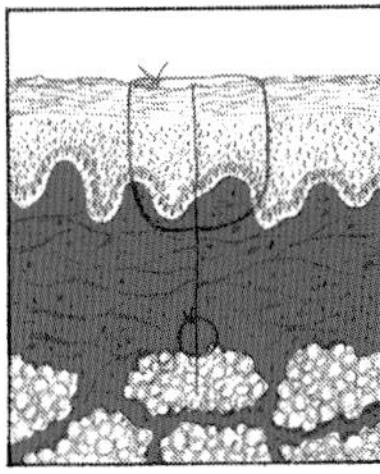

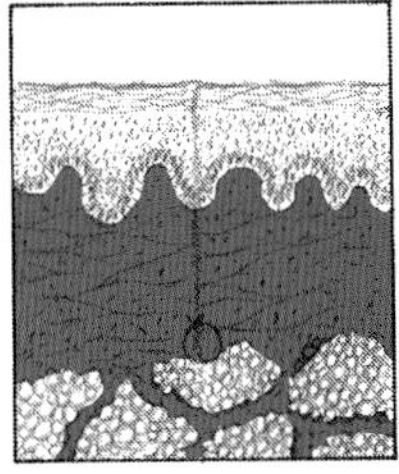

Second intention (wide, irregular wound)

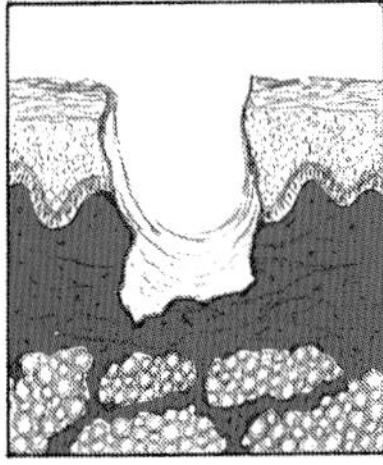

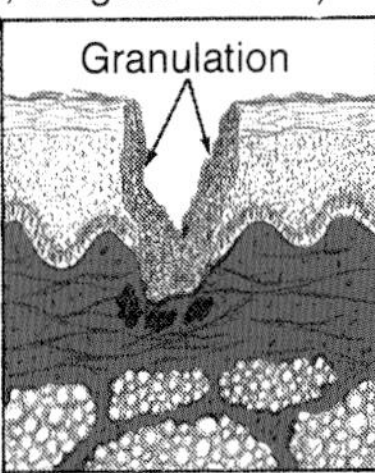

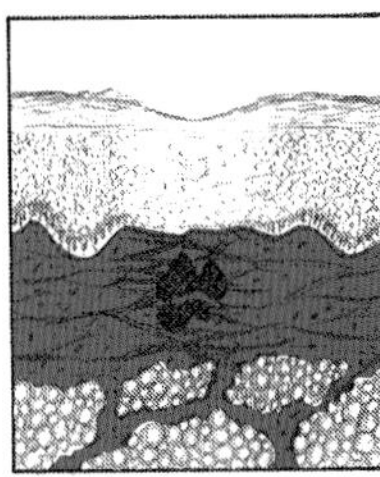

Third intention (puncture wound)

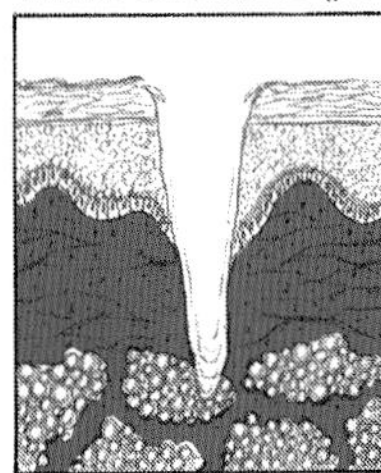

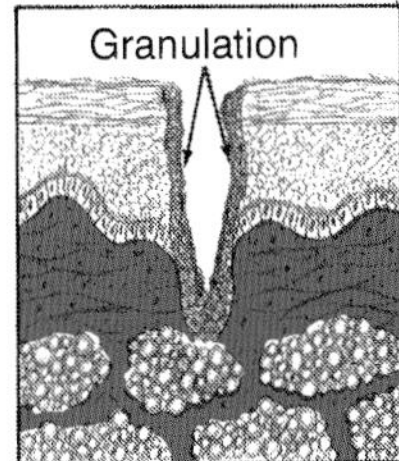

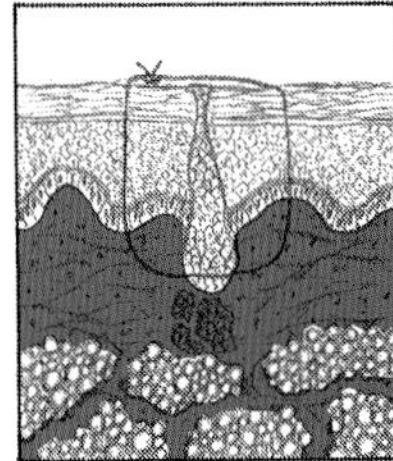

FIG. **53** Types of wound healing. Illustration shows types of wound healing as first intention (clear incision), second intention (wide, irregular wound), and third intention (puncture wound). (From Hockenberry MJ. *Nursing Care of Infants and Children*. 12th ed. St. Louis: Elsevier, 2023.)

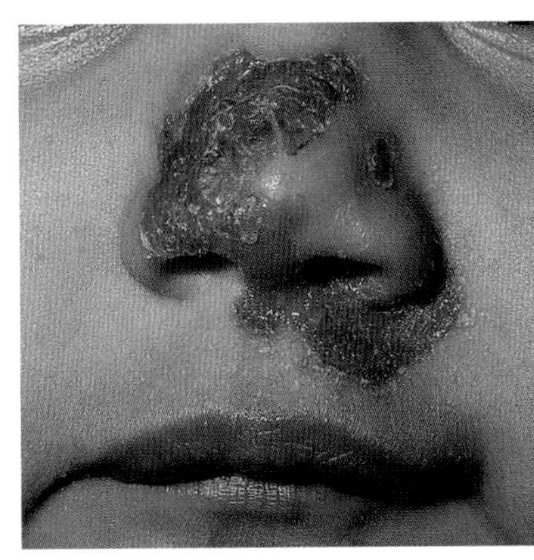

FIG. **54** Impetigo contagiosa. Close-up of child's face with reddish crusted lesion on the nose. (From Weston WL, Lane AT. *Color Textbook of Pediatric Dermatology*. 4th ed. St. Louis: Mosby; 2007.)

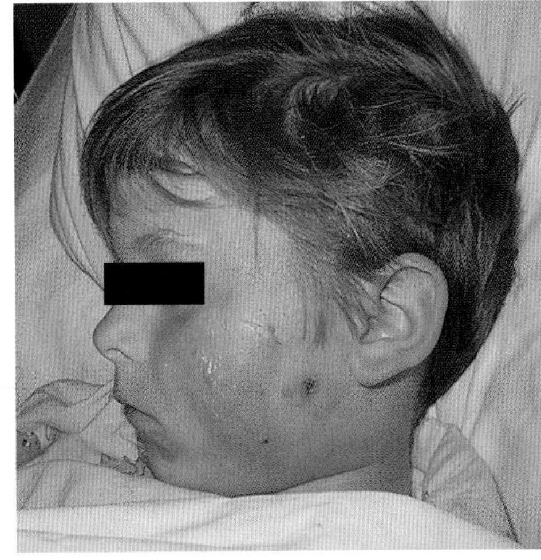

FIG. **55** Cellulitis of cheek from a puncture wound. Close-up child's face with swollen skin, filled with pus and inflammation on left cheek. (From Weston WL, Lane AT. *Color Textbook of Pediatric Dermatology*. 4th ed. St. Louis: Mosby; 2007.)

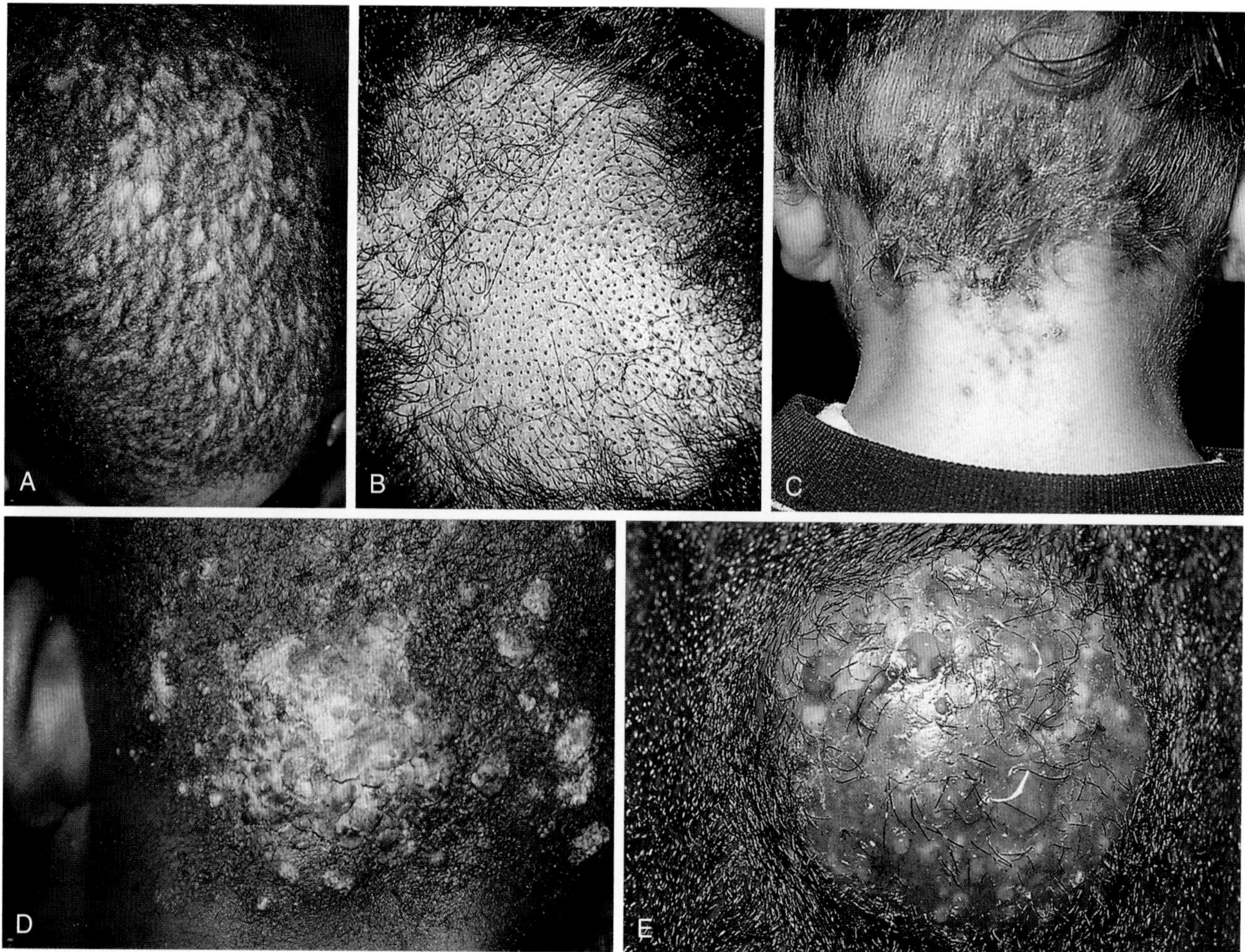

FIG. **56** Tinea capitis: superficial papules and pustules have ruptured, producing weeping and crusting lesions simulating impetigo. (From Moon M, et al., Dermatology. In: Zitelli BJ, McIntire SC, Nowalk AJ, Garrison J, eds. *Zitelli and Davis' Atlas of Pediatric Physical Diagnosis.* 8th ed. Philadelphia: Elsevier; 2023:276–341.)

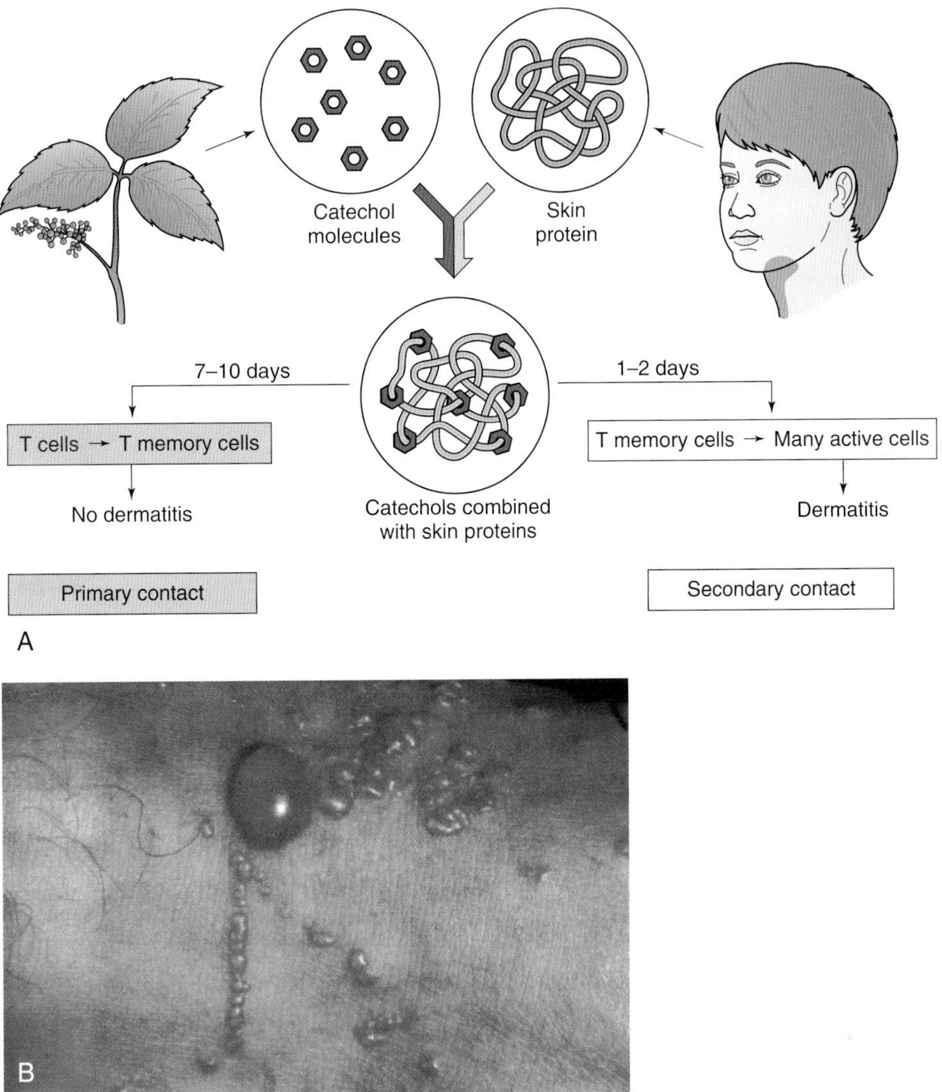

FIG. **57** (A) Development of allergic contact dermatitis. (B) Poison ivy lesions; note the "streaked" blisters surrounding one large blister. A flowchart and an image are seen. In (A) catechol molecules from plants and skin protein in a person, lead to catechols combined with skin proteins. Two situations are possible. In primary contact, within 7 to 10 days, T cells communicate to T memory cells, and there is no dermatitis. In secondary contact, within 1 to 2 days, T memory cells communicate to many active cells, and there is dermatitis. In (B) both a stretch and a rash of blisters surround one large blister on surface of skin. (A, From Damjanov I, Linder J: *Anderson's pathology*. ed 10, St. Louis: Mosby; 1996. B, From Habif TP. *Clinical Dermatology: A Color Guide to Diagnosis and Therapy.* 5th ed. St. Louis: Mosby; 2010.)

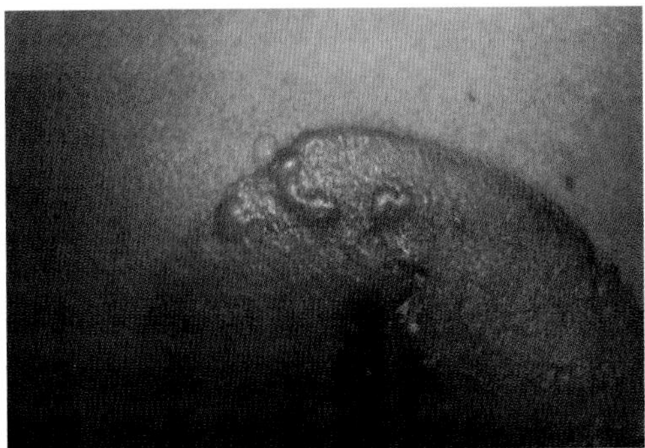

FIG. **58** Brown recluse spider bite. Note central necrosis surrounded by purplish area and blisters. Close-up of skin with fang marks, with fluid-filled blisters surrounded by red-colored boundaries. (From Weston WL, Lane AT. *Color Textbook of Pediatric Dermatology.* 4th ed. St. Louis: Mosby; 2007.)

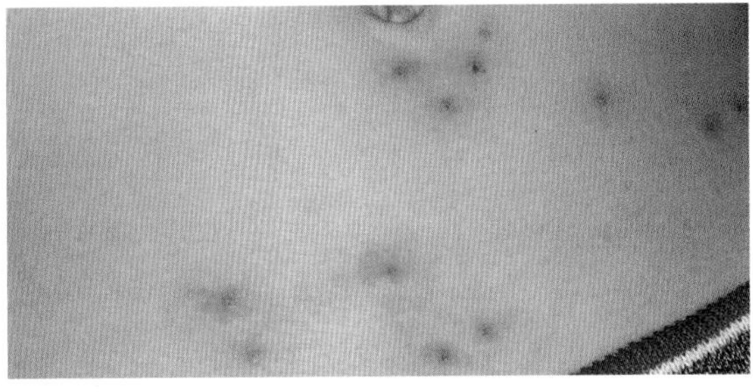

FIG. **59** Papular urticaria. Clusters of red papules surrounded by the urticarial flare due to cat fleas. (Reprinted with permission from Morelli JG, Torres-Zegarra C. *Pediatric Dermatology*. 3rd ed. St Louis: Elsevier; 2021.)

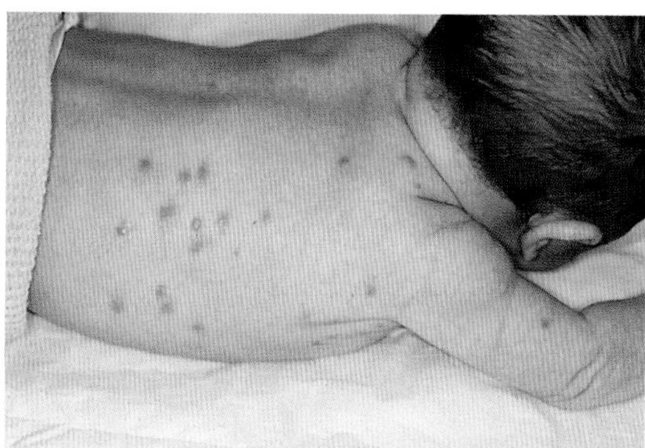

FIG. **60** Scabies. Pimple-like rash, spots on the back of infant. (Courtesy Department of Dermatology, School of Medicine, University of Utah.)

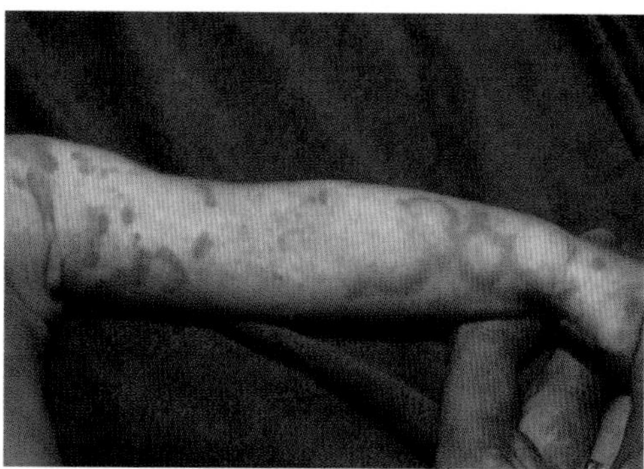

FIG. **61** Lyme disease. Note annular red rings in erythema chronicum migrans. Close-up child's hand with rash all over. (From Weston WL, Lane AT. *Color Textbook of Pediatric Dermatology*. 4th ed. St. Louis: Mosby; 2007.)

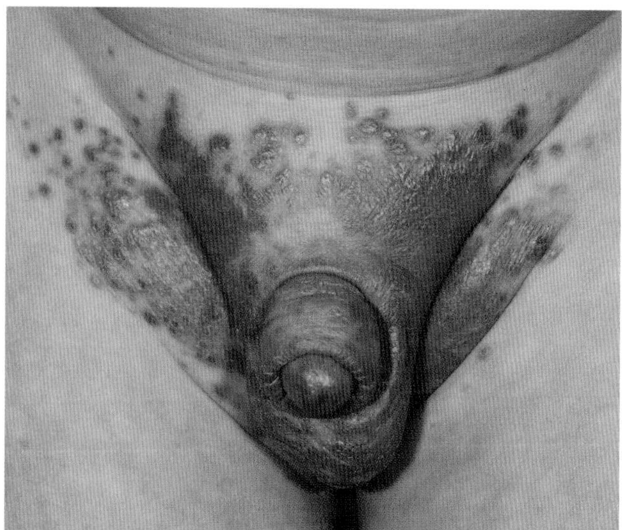

FIG. **62** Irritant diaper dermatitis. Note the sharply demarcated edges. Close up male child's genital area with severe rash all over. (From Habif TP. *Clinical Dermatology: A Color Guide to Diagnosis and Therapy*. 5th ed. St Louis: Elsevier; 2010.)

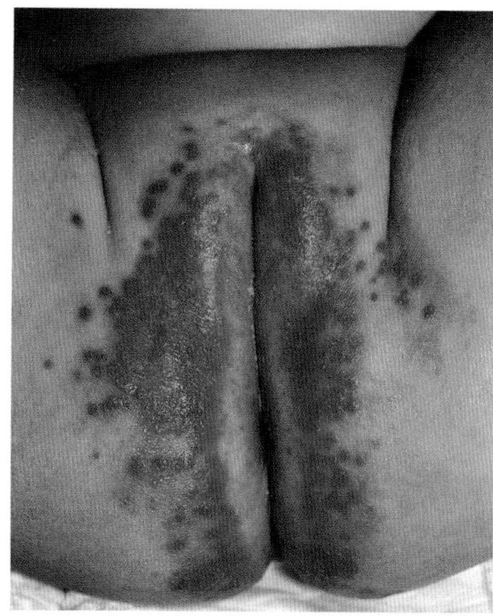

FIG. **63** Candidiasis of diaper area. Note the beefy red central erythema with satellite pustules. Close-up female child's genital area with severe rash all over. (From Paller AS, Mancini AJ. *Hurwitz Clinical Pediatric Dermatology*. 4th ed. St. Louis: Saunders Elsevier; 2011.)

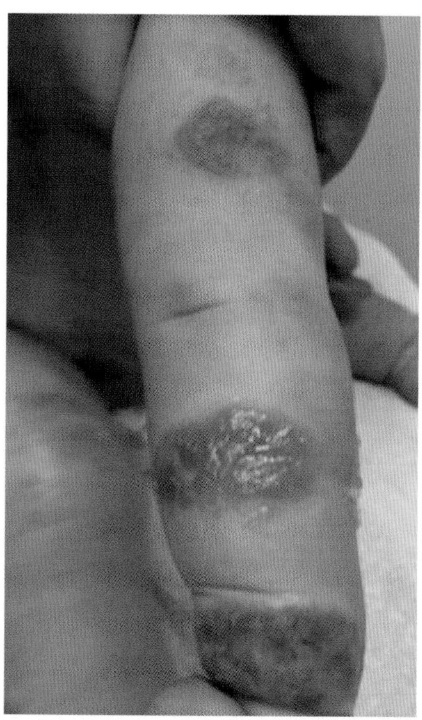

FIG. **64** Atopic dermatitis. Close-up of a child's hand with swollen and cracked skin, with clear fluid coming from affected area. (From Gupta, D. Atopic dermatitis: a common pediatric condition and its evolution in adulthood. *Med Clin North Am*. 2015;99[6]:1269–1285.)

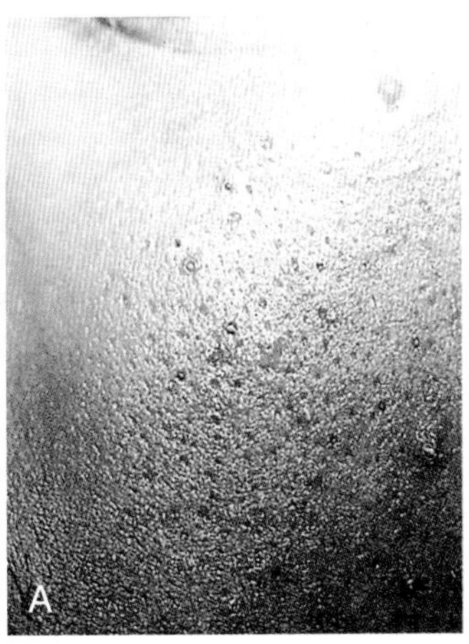

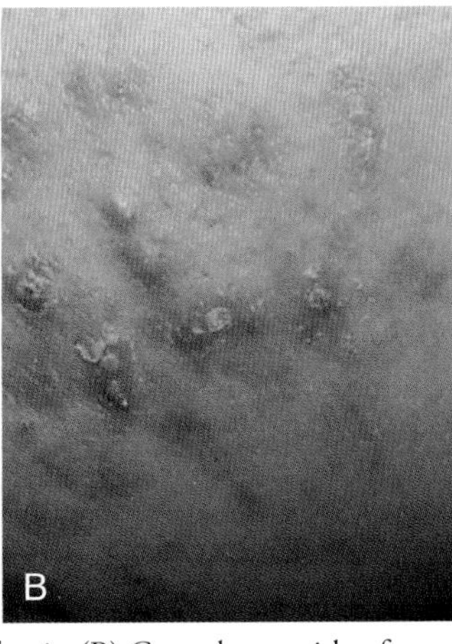

FIG. **65** Acne vulgaris. (A) Acne vulgaris. (B) Comedones with a few inflammatory pustules. (A) Close-up of otender bumps on skin. (B) Close-up of lumps on the skin. (From Zitelli BJ, McIntire SC, Nowalk AJ. *Zitelli and Davis' Atlas of Pediatric Physical Diagnosis*. 6th ed. St Louis: Saunders; 2012.)

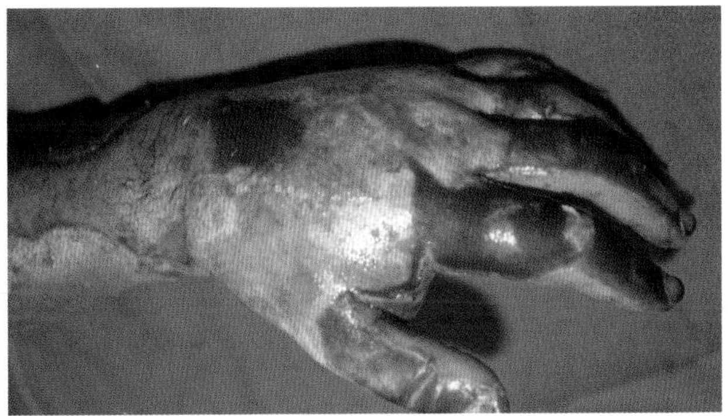
FIG. **66** Deep partial-thickness burn. (From Ignatavicius D, Workman M, Rebar C, & Heimgartner N. Medical-surgical nursing: Concepts for interprofessional collaborative care, 10th ed. St. Louis: Elsevier, 2021. p. 462.)

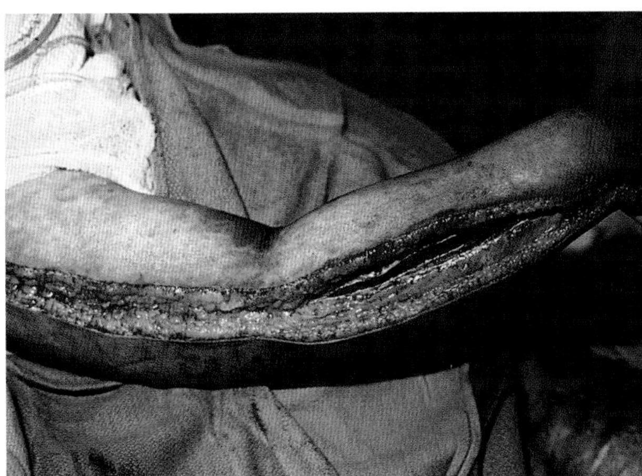
FIG. **67** Escharotomy and fasciotomy in severely burned arm. (From Rodgers CC, Wilson D, Hockenberry MJ. Wong's nursing care of infants and children, 11th ed. St Louis: Elsevier, 2018.)

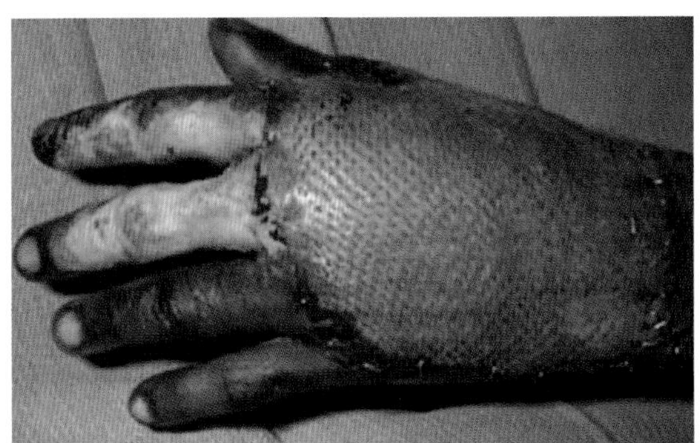
FIG. **68** Mesh graft. (From Hockenberry MJ, Wilson D. *Wong's Nursing Care of Infants and Children*. 11th ed. St Louis: Elsevier; 2018.)

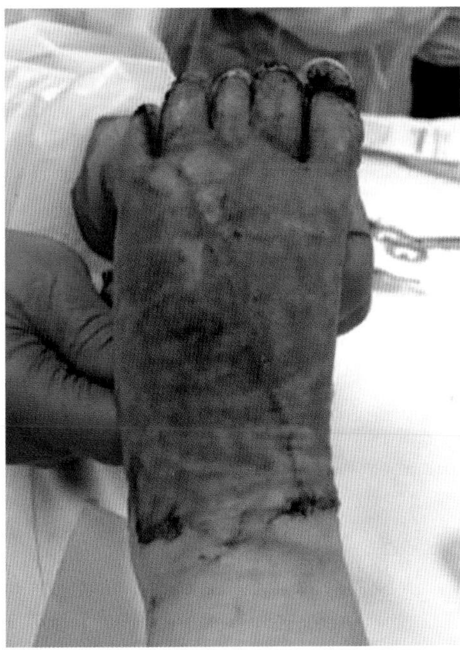
FIG. **69** Sheet graft. (From Hockenberry MJ, Wilson D. *Wong's Nursing Care of Infants and Children*. 11th ed. St Louis: Elsevier; 2018.)

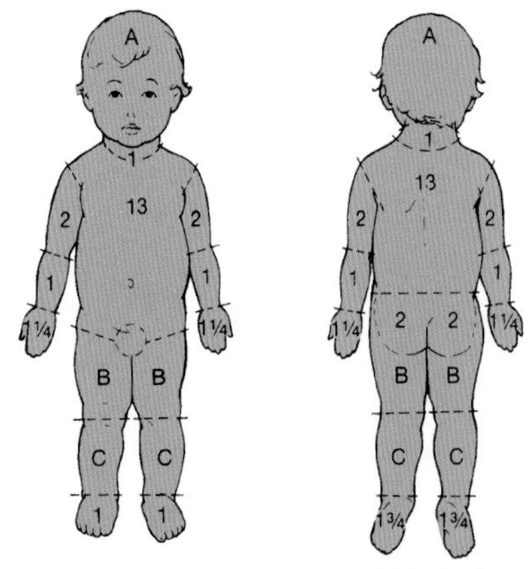

RELATIVE PERCENTAGES OF AREAS AFFECTED BY GROWTH

A

AREA	BIRTH	AGE 1 YR	AGE 5 YR
A = ½ of head	9½	8½	6½
B = ½ of one thigh	2¾	3¼	4
C = ½ of one leg	2½	2½	2¾

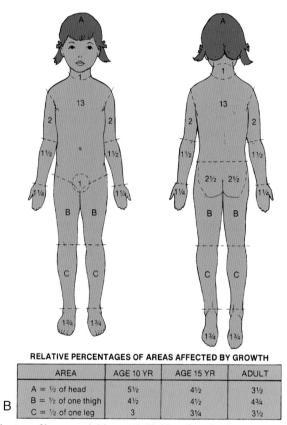

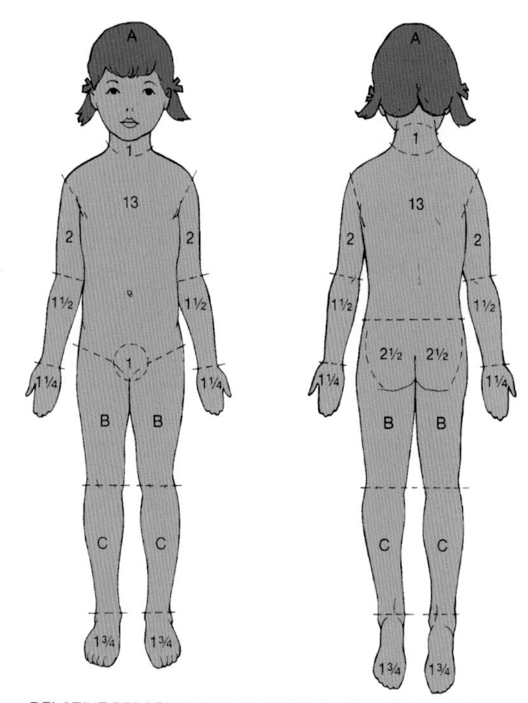

RELATIVE PERCENTAGES OF AREAS AFFECTED BY GROWTH

B

AREA	AGE 10 YR	AGE 15 YR	ADULT
A = ½ of head	5½	4½	3½
B = ½ of one thigh	4½	4½	4¾
C = ½ of one leg	3	3¼	3½

FIG. **70** Charts for estimation of distribution of burns in children. (A) Children from birth to age 5 years. (B) Older children.

EPIDERMIS: Sweat duct, Capillary

DERMIS: Sebaceous gland, Nerve endings, Hair follicle

Sweat gland, Fat, Blood vessels

Bone

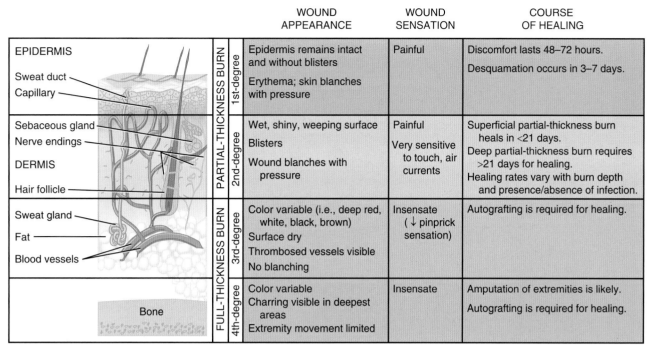

		WOUND APPEARANCE	WOUND SENSATION	COURSE OF HEALING
PARTIAL-THICKNESS BURN	1st-degree	Epidermis remains intact and without blisters Erythema; skin blanches with pressure	Painful	Discomfort lasts 48–72 hours. Desquamation occurs in 3–7 days.
	2nd-degree	Wet, shiny, weeping surface Blisters Wound blanches with pressure	Painful Very sensitive to touch, air currents	Superficial partial-thickness burn heals in <21 days. Deep partial-thickness burn requires >21 days for healing. Healing rates vary with burn depth and presence/absence of infection.
FULL-THICKNESS BURN	3rd-degree	Color variable (i.e., deep red, white, black, brown) Surface dry Thrombosed vessels visible No blanching	Insensate (↓ pinprick sensation)	Autografting is required for healing.
	4th-degree	Color variable Charring visible in deepest areas Extremity movement limited	Insensate	Amputation of extremities is likely. Autografting is required for healing.

FIG. **71** Classification of burn depth according to depth of injury. (From Black JM. *Medical-Surgical Nursing: Clinical Management for Positive Outcomes*. 8th ed. Philadelphia: Saunders; 2008.)

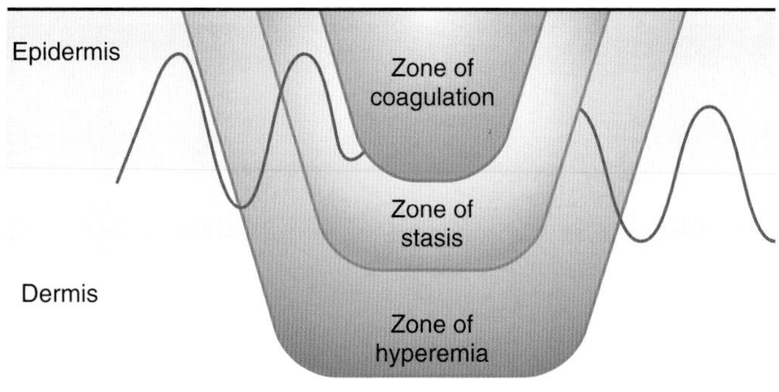

FIG. **72** Zones of injury in burn. (From Townsend DM. *Sebiston Textbook of Surgery*. 18th ed. Philadelphia: Saunders; 2007.)

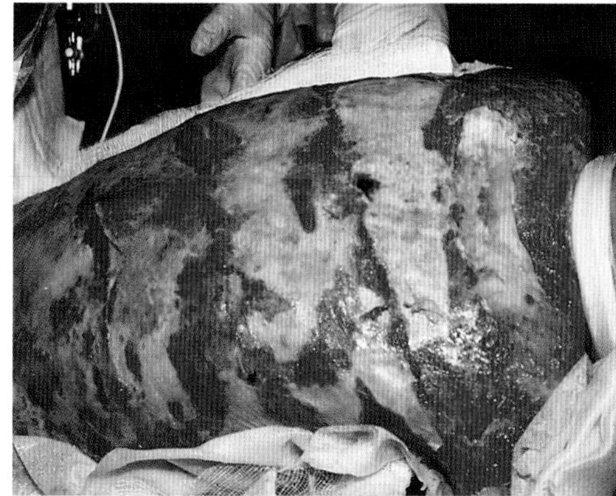

FIG. **73** Adherent allograft applied to excised full-thickness wound.

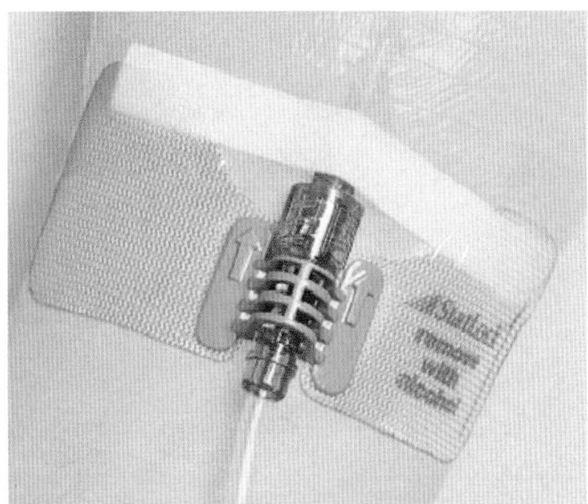

FIG. **74** StatLock securement devices enhance peripheral intravenous line dwell time and decrease phlebitis. (From Hockenberry MJ, Wilson D. *Wong's Nursing Care of Infants and Children*. 10th ed. St Louis: Elsevier; 2015.)

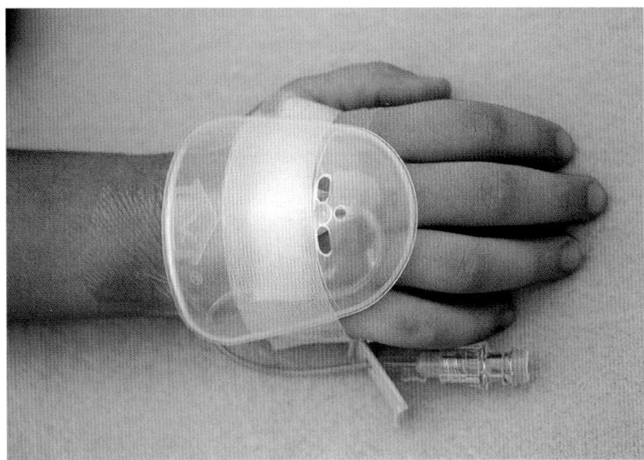

FIG. **75** I.V. house used to protect the intravenous site. (From Hockenberry MJ, Wilson D. *Wong's Nursing Care of Infants and Children*. 10th ed. St Louis: Elsevier; 2015.)

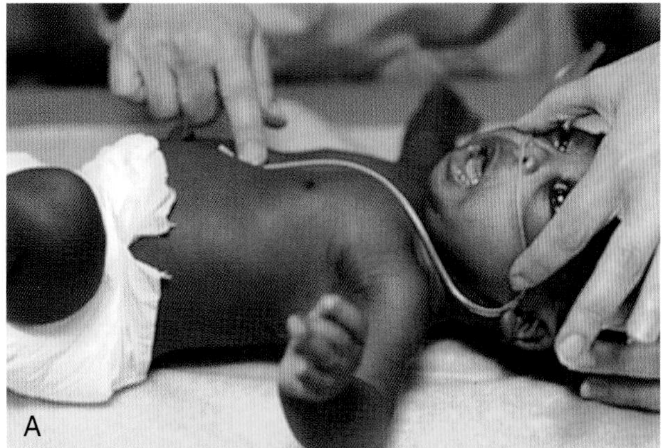

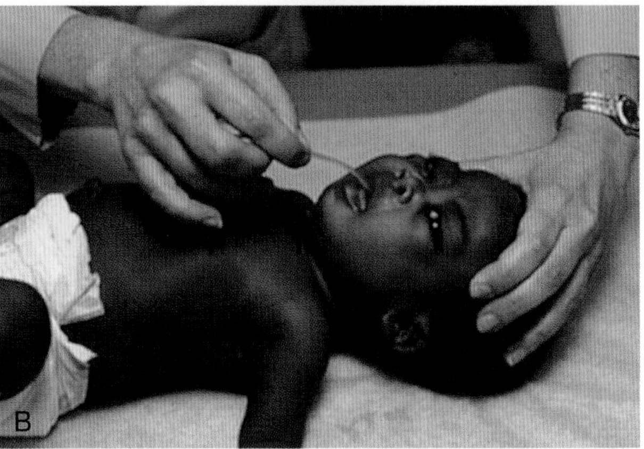

FIG. **76** Gavage feeding. (A) Measuring the tube for orogastric feeding from the tip of the nose to the earlobe and to the midpoint between the end of the xiphoid process and the umbilicus. (B) Inserting the tube. (From Hockenberry MJ, Wilson D. *Wong's Nursing Care of Infants and Children*. 10th ed. St Louis: Elsevier; 2015.)

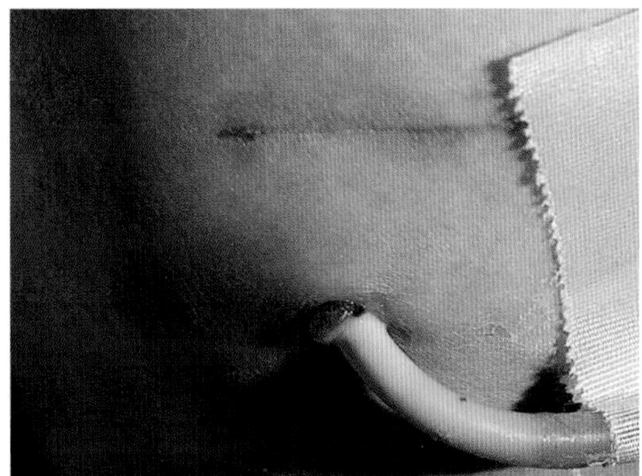

FIG. **77** Appearance of healthy granulation tissue around a stoma. (From Hockenberry MJ, Wilson D. *Wong's Nursing Care of Infants and Children*. 10th ed. St Louis: Elsevier; 2015.)

and using alcohol and other substances (e.g., marijuana, opioid ingestion) that impair judgement. Developmental characteristics of teenagers and injury prevention suggestions are listed next.

Developmental Abilities Related to Risk of Injury

Need for independence and freedom
Testing independence
Age permitted to drive a motor vehicle (varies from state to state)
Inclination for risk taking
Feeling of indestructibility
Need for discharging energy, often at expense of logical thinking and other control mechanisms
Strong need for peer approval
Attempting hazardous maneuvers
Peak incidence for practice and participation in sports
Access to more complex tools, objects, and locations
Can assume responsibility for own actions

Injury Prevention

Motor or Nonmotor Vehicles

Pedestrian

Emphasize and encourage safe pedestrian behavior.
Use crosswalks.
At night, walk with a friend.
If someone is following you, go to nearest public place with people.
Do not walk in secluded areas; take well-traveled walkways.

Passenger

Promote appropriate behavior while riding in a motor vehicle.
Refuse to ride with an impaired person or one who is driving recklessly.

Driver

Provide competent driver education; encourage judicious use of vehicle; discourage drag racing or playing chicken; maintain vehicle in proper condition (e.g., brakes, tires).
Teach and promote safety and maintenance of two- and three-wheeled vehicles.
Promote and encourage wearing of safety apparel, such as a helmet and long trousers.
Reinforce the dangers of drugs, including alcohol, when operating a motor vehicle.
Discourage distractions while driving—cell phone talking or texting, eating, smoking, or reading.

Drowning

- Teach nonswimmers to swim.
- Teach basic rules of water safety.
  Judicious selection of places to swim
  Sufficient water depth for diving
  Swimming with a companion
  No alcohol with water sports

Burns

Reinforce proper behavior in areas with burn hazards (gasoline, electric wires, and fires).
Advise against excessive exposure to natural or artificial sunlight (ultraviolet burn).
Discourage smoking.
Encourage use of sunscreen.

Poisoning

Educate in hazards of drug use, including alcohol.

Falls

Teach and encourage general safety measures in all activities.

Bodily Damage

Promote acquisition of proper instruction in sports and use of sports equipment.
Instruct in safe use of and respect for firearms and other devices with potential danger (e.g., power tools, firecrackers).
Provide and encourage use of protective equipment when using potentially hazardous devices.
Promote access to or provision of safe sports and recreational facilities.
Be alert for signs of depression (potential suicide).
Instruct regarding proper use of corrective devices (e.g., glasses, contact lenses, hearing aids).
Encourage and foster judicious application of safety principles and prevention.

Guidelines for Automobile Safety Seats

Motor vehicle injuries cause more accidental deaths in all pediatric age groups after age 1 year than any other type of injury or disease and are responsible for a significant number of all accidental deaths among children 1 to 4 years. Many of the deaths are caused by injuries within the car when restrains have not been used or have been used improperly. Unrestrained children (e.g., riding is in the arms or on the lap of another person; or in the bed of a pick-up truck) are at higher risk of injury and continues to be a major factor in fatal accidents involving children. These deaths and injuries are mostly preventable. All states have laws that require children to be properly secured in motor vehicles.

Nurses are responsible for educating parents regarding the importance of car restraints and their proper use. Five types of restraints are available: (1) infant-only devices, (2) convertible models for both infants and toddlers, (3) booster seats, (4) safety belts, and (5) devices for children with special needs.

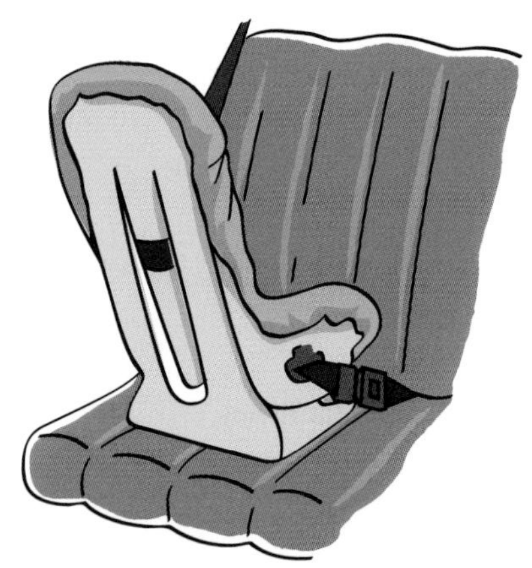

FIG. **2.1** Rear-facing infant seat in rear seat of car.

The infant-only restraint is a semireclined seat that faces the rear of the car (see Fig. 2.1). A rear-facing car seat provides the best protection for the disproportionately heavy head and weak neck of an infant. This position minimizes the stress on the neck by spreading the forces of a frontal crash over the entire back, neck, and head; the spine is supported by the back of the car seat. If the seat were faced forward, the head would whip forward because of the force of the crash, creating enormous stress on the neck. The restraint is anchored to the vehicle with the vehicle's seat belt or LATCH (lower anchor and tether for children) system that provides car seat anchors between the front cushion and backrest so that the seat belt does not have to be used. LATCH, a universal safety system, has been required in cars since 2002, and when used appropriately the top anchor prevents the child from pitching forward during a crash (see Fig. 2.2A and B on anchors/tethers). With the LATCH system in cars, all cars manufactured after 2002 will no longer need to use seat belts to anchor child safety seats.

Many infant seats have a dense plastic base that can be left in the car; the seat latches or clicks into the base so that the base does not have to be installed each time the car seat is removed.

The ***convertible restraint*** is a semireclined seat that is suitable for infants and toddlers in the rear-facing position. The AAP has recommended that all infants and toddlers ride in rear-facing car safety seats until they reach or surpass the maximum height and weight recommended for the car seat.[1] Once the child has outgrown the rear-facing seat, a forward-facing seat with a harness is recommended. Vehicles (manufactured after 1999) have tether straps that attach to anchors in the car seat to better secure the seat and minimize forward movement of the forward-facing convertible seats in the event of an accident.

Convertible restraints use different types of harness systems: a *five-point harness* that consists of a strap over each shoulder, one on each side of the pelvis, and one between the legs (all five come together at a common buckle), as well as a *padded overhead shield* that uses shoulder straps attached to a shield that is held in place by a crotch strap. With both the infant and toddler restraints, it is important not to add extra blankets, head cushions, or padding between the child and the restraint straps that did not come as original equipment because these "add-ons" create spaces of air between the child and the restraint and decrease support for the back, head, and neck. Cars with free-sliding latch plates on the lap or shoulder belt require the use of a metal locking clip to keep the belt in a tight-holding position. The locking clip is threaded onto the belt above the latch plate (Fig. 2.3A). If the car has automatic lap and shoulder belts, the parents need to have additional lap belts installed to properly secure the restraint. Children aged 2 years and older who have reached the maximum recommended height or weight for the rear-facing car seat should ride forward facing in a car safety seat with a harness as long as possible, which is recommended by the AAP.[1]

Booster seats are not restraint systems like the convertible devices because they depend on the vehicle belts to hold the child and booster seat in place. Three booster models have been approved by the National Highway Traffic Safety Administration (NHTSA): the high-back belt-positioning seat (see Fig. 2.3B), which provides head and neck support for the child riding in a vehicle seat without a head rest; the

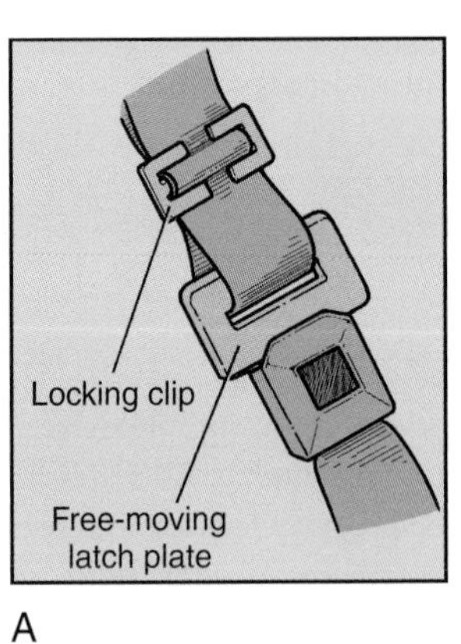

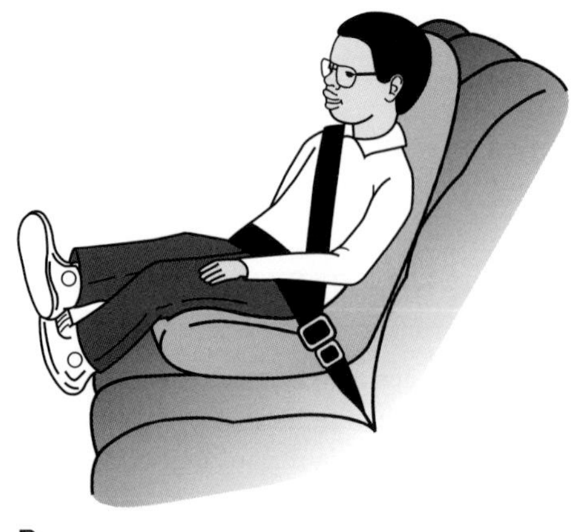

FIG. **2.2** (A) Locking clip used with free-sliding lap/shoulder belt to keep the belt in a tight holding position. (B) Automobile booster seat. Note placement of shoulder strap (away from neck and face).

[1]Durbin DR, Hoffman BD, Council on Injury, Violence, and Poison Prevention. Child passenger safety. *Pediatrics.* 2018;142(5):e20182461.

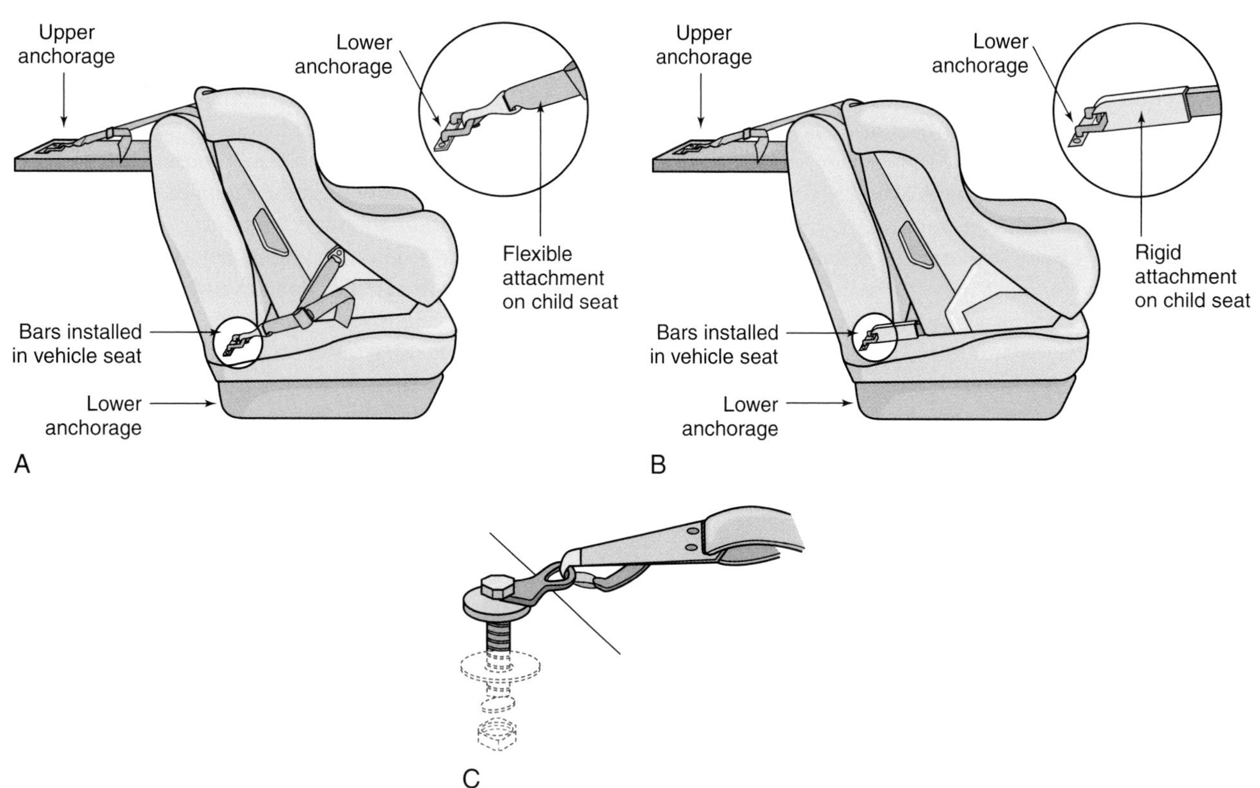

FIG. **2.3** Lower anchors and tethers for children (LATCH). (A) Flexible two-point attachment with top tether. (B) Rigid two-point attachment with top tether. (C) Top tether. (Courtesy of U.S. Department of Transportation, National Highway Traffic Safety Administration.)

no-back belt-positioning seat, which should be used only if the vehicle seat has a head rest; and a combination seat, which converts from a forward-facing toddler seat to a booster seat. This last model is equipped with a harness for use in toddlers; the harness may be removed and a shoulder-lap belt used when the child outgrows the harness. Belt-positioning booster seats are used for children who are less than 145 cm (4 feet, 9 inches) tall and who weigh 15.9 kg to 36.3 kg (35 to 80 lb, depending on the type of booster seat). In general, school-aged children should ride in a belt-positioning booster seat until approximately 7 to 8 years old. However, because children's sizes vary considerably, manufacturers' recommendations should be followed regarding weight and height. A booster seat should be used until the child is able to sit against the back of the seat with feet hanging down and legs bent at the knees. The belt-positioning booster model raises a child higher in the seat, moving the shoulder part of the belt off the neck and the lap portion of the belt off the abdomen onto the pelvis (see Fig. 2.3C).

The AAP recommended children should use specially designed car restraints until they are 145 cm (4 feet, 9 inches) in height or are 8 to 12 years old.[l] Shoulder-lap safety belts should be worn low on hips, snug, and not on the abdominal area. Children should be taught to sit up straight to allow proper fit. The shoulder belt lies across the middle of the chest and shoulder, not cross the child's neck or face.[l]

Children with disabilities may require a restraint system that secures them appropriately in the event of a crash. Examples of such devices include car bed restraints for infants who cannot tolerate a semireclining position and specially adapted molded-plastic chairs for children who have spica casts. The adjustable vest is a special safety harness especially for larger children with special needs that helps the wearer to maintain a secure upright position. Additional safety restraints and a list of distributors are available at the Safe Ride News website https://www.saferidenews.com.

The back middle seat is the safest area in the car for children. AAP strongly recommended that all children younger than 13 years should be restrained in the rear seats of vehicles for optimal protection.[l] Severe injuries and deaths in children have occurred from air bags deploying on impact in the front passenger seat. Children should not ride in the front seat of any activated air bag-equipped car, except in emergencies, and then the vehicle seat must be as far back as possible. Many newer model cars are equipped with a "smart" air bag system that allows air bag deactivation when a child is riding in the passenger seat. Parents should remember to turn the air bag switch back on once the child is no longer in the front seat. In addition, in the mid-1990s, vehicles were equipped with side-impact air bags for protection; these air bags are reported to be safe as long as the child is in a proper restraint system. The NHTSA recommends that vehicle owners with side-impact air bags check the manufacturer's recommendations for child safety. Because of a large number of adverse events involving serious injuries and even some child fatalities with air bags, some manufacturers installed air bags designed to minimize injury to adults and children at deployment yet still protect the passenger. Because diverse types of air bags continue to be in use, parents are cautioned to continue placing all children younger than age 13 years in the back seat with the proper child restraint system. Built-in safety seats are available in some cars and vans. They may be used for children who are at least 1 year of age and weigh at least 9 kg (20 lb). Built-in seats eliminate installation problems. However, weight and height limits vary. Reinforce that owners must verify with vehicle manufacturers details about built-in seats.

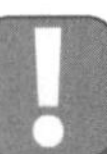

For any restraint to be effective, it must be used consistently and properly. Nurses must stress correct use of car safety restraints and rules that ensure compliance to parents. Despite widespread education and publicity regarding seat belt safety restraint and the danger of front seat air bags for children, children are still placed in potentially lethal situations of either improper seat restraint or no restraint. By 1985, all 50 states and the District of Columbia had passed laws requiring child restraints for young children. Most states have enhanced their child occupant retrain laws to include booster seat for older children. Current information on all child restraint laws in the United States is updated by the Insurance Institute of Highway Safety and can be found at https://www.iihs.org/search?query=child%20seatbelt%20laws.

PARENT RESOURCES, CAR SEAT SAFETY

American Academy of Pediatrics
345 Park Boulevard
Itasca, IL 60143
Phone: 800-433-9016
Website: https://www.aap.org/

US Department of Transportation
National Highway Traffic Safety Administration
1200 New Jersey Ave, SE, West Building
Washington, DC 20590
Phone: 888-327-4236
Website: www.nhtsa.gov

SafeKids USA
Website: www.safekids.org

Contact your local SafeKids chapter, which sponsors Seat Belt Fit clinics to ensure that seat belt restraint systems being used are adequate protection.

For children with special needs, the following is an available resource for car restraint information:

Automotive Safety Program
Indiana University School of Medicine
Fesler Hall, Room 207
1130 West Michigan Street
Indianapolis, IN 46202
Phone: 317-274-2977; 800-543-6227
Website: https://preventinjury.pediatrics.iu.edu/special-needs

Neonatal Car Seat Evaluation: The Preterm and Late-Preterm Infant[m]

The AAP (Bull, Engle, and AAP, 2009) recommends that all infants born in United States before 37 weeks of gestation have a predischarge car seat tolerance screen (CSTS) for cardiorespiratory instability events (e.g., apnea, bradycardia, and oxygen desaturation episodes) while in a semiupright safety car seat. Newer studies with stringent standardized failure criteria have reported CSTS failure between 4.6% and 9.2%, with higher retesting rates (approximately 24%) with the recommendation using an approved car bed.[m] Car beds are a restraint system that allows infants to lie flat secured with harness device with recommended CSTS retest follow-up to safely transition to car seat. Most facilities have developed policies and procedures for implementing an CSTS program; however, few evidence-based practice recommendations have been published to date delineating specific requirements for such a program. Based on the available literature, suggestions for providing a car seat evaluation of infants born before 37 weeks of gestation and/or weighing less than 2500 g at birth include the following[m]:

- Use the parents' car seat for the evaluation.
- Perform the evaluation 1 to 7 days before the infant's anticipated discharge.
- Secure the infant in the car seat per guidelines using blanket rolls on side.
- Set pulse oximeter low alarm at 88% (arbitrary).
- Set heart rate low alarm limit at 80 beats/min and apnea alarm at 20 seconds (cardiorespiratory monitor).
- Leave the infant undisturbed in car seat for 90 minutes *or* for the time parents state it takes to arrive at their home (if more than the 90 minutes).
- Document the infant's tolerance to the car seat evaluation.
- An episode of desaturation, bradycardia, or apnea (20 seconds or more) constitutes a failure, and evaluation by the practitioner must occur before discharge.
- Repeat the test after 24 hours once modifications are made to the car seat, car bed, or infant's position in either restraint system.
- It is recommended that a certified car seat technician place the infant in the car seat (or bed). The technician will demonstrate appropriate positioning of the infant in the restraint device to the parents and have the parents do a return demonstration.
- Document the interventions, the infant's tolerance, and the parents' return demonstration.

[m] Modified from Bull MJ, Engle WA, American Academy of Pediatrics. Safe transportation of preterm and low birth weight infants at hospital discharge. *Pediatrics.* 2009;123(5):1424–1429; Davis NL, Shah N. Use of car beds for infant travel: a review of the literature. *J Perinatol.* 2018;38:1287–1294; Hoffman BD, Gilbert TA, Chan K, et al. Getting babies safely home: a retrospective chart review of car safety seat tolerance screening outcomes. *Acad Pediatr.* 2021;21:1355–1362; and Magnarelli M, Shah Solanki N, Davis NL. Car seat tolerance screening for late-preterm infants. *Pediatrics.* 2020;145(1):e20191703.

Parental Guidance

Guidance During Infancy

First 6 Months

Teach car safety with use of federally approved restraint, facing rearward, in the middle of the back seat.
Understand each parent's adjustment to newborn, especially mother's postpartum emotional needs.
Teach care of infant, and help parents to understand the infant's individual needs and temperament and that the infant expresses wants through crying.
Reassure parents that infant cannot be spoiled by too much attention during the first 4 to 6 months.
Encourage parents to establish a schedule that meets needs of child and themselves.
Help parents to understand infant's need for environmental stimulation.
Support parents' pleasure in seeing child's growing friendliness and social responses, especially smiling.
Plan anticipatory guidance for safety.
Stress need for immunizations.
Prepare for introduction of solid foods.

Second 6 Months

Prepare parents for child's "stranger anxiety."
Encourage parents to allow child to cling to them and avoid long separation from either parent.
Guide parents concerning discipline because of infant's increasing mobility.
Encourage use of negative voice and eye contact rather than physical punishment as a means of discipline.
Encourage showing most attention when infant is behaving well, rather than when infant is crying.
Discuss injury prevention because of child's advancing motor skills and curiosity.
Encourage parents to leave child with suitable caregiver to allow themselves some free time.
Discuss readiness for bottle weaning.
Explore parents' feelings regarding infant's sleep patterns.

Guidance During Toddler Years

Ages 12 to 18 Months

Prepare parents for expected behavioral changes of toddler, especially negativism, and ritualism.
Assess present feeding habits, and encourage gradual weaning from bottle to cup and increased intake of solid foods.
Stress expected feeding changes of physiologic anorexia, food fads and strong taste preferences, need for scheduled routine at mealtimes, inability to sit through an entire meal, and lack of table manners.
Assess sleep patterns at night, particularly habit of a bedtime bottle, which is a major cause of early childhood dental caries, and procrastination behaviors that delay hour of sleep.
Prepare parents for potential dangers of the home and motor vehicle environment, particularly motor vehicle injuries, drowning, accidental poisoning, and falling injuries; give appropriate suggestions for childproofing the home.
Discuss need for firm but gentle discipline and ways in which to deal with negativism and temper tantrums; stress positive benefits of appropriate discipline.
Emphasize importance for both child and parents of brief, periodic separations.
Discuss toys that use developing gross and fine motor, language, cognitive, and social skills.
Emphasize need for dental supervision, types of basic dental hygiene at home, and food habits that predispose children to caries; stress importance of supplemental fluoride (if adequate amounts are not in potable [drinking] water source).

Ages 18 to 24 Months

Stress importance of peer companionship in play.
Explore need for preparation for additional sibling; stress importance of preparing child for new experiences.
Discuss present discipline methods, their effectiveness, and parents' feelings about child's negativism; stress that negativism is important aspect of developing self-assertion and independence and is not a sign of spoiling.
Discuss signs of readiness for toilet training; emphasize importance of waiting for physical and psychological readiness.
Discuss development of fears, such as of darkness or loud noises, and of habits, such as security blanket or thumb sucking; stress normalcy of these transient behaviors.
Prepare parents for signs of regression in time of stress.
Assess child's ability to separate easily from parents for brief periods under familiar circumstances.
Allow parents to express their feelings of weariness, frustration, and exasperation.
Point out some of the expected changes of the next year, such as longer attention span, somewhat less negativism, and increased concern for pleasing others.

Ages 24 to 36 Months

Discuss importance of imitation and domestic mimicry and need to include child in activities.
Discuss approaches toward toilet training, particularly realistic expectations and attitude toward accidents.
Stress uniqueness of toddlers' thought processes, especially regarding their use of language, lack of understanding

time, causal relationships in terms of proximity of events, and inability to see events from another's perspective.

Stress that discipline must still be structured and concrete and that relying solely on verbal reasoning and explanations leads to confusion, misunderstanding, and even injuries.

Discuss investigation of preschool or daycare center toward completion of second year.

Guidance During Preschool Years

Age 3 Years

Prepare parents for child's increasing interest in widening relationships.

Encourage enrollment in preschool.

Emphasize importance of setting limits.

Prepare parents to expect exaggerated tension-reduction behaviors, such as need for security blanket.

Encourage parents to offer child choices.

Prepare parents to expect marked changes at 3{½} years, when child becomes insecure, and exhibits emotional extremes.

Prepare parents for normal dysfluency in speech, and advise them to avoid focusing on the pattern.

Prepare parents to expect extra demands on their attention as a reflection of child's emotional insecurity and fear of loss of love.

Warn parents that the equilibrium of a 3-year-old will change to the aggressive, out-of-bounds behavior of a 4-year-old.

Inform parents to anticipate a more stable appetite with more food selections.

Stress need for protection and education of child to prevent injury.

Age 4 Years

Prepare parents for more aggressive behavior, including motor activity and offensive language.

Prepare parents to expect resistance to their authority.

Explore parental feelings regarding child's behavior.

Suggest some type of respite for primary caregivers, such as placing child in preschool for part of the day.

Prepare parents for child's increasing curiosity.

Emphasize importance of realistic limit setting on behavior and appropriate discipline techniques.

Prepare parents for a highly imaginative 4-year-old who indulges in tall tales (to be differentiated from lies) and develops imaginary playmates.

Prepare patients to expect nightmares or an increase in nightmares.

Provide reassurance that a period of calmness begins at 5 years of age.

Age 5 Years

Inform parents to expect tranquil period at 5 years.

Help parents to prepare the child for entrance into school environment.

Make certain that immunizations are up to date before child enters school.

Suggest that unemployed parental caregivers consider own activities when child begins school.

Guidance During School-Age Years

Age 6 Years

Prepare parents to expect child's strong food preferences and frequent refusals of specific food items.

Prepare parents to expect increasingly ravenous appetite.

Prepare parents for emotional reactions as child experiences erratic mood changes.

Help parents anticipate continued susceptibility to illness.

Teach injury prevention and safety, especially bicycle safety.

Encourage parents to respect child's need for privacy and to provide a separate bedroom for child, if possible.

Prepare parents for child's increasing interests outside the home.

Help parents understand the need to encourage child's interactions with peers.

Ages 7 to 10 Years

Prepare parents to expect improvement in child's health and fewer illnesses, but warn them that allergies may increase or become apparent.

Prepare parents to expect an increase in minor injuries.

Emphasize caution in selecting and maintaining sports equipment, and reemphasize safety.

Prepare parents to expect increased involvement with peers and interest in activities outside the home.

Emphasize the need to encourage independence while maintaining limit setting and discipline.

Prepare mothers to expect more demands at 8 years of age.

Prepare fathers to expect increasing admiration at 10 years of age; encourage father-child activities.

Prepare parents for prepubescent changes in girls.

Ages 11 to 12 Years

Help parents prepare child for body changes of pubescence.

Prepare parents to expect a growth spurt in girls.

Make certain child's sex education is adequate with accurate information.

Prepare parents to expect energetic but stormy behavior at 11 years old and child becoming more even tempered at 12 years old.

Encourage parents to support child's desire to "grow up" but to allow regressive behavior when needed.
Prepare parents to expect an increase in child's masturbation.
Instruct parents that the child may need more rest.
Help parents educate child regarding experimentation with potentially harmful activities.

Health Guidance

Help parents understand the importance of regular health and dental care for child.
Encourage parents to teach and model sound health practices, including diet, rest, activity, and exercise.
Stress the need to encourage children to engage in appropriate physical activities.
Emphasize providing a safe physical and emotional environment.
Encourage parents to teach and model safety practices.

Electronic Communication Safety

Advanced technology of wireless computers/tablets and cellular (mobile) phones with social electronic media (e.g., Facebook, Snap-chat, Instagram, emails, blogs, twitter, numerous other media) is prominent in lives of today's children, adolescents, and adults. Cellular phones offer additional means of communication (e.g., texting, instant messages, talking). With the popularity of electronic technology, children and adolescents may experience a decrease in parental or adult social interactions. The increased mobility of devices and wireless Internet allow the individual to participate in social media or video games or explore the Internet independently, which has the potential for positive (e.g., learning opportunities, network) or negative ramifications (cyber bullying, predators to harm children). *Cyber bullying* is the use of an electronic device to communicate insults, harassment, and publicly humiliating statements about a person, usually involving an adolescent. Actions that may be helpful in providing Internet safety for the child and family follow:

Following are the AAP new recommendations (2022) for screen time: available at https://www.pathwaypeds.com/american-academy-of-pediatrics-announces-new-recommendations-for-childrens-media-use/.

- Children younger than 18 months, avoid use of screen media other than video-chatting. Parents of children 18 to 24 months who want to introduce digital media should choose high-quality programing and watch it with their children to help them understand what they are seeing and apply it to the world around them.
- Children ages 2 to 5 years, limit screen use to 1 h/day of high-quality programs. Parents should co-view media with children to help them understand what they are seeing and apply it to the world around them.
- Children ages 6 and older, place consistent limits on the time spent using media and the types of media, and make sure media does not take the place of adequate sleep (8 to 12 hours depending on age), physical activity (minimal of 1 hour), and other behaviors essential to health.
- Designate media-free times together, such as dinner or driving, as well as media-free locations at home, such as bedrooms.
- Have ongoing communication about online citizenship and safety, including treating others with respect online and offline.

Other Internet Safety Actions

- Encourage clear guidelines for Internet use, and provide direct supervision. Have frank discussions of what youth may encounter in viewing media. Be mindful of own media use in the home.
- Discuss with the adolescent or child the types of services he or she accesses and what types of communication (e-mail, instant messaging) or chatrooms the child or adolescent frequents.
- Encourage discussion of the fact that not all material printed on the Internet is true.
- Stress with the child to notify parent immediately if receive messages or bulletin boards that include offensive, suggestive, obscene, or threatening information or anything that makes the child or adolescent uncomfortable.
- Discuss Internet safety rules (e.g., avoid giving out personal identifying information) with all household members, including young children
- Know the type of games children and adolescents are involved in via the Internet; some may not be harmless and may contain adult material.

Guidance During Adolescence

Encourage Parents to

Accept adolescent as a unique individual.
Respect adolescent's ideas, likes and dislikes, and wishes.
Be involved with school functions and attend adolescent's performances, whether it is a sporting events or a school play.
Listen and try to be open to adolescent's views, even when they differ from parental views.
Avoid criticism about no-win topics.
Provide opportunity for choosing options and to accept the natural consequences of these choices.
Allow adolescent to learn by doing, even when choices and methods differ from those of adults.
Provide adolescent with clear, reasonable limits.
Clarify house rules and the consequences for breaking them. Let society's rules and consequences teach responsibility outside the home.
Allow increasing independence within limitations of safety and well-being.
Respect adolescent's privacy.
Try to share adolescent's feelings of joy or sorrow.
Respond to feelings as well as to words.

Be available to answer questions, give information, and provide companionship.
Try to make communication clear.
Avoid comparisons with siblings.
Assist adolescent in setting appropriate career goals and preparing for adult roles.
Welcome adolescent's friends into the home, and treat them with respect.
Provide unconditional love and acceptance.
Be willing to apologize when mistaken.

Be Aware That Adolescents

Are subject to turbulent, unpredictable behavior.
Are struggling for independence.
Are extremely sensitive to feelings and behaviors that affect them.
May receive a different message than what was sent.
Consider friends extremely important.
Have a strong need to belong.

Play

Functions of Play

Sensorimotor Development

Improves fine motor and gross motor skills and coordination
Enhances development of all the senses
Explores the physical nature of the world
Provides for release of surplus energy
Encourages and enhances communication

Intellectual Development

Provides multiple sources of learning:

- Explores and manipulates shapes, sizes, textures, and colors and learns the significance of objects and numbers
- Develops an understanding or spatial relationships, and abstract concepts
- Practices and expands language skills

Provides opportunity to rehearse past experiences to assimilate them into new perceptions and relationships.

Helps children to comprehend the world in which they live and to distinguish between fantasy and reality.

Socialization and Moral Development

Learns adult roles, including gender role behavior
Establishes social relationships and solves the problems associated with these relationships
Encourages interaction and development of positive attitudes toward others
Learns and reinforces approved patterns of behavior and moral standards
Learns right from wrong, the standards of society and assumes responsibility for their actions

Creativity

Provides an expressive outlet for creative ideas and interests
Allows for fantasy and imagination
Enhances development of special talents and interests
Develops satisfaction in the creation of something new and different and transfers their creative interest to situations outside the world of play

Self-Awareness

Facilitates the development of self-identity
Encourages regulation of own behavior
Allows for testing of own abilities (self-mastery)
Provides for comparison of own abilities with those of others
Allows opportunities to learn how own behavior affects others

Therapeutic Value

Provides for release from tension and stress
Allows expression of emotions and release of unacceptable impulses in a socially acceptable fashion
Encourages experimentation and testing of fearful situations in a safe manner
Facilitates nonverbal and indirect verbal communication of needs, fears, and desires
Seeks acceptance and presence of adults to help control their aggressive tendencies

Morality

Allows expression of cultural values and beliefs
Adheres to the accepted codes of behavior of the culture (e.g., fairness, honesty, self-control, consideration of others)
Learns to conform to standards of the group as realizes their peers tend not to be tolerant of group rule violations

Role of Play

In play, children continually practice the complicated, stressful processes of living, communicating, and achieving satisfactory relationships with other people. Both play theories of Parten and Piaget are incorporated in the General Trends of Play during Childhood. Jean Piaget's four cognitive stages of play throughout life include: functional (explore object using senses), constructive (use objects with purpose), symbolic/fantasy (incorporate objects in imaginative play and role-plays), and games with rules (follow rules in both solitary and group play). Mildren Parten Newhall's six stages of play (known as Paten's Stages of Play) during first 5 years of life include: unoccupied (infant plays/moves with body parts), solitary (child plays alone), spectator (watch others play), parallel (plays alongside other children), associative (play together but no organization), and cooperative (organized play with other children or in a group). Play stages descriptions of Piaget and Parten were obtained from a 2022 article on Stages of play:

The play theories of Parten and Piaget from https://wellbeingswithalysia.com/stages-of-play/. Play is important, and knowing the theory behind the stages makes a more in-tune nurse. Play begins in infancy and continues throughout life.

General Trends of Play During Childhood

Age	Social Character of Play	Content of Play	Most Prevalent Type of Play	Characteristics of Spontaneous Activity	Purpose of Dramatic Play	Development of Ethical Sense
Infant	Unoccupied Solitary	Social-affective Functional	Sensorimotor	Sense-pleasure	Self-identity	
Toddler	Parallel Spectator	Imitative Constructive	Body movement	Intuitive judgment	Learning gender role	Beginning of moral values
Preschool	Associative Spectator	Imaginative Constructive Symbolic	Fantasy Informal games	Concept formation Reasonably constant ideas	Imitating social life Learning social roles	Developing concern for playmates Learning to share and cooperate
School-age	Cooperative	Competitive games and contests Fantasy and Symbolic	Physical activity Group activities Formal games Play acting	Testing concrete situations and problem solving Adding fresh information	Vicarious mastery	Peer loyalty Playing by the rules Hero worship
Adolescent	Cooperative	Competitive games and contests Daydreaming	Social interaction	Abstract problem solving	Presenting ideas	Causes and projects

Play During Infancy

Age (Months)	Visual Stimulation	Auditory Stimulation	Tactile Stimulation	Kinetic Stimulation
Suggested Activities				
Birth to 1	Hang bright, shiny object within 20–25 cm (8–10 inches) of infant's face and in midline. Hang mobiles with black-and-white designs and high-contrast colors and designs.	Talk to infant; sing in soft voice. Play music box, radio, or television. Have ticking clock or metronome nearby.	Hold, caress, and cuddle infant. Keep infant warm. Infant may like to be swaddled.	Rock infant; place in cradle. Use stroller or carrier for walks.
2–3	Provide bright objects. Make room bright with pictures or mirrors. Take infant to various rooms while doing chores. Place in infant seat for vertical view of environment.	Talk to infant. Include in family gatherings. Expose to various environmental noises other than those of home. Use rattles, interactive toys (toys that respond when handled).	Caress infant while bathing and at diaper change. Comb hair with a soft brush.	Use infant swing. Take in car for rides. Exercise body by moving extremities in swimming motion. Infant activity gym (hangs above infant so she or he can touch).

Age (Months)	Visual Stimulation	Auditory Stimulation	Tactile Stimulation	Kinetic Stimulation
4–6	Place infant in front of safety (unbreakable) mirror. Give infant brightly colored toys to hold (small enough to grasp). Give infant books made of cloth, vinyl, or thick cardboard.	Talk to infant; repeat sounds infant makes. Laugh when infant laughs. Call infant by name. Crinkle different papers by infant's ear. Place rattle or bell in hand. Introduce nursery rhymes and songs.	Give infant soft squeeze toys of various textures. Allow infant to splash in bath. Place infant nude on soft rug and move extremities. Provide interactive toys Place infant supine, and provide dangling toys a few inches above that she or he can touch; provide rattling or soft noise toys	Use swing or stroller. Bounce infant in lap while holding in standing position. Support infant in sitting position; let infant lean forward to balance self. Place infant on floor to crawl, roll over, and sit.
6–9	Give infant large toys with bright colors, and noise makers. Place unbreakable mirror where infant can see self. Play peek-a-boo, especially hiding face. Play hide and seek with toy. Make funny faces to encourage imitation.	Call infant by name. Repeat simple words, such as "dada," "mama," and "bye-bye." Speak clearly. Name parts of body, people, and foods. Tell infant what you are doing. Use "no" only when necessary. Give simple commands. Show how to clap hands, bang a drum.	Let infant play with fabrics of various textures. Have bowl with foods of different sizes and textures to feel. Let infant catch running water. Encourage water play in large bathtub or shallow pool.	Hold up-right to bear weight and bounce. Pick up, and say "up." Put down, and say "down." Place toys out of reach, and encourage infant to get them. Play pat-a-cake.
9–12	Show infant large pictures in books. Take infant to places where there are animals, many people, and different objects (e.g., shopping center). Play ball by rolling it to infant, and demonstrate throwing it back. Demonstrate building a two-block tower.	Read simple nursery rhymes to infant. Point to body parts and name each one. Imitate sounds of animals.	Give infant finger foods of different textures. Allow infant to mess up and squash food. Allow infant to feel cold (ice cube) or warm (bath water); say what temperature each is. Allow infant to feel a breeze (fan blowing).	Give infant large push-pull toys. Place furniture to encourage cruising on floor. Turn in different positions.
Suggested Toys				
Birth to 6	Nursery mobiles Books with high-contrast pictures Unbreakable mirrors Contrasting colored sheets	Music boxes Musical mobiles Small-handled clear rattle Infant activity gym	Stuffed animals Soft clothes Soft or furry quilt Soft mobiles	Rocking crib or cradle Weighted or suction toy Infant swing

Age (Months)	Visual Stimulation	Auditory Stimulation	Tactile Stimulation	Kinetic Stimulation
6–12	Various colored blocks Nested boxes or cups Books with rhymes and bright pictures Strings of big beads Simple take-apart toys Large ball Cup and spoon Large puzzles Pop-up toys (Jack-in-the-box)	Rattles of different sizes, shapes, tones, and bright colors Squeaky animals and dolls Recordings of light, rhythmic music Rhythmic musical instruments Interactive toys	Soft, different-textured animals and dolls Sponge toys, floating toys Squeeze toys Teething toys Books with textures and objects, such as fur and zippers	Activity box for crib Push-pull toys Wind-up swing

Play During Toddlerhood

Physical Development	Social Development	Mental Development and Creativity
Suggested Activities		
Provide spaces that encourage physical activity. Provide sandbox, swing, and other scaled-down playground equipment.	Provide replicas of adult tools and equipment for imitative play. Permit child to help with adult tasks. Encourage imitative play. Provide toys and activities that allow for expression of feelings. Allow child to play with some actual items used in the adult world; for example, let child help wash dishes or play with pots and pans and other utensils (check for safety).	Provide opportunities for water play. Encourage building, drawing, and coloring. Provide various textures in objects for play. Provide large boxes and other safe containers for imaginative play. Provide books with pictures of animals, cars, trucks, and trains. Read stories appropriate to age. Monitor TV viewing (1 h or less).
Suggested Toys		
Push-pull toys Rocking horse Riding toy Balls (large) Blocks (unpainted) Pounding board Slide with supervision Pail and shovel Containers Play-Doh	CD player or tape recorder Purse Housekeeping toys (broom, dishes) Toy telephone Dishes, stove, table and chairs Mirror Puppets, dolls, stuffed animals (check for safety [e.g., no button eyes])	Wooden puzzles Cloth or vinyl picture books Paper, finger paint, thick crayons Blocks (wood or plastic) Wooden shoe for lacing Appropriate TV programs, videos, music CDs Shape sorters Cause/effect toys such as pop-ups

Play During Preschool Years

Physical Development	Social Development	Mental Development and Creativity
Suggested Activities		
Provide spaces for the child to run, jump, and climb. Teach child to swim. Teach water safety. Teach simple sports and activities.	Encourage interactions with neighborhood children. Intervene when children become destructive. Enroll child in preschool.	Encourage creative efforts with raw materials. Read stories. Monitor TV viewing. Attend theater and other cultural events appropriate to child's age. Take short excursions to park, seashore, museums, zoo.

Physical Development	Social Development	Mental Development and Creativity
Suggested Toys		
Medium-height slide Adjustable swing Vehicles to ride Tricycle Wading pool Wheelbarrow Sled Wagon Roller skates, speed graded to skill	Child-sized playhouse Dolls, stuffed toys Dishes, table Ironing board and iron Cash register, toy typewriter, computer Trucks, cars, trains, airplanes Play clothes for dress-up Doll carriage, bed, high chair Doctor and nurse kits Toy nails, hammer, saw Grooming aids, play makeup, or shaving kits	Books Jigsaw puzzles Musical toys (xylophone, piano, drum, horns) Picture games Blunt scissors, paper, glue Newsprint, crayons, poster paint, large brushes, easel, finger paint Flannel board and pieces of felt in colors and shapes CDs/tapes Dry erase board Sidewalk chalk (different colors) Wooden and plastic construction sets Magnifying glass, magnets

Play During Hospitalization

Functions of Play in the Hospital

- Helps the child to feel more secure in an unfamiliar environment
- Provides diversion and brings about relaxation
- Lessen the stress of separation and the feeling of homesickness
- Provides an expressive outlet for creative ideas and interests
- Helps children have an age-appropriate understanding of illness and treatment
- Provides a means to release tension and express feelings
- Encourages interaction and development of positive attitudes toward others
- Provides a means for accomplishing therapeutic goals
- Places child in active role and provides opportunity to make choices and be in control

Therapeutic Play Activities for Hospitalized Children

Oral Fluid Intake

- Make snow cones or freezer pops using child's favorite flavor.
- Cut gelatin into fun shapes.
- Make game of taking sip when turning page of book or during games such as Simon Says.
- Use small medicine cups; decorate the cups.
- Have a tea party; pour at small table.
- Cut straw in half, and place in small container (much easier for small child to suck liquid).
- Use a decorative straw.
- Make a progress poster; give rewards for drinking a predetermined quantity.

Deep Breathing

- Blow on pinwheel, feathers, whistle, harmonica, toy horns, or party noisemakers.
- Practice on band instruments.
- Have blowing contest using boats, cotton balls, feathers, Ping-Pong balls, or pieces of paper; blow such objects over a tabletop goal line, up in the air, against an opponent, or up and down a string.
- Move paper or cloth from one container to another using suction from a straw.
- Use incentive spirometer as prescribed
- Dramatize scenes, such as "I'll huff and puff and blow your house down" from the "Three Little Pigs."
- Take a deep breath, and pretend to "blow out the candles" on a birthday cake.

Range of Motion and Use of Extremities

- Toss wadded paper into a wastebasket.
- Play tickle toes; have child wiggle them on request.
- Play games such as Twister or Simon Says.
- Do bed aerobics, shadow dancing.
- Engage in puppet play.
- Play pretend and guess games (e.g., imitate a bird, butterfly, or horse).
- Have tricycle or wheelchair races in a safe area.
- Play kickball or throw ball with a soft foam ball in a safe area.
- Position bed so that child must turn to view television or doorway.
- Have child climb wall with fingers like a spider.

Pretend to teach aerobic dancing or exercise; encourage parents to participate.
Encourage swimming if feasible.
Play video games or pinball (fine motor movement).
Play hide-and-seek game; hide toy somewhere in bed (or room, if ambulatory)
Provide clay to mold with fingers.
Have child paint or draw on large sheets of paper placed on floor or wall.
Encourage combing own hair; play beauty shop with "customer" in different positions.

Tension-Release Activities

Muscle relaxation exercises
Distraction by telling stories or singing
Breathing through party blower or pinwheel
Counting
Pillow punching
Finger painting with shaving cream, pudding, or paint
Water play (target squirting with syringes)
Make magic glitter wands
Carpentry (pounding or hammering wood pegs)
Finger paint with Play-Doh.
Looking at pop-up books
Squeezing Nerf or stress ball
Listening to music
Make imagery scrapbook of pleasant images
Throwing sponge ball at a target on wall or door
Playing handheld games
Make a foil (aluminum) sculpture
Giving detailed explanation of procedure
Soothing touches or hugs
Deep breathing
Building tower blocks and knocking them over to allow acceptable, safe outlet for aggression
Playing with Play-Doh or clay sculptures
Target squirting with syringes

Injections

Let child handle syringe (without needle), alcohol swab, and band-aid and pretend to give an injection to doll or stuffed animal.
Use syringes to decorate cookies with frosting, squirt water, or target shoot into a container.
Allow child to have a collection of syringes (without needles); make wild creative objects with syringes.
Have child count to 10 or 15 during injection or "blow the hurt away."

Oral Medication Intake

NOTE: Remember to ask the pharmacist or physician if pill/medication can be crushed, divided in half, or mixed with food or liquid.
Allow child to choose how to take medication (e.g., by spoon, syringe, or medicine cup) to allow sense of control.
Offer a favorite drink, water, juice, soft drink, or ice pop or frozen juice bar after the medication to cover the taste.
Ask the pharmacist about using a flavor additive (e.g., apple, banana, bubble gum flavors) to help medication taste better. These do not require a prescription and usually at a nominal cost.
Suck on something cold (Popsicles or crushed ice) to numb the taste buds on the tongue before giving medication.
If nausea is a problem, give carbonated beverage poured over finely crushed ice before or immediately after the medication
Inquire if it is safe to mix liquid medication in a small amount (1 tsp) of appropriate of sweet-tasting substance (e.g., flavored syrups, jam, fruit purees, sherbet, ice cream); avoid essential food items because child may later refuse to eat them.

Pill Swallowing Tips—Instruct the Child Stand Up or Sit Up Straight Prior to Pill Swallowing

Train child in small steps with success at every step (e.g., have child practice with a piece of small cake decoration, mini M&M, or Tic Tac). Practice until child accomplishes the smallest size without a problem, and then move up to something slightly larger.
Place pill or capsule into ice cream, yogurt, applesauce, or pudding, and swallow it all together (avoid this in younger child because of association with food).
Place pill on a spoon of JELLO, and slurp it right down.
Some pills are easier to swallow if cut in half. Ask pharmacist if this is acceptable and if medication does not lose its potency.
Place pill on tongue, and have child drink a glass of water through a straw.
Purchase a "pill cup" (a cup with a little pocket in it that aids pill to float down with liquid when drinking).
Crush medication, and mix with flavored syrup on spoon.

Ambulation

Give child something to push:

- Toddler—push-pull toy
- School-age child—wagon or a doll in a stroller or wheelchair
- Adolescent—decorated intravenous (IV) line stand

Have a parade; make hats, and so on.
Encourage foot pointing.
Have a treasure hunt.
Play Simon Says or Red Light/Green Light

Immobilization or Isolation

Flashlight play—Use flashlights to create designs on wall or ceiling.
Make smiling masks.
Use isolation pen pals or phone pals to provide social experience for confined children.
Unit scrapbook—View photographs of people and places on unit.
Make bed into a pirate ship or airplane with decorations.
Move patient's bed frequently, especially to playroom, hallway, or outside.
Remote control cars/truck to provide sense of motion
Velcro darts with string attached for easy retrieval

Pain Assessment and Management

Symbol ▶ indicates material that may be photocopied and distributed to families.

Procedural Assessment and Analgesia

Children's Response to Pain

Children's ability to describe pain changes as they grow older and as they cognitively and linguistically mature. Three types of measures—behavioral, physiologic, and self-report— have been developed to measure children's pain, and their applicability depends on the child's cognitive and linguistic ability.

Developmental Characteristics of Children's Responses to Pain

Preterm Infant

- The preterm infant's response may be behaviorally blunted or absent. However, there is sufficient evidence that preterm infants are neurologically capable of experiencing pain.
- Use a preterm infant pain scale.
- Assume that painful procedures in older children and adults are also painful in a preterm infant (e.g., venipuncture, lumbar puncture, endotracheal intubation, circumcision, chest tube insertion, heel puncture).

Young Infant

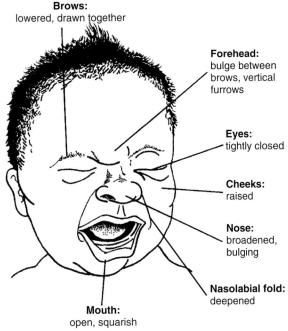

- Generalized body response of rigidity or thrashing, possibly with the local reflex withdrawal of stimulated area (Fig. 3.1)
- Loud crying
- The facial expression of pain (brows lowered and drawn together, eyes tightly closed, and mouth open and squarish)

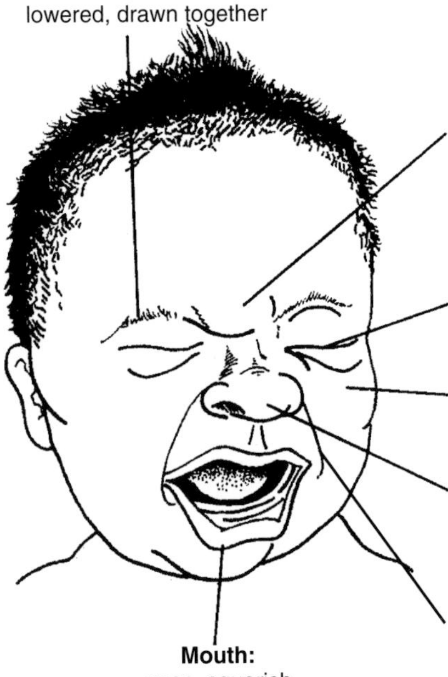

FIG. **3.1** Facial expression of physical distress is the most consistent behavioral indicator of pain in infants.

- No association demonstrated between approaching stimulus and subsequent pain

Older Infant

- Localized body response with the deliberate withdrawal of stimulated area
- Loud crying
- The facial expression of pain or anger
- Physical resistance, especially pushing the stimulus away after it is applied

Young Child

- Loud crying, screaming
- Verbal expressions such as "Ow," "Ouch," or "It hurts."
- The thrashing of arms and legs
- Attempts to push stimulus away before it is applied
- Lack of cooperation; the need for parent engagement and distraction techniques
- Requests termination of the procedure
- Clings to parent, nurse, or another significant person
- Requests emotional support, such as hugs or other forms of physical comfort
- May become restless and irritable with continuing pain
- Behaviors occurring in anticipation of actual painful procedure

School-Age Child

- May see all behaviors of a young child, especially during an actual painful procedure, but less in the anticipatory period
- Stalling behavior, such as "Wait a minute" or "I'm not ready."
- Muscular rigidity, such as clenched fists, white knuckles, gritted teeth, contracted limbs, body stiffness, closed eyes, wrinkled forehead

Adolescent

- Less vocal protest
- Less motor activity
- More verbal expressions, such as "It hurts" or "You're hurting me."
- Increased muscle tension and body control

Table 3.2 depicts various neonatal assessment scales with variables assessed and score ranges.

Category	Score		
	0	1	2
Face	No particular expression or smile	Occasional grimace or frown, withdrawn, disinterested	Frequent-to-constant quivering chin, clenched jaw
Legs	Normal position or relaxed	Uneasy, restless, tense	Kicking, or legs drawn up
Activity	Lying quietly, normal position, moves easily	Squirming, shifting back and forth, tense	Arched, rigid, or jerking
Cry	No cry (awake or asleep)	Moans or whimpers, occasional complaint	Crying steadily, screams or sobs, or frequent complaints
Consolability	Content, relaxed	Reassured by occasional touching, hugging, or being talked to, distractible	Difficult to console or comfort

Each of the five categories–(F) Face, (L) Legs, (A) Activity, (C) Cry, (C) Consolability–is scored from 0-2, which results in a total score between 0 and 10.

FIG. **3.2** FLACC Pain Rating Scale. (From Workman ML, LaCharity LA. Understanding pharmacology: Essentials for medication safety, ed 2, Elsevier; 2016.)

Nonpharmacologic Strategies for Pain Management

General Strategies

Evidence-Based Practice—Nonpharmacologic Interventions During Painful Procedures

Use nonpharmacologic interventions to supplement, not replace, pharmacologic interventions, and use for mild pain and pain that is reasonably well controlled with analgesics.

Form a trusting relationship with the child and family. Express concern regarding their reports of pain and intervene appropriately.

Use general guidelines to prepare a child for the procedure.

Prepare the child before potentially painful procedures but avoid "planting" the idea of pain. For example, instead of saying, "This is going to (or may) hurt," say, "Sometimes this feels like pushing, sticking, or pinching, and sometimes it doesn't bother people. Tell me what it feels like to you."

Use "non-pain" descriptors when possible (e.g., "It feels like heat" rather than "It's a burning pain"). This allows for variation in sensory perception, avoids suggesting pain, and gives the child control in describing reactions.

Avoid evaluative statements or descriptions (e.g., "This is a terrible procedure" or "It really will hurt a lot").

Stay with a child during a painful procedure.

Allow parents to stay with the child if the child and parent desire; encourage a parent to talk softly to the child and to remain near the child's head.

Involve parents in learning specific nonpharmacologic strategies and in assisting a child with their use.

Educate the child about the pain, especially when explanation may lessen anxiety (e.g., that pain may occur after surgery and does not indicate something is wrong); reassure the child that he or she is not responsible for the pain.

For long-term pain control, give a child a doll, which represents "the patient," and allow a child to do everything to the doll that is done to the child; pain control can be emphasized through the doll by stating, "Dolly feels better after the medicine."

Teach procedures to children and families for later use.

Specific Strategies

Distraction

Involve parent and child in identifying strong distracters.

Involve the child in play; use radio, tape recorder, CD player, or computer game; have the child sing or use rhythmic breathing.

Have the child take a deep breath and blow it out until told to stop.

Have the child blow bubbles to "blow the hurt away."

Have the child concentrate on yelling or saying "ouch," with instructions to "yell as loud or soft as you feel it hurt; that way, I know what's happening."

TABLE 3.1 Pain Rating Scales for Children

Pain Scale, Description	Instructions	Recommended Age, Comments
Wong-Baker FACES Pain Rating Scale[a]		
Consists of six cartoon faces ranging from smiling faces for "no pain" to tearful faces for "worst pain."	*Brief word instructions:* Point to each face using the words to describe the pain intensity. Ask a child to choose a face that best describes their own pain and record the appropriate number.	For children as young as 3 years old. Using original instructions without affect words, such as happy or sad, or brief words resulted in the same range of pain rating, probably reflecting the child's rating of pain intensity. For coding purposes, numbers 0, 2, 4, 6, 8, and 10 can be substituted for 0–5 system to accommodate 0–10 system. The Wong-Baker FACES Pain Rating Scale provides three scales in one: facial expressions, numbers, and words. Research supports cultural sensitivity of FACES for Caucasian, African American, Hispanic, Thai, Chinese, and Japanese children.

					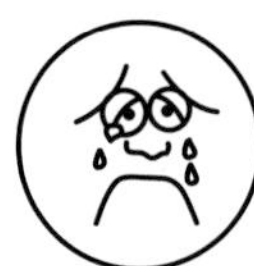
0	1 or 2	2 or 4	3 or 6	4 or 8	5 or 10
No hurt	Hurts little bit	Hurts little more	Hurts even more	Hurts whole lot	Hurts worst

Pain Scale, Description	Instructions	Recommended Age, Comments
Word-Graphic Rating Scale[b] (Tesler et al., 1991)		
Uses descriptive words (may vary in other scales) to denote varying intensities of pain	Explain to the child, "This is a line with words to describe how much pain you may have. This side of the line means no pain, and over here, the line means worst possible pain." (Point with your finger where "no pain" is, and run your finger along the line to "worst possible pain," as you say it.) "If you have no pain, you will mark like this." (Show example.) "If you have some pain, you will mark somewhere along the line, depending on how much pain you have." (Show example.) "The more pain you have, the closer to worst pain you would mark. The worst pain possible is marked like this." (Show example.) "Show me how much pain you have right now by marking with a straight, up-and-down line anywhere along the line to show how much pain you have right now." With the millimeter rule, measure from the "no pain" end to mark and record this measurement as a pain score.	For children from 4 to 17 years old.

No pain	Little pain	Medium pain	Large pain	Worst possible pain

Pain Scale, Description	Instructions	Recommended Age, Comments
Numeric Scale		
Uses straight line with endpoints identified as "no pain" and "worst pain," and sometimes "medium pain" in the middle; divisions along the line are marked in units from 0 to 10 (high number may vary)	Explain to the child that at one end of a line is 0, which means that person feels no pain (hurt). At the other end is usually a 5 or 10, which means the person feels worst pain imaginable. The numbers 1–5 or 1–10 are for very little pain to a whole lot of pain. Ask a child to choose a number that best describes their own pain.	For children as young as 5 years old, as long as they can count and have some concept of numbers and their values in relation to other numbers. The scale may be used horizontally or vertically. Number coding should be the same as other scales used in a facility.

TABLE 3.1 Pain Rating Scales for Children—cont'd

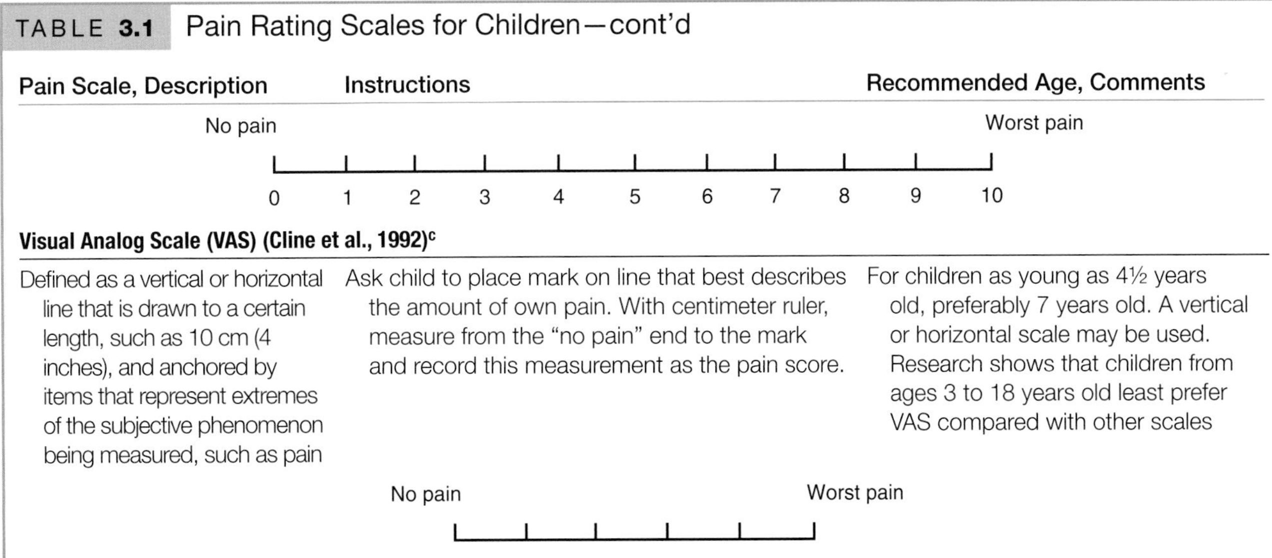

Pain Scale, Description	Instructions	Recommended Age, Comments
Visual Analog Scale (VAS) (Cline et al., 1992)[c]		
Defined as a vertical or horizontal line that is drawn to a certain length, such as 10 cm (4 inches), and anchored by items that represent extremes of the subjective phenomenon being measured, such as pain	Ask child to place mark on line that best describes the amount of own pain. With centimeter ruler, measure from the "no pain" end to the mark and record this measurement as the pain score.	For children as young as 4½ years old, preferably 7 years old. A vertical or horizontal scale may be used. Research shows that children from ages 3 to 18 years old least prefer VAS compared with other scales

[a]Wong-Baker FACES Foundation. (2020). Wong-Baker FACES Pain Rating Scale. Published with permission from http://www.WongBakerFACES.org. Originally published in Whaley & Wong's Nursing Care of Infants and Children. © Elsevier Inc.

[b]Instructions for Word-Graphic Rating Scale from Acute Pain Management Guideline Panel. (1992). Acute pain management in infants, children, and adolescents: Operative and medical procedures; Quick reference guide for clinicians. ACHPR Pub. No. 92-0020. Rockville, MD: Agency for Health Care Research and Quality, US Department of Health and Human Services. Word-Graphic Rating Scale is part of the Adolescent Pediatric Pain Tool and is available from Pediatric Pain Study, University of California, School of Nursing, Department of Family Health Care Nursing, San Francisco, CA 94143-0606; 415-476-4040.

[c]Cline ME, Herman J, Shaw ER, et al. Standardization of the visual analogue scale. *Nurs Res.* 1992;41(6):378–380.

TABLE 3.2 Summary of Pain Assessment Scales for Infants

	PIPP-revised (Stevens et al., 2014)	NIPS (Lawrence et al., 1993)	NPASS (Hummel et al., 2008)	COMFORT-neo (van Dijk et al., 2009)	CRIES (Krechel & Bildner, 1995)
Age range	25–40 weeks	26–40 weeks	23–40 weeks	24–42 weeks	32–40 weeks
Type of pain	Procedural and postoperative		Procedural and prolonged	Prolonged pain	Postoperative pain
Variables assessed	Scored at (0–3) each Heart rate Oxygen saturation Brow bulge Eye squeeze Nasolabial furrow Behavioral state	Breathing (0–1) Face (0–1) Arms (0–1) Legs (0–1) Cry (0–2) Arousal (0–1)	Scored at (0–2) each Vital signs Crying/irritability Facial expressions Behavioral state Extremities/tone	Scored at (1–5) each Alertness Calmness/agitation Respiratory response or crying Body movement Muscle tone Facial tension	Scored at (0–2) each Crying Oxygen requirement Changes to vital signs Facial expressions Sleeplessness
Score range	0–21	0–7	Pain: 0–10	6–30	0–10
Adjusted for gestational age	Yes Scored at (0–3)	No	Yes	No	No

Adapted from Harris J, Ramelet A, van Dijk M, et al. Clinical recommendations for pain, sedation, withdrawal and delirium assessment in critically ill infants and children: an ESPNIC position statement for healthcare professionals. *Intensive Care Med.* 2016;42:972–986.

References

Hummel P, Puchalski M, Creech SD. Clinical reliability and validity of the N-PASS: neonatal pain, agitation, and sedation scale with prolonged pain. *J Perinatol.* 2008;28(1):55–60.

Krechel SW, Bildner J. Cries: a new neonatal postoperative pain measurement score: initial testing of validity and reliability. *Paediatr Anaesth.* 1995;5(1):53–61.

Lawrence J, Alcock D, McGrath P, et al. The development of a tool to assess neonatal pain. *Neonatal Netw.* 1993;12(6):59–66.

Stevens BJ, Gibbins S, Yamada J, et al. The premature infant pain profile-revised (PIPP-R): initial validation and feasibility. *Clin J Pain.* 2014;30(3):238–243.

van Dijk M, Roofthooft DW, Anand KJ, et al. Taking up the challenge of measuring prolonged pain in (premature) neonates: the COMFORTneo scale seems promising. *Clin J Pain.* 2009;25(7):607–616.

Have the child look through a kaleidoscope (the type with glitter suspended in a fluid-filled tube) and encourage him or her to concentrate by asking, "Do you see the different designs?"
Use humor, such as watching cartoons, telling jokes or funny stories, or acting silly with children.
Have the child read, play games, or visit with friends.

Relaxation

With an infant or young child:
Hold in a comfortable, well-supported position, such as vertically against the chest and shoulder.
Rock in a wide, rhythmic arc in a rocking chair or sway back and forth rather than bouncing a child.
With a slightly older child:
Ask a child to take a deep breath and "go limp as a rag doll" while exhaling slowly; then, ask a child to yawn (demonstrate if needed).
Help the child assume a comfortable position (e.g., pillow under neck and knees).
Begin progressive relaxation: starting with the toes, systematically instruct a child to let each body part "go limp" or "feel heavy"; if a child has difficulty relaxing, instruct a child to be tense or tighten each body part and then relax it.
Allow the child to keep eyes open since children may respond better if their eyes are open rather than closed during relaxation.

Guided Imagery

Have the child identify some highly pleasurable real or imaginary experience.
Have the child describe details of the event, including as many senses as possible (e.g., "feel the cool breezes," "see the beautiful colors," "hear the pleasant music").
Have a child write down or tape-record the script.
Encourage the child to concentrate only on the pleasurable event during the painful time; enhance the image by recalling specific details through reading the script or playing the tape.
Combine with relaxation and rhythmic breathing.

Positive Self-Talk

Teach child positive statements to say when in pain (e.g., "I will be feeling better soon," "When I go home, I will feel better, and we will eat ice cream").

Thought Stopping

Identify positive facts about the painful event (e.g., "It does not last long").
Identify reassuring information (e.g., "If I think about something else, it does not hurt as much").
Condense positive and reassuring facts into a set of brief statements, and have the child memorize them (e.g., "Short procedure, good veins, a little hurt, nice nurse, go home").
Have the child repeat the memorized statements whenever thinking about or experiencing the painful event.

Analgesic Drug Administration

Routes and Methods

Oral

The oral route preferred because of its convenience, cost, and relatively steady blood levels
Higher dosages of an oral form of opioids are required for equivalent parenteral analgesia
Peak drug effect occurs after 1 to 2 hours for most analgesics
Delay in onset is a disadvantage when rapid control of severe pain or of fluctuating pain is desired
In young infants, oral sucrose can provide analgesia for painful procedures.

Sublingual, Buccal, or Transmucosal

Tablet or liquid placed between cheek and gum (buccal) or under the tongue (sublingual)
Highly desirable because more rapid onset than the oral route
Produces less first-pass effect through the liver than oral route, which normally reduces analgesia from oral opioids (unless a sublingual or buccal form is swallowed, which often occurs in children)
Few drugs commercially available in this form
Many drugs can be compounded into sublingual troche or lozenge.

Intravenous (IV) (Bolus)

Preferred for rapid control of severe pain
Provides the most rapid onset of effect, usually in about 5 minutes
Advantages for acute pain, procedural pain, and breakthrough pain
Needs to be repeated hourly for continuous pain control
Drugs with a short half-life (morphine, fentanyl, hydromorphone) are preferable to avoid a toxic accumulation of the drug

IV (Continuous)

Preferred over bolus and intramuscular injection for maintaining control of pain
Provides steady blood levels
Easy to titrate dosage

EVIDENCE-BASED PRACTICE

Reduction of Minor Procedural Pain in Infants

Ask the Question

Question

In newborns and infants, does sucrose provide adequate analgesia during minor painful procedures? Are the effects age-dependent?

Search for the Evidence

Search Strategies

Search selection criteria included English publications within the past 10 years and research-based articles (level 1 or lower) on neonates or infants undergoing venipuncture or immunizations.

Databases Used

PubMed, Cochrane Collaboration, MD Consult, Joanna Briggs Institute, National Guideline Clearinghouse (AHQR), TRIP Database Plus, PedsCCM, BestBETs

Critically Analyze the Evidence

Grade criteria: Evidence quality high; recommendation strong (Guyatt et al., 2008)

Sucrose for analgesia in newborn infants undergoing painful procedures

A systematic review of the effectiveness of sucrose in providing pain relief in neonates and newborn infants during painful procedures included 74 randomized controlled trials that included over 7000 infants using the standard Cochrane Neonatal methodology (Stevens et al., 2016). The main outcome measures were composite pain scores, with secondary outcomes including physiological and behavioral pain indicators. There was high-quality evidence for the beneficial effects of sucrose in reducing procedural pain related to heel lance, venipuncture, and intramuscular injections.

Minimally effective dose of sucrose for neonatal procedural pain relief

In a randomized controlled study, investigators sought to identify the minimally effective dose of 24% sucrose for reducing pain in hospitalized infants undergoing heel lance (Stevens et al., 2018). The researchers included 245 neonates from 4 tertiary NICUs in Canada who were between the ages of 24 and 42 weeks of gestational age. Infants were randomized to three doses of 24% sucrose plus non-nutritive sucking/pacifier for 2 min prior to heel lance. Sucrose dose levels were 0.1 mL (81), 0.5 mL (81) and 1.0 mL (83). Pain levels were measured using the Premature Infant Pain Profile—Revised. There were five reported adverse effects (three neonates with gagging/choking, one with oxygen desaturation to less than 80%, and one with decreased HR <80%. All events resolved spontaneously without medical intervention. There were no statistically different pain findings across the three groups, and the investigators determined the minimally effective dose of sucrose to be 0.1 mL.

Sucrose for pain management in newborn infants undergoing casting for club foot

In a double-blind, randomized controlled trial, researchers evaluated the effectiveness of sucrose for pain management during clubfoot casting and manipulation (Milbrandt et al., 2018). Infants from birth to 6 months (ave age 17.94 days old) who were treated with a Ponseti clubfoot manipulation and casting were randomized to a 2 oz bottle of 20% sucrose solution, water, or milk (breast or other) during each casting. Thirty-three infants underwent 131 casting procedures. Providers were blinded to the type of solution the infants received. The pain was measured by the Neonatal Infant Pain Score (NIPS). Infants who received water had the highest NIPS score ($P < .5$), while children receiving sucrose had the lowest pain score ($P = .08$). The investigators found that infants undergoing Ponseti manipulation and casting had lower pain scores when given sucrose solution or breast milk/milk during the procedure.

Skin-to-skin care versus sucrose for preterm neonatal pain

In a randomized, blinded crossover trial, investigators compared skin-to-skin care (SSC) to sucrose for preterm neonatal pain during heel stick procedure (Nimbalkar et al., 2020). The pain was assessed using the premature infant pain profile. One hundred neonates were randomized into two groups. Group A neonates received SSC 15 min prior to the heel stick and sucrose 2 min before the second heel stick. Group B neonates received sucrose 15 min before the first heel-stick and SSC 15 min before the second heel-stick. Oral sucrose had a small statistical but not clinically significant difference in the reduction of PIPP scores. Heart rate and behavioral state were found to be lower than the sucrose group but were not statistically significant. The authors cite concerns related to developmental outcomes related to frequent sucrose use and recommend SSC as the first line of prevention for pain control with oral sucrose in settings where SSC is not feasible.

Breastfeeding for procedural pain in infants beyond the neonatal period

A systematic review of the literature using Cochrane methodology standards was conducted to determine the effect of breastfeeding on procedural pain in infants beyond the neonatal period (Harrison et al., 2016). Ten studies with a total of 166 infants included were aged 1–12 months who received breastfeeding during painful procedures. Comparison studies included oral administration of water, sweet-tasting solutions, expressed breast milk or formula, pacifiers, cuddling, distraction, topical anesthetics, and skin-to-skin care. Procedures included subcutaneous/intramuscular injection, venipuncture, intravenous line insertion, and heel finger lance. In summary, breastfeeding reduced behavioral pain responses during vaccination compared to no treatment, water, and other interventions. The authors conclude that breastfeeding before and during vaccination injections reduces pain in most babies up to the age of 1 year.

Analgesic effects of breast and formula feeding during routine childhood immunizations up to 1 year of age

In a non-randomized, non-blinded study, pain parameters (latency, duration of crying, and pain scores) in three groups of children (breastfed, formula-fed, and unfed controls during immunization (Viggiano et al., 2021). The Neonatal Infant Pain Scale (NIPS) and Face, Legs, Activity, Cry, Consolability Scale (FLACC) was used to evaluate pain. The authors found that infants that were breastfed during immunizations had a longer time to initiate crying than infants who were formula feed or received no feeding, suggesting that breastfeeding provides better pain relief during immunizations than formula feed infants or those who do not feed during immunization.

Apply the Evidence and Nursing Implications

Sucrose

- Sucrose is effective in reducing pain response in neonates and infants up to 1 year of age undergoing minor acute painful procedures.
- Adverse effects in reported studies have been minimal and resolved without intervention.
- The minimum effective dose has been determined to be 0.1 mL of 24% solution given at least 2 min before a procedure.
- The analgesic effect of sucrose in combination with sucking a bottle or pacifier appears to be enhanced.
- Studies of older infants have used both sucrose and breastfeeding.
- Sucrose, in combination with nonpharmacologic support during a procedure, may increase the analgesic response even with lower concentrations of sucrose. Interventions include pacifier, holding, swaddling, skin-to-skin contact, and rocking.

Continued

EVIDENCE-BASED PRACTICE—cont'd

- Administration can be by labeled oral syringes, dipped pacifiers, or bottles, depending on the infant's ability and age.
- The advantages of minimum wait time, low cost, and decreased risk of adverse effects were significant.
- The effects of repeated dosing over time and dosing of infants younger than 27 weeks are not known.

References

Harrison D, Reszel J, Bueno M, et al. Breastfeeding for procedural pain in infants beyond the neonatal period. *Cochrane Database Syst Rev.* 2016;10(10):Cd011248.

Milbrandt T, Kryscio R, Muchow R, et al. Oral sucrose for pain relief during clubfoot casting: a double-blinded randomized controlled trial. *J Pediatr Orthop.* 2018;38(8):430–435.

Nimbalkar S, Shukla VV, Chauhan V, et al. Blinded randomized crossover trial: skin-to-skin care vs. sucrose for preterm neonatal pain. *J Perinatol.* 2020;40(6):896–901.

Stevens B, Yamada J, Campbell-Yeo M, et al. The minimally effective dose of sucrose for procedural pain relief in neonates: a randomized controlled trial. *BMC Pediatr.* 2018;18(1):85.

Stevens B, Yamada J, Ohlsson A, et al. Sucrose for analgesia in newborn infants undergoing painful procedures. *Cochrane Database Syst Rev.* 2016;7(7):Cd001069.

Viggiano C, Occhinegro A, Siano MA, et al. Analgesic effects of the breast- and formula feeding during routine childhood immunizations up to 1 year of age. *Pediatr Res.* 2021;89(5):1179–1184.

Subcutaneous (SC) (Continuous)

Used when oral and IV routes are not available

Provides equivalent blood levels to continuous IV infusion

Suggested initial bolus dose to equal 2-hour IV dose; total 24-hour dose usually requires concentrated opioid solution to minimize infused volume; use smallest-gauge needle that accommodates infusion rate

Patient-Controlled Analgesia (PCA)

Generally refers to self-administration of drugs, regardless of route

Typically uses a programmable infusion pump (IV, epidural, SC) that permits self-administration of boluses of medication at preset dose and time interval (lockout interval is the time between doses)

PCA bolus administration often combined with an initial bolus and continuous (basal or background) infusion of opioid

Optimum lockout interval is not known but must be at least as long as the time needed for the onset of the drug

Should effectively control pain during movement or procedures

A longer lockout provides a larger dose

Family-Controlled Analgesia

One family member (usually a parent) or other caregiver is designated as the child's primary pain manager with responsibility for pressing the PCA button

Guidelines for selecting a primary pain manager for family-controlled analgesia:

- Spends a significant amount of time with the patient
- Is willing to assume responsibility of being the primary pain manager
- Is willing to accept and respect patient's reports of pain (if able to provide) as best indicator of how much pain the patient is experiencing; knows how to use and interpret a pain rating scale
- Understands the purpose and goals of the patient's pain management plan
- Understands the concept of maintaining a steady analgesic blood level
- Recognizes signs of pain and side effects and adverse reactions to opioid

Nurse-Activated Analgesia

The child's primary nurse is designated as the primary pain manager and is the only person who presses the PCA button during that nurse's shift.

Guidelines for selecting a primary pain manager for family-controlled analgesia also applicable to nurse-activated analgesia

It may be used in addition to a basal rate to treat breakthrough pain with bolus doses; patients are assessed every 30 minutes for the need for a bolus dose

It may be used without a basal rate as a means of maintaining analgesia with around-the-clock bolus doses

Intramuscular

NOTE: Not recommended for pediatric pain control; not current standard of care

Intradermal

Used primarily for skin anesthesia (e.g., before lumbar puncture, bone marrow aspiration, arterial puncture, skin biopsy)

Local anesthetics (e.g., lidocaine) cause a stinging, burning sensation

The duration of stinging is dependent on the type of "caine" used

To avoid stinging sensation associated with lidocaine:

- Buffer the solution by adding 1 part sodium bicarbonate (1 mEq/ml) to 9 to 10 parts 1% or 2% lidocaine with or without epinephrine

3 PAIN ASSESSMENT AND MANAGEMENT

EVIDENCE-BASED PRACTICE

Needle-Free Injection System: J-Tip to Administer Buffered Lidocaine

Ask the Question

Question

In pediatrics, are needle-free injection systems (e.g., J-Tip) effective and safe in relieving pain during peripheral intravenous (PIV) cannulation?

Search for the Evidence

Search Strategies

English language research-based publications on jet injectors for delivery of lidocaine during PIV cannulation without time limitation were included. Exclusions included dental products, insulin, growth factor, and medications other than lidocaine.

Databases Used

Cochrane Collaboration Database, Joanna Briggs Institute, National Guideline Clearinghouse (AHRQ), PubMed, SUMSearch, CINAHL, Scopus, UpToDate, BestBETs, manufacturers' or distributors' websites (National Medical Products, Bioject, and Injex)

Critically Analyze the Evidence

Grade criteria: Evidence quality moderate, recommendations weak (Guyatt et al., 2008)

Jet injected lidocaine to reduce venipuncture reduce pain in young children

In a randomized, single-dose clinical trial of jet injected lidocaine for venipuncture (Lunoe et al., 2015), 205 children aged 1–6 years were randomized into three groups: J-tip, Vapocoolant spray (Control), and vapor coolant and "pop" of an empty J-tip. The procedure was videotaped, and the pain was scored by the FLACC pain tool. Children were randomized to intervention (0.2 mL 1% buffered lidocaine), control (vapor coolant), or sham group empty J-tip and vapor coolant). The study group was blinded to group randomizations. Results demonstrated that children who received the J-tip intervention had no significant increase in pain at needle insertion and 45% had no or mild pain at the time of venipuncture. There were no group differences in the first attempt venipuncture success, with all groups in the 90% range.

Needle-free injection systems to transform intravenous catheter placement in pediatrics

In an observational, prospective, cohort case-control study, 85 patients enrolled in the study, with 41 patients being assigned to the needle-free injected lidocaine pretreatment prior to IV insertion and 44 with usual IV insertion practice (Kelly et al., 2017). The same nurses were used to insert IVs in both groups of patients. The mean pain score for patients who received needle free injected lidocaine was 2.45, compared to patients who received no local anesthetic having a mean pain score of 5.83 ($P < .001$). The authors demonstrated a statistically significant decrease in pain for patients receiving pretreatment with needle-free injected lidocaine prior to IV insertion, suggesting implications for improving pain management related to IV insertion.

Comparison of children's venipuncture fear and pain

In a prospective, randomized trial, children's self-report of pain and fear related to IV insertion were evaluated by comparing a topical cream anesthetic (EMLA) and a needless lidocaine injection system (J-Tip) (Stoltz & Manworren, 2017). One hundred fifty consecutive patients were assigned 1:1 to treatment groups. The patient's self-report of pain was measured using a visual analog scale (VAS), and fear was measured by the Children's Fear Scale (CFS). Children who received EMLA had a lower VAS pain score, suggesting less pain; however, the magnitude of the difference was moderate. The main effect comparing the two interventions was not significant—suggesting no difference in the effectiveness of the two interventions for reducing fear. The authors conclude that when IV insertion can be delayed the required 60–90 min, EMLA should be used. If a delay is contraindicated, J-tip is a reasonable alternative to minimize IV insertion pain.

Needle-free injected lidocaine versus topical anesthesia for infant lumbar puncture

A randomized, double-blind trial of a needless lidocaine injection system (J-tip) and topical anesthetic evaluated pain response in infants aged 0–4 months undergoing lumbar puncture in the emergency department (Caltagirone et al., 2018). Fifty-eight infants (29 in each group) were consented and randomized to J-tip or a topical anesthetic. The pain was evaluated using the Neonatal Facial Coding System (NFCS), which evaluates cry, brow bulge, eye squeeze, nasolabial furrow, and open mouth. NFCS scores were similar in both groups across all time points. The authors found that procedures performed with J-tip were twice as likely to be successful compared to procedures using TA cream. The authors conclude that it may be difficult to mitigate the stress of infant LPs and suggest that other adjuncts, such as oral sucrose, may be added to provide additional comfort.

Apply the Evidence and Nursing Implications

The overall evidence for the use of needle-free injectable lidocaine products is moderate.

Current studies demonstrate the utility of needle-free injectable lidocaine products for pain management strategies. Further studies are needed to increase the evidence base for needle-free injectable lidocaine in infants and children.

References

Caltagirone R, Raghavan VR, Adelgais K, et al. A Randomized double blind trial of needle-free injected lidocaine versus topical anesthesia for infant lumbar. *Acad Emerg Med.* 2018;25(3):310–316.

Harrison D, Reszel J, Bueno M, et al. Breastfeeding for procedural pain in infants beyond the neonatal period. *Cochrane Database Syst Rev.* 2016;10(10):Cd011248.

Kelly S, Russell J, Devgon P, et al. Transformation of the peripheral intravenous catheter placement experience in pediatrics. *J Vasc Access.* 2017;18(3):259–263.

Lunoe MM, Drendel AL, Levas MN, et al. A randomized clinical trial of jet-injected lidocaine to reduce venipuncture pain for young children. *Ann Emerg Med.* 2015;66(5):466–474.

EVIDENCE-BASED PRACTICE

Ask the Question

Question

Does the use of an external cold and vibration product offer additional analgesic advantages (less time, ease of use, lower cost, higher effectiveness, decreased anxiety) in relieving pain during peripheral intravenous (PIV) cannulation in children compared with LMX (lidocaine) cream, buffered lidocaine via injection and other strategies?

Search for the Evidence

Search Strategies

English research-based publications on lidocaine-tetracaine patches for venipuncture without time limitations were included. Exclusions included epidural use, dermatologic procedures, and S-Caine Peel.

Databases Used

Cochrane Collaboration Database, Joanna Briggs Institute, National Guideline Clearinghouse (AHRQ), PubMed, SUMSearch, CINAHL, Scopus, Micromedex, UpToDate, BestBETs, manufacturer's websites (Endo Pharmaceuticals, ZARS Pharma)

Critically Analyze the Evidence

Grade criteria: Evidence quality low to very low; recommendation weak (Guyatt et al., 2008)

Analgesia by cooling vibration during venipuncture in cognitively impaired children

A prospective randomized controlled trial sought to assess if a cooling vibration device (Buzzy) decreased pain during venipuncture and intravenous cannulation in children with cognitive impairment (Schreiber et al., 2016). Seventy non-verbal children aged 4–17 years of age with cognitive impairment were randomized to Buzzy, frozen ice pack, or no intervention. Procedural pain was measured using the Noncommunicating Children's Pain Checklist—postoperative version. Children receiving venipuncture with the Buzzy product demonstrated significantly lower pain scores than children who received an ice pack or no intervention. There was no difference in procedural success rate in the Buzzy group and the no intervention group. Findings demonstrated that Buzzy could significantly lower procedural pain in children with cognitive impairment.

Audiovisual distraction and external cold vibration for children undergoing venipuncture

In a randomized clinical trial, 150 children aged 5–12 years who were scheduled for venipuncture were randomized into four groups—animated cartoons, Buzzy device, animated cartoons, and Buzzy, and no intervention (Bergomi et al., 2018). Venipuncture was conducted by experienced pediatric nurses using a 21 gauge needle and vacutainer. The pain was rated using the Won-Baker Faces Pain Rating Scale WBFP, and child anxiety was measured using the Children's Emotional Manifestation Scale (CEMS). Parents were asked to rate their anxiety by estimating their anxiety with a number rating from 0 to 10. Findings showed that children in the intervention groups had less pain during venipuncture than children with no intervention. Children in the cartoon intervention had significantly less pain during venipuncture than other groups. The secondary analysis demonstrated that Buzzy was highly effective in children less than nine years, and there was a significant effect in the Buzzy and cartoon group. Lastly, children's and parent's anxiety decreased more in the intervention groups versus the no-intervention group. The authors suggest that the use of non-pharmacologic interventions reduces the perception of pain and that the Buzzy was found to be particularly effective for younger children.

Pain relief during venipuncture in children using the Buzzy system

The efficacy of the Buzzy system for reducing pain was evaluated in a randomized, controlled trial comparing Buzzy with distraction cards to a "magic glove" intervention (Susam et al., 2018). Sixty-four children aged 3–10 who were scheduled for venipuncture participated in the trial. Parents were provided a 5-point Likert scale questionnaire regarding their experience of using the Buzzy. Children in the Buzzy and distraction card group had significantly lower pain scores than the magic glove group ($P = .39$). Parents rated the Buzzy system as positive or very positive, with 71.9% of parents indicating they would reuse the Buzzy system in a future venipuncture.

Systematic Review and Meta-Analysis of the efficacy of the Buzzy Device for needle-related procedures

A systematic review and meta-analysis were conducted to assess the efficacy of the Buzzy device combining cold and vibration for needle-related procedures and to update and expand the knowledge on this topic (Ballard et al., 2019). The authors utilized the Preferred Reporting Items for Systematic Reviews and Meta-Analysis (PRISMA), and the protocol was registered in the PROSPERO database and published in the Systematic Reviews Journal. Primary outcomes were needle-related procedural pain intensity via self-report, parent report, or observer report. Secondary outcomes included procedural anxiety and success of needle-related procedures at the first attempt for venipuncture or IV catheter insertions. A total of 7 trials were included in the analysis and synthesized the evidence of 9 RCTs involving 1145 children and adolescents. Findings demonstrated that Buzzy demonstrated a statistically significant effect on reducing self-reported procedural pain and anxiety, as well as parent-reported procedural pain and anxiety during needle-related procedures. Although many trials included in the analysis support the efficacy of the Buzzy device for reducing pain and anxiety during needle procedures, the quality of evidence was rated as very low due to issues with study design and rigor.

Thermomechanical stimulation (Buzzy) for vaccination pain in adults

In a prospective, randomized controlled trial, 497 employee volunteers 18 years or older undergoing annual mandatory influenza vaccination were consented and randomized to either a Buzzy intervention or no-intervention group (Redfern et al., 2019). Post-vaccine pain report was measured by a 10-cm visual analog scale. Secondary outcome measures were self-reported anxiety levels measured by VAS and satisfaction with injection measured by a 10-point Likert scale. Demographic information and history with needles and vaccinations were obtained. Participants receiving the Buzzy device during injection rated post-procedure pain significantly lower than the control group ($P = .035$). Reported satisfaction did not vary across experimental and control groups. However, those in the Buzzy group reported the injection was better than previous experiences. A post-hoc evaluation of Buzzy between low and high anxiety participants demonstrated that a significant reduction in pain was reported for the high pre-procedure anxiety group.

Apply the Evidence and Nursing Implications

The overall evidence for the use of the Buzzy cold/vibration device demonstrates efficacy in reducing needle-related procedural pain in a variety of populations of patients.

Further studies are needed to increase the evidence base for the Buzzy cold/vibration device.

References

Ballard A, Khadra C, Adler S, et al. Efficacy of the buzzy device for pain management during needle-related procedures: a systematic review and meta-analysis. *Clin J Pain.* 2019;35(6):532–543.

EVIDENCE-BASED PRACTICE—cont'd

Bergomi P, Scudeller L, Pintaldi S, et al. Efficacy of non-pharmacological methods of pain management in children undergoing venipuncture in a pediatric outpatient clinic: a randomized controlled trial of audiovisual distraction and external cold and vibration. *J Pediatr Nurs.* 2018;42:e66–e72.

Caltagirone R, Raghavan VR, Adelgais K, Roosevelt GE. A randomized double blind trial of needle-free injected lidocaine versus topical anesthesia for infant lumbar puncture. *Acad Emerg Med.* 2018;25(3):310–316.

Harrison D, Reszel J, Bueno M, et al. Breastfeeding for procedural pain in infants beyond the neonatal period. *Cochrane Database Syst Rev.* 2016;10(10):Cd011248.

Kelly S, Russell J, Devgon P, et al. Transformation of the peripheral intravenous catheter placement experience in pediatrics. *J Vasc Access.* 2017;18(3):259–263.

Lunoe MM, Drendel AL, Levas MN, et al. A randomized clinical trial of jet-injected lidocaine to reduce venipuncture pain for young children. *Ann Emerg Med.* 2015;66(5):466–474.

Milbrandt T, Kryscio R, Muchow R, et al. Oral sucrose for pain relief during clubfoot casting: a double-blinded randomized controlled trial. *J Pediatr Orthop.* 2018;38(8):430–435.

Nimbalkar S, Shukla VV, Chauhan V, et al. Blinded randomized crossover trial: skin-to-skin care vs. sucrose for preterm neonatal pain. *J Perinatol.* 2020;40(6):896–901.

Redfern RE, Micham J, Seegert S, et al. Influencing vaccinations: a buzzy approach to ease the discomfort of a needle stick-a prospective, randomized controlled trial. *Pain Manag Nurs.* 2019;20(2):164–169.

Schreiber S, Cozzi G, Rutigliano R, et al. Analgesia by cooling vibration during venipuncture in children with cognitive impairment. *Acta Paediatr.* 2016;105(1):e12–e16.

Stevens B, Yamada J, Campbell-Yeo M, et al. The minimally effective dose of sucrose for procedural pain relief in neonates: a randomized controlled trial. *BMC Pediatr.* 2018;18(1):85.

Stevens B, Yamada J, Ohlsson A, et al. Sucrose for analgesia in newborn infants undergoing painful procedures. *Cochrane Database Syst Rev.* 2016;7(7):Cd001069.

Stoltz P, Manworren RCB. Comparison of children's venipuncture fear and pain: randomized controlled trial of EMLA® and J-tip needleless injection system®. *J Pediatr Nurs.* 2017;37:91–96.

Susam V, Friedel M, Basile P, et al. Efficacy of the Buzzy System for pain relief during venipuncture in children: a randomized controlled trial. *Acta Biomed.* 2018;89(6-s):6–16.

Viggiano C, Occhinegro A, Siano MA, et al. Analgesic effects of breast- and formula feeding during routine childhood immunizations up to 1 year of age. *Pediatr Res.* 2021;89(5):1179–1184.

Transdermal fentanyl (Duragesic)

Available as a patch for continuous pain control

Safety and efficacy not established in children younger than age 12 years

Not appropriate for initial relief of acute pain because of a long interval to peak effect (12 to 24 hours); for rapid onset of pain relief, give an immediate-release opioid.

Orders for "rescue doses" of an immediate-release opioid recommended for breakthrough pain, a flare of severe pain that breaks through the medication being administered at regular intervals for persistent pain

Has a duration of up to 72 hours for prolonged pain relief

If respiratory depression occurs, there is a possible need for several doses of naloxone

Vapocoolant

Use of prescription spray coolants, such as Fluori-Methane or ethyl chloride (Pain-Ease); applied to the skin for 10 to 15 seconds immediately before the needle puncture; anesthesia lasts about 15 seconds.

Cold is disliked by some children; it may be less uncomfortable to spray coolant on a cotton ball and then apply this to the skin

The application of ice to the skin for 30 seconds was found to be ineffective.

Rectal

Alternative to oral or parenteral routes

Variable absorption rate

Generally disliked by children

Many drugs able to be compounded into rectal suppositories*

Regional Nerve Block

Use of long-acting local anesthetic (bupivacaine or ropivacaine) injected into nerves to block pain at the site

Provides prolonged analgesia postoperatively, such as after inguinal herniorrhaphy

It may be used to provide local anesthesia for surgery, such as dorsal penile nerve block for circumcision or for reduction of fractures

Inhalation

Use of anesthetics, such as nitrous oxide, to produce partial or complete analgesia for painful procedures

Side effects (e.g., headache) possible from occupational exposure to high levels of nitrous oxide

Epidural or Intrathecal

Involves catheter placed into epidural, caudal, or intrathecal space for continuous infusion or single or intermittent administration of opioid with or without a long-acting local anesthetic (e.g., bupivacaine, ropivacaine)

Analgesia primarily from the drug's direct effect on opioid receptors in the spinal cord

Respiratory depression is rare but may have slow and delayed onset; it can be prevented by checking the level of sedation and respiratory rate and depth hourly for initial 24 hours and decreasing the dose when excessive sedation is detected

Nausea, itching, and urinary retention are common dose-related side effects of the epidural opioid.

Mild hypotension, urinary retention, and temporary motor or sensory deficits are common unwanted effects of the local epidural anesthetic.

Catheter for urinary retention inserted during surgery to decrease trauma to a child; if inserted when a child is awake, anesthetize urethra with lidocaine

TABLE 3.3 Nonsteroidal Antiinflammatory Drugs for Children

Drug	Dosage	Comments
Choline magnesium trisalicylate (Trilisate)	10–15 mg/kg q8–12h PO Maximum dose 3000 mg/day	Available in suspension, 500 mg/5 mL Prescription
Ibuprofen (children's Motrin, children's Advil)	Children >6 months old: 5–10 mg/kg/dose q6–8h Maximum dose 30 mg/kg/day or 3200 mg/day	Available in numerous preparations Available in suspension, 100 mg/5 mL, and drops, 100 mg/2.5 mL Nonprescription
Naproxen (Naprosyn)	Children >2 years old: 5–10 mg/kg/dose every 12 h Maximum 20 mg/kg/day or 1250 mg/day	Available in suspension, 125 mg/5 mL, and several different dosages for tablets Prescription
Indomethacin	1 mg/kg q6–12h Maximum 3 g/kg/day or 150 mg/day	Available in 25-mg and 50-mg capsules and suspension 25 mg/5 mL Prescription
Diclofenac	1–2 mg/kg q6–12h PO Maximum 3 mg/kg/day or 150 mg/day	Available in 50-mg tablet and extended-release 100-mg tablets Prescription

PO, By mouth.
Data from American Pain Society. (2016). *Principles of analgesic use* (7th ed.). Chicago.

TABLE 3.4 Starting Dosages for Opioid Analgesics in Opioid-Naive Children (for Infants, Start at 25% to 33% of Dose and Titrate Analgesia and Sedation)

Medicine	Route of Administration	Starting Dosage
Morphine	Oral (immediate release)	0.3 mg/kg q3–4h PO
	Oral (prolonged release)	0.3–0.9 mg/kg q8–12h PO
	IV injection[a]	0.1 mg/kg q1–2h IV or SC
	SC injection	
	IV infusion	0.02 mg/kg/h
	SC infusion	
Fentanyl	IV injection	0.5–1 mcg/kg,[a] repeated q30–60min
	IV infusion	0.5–1 mcg/kg[a]
Hydromorphone[c]	Oral (immediate release)	60 mcg/kg q3–4h (maximum: 2–4 mg/dose)
	IV injection[a] or SC injection	15 mcg/kg q2–3h
Methadone	Oral (immediate release)	0.1 mg/kg
	IV injection[b] or SC injection	Every 4 h for the first two to three doses, then as analgesia duration increases, wean to q6–8h; intervals of analgesia beyond q8h are rare, but it may be dosed q12–24h to treat withdrawal[d]
Oxycodone	Oral (immediate release)	0.2 mg/kg q3–4h (maximum: 10 mg/dose)
	Oral (prolonged release)	0.2–0.6 mg/dose or 10 mg q12h

[a]Administer IV opioids over 3 to 5 minutes.
[b]Due to the complex nature and wide interindividual variation in the pharmacokinetics of methadone, methadone should be commenced only by practitioners experienced with its use.
[c]Hydromorphone is a potent opioid, and significant differences exist between oral and IV dosing. Use extreme caution when converting from one route to another.
[d]Methadone initially should be titrated like other strong opioids. The dosage may need to be reduced by 50% 2 to 3 days after the effective dose has been found to prevent adverse effects due to methadone accumulation. From then on, dosage increases should be performed at intervals of 1 week or longer and with a maximum increase of 50%.
IV, Intravenous; *PO*, by mouth; *SC*, subcutaneous.
Data from American Pain Society. *Principles of Analgesic Use*. 7th ed. Chicago, IL: Author; 2016.

Side Effects of Opioids

General

a. Constipation (possibly severe)
b. Respiratory depression
c. Sedation
d. Nausea and vomiting
e. Agitation, euphoria
f. Mental clouding
g. Hallucinations
h. Orthostatic hypotension
i. Pruritus
j. Urticaria
k. Sweating
l. Miosis (may be a sign of toxicity)
m. Anaphylaxis (rare)

Signs of Tolerance

a. Decreasing pain relief
b. Decreasing duration of pain relief

Signs of Withdrawal Syndrome in Patients With Physical Dependence

1. Initial signs of withdrawal
   a. Lacrimation
   b. Rhinorrhea
   c. Yawning
   d. Sweating
2. Later signs of withdrawal
   a. Restlessness
   b. Irritability
   c. Tremors
   d. Anorexia
   e. Dilated pupils
   f. Gooseflesh
   g. Nausea, vomiting

GUIDELINES

Managing Opioid-Induced Respiratory Depression

Assess sedation level
If sedated, stimulate patient (shake shoulder gently, call by name, ask to breathe).
Stop or reduce opioid.
Monitor closely for pain and progressive sedation and respiratory depression.
If patient cannot be aroused and respirations are depressed or patient is apneic:
Stop or reduce opioid.
Administer oxygen.
Support respirations.
Initiate resuscitation efforts as appropriate.
Administer naloxone (Narcan):
- For children weighing less than 40 kg (88 lb), dilute 0.1 mg naloxone in 10 ml sterile saline to make 10 mcg/ml solution and give up to 0.5 mcg/kg.
- For children weighing more than 40 kg (88 lb), dilute 0.4-mg ampule in 10 ml sterile saline (usually only 40 to 50 mcg are needed except with unwitnessed acute intoxication such as in emergency department).

Administer bolus by slow intravenous push until effect is obtained.
Closely monitor patient. Naloxone's duration of antagonist action may be shorter than that of the opioid, requiring repeated doses of naloxone.
Note: Respiratory depression caused by benzodiazepines (e.g., diazepam [Valium] or midazolam [Versed]) can be reversed with flumazenil (Romazicon). Pediatric dosing experience suggests 0.01 mg/kg (0.1 ml/kg); if no (or inadequate) response after 1 to 2 minutes, administer same dose and repeat as needed at 60-second intervals for maximum dose of 1 mg (10 ml).

GUIDELINES

Applying a Topical Anesthetic

There are several topical anesthetics available; the time it takes the medication to actually "work" and numb the site varies. LMX4 is a 4% liposomal lidocaine preparation that is applied just like EMLA; the main difference is that LMX4 is reported to numb the skin within 30 min. Do not use any alcohol-based product before the application of this anesthetic. See Evolve Evidence-Based Practice: EMLA versus LMX for pain reduction during peripheral IV access in children.

Equipment

EMLA cream or LMX4 cream
Transparent dressing
Plastic film and tape (if needed)
Ballpoint pen or marker
Tissue or paper towel

Instructions for EMLA Cream and LMX4 Cream

1. Unscrew the cap, and puncture the metal covering of the tube with the point on the top of the cap.
2. EMLA: Apply ½ of the 5-g tube in a thick layer to about a 2-inch by 2-inch area of skin where the procedure will be done. If the puncture area is very small, such as a finger stick, you can use ½ of the tube.
   LMX4: Apply a pea-sized amount to the area of skin to be numbed, and rub it in for approximately 30 s. Then apply a larger dollop

Continued

GUIDELINES—cont'd

(approximately 2.5 g or ½ of a 5-g tube) over the area and apply the dressing.

3. Remove the center cutout piece of the transparent dressing.
4. Peel the paper liner from the paper-framed dressing.
5. Cover the topical anesthetic cream so that you get a thick layer underneath. Do not spread out the cream. Smooth down the dressing edges carefully, and be sure it is secure to avoid leakage.
6. Remove the paper frame. Mark directly on the occlusive dressing the time you applied the cream.
7. To remove the transparent dressing, grasp opposite sides of the film and pull the sides away from each other to stretch and loosen the film. After the film begins to loosen, grasp the other two sides of the film and pull. This method is easier and more comfortable than pulling the dressing up and off the skin.
8. Wipe off the topical anesthetic cream with a tissue. The numbing effect can last 1 h or more after removing the dressing.

EMLA Cream is a registered trademark of Abraxis BioScience, Inc., and is manufactured by Abraxis BioScience, Inc., for use in the United States only.

GUIDELINES

Administering Buffered Lidocaine

Procedures: Per Procedural Pain Protocol, may be used prior to peripheral intravenous (PIV) insertion, venipuncture, arterial puncture, or AV graft/AV fistula access.

Contraindications: Known hypersensitivity to xylocaine or other amide-type local anesthetics such as prilocaine, mepivacaine, bupivacaine, or etidocaine.

Dosage: Inject 0.1 mL intradermally ½ cm below the proposed PIV insertion site.

Administration: Buffered lidocaine 1% prefilled syringes must be refrigerated. Allow the medication to warm to room temperature just prior to administration (rolling the syringe between hands to warm the contents is allowable). Insert 30-gauge needle intradermally ½ cm below the proposed insertion site. Aspirate the plunger of the syringe to verify that the vein has not been entered. Instill buffered lidocaine 0.1 mL at a constant rate to form a small wheal. Buffered lidocaine may be used in up to three potential sites (maximum of three 0.1 mL injections may be given within 2 h). Wait at least 1 min before attempting the insertion/puncture. Perform needlestick with the needle entering the skin within the wheal.

Sedation for Painful Procedures

Pain associated with invasive procedures and anxiety associated with diagnostic imaging can be managed with sedation and analgesia. Sedation involves a wide range of levels of consciousness and is listed in categories found below.

Sedation Categories

Minimal Sedation (Anxiolysis)

The patient responds to verbal commands
Cognitive function may be impaired
Respiratory and cardiovascular systems unaffected

Moderate Sedation (Previously Conscious Sedation)

The patient responds to verbal commands but may not respond to light tactile stimulation
Cognitive function is impaired

Respiratory Function Adequate; Cardiovascular Unaffected

Deep Sedation

Patient cannot be easily aroused except with repeated or painful stimuli
Ability to maintain airways may be impaired

Spontaneous Ventilation May Be Impaired; Cardiovascular Function Is Maintained

General Anesthesia

Loss of consciousness, a patient cannot be aroused by painful stimuli
Airway cannot be maintained adequately, and ventilation is impaired

Cardiovascular Function May Be Impaired

GUIDELINES

Pain Management During Neonatal Circumcision[a]

Pharmacologic Interventions

Use of Topical Anesthetic Only

1. One hour before the procedure, administer acetaminophen (e.g., Tylenol 10–15 mg/kg) as ordered by the practitioner.
2. Cover the penis with a "finger cot" that is cut from a vinyl or latex glove or a piece of plastic wrap, and secure the bottom of the covering with tape. Avoid using Tegaderm or large amounts of tape on the skin because removing the adhesive causes pain and can irritate the fragile skin.
3. If the infant urinates during the time EMLA is applied (1 h) and a significant amount of EMLA is removed, reapply the cream and covering. The total application of EMLA should not exceed a surface area of 10 cm^2 (1.25 × 1.25 inches). Place a thick layer (1 g) of EMLA[b] or LMX4[c] cream around the penis where the prepuce (foreskin) attaches to the glans. Avoid placing cream on the tip of the penis where it may come in contact with the urethral opening.
4. Remove cream with clean cloth or tissue. Blanching of skin is an expected reaction to EMLA's application under an occlusive dressing; erythema and some edema may occur also.
5. Two minutes before starting the procedure, give the infant a sucrose solution; 24% (weight/volume) sucrose solution is available commercially from Children's Medical Ventures (800-345-6443), or it may be easily made by a hospital pharmacy. Use this solution to coat the pacifier (recoat several times before and during the procedure).
6. After the procedure, apply petrolatum or A&D ointment on a 2 × 2-inch dressing before diapering the infant to prevent the wound from adhering to the dressing or diaper.
7. Administer acetaminophen as ordered by the practitioner 4 h after the initial dose; give additional doses as needed but not to exceed five doses in 24 h or a maximum dose of 75 mg/kg/day.

Use of Dorsal Penile Nerve Block (DPNB) or Ring Block

1. One hour before the procedure, administer acetaminophen as ordered by the practitioner.
2. One hour before the procedure, apply EMLA. For the DPNB, apply EMLA to the prepuce as described previously and at the penile base. For the ring block, apply EMLA to the prepuce as described previously and to the shaft of the penis. Use a topical anesthetic in conjunction with the DPNB or ring block to avoid the pain of injecting the anesthetic.
3. Use a 30-gauge needle to administer the lidocaine. For the DPNB, 0.4 mL of the lidocaine is infiltrated at the 10:30 and 1:30 o'clock positions in Buck fascia at the penile base. For the ring block, 0.4 mL of lidocaine is infiltrated subcutaneously on each side of the shaft of the penis below the prepuce.
4. For maximum anesthesia, wait 5 min after the injection of lidocaine. An alternative anesthetic agent is a chloroprocaine, which is as effective as lidocaine after 3 min.
5. Approximately 2 min before the circumcision, administer concentrated oral sucrose solution as described previously.
6. After the procedure, apply A&D ointment or petrolatum and administer acetaminophen as described previously.

Nonpharmacologic Interventions

In addition to the preceding pharmacologic interventions:

- If using a Circumstraint board, pad with blankets or other thick, soft material such as "lamb's wool." A more comfortable, padded, and physiologic restraint that places the infant semi-reclining can also decrease distress (Stang et al., 1997).
- Provide the parents, caregiver, or another staff member with the option to hold the infant during the procedure or to be present during the circumcision.
- Swaddle the upper body and legs to provide warmth and containment and to reduce movement.
- If the patient is not swaddled and is unclothed, use a radiant warmer to prevent hypothermia. Shield the infant's eyes from overhead lights.
- Prewarm any topical solutions to be used in sterile preparation of the surgical site by placing them in a warm blanket or towel.
- Play infant relaxation music before, during, and after the procedure; allow parents or other caregivers the option of choosing the music.

After the procedure, remove restraints and swaddle. Immediately have the parent, other caregivers, or nursing staff holds the infant. Continue to have the infant suck on a pacifier or offer to feed.

References

Labban M, Menhem Z, Bandali T, et al. Pain control in neonatal male circumcision: a best evidence review. *J Pediatr Urol.* 2021;17(1):3–8.

Omole F, Smith W, Carter-Wicker K. Newborn circumcision techniques. *Am Fam Physician.* 2020;101(11):680–685.

Rossi S, Buonocore G, Bellieni CV. Management of pain in newborn circumcision: a systematic review. *Eur J Pediatr.* 2021;180(1):13–20.

Zeitler M, Rayala B. Neonatal circumcision. *Prim Care.* 2021;48(4):597–611.

[a]There is sufficient evidence and support for the use of a combination of pharmacologic and nonpharmacologic interventions to holistically manage neonatal circumcision pain. Combined analgesia, nonpharmacologic interventions (such as swaddling), and local anesthesia may be used during the procedure to provide holistic pain management.

[b]On March 11, 1999, the US Food and Drug Administration approved the use of EMLA in infants age 37 weeks of gestation, provided practitioners followed recommendations regarding maximal dose and limits for exposure time to the medication. In addition, practitioners are advised not to use EMLA with infants who are receiving methemoglobinemia-inducing medications such as acetaminophen or phenobarbital. Although the package insert warns that patients taking acetaminophen are at greater risk for developing methemoglobinemia, there have been no reported cases of this complication in children taking acetaminophen and using EMLA.

[c]LMX4 (previously Ela-Max) is a 4% lidocaine cream reported to be effective within 30 minutes of application for venipuncture. There is no need to apply an occlusive dressing over LMX4 cream as recommended for EMLA (Wong, 2003). The use of LMX4 for pain relief of pediatric meatotomy has been reported previously (Smith and Gjellum, 2004). Despite anecdotal reports of its use in neonatal circumcision, at this time, no studies are available regarding the use or effectiveness of LMX4 for neonatal circumcision analgesia.

[e]For information on Stang Circ Chair, contact Pedicraft, 4134 Saint Augustine Rd, Jacksonville, FL 32207, 800-223-7649; e-mail: info@pedicraft.com; www.pedicraft.com

[f]Suggested infant relaxation music: Heartbeat Lullabies by Terry Woodford. Available from Baby-Go-To-Sleep Center, Audio-Therapy Innovations, Inc., PO Box 550, Colorado Springs, CO 80901, 800-537-7748.

TABLE 3.5 Coanalgesic Adjuvant Drugs

Drug	Dosage	Indications	Comments
Antidepressants			
Amitriptyline	0.05–1mg/kg/day mg/kg PO hs Titrate upward by 0.25 mg/kg q5–7days prn Available in 10- and 25-mg tablets Usual starting dose: 10–25 mg	Continuous neuropathic pain with burning, aching, dysesthesia with insomnia	Provides analgesia by blocking the reuptake of serotonin and norepinephrine, possibly slowing the transmission of pain signals Helps with pain related to insomnia and depression (use nortriptyline if a patient is oversedated) Analgesic effects were seen earlier than antidepressant effects
Nortriptyline	0.05–1.0 mg/kg PO AM or bid Titrate up by 0.5 mg q5–7days Maximum: 25 mg/dose	Neuropathic pain as above without insomnia	Side effects include dry mouth, constipation, urinary retention
Anticonvulsants			
Gabapentin	Initially 2 mg/kg/day, titrate to 5–30 mg/kg/day orally in 3 divided doses Maximum: 300 mg/day	Neuropathic pain	Mechanism of action unknown Side effects include sedation, ataxia, nystagmus, dizziness
Carbamazepine	Initially, 10 mg/kg/day orally in 2 or 3 divided doses May increase dose by 100 mg/day at weekly intervals as needed Do not exceed 30 mg/kg/day	Sharp, lancinating neuropathic pain Peripheral neuropathies Phantom limb pain	Similar analgesic effect to amitriptyline Monitor blood levels for toxicity only Side effects include decreased blood counts, ataxia, gastrointestinal irritation
Anxiolytics			
Lorazepam	0.02–0.09 mg/kg tid Maximum: 2 mg/dose	Muscle spasm Anxiety	May increase sedation in combination with opioids Can cause depression with prolonged use
Diazepam	For skeletal muscle spasm: Adjunct: 6 months or older, initial, 1–2.5 mg orally 3–4 times daily, may increase gradually as needed Maximum: 10 mg/dose		
Corticosteroids			
Dexamethasone	Dose dependent on clinical situation; higher bolus doses in cord compression, then lower daily dose 0.02–0.3 mg/kg/day in 3 or 4 divided doses	Pain from increased intracranial pressure Bony metastasis Spinal or nerve compression	Side effects include edema, gastrointestinal irritation, increased weight, acne Use gastro protectants such as H_2-blockers (ranitidine) or proton pump inhibitors, such as omeprazole for long-term administration of steroids or NSAIDs in end-stage cancer with bony pain
Others			
Clonidine	2–5 mcg/kg PO q4–6h May also use a 100-mcg transdermal patch q7days for patients >40 kg (88 pounds)	Neuropathic pain Lancinating, sharp, electrical, shooting pain Phantom limb pain	α_2-Adenoreceptor agonist modulates ascending pain sensations Routes of administration: oral, transdermal, and spinal Management of withdrawal symptoms Monitor for orthostatic hypertension decreased heart rate Sedation common

TABLE 3.5 Coanalgesic Adjuvant Drugs—cont'd

Drug	Dosage	Indications	Comments
Mexiletine	Initially, 150 mg at hs; titrate to 10–15 mg/kg Maximum: 300 mg/dose		Similar to lidocaine, longer acting Stabilizes sodium conduction in nerve cells, reduces neuronal firing Can enhance the action of opioids, antidepressants, anticonvulsants Side effects include dizziness, ataxia, nausea, vomiting May measure blood levels for toxicity

bid, Twice a day; *hs,* at bedtime; *IV,* intravenous; *NSAID,* nonsteroidal antiinflammatory drug; *PO,* by mouth; *prn,* as needed; *q,* every; *tid,* three times a day.

TABLE 3.6 Management of Opioid Side Effects

Side Effect	Adjuvant Drugs	Nonpharmacologic Techniques
Constipation	Senna and docusate sodium *Tablet:* 2–6 years old: Start with ½ tablet once a day; maximum: 1 tablet twice a day 6–12 years old: Start with 1 tablet once a day; maximum: 2 tablets twice a day >12 years old: Start with 2 tablets once a day; maximum: 4 tablets twice a day *Liquid:* 1 month–1 year old: 1.25–5 mL q hs 1–5 years old: 2.5–5 mL q hs 5–15 years old: 5–10 mL q hs >15 years old: 10–25 mL q hs Casanthranol and docusate sodium *Liquid:* 5–15 mL q hs *Capsules:* 1 cap PO q hs Bisacodyl: PO or PR 3–12 years old: 5 mg/dose/day >12 years old: 10–15 mg/dose/day Lactulose 7.5 mL/day after breakfast Adult: 15–30 mL/day PO Mineral oil: 1–2 tsp/day PO Magnesium citrate <6 years old: 2–4 mL/kg PO once 6–12 years old: 100–150 mL PO once >12 years old: 150–300 mL PO once Milk of magnesia <2 years old: 0.5 mL/kg/dose PO once 2–5 years old: 5–15 mL/day PO 6–12 years old: 15–30 mL PO once >12 years old: 30–60 mL PO once	Increase water intake Prune juice, bran cereal, vegetables Exercise
Sedation	Caffeine: Single dose of 1–1.5 mg PO Dextroamphetamine: 2.5–5 mg PO in AM and early afternoon Methylphenidate: 2.5–5 mg PO in AM and early afternoon Consider opioid switch if sedation persists	Caffeinated drinks (e.g., Mountain Dew, cola drinks)
Nausea, vomiting	Ondansetron: 0.1–0.15 mg/kg IV or PO q4h; maximum: 8 mg/dose Granisetron: 10–40 mcg/kg q2–4h; maximum: 1 mg/dose Droperidol: 0.05–0.06 mg/kg IV q4–6h; can be very sedating	Imagery, relaxation Deep, slow breathing

Continued

TABLE 3.6 Management of Opioid Side Effects—cont'd

Side Effect	Adjuvant Drugs	Nonpharmacologic Techniques
Pruritus	Diphenhydramine: 1 mg/kg IV or PO q4–6h prn; maximum: 25 mg/dose Hydroxyzine: 0.6 mg/kg/dose PO q6h; maximum: 50 mg/dose Naloxone: 0.5 mcg/kg q2min until pruritus improves (diluted in solution of 0.1 mg naloxone per 10 mL saline) Butorphanol: 0.3–0.5 mg/kg IV (use cautiously in opioid-tolerant children; may cause withdrawal symptoms); maximum: 2 mg/dose because mixed agonist-antagonist	Oatmeal baths, good hygiene Exclude other causes of itching Change opioids
Respiratory depression—mild to moderate	Hold dose of opioid Reduce subsequent doses by 25%	Arouse gently, give oxygen, and encourage to deep breathe
Respiratory depression—severe	Naloxone During disease pain management: 0.5 mcg/kg in 2-min increments until breathing improves (Pasero & McCaffrey, 2011) Reduce opioid dose if possible Consider opioid switch During sedation for procedures: 5–10 mcg/kg until breathing improves Reduce opioid dose if possible Consider opioid switch	Oxygen, bag, and mask, if indicated
Dysphoria, confusion, hallucinations	Evaluate medications, and eliminate adjuvant medications with central nervous system effects as symptoms allow Consider opioid switch if possible Haloperidol (Haldol): 0.05–0.15 mg/kg/day divided in two to three doses; maximum: 2–4 mg/day	Rule out other physiologic causes
Urinary retention	Evaluate medications, and eliminate adjuvant medications with anticholinergic effects (e.g., antihistamines, tricyclic antidepressants) Occurs more frequently with spinal analgesia than with systemic opioid use Oxybutynin 1-year old: 1 mg tid 1–2 years old: 2 mg tid 2–3 years old: 3 mg tid 4–5 years old: 4 mg tid >5 years old: 5 mg tid	Rule out other physiologic causes In/out or indwelling urinary catheter

hs, At bedtime; *IV,* intravenous; *PO,* by mouth; *PR,* by rectum; *prn,* as needed; *q,* every; *tid,* three times a day.

TABLE 3.7 Approximate Equianalgesia Ratios for Switching Between Parenteral and Oral Dosage Forms

Medicine	Dosage Ratio Parenteral	Dosage Ratio Oral
Morphine	1	3
Hydromorphone	0.15	0.6
Fentanyl	0.01	—
Hydrocodone	—	3
Oxycodone	—	2

Data from American Pain Society. *Principles of Analgesic Use.* 7th ed. Chicago, IL: Author; 2016.

TABLE 3.8 Initial Patient-Controlled Analgesia Settings for Opioid-Naive Children

Drug	Continuous Infusion Dosage	Bolus Dosage/Frequency
Morphine	0–0.02 mg/kg/h	0.02 mg/kg q15–30min
Hydromorphone	0–0.004 mg/kg/h	0.004 mg/kg q15–30min
Fentanyl	0–0.5 to 1 mcg/kg/h	0.5–1 mcg/kg q10–15min

TABLE 3.9 Needlestick Pain Prevention Products

Product	Onset	Duration	Appropriate Age/Weight	Potential Adverse Effects; Contraindications
EMLA	1 h	4 h	Approved by FDA for use in neonates over 27 weeks of gestation Has been used in preterm infants <37 weeks; safety of repeated dosages in preterm infants not established (Biran et al., 2011)	Blanching, erythema Methemoglobinemia
LMX4	30 min	1 h	Not recommended for use <1 month of age	Redness, irritation at the site of the cream Swelling, abnormal sensation at the site of the cream
Needle-free jet injection with buffered lidocaine	10–30 s	1–4 h	Theoretic safety for ≥37 weeks of gestation but no published research Safety established for use in children ≥1 year of age (Lunoe et al., 2015)	Blanching, erythema, bleeding with improper placement; do not use in children with bleeding disorders or especially fragile skin
Sucrose pacifier	2 min	10 min	Newborn to 6 months	
Cold vibration device	15 s	Limit use to 3 min	≥1 year of age; assess cold tolerance before use	Blanching, erythema

FDA, US Food and Drug Administration.

Evidence-Based Pediatric Nursing Interventions

Symbol ▶ indicates material that may be photocopied and distributed to families.

Preparing Children for Procedures Based on Developmental Characteristics

Infancy: Developing a Sense of Trust and Sensorimotor Thought

Attachment to Parent

Involve parent in procedure if desired.

Keep parent in infant's line of vision.

If parent is unable to be with infant, place a familiar object or comfort/security item with infant (e.g., stuffed toy, pacifier, or blanket).

Stranger Anxiety

Have usual caregivers perform or assist with procedure.

Make advances slowly and in a nonthreatening manner.

Limit the number of strangers entering room during procedure.

Sensorimotor Phase of Learning

Use sensory soothing measures during procedure (e.g., stroking skin, talking softly, giving a pacifier).

Use analgesics (e.g., topical anesthetic, intravenous opioid) to control discomfort.

Cuddle and hug infant after a stressful procedure; encourage family to comfort infant.

Increased Muscle Control

Expect older infants to resist.

Restrain adequately.

Keep harmful objects out of reach.

Memory for Past Experiences

Realize that older infants may associate objects, places, or persons with prior painful experiences and will cry and resist at the sight of them.

Keep frightening objects out of view.

Perform painful procedures in a separate room (not in crib or bed).

Use nonintrusive procedures whenever possible (e.g., axillary temperature, oral medication).*

Imitation of Gestures

Model desired behavior (e.g., opening mouth).

Toddler: Developing a Sense of Autonomy and Sensorimotor to Preoperational Thought

Use the same approaches as for infant in addition to the following.

Egocentric Thought

Explain procedure in relation to what the child will see, hear, taste, smell, and feel.

Emphasize those aspects of the procedure that require cooperation (e.g., lying still).

Tell child it is acceptable to cry, yell, or use other means to express discomfort verbally.

Designate one health care person to speak during procedure. Hearing more than one can be confusing to child.

Negative Behavior

Expect treatments to be resisted; child may try to run away.

Use a firm, direct approach.

Ignore temper tantrums.

Use distraction techniques (e.g., singing a song with child).

Restrain adequately.

Animism

Keep frightening objects out of view. (Young children believe objects have lifelike qualities and can harm them.)

Limited Language Skills

Communicate using behaviors.

Use a few simple terms familiar to child.

Give one direction at a time (e.g., "Lie down," then "Hold my hand").

Use small replicas of equipment; allow child to handle the equipment.

Use play; demonstrate on a doll but avoid child's favorite doll, because child may think the doll is really feeling the procedure.

Prepare parents separately to avoid the child misinterpreting words.

Limited Concept of Time

Prepare child shortly or immediately before procedure.

Keep teaching sessions short (about 5 to 10 minutes).

Have preparations completed before involving child in procedure.

Have extra equipment nearby (e.g., alcohol swabs, new needles, adhesive bandages) to avoid delays.

Tell child when procedure is completed.

Striving for Independence

Allow choices when they exist but realize that child may still be resistant and negative.

Allow child to participate in care and to help whenever possible (e.g., drink medicine from a cup, hold a dressing).

Provide opportunities/choices for coping/distraction (e.g., bubbles, music, books) before procedure begins.

Preschooler: Developing a Sense of Initiative and Preoperational Thought

Egocentric

Explain procedure in simple terms and in relation to how it affects child (as with a toddler, stress sensory aspects).

Demonstrate the use of equipment.

Allow child to play with miniature or actual equipment.

Encourage playing out the experience on a doll both before and after procedure to clarify misconceptions.

Use neutral words to describe the procedure (Table 4.1).

Increased Language Skills

Use verbal explanation, but avoid overestimating child's comprehension of words.

Encourage child to verbalize ideas and feelings.

Rephrase questions to make sure of what child is asking.

Concept of Time and Frustration Tolerance Still Limited

Implement the same approaches as for a toddler, but may plan longer teaching session (10 to 15 minutes); may divide information into more than one session.

Illness and Hospitalization May Be Viewed as Punishment

Clarify why each procedure is performed; a child will find it difficult to understand how medicine can taste bad and make him or her feel better at the same time.

Ask for child's thoughts regarding why a procedure is performed.

State directly that procedures are never a form of punishment.

Animism

Keep equipment out of sight, except when shown to or used on child.

Fears of Bodily Harm, Intrusion, and Castration

Point out on drawing, doll, or child where the procedure will be performed.

Emphasize that no other body part will be involved.

Use nonintrusive procedures whenever possible (e.g., axillary temperatures, oral medication).

Apply an adhesive bandage over the puncture site.

Encourage parental presence.

Realize that procedures involving genitalia produce anxiety.

Allow child to wear underpants with gown.

Explain unfamiliar situations, especially noises or lights.

Striving for Initiative

Involve child in care whenever possible (e.g., to hold equipment, remove dressing).

Give choices when they exist, but avoid excessive delays.

Praise child for helping and for attempting to cooperate; never shame child for lack of cooperation.

TABLE 4.1 Selecting Nonthreatening Words or Phrases

Words and Phrases to Avoid	Suggested Substitutions
Shot, bee sting, stick	Medicine under the skin
Organ	Special place in body
Test	See how (specify body part) is working
Incision, cut	Special opening
Edema	Puffiness, swelling
Stretcher, gurney	Rolling bed
Stool	Child's usual term
Dye	Special medicine
Pain	Hurt, discomfort, "owie," "boo-boo," sore, achy
Deaden	Numb, make sleepy
Fix	Make better
Take (as in "take your temperature or blood pressure")	See how warm you are; check your pressure; hug your arm
Put to sleep, anesthesia	Special sleep so you won't feel anything
Catheter	Tube
Monitor	TV screen
Electrodes	Stickers, ticklers
Burn	Warm
Dressings, dressing change	Bandages

School-Age Child: Developing a Sense of Industry and Concrete Thought

Increased Language Skills; Interest in Acquiring Knowledge

Explain procedures using correct scientific or medical terminology.
Explain reason for the procedure using simple diagrams of anatomy and physiology.
Explain function and operation of equipment in concrete terms.
Allow child to manipulate equipment; use a doll or another person as a model to practice using equipment whenever possible (doll play may be considered childish by older school-age child).
Allow time before and after procedure for questions and discussion.

Improved Concept of Time

Plan for longer teaching sessions (about 20 minutes).
Prepare before procedure.

Increased Self-Control

Gain child's cooperation.
Tell child what is expected.
Suggest ways of maintaining control (e.g., deep breathing, relaxation, counting).

Striving for Industry

Allow responsibility for simple tasks (e.g., collecting specimens).
Include in decision making (e.g., what time of day to perform procedure, the preferred site).
Encourage active participation (e.g., removing dressings, handling equipment, opening packages).

Developing Relationships with Peers

May prepare two or more children for the same procedure or encourage one peer to help prepare another.
Provide privacy from peers during procedure to maintain self-esteem.

Adolescent: Developing a Sense of Identity and Abstract Thought

Increasingly Capable of Abstract Thought and Reasoning

Supplement explanations with reasons why procedure is necessary or beneficial.
Explain the long-term consequences of procedures.
Realize that adolescents may fear death, disability, or other potential risks.
Encourage questioning regarding fears, options, and alternatives.

Conscious of Appearance

Provide privacy.
Discuss how procedure may affect appearance (e.g., scar) and what can be done to minimize it.
Emphasize any physical benefits of procedure.

Concerned More With Present Than With Future

Realize that the immediate effects of procedure are more significant than future benefits.

Striving for Independence

Involve in decision making and planning (e.g., time and place; individuals present during procedure; clothing; whether they will watch procedure).
Impose as few restrictions as possible.
Suggest methods of maintaining control.
Accept regression to more childish methods of coping.
Realize that adolescents may have difficulty accepting new authority figures and may resist complying with procedures.

Developing Peer Relationships and Group Identity

Same as for school-age child but assumes even greater significance.
Allow adolescents to talk with other adolescents who have had the same procedure.

Preparing the Family

The process of patient education involves giving the family information about the child's condition, the regimen that must be followed and why, and other health teachings as indicated. The goal of this education is to enable the family to modify behaviors and adhere to the regimen that has been mutually established.

General principles of family education are as follows:

1. Establish a rapport with the family.
2. Avoid using any specialized terms or jargon. Clarify all terms with the family.
3. When possible, allow family members to decide how they want to be taught (e.g., all at once or over a day or two). This gives the family a chance to incorporate the information at a rate that is comfortable.

4. Provide accurate information to the family about the illness.
5. Assist family members in identifying obstacles to their ability to comply with the regimen and in identifying the means to overcome those obstacles. Then help family members find ways to incorporate the plan into their daily lives.

If equipment will be needed at home (e.g., suction machines, syringes), begin making the necessary arrangements in advance so that discharge can proceed smoothly. Whenever possible, make arrangements for the family to use the same equipment in the home that they are using in the hospital. This allows them to become familiar with the items. In addition, the staff can help troubleshoot the equipment in a controlled environment. Plan the teaching sessions well in advance of the time the family will be responsible for performing the care. The more complex the procedure, the more time is needed for training.

Review the instructions with family members. Encourage note-taking if they desire. Allow ample practice time under supervision. At least one family member, but preferably two members, should demonstrate the procedure before they are expected to care for the child at home. Provide the family with the telephone numbers of resource individuals who are available to assist them in the event of a problem.

GUIDELINES

Family Preparation for Procedures

Family education for specific procedures are included throughout this unit. General concepts applicable to most family education sessions include the following:

1. Name of the procedure
2. Purpose of the procedure
3. Length of time anticipated to complete the procedure
4. Anticipated effects
5. Signs of adverse effects
6. Assess the family's level of understanding
7. Demonstrate and have family return demonstration (if appropriate)

Skin Care and General Hygiene

Skin Care

General Guidelines

Keep skin free of excess moisture (e.g., urine or fecal incontinence, wound drainage, excessive perspiration).

Cleanse skin with gentle soap (e.g., Dove) or cleanser (e.g., Cetaphil). Rinse well with plain, warm water.

Provide daily cleansing of eyes, oral area, diaper or perineal area, and any areas of skin breakdown.

Apply non–alcohol-based moisturizing agents after cleansing to retain moisture and rehydrate skin.

Use minimum tape and adhesives. On very sensitive skin, use a protective, pectin-based, or hydrocolloid skin barrier between skin and tape and adhesives.

Place pectin-based or hydrocolloid skin barriers directly over excoriated skin. Leave the barrier undisturbed until it begins to peel off. With wet, oozing excoriations, place a small amount of stoma powder (as used in ostomy care) on site, remove excess powder, and apply a skin barrier. Hold the barrier in place for several minutes to allow the barrier to soften and mold to the skin surface. See Table 4.2 for common wound care products.

Alternate electrode and probe placement sites and thoroughly assess underlying skin, typically every 8 to 24 hours.

Eliminate pressure secondary to medical devices such as tracheostomy tubes, wheelchairs, braces, and gastrostomy tubes.

Be certain fingers or toes are visible whenever an extremity is used for an IV or arterial line.

Reduce friction by keeping skin dry (may apply absorbent powder such as cornstarch) and using soft, smooth bed linens and clothes.

Use a draw sheet to move a child in bed or onto a stretcher to reduce friction and shearing injuries; do not drag the child from under the arms.

Position in neutral alignment; pillows, cushions, or wedges may be needed to prevent hip abduction and pressure to bony prominences, such as heels, elbows, and sacral and occipital areas. When the child is positioned laterally, pillows/cushions between the knees, under the head, and under the upper arm will help promote neutral body alignment. Avoid donut cushions because they can cause tissue ischemia. Elevate the head of the bed 30 degrees or less to reduce pressure, unless contraindicated

Do not massage reddened, bony prominences because this can cause deep tissue damage; provide pressure relief to these areas instead.

Routinely assess the child's nutritional status. A child who is on nothing by mouth (NPO) status for several days and who is receiving only IV fluids is nutritionally at risk. This can also affect the skin's ability to maintain its integrity. Hyperalimentation (TPN, TNA) should be considered for these children at risk.

Identify children who are at risk for skin breakdown before it occurs. Employ measures such as pressure-reducing devices (reduce pressure more than would usually occur on a regular hospital bed or chair) or pressure-relieving devices (maintain pressure below that which would cause capillary closing) to prevent breakdown (Table 4.3).

Adhesives

Decrease use as much as possible.

EVIDENCE-BASED PRACTICE

Wound Care

Ask the Question

In children, what dressings are more effective in reducing healing time and pain?

Search the Evidence

Search Strategies

Search selection criteria included English-language publications and research-based articles on wound care in the neonatal and pediatric population through 2022.

Databases Used

National Guideline Clearinghouse (AHRQ), Cochrane Collaboration, PubMed, Medscape

Critically Analyze the Evidence

Grade criteria: Evidence quality low; recommendation strong (Guyatt et al., 2008)

- The studies that were consulted (Benbow, 2008; Berger et al., 2000; Dickson and Bodnaryk, 2006; Lund et al., 2001; Nuutila and Eriksson, 2021; Ovington, 2001; Valencia, 2001; Vermeulen et al. 2004) found that moist wound healing is two or three times faster than when wounds are left open to the air. Moisture-retentive dressings such as transparent and hydrocolloid dressings accelerate wound healing, protect the wound, decrease bacterial wound contamination and infection, and reduce scarring. Comparatively, wet-to-dry dressings are associated with increases in labor costs, dressing change frequency, wound healing time, infection rates, pain, disruption of newly formed healthy tissue, and dispersal of bacteria on removal.
- Dressing type and dressing change frequency should be based on the wound type and location, phase of wound healing, and amount of exudate. Many of the newer dressings allow for reduced dressing changes because they absorb more drainage and promote a moist wound-healing environment. In addition, wound gels provide moisture to a wound bed while eliminating dead space. If a wound is infected or bacterial colonization is suspected, antibacterial ointments are indicated to reduce the bacterial bioburden and promote moist wound healing.
- Packing wounds with absorptive materials reduces wound exudate and abscess development and prevents skin maceration. There is insufficient evidence to suggest whether one dressing or topical product is more effective at healing a wound than another. There is evidence to suggest that wet-to-dry gauze dressings are more painful to patients on removal (Vermeulen et al., 2004).
- Premature and newborn infants are prone to epidermal stripping and skin tears secondary to an immature epidermal-dermal bond. Avoid tape when possible. Secure dressings with a stretchy overwrap or use Montgomery straps. Frame wounds with a barrier dressing and adhere tape to the barrier. Apply non–alcohol-based skin preparation barriers under tape and dressings (AWHONN, 2007).

Apply the Evidence: Nursing Implications

- Apply dressings that provide a moist wound environment.
- Pack wounds to eliminate dead space, absorb exudate, and prevent abscess formation.
- Dressing change frequency should be based on wound type and location, amount of pain and exudate, and the need for wound assessment. Most wounds require a daily dressing change.
- Protect the periwound skin with a barrier dressing or protective wipe to prevent epidermal injury.
- Avoid tape and secure dressings with stretchy wraps.

References

Association of Women's Health, Obstetric and Neonatal Nurses. Neonatal Skin Care. In: *Evidence-Based Clinical Practice Guideline.* 2nd ed. Washington, DC: The Association; 2007.

Benbow M. Exploring the concept of moist wound healing and its application in practice. *Br J Nurs.* 2008;17(15):S4,S6,S8 passim.

Berger RS, Pappert AS, Van Zile PS, et al. A newly formulated topical triple-antibiotic ointment minimizes scarring. *Cutis.* 2000;65(6):401–404.

Dickson D, Bodnaryk K. Neonatal intravenous extravasation injuries: evaluation of a wound care protocol. *Neonatal Netw.* 2006;25(1):13–19.

Guyatt GH, Oxman AD, Vist GE, et al. GRADE: an emerging consensus on rating quality of evidence and strength of recommendations. *BMJ.* 2008;336(7650):924–926.

Lund C, Osborne J, Kuller J, et al. Neonatal skin care: clinical outcomes of the AWHONN/NANN evidence-based clinical practice guideline. Association of Women's Health, Obstetric and Neonatal Nurses and the National Association of Neonatal Nurses. *J Obstet Gynecol Neonatal Nurs.* 2001;30(1):41–51.

Nuutila K, Eriksson E. Moist wound healing with commonly available dressings. *Adv Wound Care (New Rochelle).* 2021;10(12):685–698.

Ovington L. Hanging wet to dry dressings out to dry. *Home Healthc Nurse.* 2001;19(8):477–484.

Valencia I. New developments in wound care for infants and children. *Pediatr Ann.* 2001;30(4):211–218.

Vermeulen H, Ubbink D, Goossens A, et al. Dressings and topical agents for surgical wounds healing by secondary intention. *Cochrane Database Syst Rev.* 2004;1:CD003554.

Use transparent adhesive dressings to secure IV lines, catheters, and central lines.

Consider the use of hydrogel electrodes.

Consider pectin barriers (Hollihesive, DuoDerm) beneath adhesives to protect the skin.

Secure pulse oximeter probe or electrodes with elasticized dressing material (carefully avoid restricting blood flow).

Do not use adhesive remover, solvents, and bonding agents. Adhesive removal can be facilitated using water, mineral oil, petrolatum, or alcohol-based foam hand cleanser.

Remove adhesives or skin barriers slowly, supporting the skin underneath with one hand and gently peeling away the product from the skin with the other hand. (CAUTION: Do not use scissors for tape or dressing removal because of the hazard of cutting the skin or amputating tiny digits.)

Treating Skin Breakdown

Numerous studies have demonstrated that normal saline (NS) is the least damaging cleanser to cells because it has a neutral pH. Other antiseptics such as povidone-iodine, hydrogen peroxide, Dakin's solution, and alcohol should not be used in open wounds, particularly at full strength, because they are toxic to white cells and fibroblasts and can impair wound healing. Study suggestions (Baranoski and Ayello, 2004; Bryant, 2002; Fernandez et al. 2002; Moore and Cowman, 2005) also include the following:

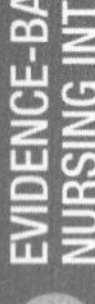

TABLE 4.2 Wound Dressing Category Definitions and Product Examples

Category	Description	Examples
Gauze or sponge for external use	Nonresorbable	Pads
	Sterile or nonsterile	Island dressings
	Strip, piece, or pad	
	Woven or nonwoven mesh cotton cellulose	
	Simple chemical derivatives of cellulose	
	Intended for medical purposes	
Hydrophilic wound dressing	Sterile or nonsterile	Alginate dressings
	Nonresorbable	Foam dressings
	Material with hydrophilic properties	Hydropolymer dressings
	No added drugs or biologics	Sheet gel dressings
	Intended to cover wound and absorb exudate	Hydrocolloid dressings
		Composite dressings
		Hydrogel dressings
Occlusive wound dressing	Sterile or nonsterile	Transparent adhesive dressings
	Nonresorbable	Thin film dressings
	Synthetic polymeric material with or without adhesive backing	Foam dressings
		Hydrocolloid dressings
	Intended to cover wound, provide or support moist wound environment, and allow exchange of gases	Composite dressings
		Hydropolymer dressings
Hydrogel wound dressing	Sterile or nonsterile	Alginate dressings
	Nonresorbable	Hydropolymer dressings
	Matrix of hydrophilic polymers or other material combined with at least 50% water	Hydrogel dressings
		Gauze dressings impregnated with hydrogel (without active ingredients)
	Intended to cover wound, absorb wound exudates, control bleeding or fluid loss, and protect against abrasion, friction, desiccation, contamination	
Porcine wound dressing	Made from pigskin	
	Temporary burn dressing	

- Cleanse all wounds with NS or a saline-based wound cleanser with surfactant.
- Cleansing with drinkable tap water may be as effective as cleansing with sterile water or sterile saline.
- For intact periwound skin, soap and water may be used.

Irrigate wound every 4 to 8 hours with warm NS using a 30-mL or larger syringe and 20-gauge catheter.

Culture wound and treat if signs of infection are present (excessive redness, swelling, pain on touch, heat, resistance to healing).

Use transparent adhesive dressing for uninfected wounds.

Use hydrocolloid for deep, uninfected wounds (leave in place for 5 to 7 days); warm barrier in hand for several minutes to soften before applying to skin.

Apply hydrogel with or without antibacterial or antifungal ointments (as ordered) for infected wounds (may need to moisten before removal).

Debride wounds of necrotic, devitalized tissue (exception: do not debride stable, dry eschar on feet and heels and on patients at risk for poor wound healing because of

TABLE 4.3 Pressure Reduction and Relief Devices[a]

Description	Advantages	Disadvantages
Overlay[b]		
Foam: Varying density; 3- to 4-inch convoluted and nonconvoluted	Primarily pressure reduction, although in children may have pressure relief advantages; can be cut to fit cribs	Can be soiled by incontinent patient; inability to reduce skin moisture because of lack of airflow
Gel or water filled: Pressure reduction; water or gel conforms to patient's contours	One-time charge; low cost for water; gels are expensive Relieves pressure and shear; nonpowered, easy cleaning	Mattress is a dense collection of viscous fluid cells; there have been reports that the mattress is cold to the touch; patients may have to spare vital calories to warm the mattress Heavy
Alternating-pressure mattress: An overlay with rows of air cells and pump; pump cycles air to provide inflation and deflation over pressure points	Intent is to relieve pressure points to create pressure gradients that enhance blood flow	Studies show inconsistent results; some have reported very low deflation interface pressures, but only the deflation pressures were used for analysis; tissue interface pressures during inflation are consistently higher and must be incorporated into the statistical analysis; clinical trials indicate higher pressure ulcer incidence rates when compared with other products
Static air: Designed with interlocking air cells that provide dry flotation; inflated with a blower	Mattress overlays that are designed with multiple chambers, allowing air exchange between the compartments	Pressure reduction depends on adequate air volume and periodic reinflation
Low–air-loss specialty overlay: Multiple airflow cushions that cover the entire bed; pressures can be set and controlled by a blower	Surface materials are constructed to reduce friction and shear and to eliminate moisture; pressure relief; can be used for prevention and/or treatment of ulcers	Surface mattress and pump are a rental item; not available for cribs
Specialty Beds[c]		
Low–air-loss beds: Bed surface consists of inflated air cushions; each section is adjusted for optimum pressure relief for patient's body size; some models have built-in scales	Provides pressure relief in any position; treatment for stages III and IV pressure ulcers; available in pediatric crib sizes	Bed is more bulky than a hospital bed, and some homes may not be able to accommodate its size; reimbursement is questionable
Low–air-loss mattress replacements	Provides pressure relief in any position; fits on hospital frame	Requires mattress storage
Air-fluidized beds: Air is blown through beads to "float" patient	Provides pressure relief for oncology patients and for treatment of full-thickness pressure ulcers, postoperative flaps, burns; lighter-weight home care units available	Can be difficult to transfer patient
Kinetic therapy: Therapy surfaces that provide continuous gentle side-to-side rotation of 40 degrees or more on each side; table-based or cushion-based	Has been demonstrated to improve mucous transport, redistribute pulmonary blood flow, and mobilize pulmonary interstitial fluid; has been used for trauma victims and unstable spinal cord injuries (should use table-based; once stabilized, may use cushion-based)	Used only in acute care settings
Continuous lateral rotation beds (CLRT): Less than 40 degrees side-to-side rotation	Helps reposition unstable spinal cord injury patient; promotes comfort and shifts pressure points	

[a]This list is a representative sampling of products and is not intended to be all-inclusive. No endorsement of any product is intended. Within each category, products must be individually evaluated on their efficacy as comfort, pressure-reducing, or pressure-relieving devices. All products within a category do not necessarily perform equally.
[b]A device that is made to fit over a regular hospital mattress.
[c]High-tech beds used in place of the standard hospital bed. These are normally used on a rental basis and are intended for short-term use. They usually provide pressure relief and eliminate shear, friction, and maceration.

GUIDELINES

Incontinence-Associated Diaper Dermatitis (IDD)

Definition: Inflammation of the skin within the diaper area

Etiology

- Contact irritants (enzyme activity of urine/stool, increased pH, medications)
- Friction
- Infection (bacterial, viral, fungal; primarily Candida)
- Underlying medical conditions (e.g., incontinence, gastroenteritis, neurogenic bladder/bowel, ileostomy/colostomy closure, short gut syndrome)

Clinical Features

Signs and Symptoms

- Erythema in diaper area
- Pruritis
- Irritability

Complications

- Candida infection (well-demarcated lesions; papule or pustule satellite lesions)
- Denuded skin

IDD Grading

- **Mild:** slight erythema in diaper area; intact skin
- **Moderate:** shiny erythema in diaper area; patchy denuded areas
- **Severe:** severe erythema in diaper area; large denuded areas; macerated skin; bleeding; ulcerations

Prevention

A—Air

- Schedule time for diaper area to air-dry (20 min 2–3 times a day).

B—Barrier

- Apply layer of skin barrier with every diaper change.
- Use petroleum jelly–based product or zinc oxide–based product or nonalcohol barrier film (e.g., Aloe Vesta Skin Protectant, Sensicare, Desitin, 3M No Sting Barrier).
- 3M No Sting Barrier must be allowed to dry before applying other barrier product; can be applied to skin only 1–2 times per day; not approved for infants younger than 30 days of age.

C—Cleanser

- Use pH-balanced, no-rinse product (e.g., Aloe Vesta Cleansing Foam) or mild soap (unscented Dove, Cetaphil).
- Infants/young children: Use mild soap and water with disposable nonwoven washcloths or unscented, alcohol-free baby wipes or Aloe Vesta Cleansing Foam with disposable nonwoven washcloths.
- Older children: Use perineal wipes with dimethicone moisture barrier[a] (Shield Barrier Cloths) or Aloe Vesta cleansing foam with disposable nonwoven washcloths or mild soap and water with disposable nonwoven washcloths.

D—Diapers

- Use super-absorptive diapers
- Change at least every 3–4 h

E—Education

- Provide verbal and written family education.

Management

A—Air

- Schedule time for diaper area to air-dry (20 min 2–3 times a day).

B—Barrier

- Mild:
  - Apply thick layer of skin barrier with every diaper change.
  - Use petroleum jelly–based product or zinc oxide–based product or nonalcohol barrier film (Aloe Vesta Skin Protectant, Sensicare, Desitin, 3M No Sting Barrier).
  - 3M No Sting Barrier must be allowed to dry before applying other barrier product; can be applied to skin only 1–2 times per day; not approved for infants younger than 30 days of age
  - If *Candida* is present, apply nystatin ointment or Aloe Vesta with miconazole 2% directly to skin before applying barrier; medical order is required.
- Moderate:
  - Apply thick layer of zinc oxide–based product (Sensicare) with every diaper change.
  - May seal ulcers with nonalcohol barrier film (3M No Sting Barrier); must be allowed to dry before applying other barrier product; can be applied to skin only 1–2 times per day; not approved for infants younger than 30 days of age.
  - If Candida is present, apply nystatin ointment or Aloe Vesta with miconazole 2% directly to skin before applying barrier; medical order required.
- Severe:
  - Apply thick layer of zinc oxide–based product (e.g., Sensicare, Criticaid Paste, Ilex Skin Protectant Paste) with every diaper change; apply like "icing" and only remove soiled product to minimize mechanical trauma.

    Sensicare—Apply if not used in previous IDD grade.

    Critic-Aid—Apply ostomy powder, followed by Critic-Aid, followed by ostomy powder (ostomy powder holds paste to moist skin and prevents removal by diaper).

    Ilex—Apply directly to skin, followed by layer of petroleum jelly to prevent the buttocks from sticking together.
  - May seal ulcers with nonalcohol barrier film (3M No Sting Barrier); must be allowed to dry before applying other barrier product; can be applied to skin only 1–2 times per day; not approved for infants younger than 30 days of age.
  - If Candida is present, apply nystatin powder directly to skin before applying barrier; medical order required.

C—Cleanser

- Use pH balanced, no-rinse product (e.g., Aloe Vesta Cleansing Foam) or mild soap (e.g., unscented Dove, Cetaphil).
- Infants/Young Children: Use mild soap and water with disposable nonwoven washcloths or unscented, alcohol-free baby wipes or Aloe Vesta Cleansing Foam with disposable nonwoven washcloths.
- Older Children: Perineal wipes with dimethicone moisture barrier[a] (Shield Barrier Cloths) or Aloe Vesta cleansing foam with disposable nonwoven washcloths or mild soap and water with disposable nonwoven washcloths
- Once a day bathe child to soak off all product; may use mineral oil to help remove product.

D—Diapers

- Use super absorptive diapers.
- Change every 2 h at a minimum.

E—Education

- Provide verbal and written family education.

Bibliography

Adam R. Skin care of the diaper area. *Pediatr Dermatol.* 2008;25(4):427–433.
Atherton DJ. A review of the pathophysiology, prevention and treatment of irritant diaper dermatitis. *Curr Med Res Opin.* 2004;20(5):645–649.

Continued

GUIDELINES

Incontinence-Associated Diaper Dermatitis (IDD)—cont'd

Atherton D, Mills K. What can be done to keep babies' skin healthy? *RCM Midwives.* 2004;7(7):288–290.

Blume-Peytavi U, Hauser M, Lünnemann L, et al. Prevention of diaper dermatitis in infants—a literature review. *Pediatr Dermatol.* 2014;31(4):413–429.

Eichenfield DZ. Evidence-based skin care in preterm infants. *Pediatr Dermatol.* 2019;36(1):16–23.

Esser MS, Johnson TS. An integrative review of clinical characteristics of infants with diaper dermatitis. *Adv Neonatal Care.* 2020;20(4):276–285.

Gupta AK, Skinner AR. Management of diaper dermatitis. *Int J Dermatol.* 2004;43(11):830–834.

Humphrey S, Bergman JN, Au S. Practical management strategies for diaper dermatitis. *Skin Therapy Lett.* 2006;11(7):1–6. [a].

Junkin J, Selekof JL. Prevalence of incontinence and associated skin injury in the acute care inpatient. *J Wound Ostomy Continence Nurs.* 2007;334(3):260–267.

Kusari A, Han AM, Virgen CA, et al. Incontinence-associated dermatitis: a consensus. *J Wound Ostomy Continence Nurs.* 2007;34(1):45–54.

McLane KM, Bookout K, McCord S, et al. The 2003 national pediatric pressure ulcer and skin breakdown prevalence survey, a multisite study. *J Wound Ostomy Continence Nurs.* 2004;31(4):168–178.

Nield LS, Kamat D. Prevention, diagnosis, and management of diaper dermatitis. *Clin Pediatr.* 2007;46(6):480–486.

Noonan C, Quigley S, Curley MAQ. Skin integrity in hospitalized infants and children, a prevalence survey. *J Pediatric Nurs.* 2006;21(6):445–453.

Odio M, Streicher-Scott J, Hanson RC. Disposable baby wipes: efficacy and skin mildness. *Dermatol Nurs.* 2001;13(2):107–121.

Ratliff C, Dixon M. Treatment of incontinence-associated dermatitis (diaper rash) in a neonatal unit. *J Wound Ostomy Continence Nurs.* 2007;34(2):158–162.

Scheinfeld N. Diaper dermatitis: a review and brief summary of eruptions of the diaper area. *Am J Clin Dermatol* 2005;6(5):273–281.

[a]Dimethicone moisture barrier (Shield Barrier Cloths) can be used for any age child; however, the product is five times more expensive than alcohol-free baby wipes.

diabetes, immunocompromise, ischemia, poor circulation, or poor nutrition).
(King et al., 2014)

Neonatal Guidelines[a]

General Skin Care

Assessment

Assess skin every day or once per shift for redness, dryness, flaking, scaling, rashes, lesions, excoriation, or breakdown. Standardized scales, such as the Neonatal Skin Condition Score (NSCS) measure skin condition objectively but may not be clinically relevant as they typically remain the same from day to day.

Evaluate and report abnormal skin findings, and analyze for possible causation.

Intervene according to interpretation of findings or as ordered.

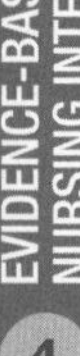

Bathing

Initial Bath

- Assess for stable temperature and vital signs; may take 2 to 4 hours.
- Use cleansing agents with neutral pH and minimal dyes or perfume, in water.
- Do not remove vernix; allow to wear off with normal care and handling.
- Bathe preterm infant less than 32 weeks in warm water alone.
- Wear gloves.

Routine

- Decrease the frequency of baths to every second or third day by daily cleansing of eye, oral, and diaper areas and pressure points.
- Use cleanser or soaps no more than two or three times a week.
- Avoid rubbing skin during bathing or drying.
- Immerse stable infants fully except the head and neck to decrease evaporative heat loss.
- Immediately after bathing, dry the newborn and place in a diaper and cap and wrap in two warm blankets; after 10 minutes, dress the infant and apply a dry cap and blankets.

Emollients

- Apply petroleum-based ointment without preservatives, perfume, or dye sparingly to the body (avoid face, and head) for dry, flaking, or fissured areas every 12 hours or as needed.
- Emollients may be used for infants on warmers or receiving phototherapy.

Disinfectants

All disinfectants have the potential to cause irritation or burns in newborns and should be removed with water or saline after an invasive procedure is performed.

- For infants less than 34 weeks gestation, use 2% aqueous chlorhexidine gluconate (CHG) or povidone-iodine. CHG with alcohol is approved for use in infants older than age 2 months, and use in neonates is considered off-label use. Avoid the use of alcohol as the primary disinfectant or to remove other disinfectants.
- Apply CHG for 30 seconds or with two applications. Aqueous CHG will not dry and can be removed with sterile gauze. Apply povidone-iodine with two applications and allow to dry.

Transepidermal Water Loss

Minimize transepidermal water loss (TEWL) and heat loss in small premature infants younger than 30 weeks by:

- Using humidified incubators (70% to 90% first 7 days, then 50% until 28 days of life).
- Applying transparent dressings to the chest, abdomen, and back.
- Using heated water pads or mattresses.

Skin Breakdown Prevention

Decrease pressure from externally applied forces using water, air, or gel mattresses, sheepskin, or cotton bedding.

Provide adequate nutrition, including protein, fat, and trace minerals such as zinc.

Apply transparent adhesive dressings to protect elbows and knees from friction injury.

Use tracheostomy and gastrostomy dressings for drainage and relief of pressure from tracheostomy or gastrostomy tube (Hydrasorb or Lyofoam).

Use emollient in the diaper area (groin, thighs) of very low–birth-weight infants to reduce urine irritation.[a]

Other Skin Care Concerns

Use of Substances on Skin

Evaluate all substances that come in contact with infant's skin.

Before using any topical agent, analyze the components of preparation and:

- Use sparingly and only when necessary.
- Confine use to smallest possible area.
- Whenever possible and appropriate, wash off with water
- Monitor infant carefully for signs of toxicity and systemic effects.

Use of Thermal Devices

Avoid heat lamps because of the increased potential for burns.

If needed, measure actual temperature of exposed skin every 15 minutes.

When using heating pads:

- Change infant's position every 15 minutes initially, then every 1 to 2 hours.
- Preset temperature of heating pads to less than 40°C (<104°F).

When using preheated transcutaneous electrodes:

- Avoid use on infants less than 1000 g.
- Set at the lowest possible temperature (<44°C [<111.2°F]), and secure with plastic wrap.
- Use pulse oximetry rather than transcutaneous monitoring whenever possible.

When prewarming heels before phlebotomy, avoid temperatures greater than 40°C (>104°F).

Warm ambient humidity, direct away from infant; use aerosolized sterile water, and maintain ambient temperature so as not to exceed 40°C.

[a]Modified from Association of Women's Health, Obstetric and Neonatal Nurses. *Neonatal Skin Care 2nd Edition Evidence-based Clinical Practice Guideline*. Washington, DC: The Association; 2007. Skin Care Special Issue: Diaper Dermatitis and Extremely Preterm Infant Skin Care. *Adv Neonatal Care*. 2016;16(Suppl 5S):E1-E2.
Kusari A, Han AM, Virgen CA, et al. Evidence-based skin care in preterm infants. *Pediatr Dermatol.* 2019;36(1);16–23.

Bathing

Never leave infant or small child unattended in a bathtub.

Hold infant who is unable to sit alone.

Support infant's head securely with one hand or grasp the infant's farther arm firmly and rest the head comfortably on your wrist.

Closely supervise the infant or child who is able to sit without assistance.

Place a pad in the bottom of the tub to prevent slipping and loss of balance.

Offer older children the option of a shower, if available.

Use judgment regarding the amount of supervision older children require.

Children with mental and/or physical limitations such as severe anemia or leg deformities and suicidal or psychotic children (who may commit bodily harm) require close supervision.

Clean the ears, between skinfolds, the neck, the back, and the genital area carefully.

Retract the foreskin of uncircumcised boys gently once it is mobile (usually older than age 3 years), clean the exposed surfaces, and replace the foreskin. Never forcefully retract the foreskin.

Provide more extensive assistance with bathing and other aspects of hygienic care to children who are debilitated: Encourage them to perform as much as they are capable of without overtaxing their energies.

Expect increasing involvement with improved strength and endurance.

Hair Care

Brush and comb hair, or help children with hair care at least once daily.

For African American children with curly hair, use a comb with widely spaced teeth. Comb, braid, plait, or weave loosely after shampooing when hair is wet.
Use special hair dressing or pomade by rubbing on the hands and transferring to hair; consult parents regarding the usual preparation. Petroleum jelly should not be used.

Style hair for comfort and in a manner pleasing to the child and parents.

Do not cut hair without parental permission, although clipping hair to provide access to the scalp vein for needle insertion is permissible.

Shampoo hair in the tub or shower, or transport the child by stretcher to an accessible sink or washbasin. If the child is unable to be transported, shampoo in the bed with adequate protection and/or with specially adapted equipment or positioning.

Wash hair of the newborn every 2 to 3 days as part of the bath.

Wash hair and scalp as needed in later infancy and childhood.

Teenagers may need more frequent hair care and shampoos.

Use commercial dry shampoo products on a short-term basis.

Skin Closure (Suture or Staple) Removal Procedure

Determine that sutures have been in place for an adequate length of time. This length of time varies depending on the area of the body sutured. Some guidelines are 3 days for the eyelids; 3 to 4 days for the neck; 5 days for the face and scalp; 7 days for the trunk and upper extremities; and 8 to 10 days for the lower extremities.

Position patient to allow access to stitches without putting undue tension on the incision.

Assess the wound for any signs of infection (redness, swelling, heat, drainage) or of the wound not healing (dehiscence).

Clean the wound with NS or antiseptic. Hydrogen peroxide may be used to remove any scabs over stitches.

Remove stitches (technique varies based on the type of stitch).

Simple Interrupted Sutures

Simple interrupted sutures are the most widely used type of stitch; each stitch is placed and tied individually.

Use forceps to firmly grasp knot and pull taught to expose underside of knot. Insert scissors underneath stitch to side of knot. Clip stitch with scissors while continuing to pull on knot with forceps. Gently pull knot with forceps to remove stitch completely. To minimize infection, cut stitch as close to skin as possible so that external parts of stitch do not pass through the wound. Repeat process for additional sutures.

Simple Continuous Sutures

Simple continuous sutures consist of a series of stitches; only the first and last stitches are tied.

Use forceps to firmly grasp knot and pull taught to expose underside of knot. Insert scissors underneath stitch to side of knot. Clip stitch with scissors. To minimize infection, stitch should be cut as close to skin as possible so that external parts of stitch do not pass through the wound. Move down to the next suture in line, keeping on the same side of the wound. Clip this stitch with scissors. Gently pull stitch with forceps to remove. Continue this process of cutting and removing stitches, working down the same side of the wound.

Staples

Insert lower jaw of staple extractor underneath first staple. Push jaws of staple remover together. Once jaws are firmly closed, pull extractor toward you to remove staple. Continue this process, removing every other staple, and then remove the remainder.

Assess for possible complications. If incision begins to separate, leave remainder of stitches in place and use skin closure strips (Steri-Strips) to secure the opening area of the wound. Notify physician.

Use dressing as needed if the wound is draining.

Procedures Related to Maintaining Safety

Ensure that environmental safety measures are in operation, such as the following:

- Good illumination
- Floors clear of fluid or objects that might contribute to falls
- Nonskid surfaces in showers and tubs
- Furniture that is scaled to the child's proportions and sturdy and well-balanced to prevent tipping over
- Beds of ambulatory patients locked in place and at a height that allows easy access to the floor
- Electrical equipment maintained in good working order, used only by personnel familiar with its use, and not in contact with moisture or near tubs
- Electrical outlets covered to prevent burns
- A well-organized fire plan known to all staff members
- All windows secure
- Blind and curtain cords out of reach with split cords to prevent strangulation
- Proper care and disposal of small objects, such as syringes, caps, needle covers, and temperature probes

Be sure child is wearing a proper identification band.

Check bath water carefully before placing child in the bath.

Securely strap infants and small children into infant seats, feeding chairs, and strollers.

Do not leave infants, young children, and children who are agitated or cognitively impaired unattended on treatment tables, on scales, or in treatment areas.

Keep portholes in incubators securely fastened when not attending the infant.

Do not use baby walkers; they provide access to hazards or may tip over, causing injury.

Keep crib sides up and fastened securely. Use cribs that meet federal safety standards (www.cpsc.gov/info/cribs/index.html.)

- Leave crib sides up regardless of child's ability to get out, and even when the crib is unoccupied, to remove the temptation for the child to climb in.
- Never turn away from an infant or small child in a crib that has the sides down without maintaining contact with the child's back or abdomen to prevent rolling, crawling, or jumping from the open crib.

Place the child who may climb over the side of the crib in a specially constructed crib with a cover or one that has a safety net placed over the top.

- Tie net to the frame in such a manner that there is ready access to the child in case of emergency.
- Never tie nets to the movable crib sides or use knots that do not permit quick release.

Do not tie balloons or other objects with long ties or strings to cribs because they can pose an entanglement hazard.
Do not tie pacifiers around the infant's neck or attach them to the infant with a string.
Do not place cribs within reach of heating units, appliances, dangling cords, outlets, or other objects that can be reached by curious hands.
Pillows should not be placed in cribs with children chronologically or developmentally less than age 12 months except to therapeutically position a patient per medical orders.
Assess the safety of toys brought to the hospital for children, and determine whether they are appropriate to the child's age and condition. Electrical or friction toys should not be allowed for children receiving oxygen therapy since sparks can cause oxygen to ignite.
Inspect toys to make certain they are allergy-free, washable, and unbreakable and that they have no small removable parts that can be aspirated or swallowed.
All objects within reach of children younger than age 3 years should pass the choke tube test. A toilet paper roll is a handy guide. If a toy or object fits into the cylinder (items less than 1¼ inches across or balls smaller than 1¾ inches), it is a potential choking danger to the child.
Latex balloons pose a choking hazard to children of all ages; if a balloon breaks, latex can be aspirated or swallowed, resulting in choking.
Set limits for the child's safety.
Make sure children understand where they are permitted to go and what they are permitted to do in the hospital.
Prevent child's access to tubs, laundry bags or chutes, elevators, medication rooms, and medication and cleaning carts.
Enforce the limitations consistently, and repeat them as frequently as necessary to make certain that they are understood.

Transporting

Carry infants and small children for short distances within the unit:

- In the horizontal position, hold or carry small infants with the back supported and the thighs grasped firmly by the carrying arm (Fig. 4.1A).
- In the football hold, support the infant on the nurse's arm with the head supported by the hand and the body held securely between the body and elbow (see Fig. 4.1B).
- In the upright position, hold the infant with the buttocks on the nurse's forearm and the front of the body resting against the chest. Support the infant's head and shoulders with the other arm to allow for any sudden movement by the infant (see Fig. 4.1C).

For more extended trips, use a suitable conveyance:

- Determine the method of transporting children by considering their age, condition, and destination.
- Use appropriate safety belts and/or raised sides to secure the child.
- Transport infants in their incubators, cribs, strollers, or in wagons with raised sides.

Use wheelchairs or stretchers with side rails for older children.
Ambulation may be appropriate for children who are not on cardiac or pulse oximetry monitors.
Critically ill children should always be transported on a stretcher or bed by at least two staff members with monitoring continuing during transport. A blood pressure monitor (or standard blood pressure cuff), pulse oximeter, cardiac monitor/defibrillator, airway equipment, and emergency medications should accompany the patient.

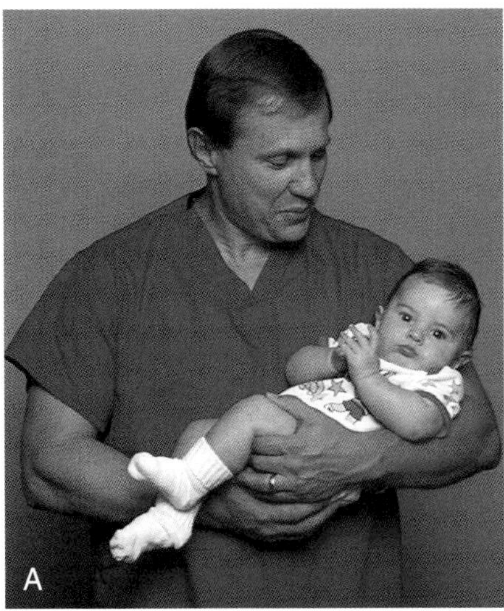

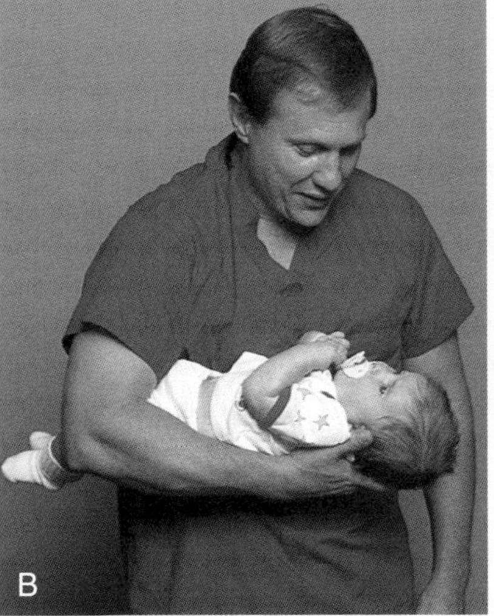

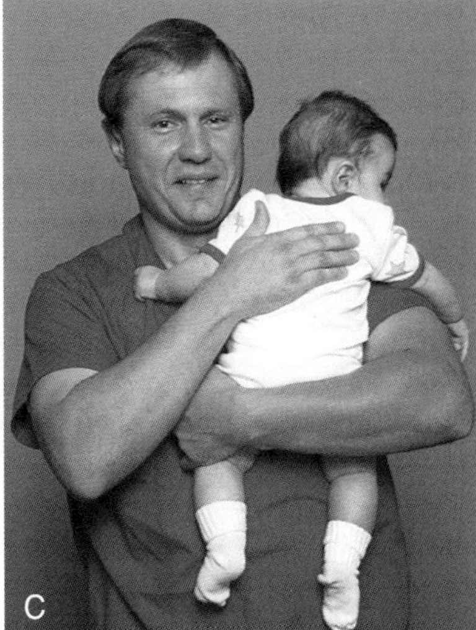

FIG. **4.1** Transporting infants. (A) Infant's thigh firmly grasped in nurse's hand. (B) Football hold. (C) Back supported.

Preventing Falls

Multiple interventions are needed to minimize pediatric patients' risk of falling. Once individual children are identified as at risk for falling, visual identification and communication of the risk among all health care providers is essential. Reduce the risk of falling through patient, family, and staff education.

Identify children at risk for falling. Perform a fall risk assessment on patients on admission and throughout hospitalization to identify patients at high risk for falls. Risk factors for hospitalized children include the following:

- Medication effects: postanesthesia or sedation; analgesics or narcotics, especially in those who have never had narcotics in the past and in whom effects are unknown
- Altered mental status: secondary to seizures, brain tumors, or medications
- Altered or limited mobility: reduced skill at ambulation secondary to developmental abilities, disease process, tubes, drains, casts, splints, or other appliances; new to ambulating with assistive devices such as walkers or crutches
- Postoperative children: risk of hypotension or syncope secondary to large blood loss, a heart condition, or extended bed rest
- History of falls
- Infants or toddlers in cribs with side rails down or on the daybed with family members

Visually identify patients at risk with one or more of the following:

- Post signs on the door and at the bedside.
- Apply a special armband labeled "Fall Precautions."
- Label the chart with a sticker.
- Document information on the chart.

Alter the environment:

- Keep bed in the lowest position, breaks locked, and side rails up.
- Place call bell within reach.
- Ensure that all necessary and desired items are within reach (e.g., water, glasses, tissues, snacks).
- Offer toileting on a regular basis, especially if patient is on diuretics or laxatives.
- Keep lights on at all times, including dim lights while sleeping.
- Lock wheelchairs before transferring patients.
- Ensure that patient has an appropriate size gown and nonskid footwear. Do not allow gowns or ties to drag on the floor when ambulating.
- Keep floor clean and free of clutter. Post "wet floor" sign if floor was recently mopped or is wet.
- Ensure that patient has glasses on if he or she normally wears them.

Educate patients and family members:

- Patients (as age appropriate):
  - Assist with ambulation even though the child may have ambulated well before hospitalization.
  - Patients who have been lying in bed will need to get up slowly, sitting on the side of the bed before standing.
- Family members:
  - Call the nursing staff for assistance, and do not allow patients to get up independently.
  - Keep the side rails of the crib or bed up whenever patient is in the crib or bed.
  - Do not leave infants on the daybed; put them in the crib with the side rails up.
  - When all family members need to leave the bedside, notify the nursing staff before leaving and ensure that the patient is in the bed or crib with side rails up and call bell within reach (if appropriate).

Restraining Methods and Therapeutic Holding

The Joint Commission (2021) defines physical holding of children and youth as a 'method of restraint in which a child's or youth's freedom of movement or normal access to his or her body is restricted by means of staff physically holding the child or youth for safety reasons. Restraint in children is defined as "any method, physical or mechanical, which restricts a person's movement, physical activity, or normal access to his or her body." Before initiating restraints, the nurse completes a comprehensive assessment of the patient to determine whether the need for a restraint outweighs the risk of not using one. Restraints can result in loss of dignity, violation of patient rights, psychological harm, physical harm, and even death.

Alternative methods should first be considered and documented in the patient's record. Some examples of alternative measures include bringing a child to the nurses' station for continuous observation, providing diversional activities such as music, encouraging the participation of the parents, or therapeutic holding. Therapeutic holding is the use of a secure, comfortable, temporary holding position that provides close physical contact with the parent or caregiver for 30 minutes or less. The use of restraints can often be avoided with adequate preparation of the child; parental or staff supervision of the child; or adequate protection of a vulnerable site, such as an infusion device. The nurse needs to assess the child's development, mental status, potential to hurt others or self, and safety. The nurse is responsible for selecting the least restrictive type of restraint (Fig. 4.2). Using less restrictive restraints is often possible by gaining the cooperation of the child and parents. Examples of less restrictive restraints are in Table 4.4.

The two types of restraints used with children are classified as medical-surgical and behavioral restraints. When a standard or protocol states that immobilization is required 100% of the time as a part of the procedure or postprocedural care process, the restraint device is considered a part of routine care. For example, the postoperative use of elbow restraints after a cleft lip repair, if written in the protocol or standard of care and used in 100% of patients, would not fall under the Joint Commission or Centers for Medicare and Medicaid Services mandates for restraints.

Medical-surgical restraints are used for children with an artificial airway or airway adjunct for delivery of oxygen, indwelling catheters, tubes, drains, lines, pacemaker wires, or suture sites. The medical-surgical restraint is used to ensure that safe care is given to the patient. The potential risks of the restraint are offset by the potential benefit of providing safer care. Criteria have been developed that outline when medical-surgical restraints may be instituted. These situations include the following:

- Risk for interruption of therapy used to maintain oxygenation or airway patency
- Risk of harm if indwelling catheter, tube, drain, line, pacemaker wire, or sutures are removed, dislodged, or ruptured
- Patient confusion, agitation, unconsciousness, or developmental inability to understand direct requests or instructions

Medical-surgical restraints can be initiated by an individual order or by protocol; the use of the protocol must be authorized by an individual order. Continued use of restraints must be renewed each day. Patients are monitored at least every 2 hours.

Behavioral restraints are limited to situations with a significant risk of patients physically harming themselves or others because of behavioral reasons and when nonphysical interventions are not effective. Before initiating a behavioral restraint, the nurse should assess the patient's mental, behavioral, and physical status to determine the cause of the child's behavior that may be harmful to the patient or others. If behavioral restraints are indicated, a collaborative approach involving the patient, if appropriate, the family, and the health care team should be used. An order must be obtained as soon as possible, but no longer than 1 hour after the initiation of behavioral restraints. Behavioral restraints for children must be reordered every 1 to 2 hours, based on age. A Licensed Independent Practitioner (LIP) must conduct an in-person evaluation within 1 hour and again every 4 hours until restraints are discontinued. Children in behavioral restraints must be continuously observed and assessed every 15 minutes. Assessment components include signs of injury associated with applying restraint, nutrition/hydration, circulation and range-of-motion of extremities, vital signs, hygiene and elimination, physical and psychological status and comfort, and readiness for discontinuation of restraint. Use clinical judgment in setting a schedule of when each of these parameters needs to be evaluated because every parameter must be assessed during each 15-minute physical assessment.

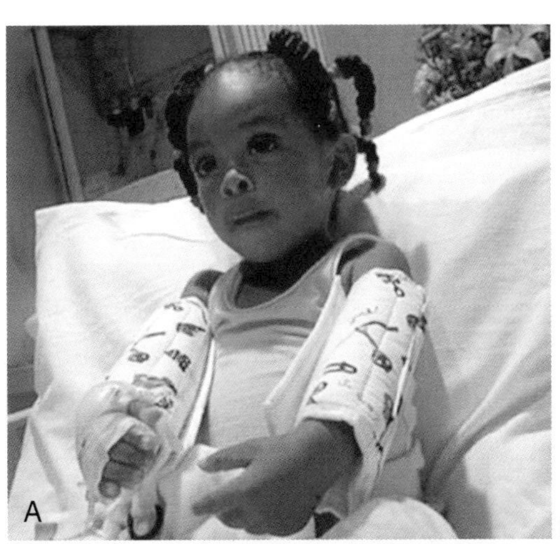

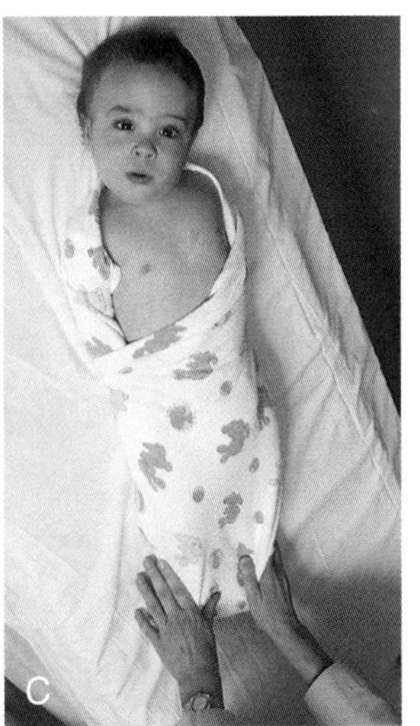

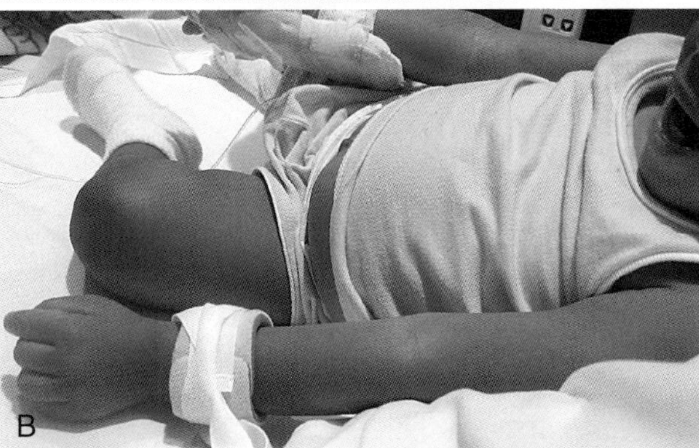

FIG. **4.2** Restraint examples from least restrictive to most restrictive. (A) Elbow restraints. (B) Wrist restraints. (C) Mummy restraint.

TABLE 4.4 Restraining Children: Less Restrictive to More Restrictive Techniques

Technique or Device	LESS RESTRICTIVE TO MORE RESTRICTIVE						
Extremities							
Sleeves		X					
Hand mitts/mittens		X					
Stockinette			X				
Elbows (no-no's)				X			
Arm board					X		
1–2 Limbs						X	
3–4 Limbs							X
Chest/Body							
Belts/safety belts	X						
Posey vest/safety jacket				X			
Mummy restraint							X
Papoose board							X
Environment							
Side rails			X				
Crib tops			X				
Seclusion							X
Other							
Chemical						X	

Restraints with ties must be secured to the bed or crib frame, not the side rails. Suggestions for increasing safety and comfort while the child is in a restraint include leaving one finger breadth between the skin and the device; tying knots that allow for quick release; ensuring the restraint does not tighten as the child moves; decreasing wrinkles or bulges in the restraint; placing jacket restraints over an article of clothing; placing limb restraints below waist level, below knee level, or distal to the IV; and tucking in dangling straps.

Positioning for Procedures

Placing a child in a comfortable or nonthreatening position (with a trusted adult) provides the child with a sense of control and minimizes anxiety. Comfort positioning encourages opportunities for the child to cope more effectively and promotes cooperation and success with procedures. Concepts of positioning include the following:

- Ensure patient and staff safety.
- Provide a secure, comforting, hugging hold with firm control of a limb or access area.
- Facilitate close physical contact with parent or caregiver.
- Allow the child to have a sense of control, as appropriate to the situation; sitting upright enhances the sense of control.
- Offer the child choices, such as the type of distraction to use (e.g., book, counting, or singing).
- Family members should provide positive support, not negative restraint.

Extremity Venipuncture or Injection

Place child on parent's (or assistant's) lap, with the child facing toward the parent and in the straddle position (Fig. 4.3A).

For venipuncture, place child's arm on a firm surface such as the treatment table (for support) and on top of a soft cloth or towel.

Have assistant or parent immobilize child's arm for venipuncture.

Have parent hug the child around the back to hold the child's free arm.

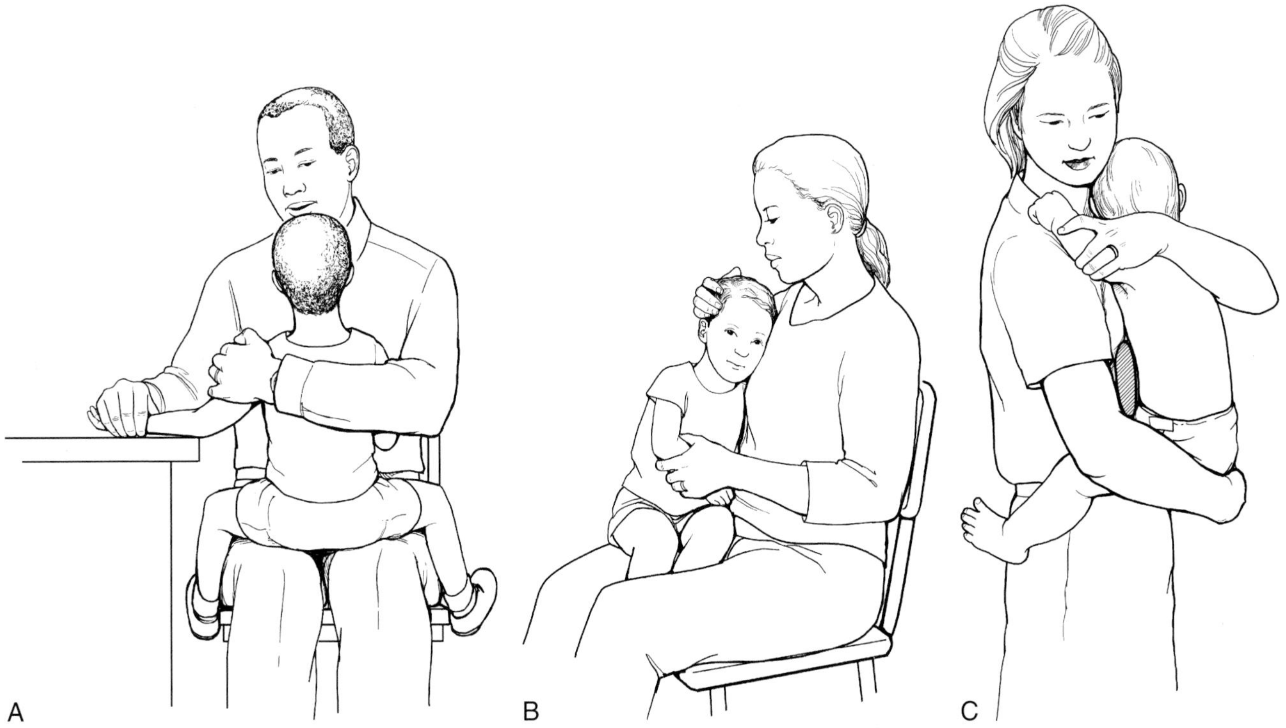

FIG. **4.3** Procedural positioning. (A) Chest-to-chest straddle position. (B) Side-sitting position with head and legs secured. (C) Chest-to-chest straddle standing position.

Place child on parent's (or assistant's) lap, with the child facing away from the parent.

To hold the child's legs still, place them between the parent's legs. This position is appropriate for an injection into the thigh; or, for an injection into the arm, place child in parent's (or assistant's) lap, with the child facing sideward (see Fig. 4.3B).

Place the child's arm closest to the parent under the parent's arm, and wrap it toward the back.

Have the parent hold the arm receiving the injection against the child's body.

ATRAUMATIC CARE

Analgesia and Sedation

For painful procedures, the child should receive adequate analgesia or sedation to minimize pain and the need for excessive restraint. For local anesthesia, use buffered lidocaine to reduce the stinging sensation, or apply a numbing cream. (See Evidence-Based Practice boxes.)

Some painful procedures, such as bone marrow tests, can be performed without restraint using general anesthesia with proper anesthesia monitoring availability (e.g., propofol [Diprivan]).

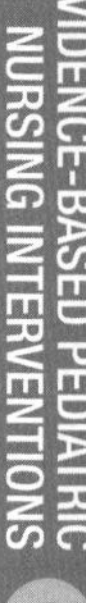

Femoral Venipuncture

Place infant supine with legs in frog position to provide extensive exposure of the groin.

Restrain legs in frog position with hands while controlling the child's arm and body movements with downward and inward pressure of forearms.

Cover genitalia to protect the operator and the venipuncture site from contamination if the child urinates during the procedure.

Site is not advisable for long-term venous access in a mobile child because of the risk of infection and trauma to the flexion area.

Subdural Puncture (Through Fontanel or Bur Holes)

Place active infant in mummy restraint.

Position supine with head accessible to the examiner.

Control head movement with a firm hold on each side of the head.

Lumbar Puncture

Infant

Place infant in sitting position with buttocks extended over the edge of the table and head in neutral position (Fig. 4.4).

In neonates, use side-lying position with modified head extension to decrease respiratory distress during procedure. Pulse oximetry and heart rate monitoring are advisable.

Hold infant at the shoulders (not the head or neck), and immobilize arms and legs with nurse's hands.

Observe infant for difficulty in breathing.

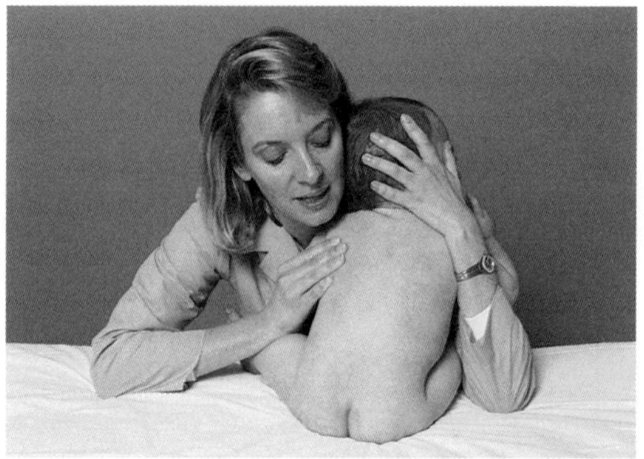

FIG. **4.4** Infant sitting position allows flexion of lumbar spine.

Child

A flexed sitting or side-lying position may be used, depending on the child's ability to cooperate and whether sedation will be used. In the sitting position with the hips flexed, the interspinous space is maximized.

Neck flexion is not necessary.

For sedated children and those who are unable to safely sit throughout the procedure, place child on side with back close to or extended over the edge of examining table, head flexed, and knees drawn up toward the chest.

Reach over the top of the child, and place one arm behind child's neck and the other behind the knees.

Stabilize this position by clasping own hands in front of the child's abdomen.

Take care that excessive pressure does not compromise circulation or breathing and that the nose and mouth are not covered by the restrainer's body.

Bone Marrow Aspiration or Biopsy

The position for a bone marrow aspiration or biopsy depends on the chosen site. In children, the posterior or anterior iliac crest is most frequently used, although in infants the tibia may be selected because of easy access to the site and holding of the child.

If the posterior iliac crest is used, position the child prone. Sometimes a small pillow or folded blanket is placed under the hips to facilitate obtaining the bone marrow specimen. Children should receive adequate analgesia or anesthesia to relieve pain. If the child may awaken, holding may be needed and is best done with two people—one person to immobilize the upper body and a second person to immobilize the lower extremities.

Nose and/or Throat Access

Position child supine with face accessible to examiner.

Control head and arms by holding child's extended arms over and close to the head, thus immobilizing both head and arms.

Ear Access

Place child in parent's (or assistant's) lap with the child's body sideways and the ear to be examined away from the parent (see Fig. 4.3B). Place the child's arm closest to the parent under the parent's arm, and wrap it toward the back.

Have the parent hold the other arm against the child's body and use the free arm to hold the head against the parent's chest.

To hold the child's legs still, place them between the parent's legs.

This can also be performed with the parent standing (see Fig. 4.3C).

Collection of Specimens

Fundamental Procedure Steps Common to all Procedures

The following steps are very important for every procedure and should be considered fundamental aspects of care. These steps, while important, are not listed in each of the specimen collection procedures.

1. Assemble necessary equipment.
2. Identify the child using two patient identifiers (e.g., patient name and medical record or birth date; neither can be a room number). Compare the same two identifiers to the specimen container and order.
3. Perform hand hygiene, maintain an aseptic technique, and follow Standard Precautions.
4. Explain procedure to parents and child according to the developmental level of the child; reassure child that the procedure is not punishment.
5. Provide atraumatic care, and position the child securely.
6. Prepare area with antiseptic agent.
7. Place specimens in appropriate containers, and apply a patient identification label to the specimen container in the presence of the child and family.
8. Discard the puncture device in puncture-resistant container near the site of use.
9. Wash procedural preparation agent off if povidone-iodine is used, if skin is sensitive, and for infants.
10. Remove gloves, and perform hand hygiene after the procedure. Have children wash their hands if they have helped.
11. Praise the child for helping.
12. Document pertinent aspects of the procedure, such as number of attempts, site and amount of blood/urine withdrawn, as well as type of test performed.

Urine

See Safety Alert.

> **SAFETY ALERT**
>
> Urine collected by the bag can be used to determine whether it is necessary to obtain a catheterized urine specimen for culture. For best results, the perineal area should be washed thoroughly before applying the urine collection bag, with prompt removal of the bag as soon as voiding occurs. Leaving the device in situ for more than 1 h is more likely to yield a contaminated urine specimen.

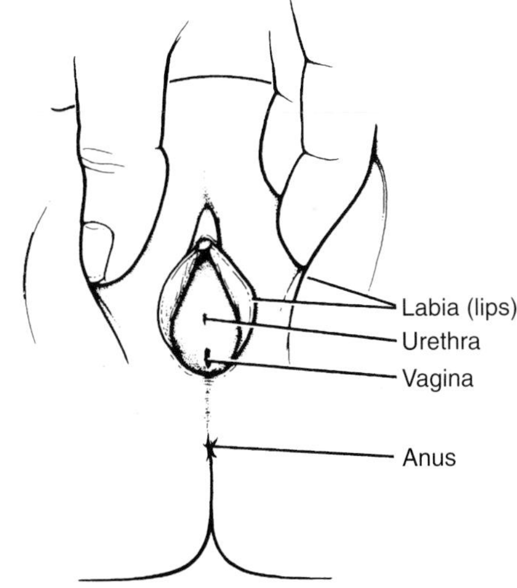

FIG. **4.5** Finger position to spread labia for cleaning before obtaining a urine sample.

Non–Toilet-Trained Child

Materials Needed to Use a Urine Collection Bag

Urine specimen cup
Urine collection bag
Soap and water
Washcloths or diaper/perineal wipes
Clean diaper

Instructions

If the child is very active, you will need help to put on the urine bag.

1. Place the child supine.
2. Remove the child's diaper.
3. Clean the child's genital area with soap and water or a diaper/perineal wipe. For girls, spread the child's labia with your fingers and wash from front to back (Fig. 4.5). For boys, wash the tip of the penis; if uncircumcised, pull back the foreskin only as far as it will easily go, cleanse, and push the foreskin back toward the tip after cleansing.
4. Have your helper hold the child's legs apart while you apply the bag.
5. Hold the urine collector with the bag portion downward.
6. Remove the bottom half of the adhesive protector.
7. For girls, spread the labia and buttocks, keeping the skin tight (Fig. 4.6). For boys, place the boy's penis and scrotum into the bag if possible (Fig. 4.7). If only the penis fits in the bag, put the sticky part of the bag on the scrotum.
8. Begin with the bottom of the adhesive. Place the sticky portion of the bag as flat as possible against the skin.
9. Smooth the plastic to avoid any wrinkles.
10. Remove the top half of the adhesive protector, and smooth it also on the skin, taking care to avoid making any wrinkles.

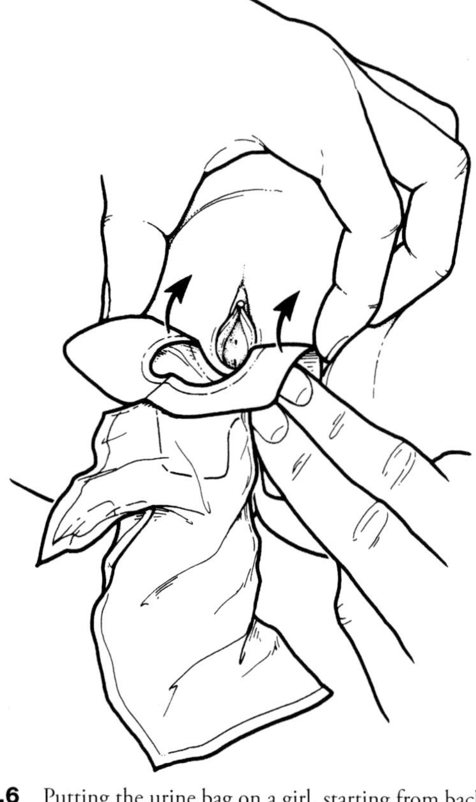

FIG. **4.6** Putting the urine bag on a girl, starting from back and proceeding to front.

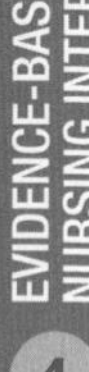

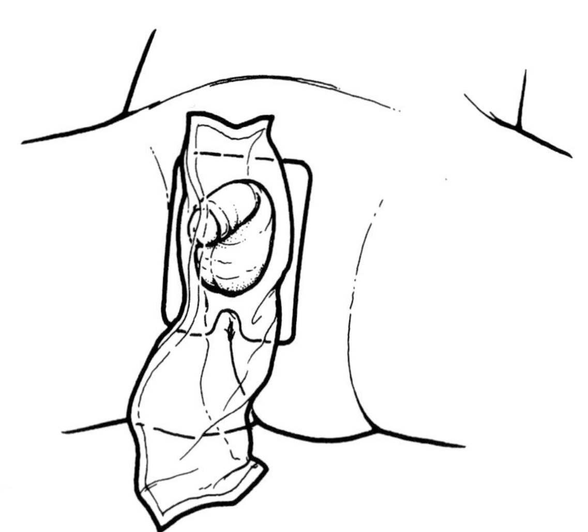

FIG. **4.7** Putting the urine bag on a boy, with the penis and scrotum inside the bag.

11. Cut a small slit in the diaper, and pull the bag through to allow room for urine to collect and to facilitate checking the contents. Check the bag often, and remove it as soon as the child urinates.
12. To remove the bag, hold it against the child's skin at the bottom and carefully peel it off by pulling the sticky part parallel to the skin.
13. Pour the urine into the specimen cup after opening the specimen drain or cutting the bag.

Small amounts of urine can be obtained using a syringe without a needle to aspirate urine directly from the diaper; if diapers with absorbent gelling material that traps urine are used, place a small gauze dressing, pad, or some cotton balls inside the diaper to collect urine, and then aspirate the urine with a syringe.

Urine should be tested within 30 minutes, refrigerated, or placed in a sterile container with a preservative.

Toilet-Trained Child

Children who are 8 years of age and older may be able to obtain the sample by themselves. Children under 8 years of age will need help. Young children may not be able to urinate on request. To help the child urinate, have her blow through a straw or listen to running water while the specimen cup is held for her. Do not give the child more than one glass of liquid to drink. Large amounts of liquid can affect the result of the urine test.

Materials Needed

Urine specimen cup
Potty chair, potty hat, or toilet
Soap and water
Washcloth or diaper/perineal wipes

Routine Urine Sample (Boys and Girls)

1. Put on nonsterile gloves. If the child is able to obtain the sample of urine, have the child wash her hands.
2. Open the urine container, taking care not to touch the inside of the cup or lid.
3. If a clean-catch specimen is needed:
   - For boys, wash the tip of the penis with a wipe or soap and water. If uncircumcised, pull back the foreskin only as far as it will easily go, then wash the tip of the penis. Rinse well if soap is used. Make sure the foreskin is pushed back toward the tip after cleaning.
   - For girls, spread the child's labia with your fingers. Wash the area from front to back with a wipe or soap and water. Rinse well if soap is used.
   - Have the child begin to urinate in the potty chair or toilet.
   - Tell the child to stop the stream. If he cannot stop the flow of urine, place the urine cup so that you can catch some of the urine.
4. Have the child urinate directly into the cup (or potty hat if more convenient for females and clean-catch not needed).
5. Replace the lid on the cup.

Bladder Catheterization

Bladder catheterization is employed for the following reasons:

- Collection of a urine specimen
- Diagnostic testing
- Continuous urinary drainage
- Intravesical instillation of medications or chemotherapeutic agents

Materials Needed

Sterile gloves (Safety Alert)
Catheter (see Safety Alert)

SAFETY ALERT

Nonlatex catheters and sterile gloves should be used for all infants and children with known latex allergy, with latex sensitivity, or on latex precautions (e.g., children with conditions associated with frequent exposure to latex-containing products).

- Select a catheter based on the purpose of the procedure, the age and gender of the child, and any history of prior urologic surgery.
- When collecting a urine specimen or completing a diagnostic test requiring catheterization for a brief period, use:
  - A 4–5 French catheter for the infant
  - A 5–8 French catheter for the toddler or school-age child
  - An 8–12 French in-and-out catheter for the adolescent girl
  - An 8–12 French, straight-tipped or coudé-tipped in-and-out catheter for the adolescent boy
- When placing an indwelling catheter, use:
  - A 6–8 French Foley catheter with a 3-mL retention balloon for the infant
  - A 6–8 French Foley catheter with a 3- to 5-mL retention balloon for the toddler or school-aged child
  - An 8–12 French Foley catheter with a 5-mL retention balloon for the adolescent girl
  - An 8–16 French Foley catheter with a 5-mL retention balloon for the adolescent boy
  - Larger French sizes (14–16) are reserved for older adolescents with more fully developed prostates. A coudé-tipped catheter is selected for the adolescent boy with a history of urologic surgery.

Catheter tray

- Catheter insertion trays are available that provide a cost-effective alternative to gathering individual supplies for catheterization. These kits may come with or without a catheter, and both should be available for use with children. When a tray is not accessible, the following materials are needed in addition to the catheter: Betadine cleanser with cotton balls, sterile draping, a syringe with 5 mL of sterile water, and sterile, water-soluble lubricating jelly.

Container for urine collection

- When collecting a specimen or completing a diagnostic test, an appropriate urine specimen container and 500-mL basin are used; when inserting an indwelling catheter, a bedside drainage bag is obtained before the procedure. When inserting a Foley catheter, it is preferable to use a preconnected (closed) system containing catheter and bedside drainage bag.

Procedure

1. Special procedural explanation considerations
   - Explain before preparation of the perineum.
   - Reassure parents that catheterization will not harm their child or damage the urethra or hymen.
   - Reassure child that insertion of the catheter will not feel like having a sharp object inserted but will produce a feeling of pressure and desire to urinate.
   - Give instruction on pelvic muscle relaxation whenever possible.
   - Young child is taught to blow (using a pinwheel is helpful) and to press the hips against the bed or procedure table during catheterization in order to relax the pelvic and periurethral muscles.
   - Older child or adolescent is taught to contract and relax the pelvic muscles, and the relaxation procedure is repeated during catheter insertion. If the child vigorously contracts the pelvic muscles when the catheter reaches the striated sphincter (proximal urethra in boys and mid-urethra in girls), catheter insertion is temporarily stopped. The catheter is neither removed nor advanced; instead, the child is assisted to press the hips against the bed or examining table and relax the pelvic muscles. The catheter is then gently advanced into the bladder.
2. Place the infant or child in a supine position with the perineum adequately exposed. Girls may bend the knees and abduct the legs in a froglike position; boys should lie with the penis lying above the upper thighs. Use rolled towels or blankets to support the legs. As an alternative, for a young child, have the parent sit on the bed or examining table with a back support. Place the child leaning back in the parent's lap with the parent's arms hugging the child's upper body. When the child's legs are in the frog position, the parent's legs can be placed over the child's to stabilize them. In this comfortable position, the perineum is exposed for the procedure and the child is helped to lie still.
3. Put on a pair of sterile gloves. (See Safety Alert.)
4. Place a sterile drape over the perineum of girls, ensuring that the vagina, labia, and urethral meatus remain exposed. Most catheter insertion kits provide a sterile drape with a diamond-shaped hole in the middle to assist with this. For boys, the sterile drape is placed over the upper aspect of the thighs.
5. Place 5 mL of sterile lubricating jelly on the sterile drape. During catheterization of an adolescent or child accustomed to the procedure, the catheter may be placed on the sterile drape laid over the perineum. When an anxious child is being catheterized, the catheter should remain on a sterile field that will not be upset should the child move during the procedure.
6. Cleanse the perineum of girls, including the labia, vaginal introitus, and urethral meatus. Use a new cotton ball for each wipe, moving in a front-to-back motion along each side of the labia minora, along the sides of the urinary

meatus, and finally straight down over the urethral opening. For boys, cleanse the entire glans penis in an outward circular fashion, using one cotton ball for each wipe. The foreskin is retracted in the uncircumcised boy just far enough to visualize the urethral opening. If the foreskin cannot be easily retracted, particular care is taken to ensure that the glans penis is adequately cleaned before catheter insertion.

7. Wipe the cleanser from the skin using sterile cotton balls.
8. Girls: Spread the labia (if necessary) using one hand in order to clearly visualize the urethral meatus. With the other hand, grasp the catheter and apply a small amount of sterile lubricant from the sterile field onto the tip of the catheter. (It is rarely necessary to spread the labia in infants; instead, locate the urethra, which often appears as a dimple above the hymen.) Gently insert the catheter until urine return is seen. If inserting an indwelling catheter, advance the catheter an additional 1 to 2 inches before attempting to fill the retention balloon.
9. Boys: Hold the penile shaft just under the glans to prevent the foreskin from contaminating the area. Grasp the catheter with the other hand, and apply a small amount of sterile lubricant from the sterile field onto the tip of the catheter. Insert the catheter while gently stretching the penis and lifting it to a 90-degree angle to the body. Resistance may occur when the catheter meets the urethral sphincter. Ask the patient to inhale deeply and advance the catheter at that time. Insert the catheter until urine return occurs; this may take several seconds longer because of the additional lubricant present in the urethra. If inserting an indwelling catheter, advance until urine return is noted and then advance to the bifurcation of the filling port before filling the retention balloon.
10. When catheterizing for specimen collection, allow 15 to 30 mL for urinalysis and urine culture. Drain bladder, and record postvoid urinary volume if collected soon after urination. Cap the specimen, label it and send it to the laboratory.
11. When inserting an indwelling catheter, gently pull the catheter back until resistance is met; this ensures that the retention balloon lies just above the bladder neck. Tape tubing to the leg to avoid pulling, or use a commercially available catheter securement device. Hang drainage apparatus to bed frame (avoid bed rails to prevent pulling on catheter).

SAFETY ALERT

Do not advance the catheter too far into the bladder. Knotting of catheters and tubes within the bladder has been reported in several case studies. Feeding tubes should not be used for urinary catheterization as they are more flexible, longer, and prone to knotting compared to commercially designed urinary catheters (Kilbane, 2009; Lodha et al., 2005; Levison and Wojtulewicz, 2004; Turner, 2004).

24-Hour Urine Collection

Begin and end collection with an empty bladder:

- At time collection begins, instruct child to void, and discard specimen.
- Twenty-four hours after that specimen was discarded, instruct child to void for last specimen.

Save all voided urine during the 24 hours in a refrigerated container marked with date, total time, and child's name.

Non–Toilet-Trained Child

Prepare skin with thin coating of skin sealant (unless contraindicated, such as in premature infant or on irritated and/or nonintact skin), and apply a urine collection bag with a collection tube that allows urine to drain into a large receptacle.

If a collection tube is not available, insert a small feeding tube through a puncture hole at the top of the bag; use a syringe without a needle to aspirate urine through the feeding tube.

Stool

Collect stool without urine contamination, if possible.

Non–Toilet-Trained Child

Put on nonsterile gloves.

Apply a urine collection bag, and apply diaper over bag. Stool specimens may also be collected directly from the diaper.

After bowel movement, use a gloved hand and tongue blade or specimen stick to collect stool. If the stool is liquid, collect as many small pieces of fecal matter as possible, using a disposable spoon. If liquid stool soaks into diaper, line the inside of a clean diaper with plastic wrap. Place the clean diaper on the child and collect the next stool sample from the plastic liner.

Place specimen in specimen container. Replace the lid on the cup.

Wash child's diaper area with warm water and soap after each stool to prevent skin irritation.

Toilet-Trained Child

Children who are aged 8 years and older may be able to obtain the sample by themselves. Tell the child how to clean herself and how to obtain the sample. Young children may not be able to defecate on request. Use the child's words and usual place for defecating to obtain the sample, if possible. Have the child tell the parent when they think they are going to have a bowel movement. To help the child defecate, have the child bear down or hold his or her breath to facilitate evacuation of the stool.

Have child urinate, and then flush the toilet.

Perform hand hygiene, and put on nonsterile gloves.

Have child defecate into bedpan or potty hat in reverse position in the toilet.

After bowel movement, use tongue depressor or specimen stick to collect stool.

Place specimen in specimen container. Replace the lid on the cup.

Apply a patient identification label to the cup.

Remove gloves, and perform hand hygiene. Have the child wash his or her hands.

Praise the child for helping.

EVIDENCE-BASED PRACTICE

The Use of Lidocaine Lubricant for Urethral Catheterization

Ask the Question

In children, does a lidocaine lubricant decrease the pain associated with urethral catheterization?

Search for the Evidence

Search Strategies

Search selection criteria included English-language publications, research-based studies, and review articles on the use of the lidocaine lubricant before urethral catheterization.

Databases Used

Cochrane Collaboration, PubMed, MD Consult, BestBETs, American Academy of Pediatrics

Critically Analyze the Evidence

- Gray (1996) published a review of strategies to minimize distress associated with urethral catheterization in children and supported intraurethral instillation of a local anesthetic that contains 2% lidocaine before catheter insertion.
- One prospective, double-blind, placebo-controlled trial evaluated the use of lidocaine lubricant for discomfort in 20 children before urethral catheterization. Two doses of lidocaine lubricant instilled into the urethra 5 min apart significantly reduced pain and distress during urethral catheterization (Gerard et al., 2003).
- Boots and Edmundson (2010) conducted a randomized controlled trial in 200 children in a follow-up to the study by Gerard and colleagues. Conclusions were that a topical application of 2% lidocaine gel followed by urethral instillation of lidocaine gel is effective in reducing discomfort before urinary catheterization, and two urethral instillations offered no significant difference over a single instillation.
- Mularoni et al. (2009) found in a three-armed placebo-controlled, double-blind, randomized controlled trial of 43 children younger than 2 years of age that topical and intraurethral lidocaine lubricant was superior to the placebos of topical aqueous lubricant alone and topical and intraurethral aqueous lubricant in lowering distress, but it did not fully alleviate pain.
- A placebo-controlled, double-blind, randomized controlled trial of 115 children younger than 2 years of age found no significant difference when 2% lidocaine gel was compared with a nonanesthetic lubricant. The lubricant was applied to the genital mucosa for 2–3 min and liberally applied to the catheter but not instilled into the urethra (Vaughn et al., 2005).
- A randomized controlled trial of 126 children ages 4 days to 23 months found a significant decrease in pain response in children who received topical and intraurethral 2% lidocaine gel compared with children who received a nonanesthetic lubricant (Castelo et al., 2014).
- A randomized controlled trial of 133 children ages 0–24 months found no difference in pain response in children who received intraurethral 2% lidocaine gel lubricant compared with children who received a nonanesthetic lubricant during urethral catheterization. However, there was a significantly increased pain response in children during instillation of the lidocaine lubricant compared with the nonanesthetic lubricant. Additionally, there was no difference in parent satisfaction scores between the nonanesthetic lubricant and lidocaine lubricant (Poonai et al., 2015).
- A systematic review and meta-analysis sought to compare the efficacy and safety of lidocaine gel to non-analgesic gel for children undergoing transurethral bladder catheterization (TUBC) (Chua et al., 2017). The review included 5 randomized controlled trials representing 369 children. Overall, lidocaine gel has no significant benefit in decreasing pain during TUBC in children under 4 years of age.
- In a randomized clinical trial of children aged 0–36 months of age who were undergoing TUBC (Uspal et al., 2018) received either intraurethral 2% lidocaine or usual care (no analgesia). Procedures were videotaped and reviewed by trained, independent blinded reviewer. Pain was scored using the Face, Legs, Arms, Cry, Consolability and the Modified Behavioral Pain Score scales. Intraurethral lidocaine did not improve procedural pain scores, which were high across all groups.
- A systematic review and meta-analysis of lidocaine gel for pain management during TUBC (Long and April, 2018) in children under 18 years of age. Findings demonstrated that lidocaine gel does not reduce pain associated with TUBC. Authors determined this evidence is of very low quality due to risk of bias and imprecision of treatment effect.

Apply the Evidence: Nursing Implications

- There is low-quality evidence with weak recommendations (Guyatt et al., 2008) for using a lidocaine lubricant to decrease pain associated with urethral catheterization.
- Four published research studies were found to support the use of anesthetic before urethral catheterization, one found topical application alone insufficient to reduce pain, and one found no difference in pain response between anesthetic and nonanesthetic application. However more recent RCTs and meta-analyses found that lidocaine instillation prior to TUBC. Several publications support the effectiveness of lidocaine gel lubricant in clinical practice. Further studies using robust methodology are necessary to strengthen the current evidence to better manage pain and discomfort during TUBC.

EVIDENCE-BASED PEDIATRIC NURSING INTERVENTIONS 4

Continued

TRANSLATING EVIDENCE INTO PRACTICE

The Use of Lidocaine Lubricant for Urethral Catheterization—cont'd

References

Boots BK, Edmundson EE. A controlled, randomised trial comparing single to multiple application lidocaine analgesia in paediatric patients undergoing urethral catheterisation procedures. *J Clin Nurs.* 2010;19(5–6):744–748.

Castelo M, Li J, Taddio A, et al. A randomized controlled trial of 2% lidocaine gel compared to current standard of care in infants undergoing urinary catheterization. *Ann Emerg Med.* 2014;64(suppl 4):S105.

Chua ME, Firaza PNB, Ming JM, et al. Lidocaine gel for urethral catheterization in children: a meta-analysis. *J Pediatr.* 2017;190:207–214.e201.

Gerard LL, Cooper CS, Duethman KS, et al. Effectiveness of lidocaine lubricant for discomfort during pediatric urethral catheterization. *J Urol.* 2003;170:564–567.

Gray M. Atraumatic urethral catheterization of children. *Pediatr Nurs.* 1996;22(4):306–310.

Guyatt GH, Oxman AD, Vist GE, et al. GRADE: an emerging consensus on rating quality of evidence and strength of recommendations. *Br Med J.* 2008;336:924–926.

Long B, April MD. Does lidocaine gel decrease procedural pain for pediatric urethral catheterization? *Ann Emerg Med.* 2018;72(5):588–590.

Mularoni PP, Cohen LL, DeGuzman M, et al. A randomized clinical trial of lidocaine gel for reducing infant distress during urethral catheterization. *Pediatr Emerg Care.* 2009;25(7):439–443.

Poonai N, Li J, Langford C, et al. Intraurethral lidocaine for urethral catheterization in children: A randomized controlled trial. *Pediatrics.* 2015;136(4):880–886.

Vaughn H, Paton EA, Bush A, et al. Does lidocaine gel alleviate the pain of bladder catheterization in young children? A randomized, controlled trial. *Pediatrics.* 2005;116(4):917–920.

Uspal NG, Strelitz B, Gritton J, et al. Randomized clinical trial of lidocaine analgesia for transurethral bladder catheterization delivered via blunt tipped applicator in young children. *Pediatr Emerg Care.* 2018;34(4):273–279.

Respiratory (Nasal) Secretions

To obtain nasal secretions using a nasal washing:

- Place child supine if maximal restraint needed; upright or semi-reclining allows the child more control and causes less anxiety.
- Instill 1 to 3 mL sterile NS with a sterile syringe (without needle or with 2 inches of 18- or 20-gauge tubing) into one nostril.
- Aspirate contents with a small, sterile bulb syringe.
- Place in sterile container.

Sputum

Older children and adolescents are able to cough as directed and supply specimens when given proper direction.

Specimens can sometimes be collected from infants and young children who have an endotracheal (ET) tube or tracheostomy by means of tracheal aspiration with a mucous trap or suction apparatus.

Blood

Heel or Finger

Heel lancing has been shown to be more painful than venipuncture; consider venipuncture when the amount of blood from the heel would require much squeezing (e.g., genetic tests).

Puncture should be no deeper than 2 mm.

To increase blood flow, warm heel by using a commercial heel warmer for 3 minutes before puncture. May hold finger under warm water for a few seconds before puncture.

Prepare area for puncture with an antiseptic agent.

Perform puncture on heel or finger in proper location with an automatic lancet device:

- Usual site for heel puncture is outer aspects of heel (Fig. 4.8A). Boundaries can be marked by an imaginary line extending posteriorly from a point between the fourth and fifth toes and running parallel to the lateral aspect of the heel and another line extending posteriorly from the middle of the great toe and running parallel to the medial aspect of the heel.
- Usual site for finger puncture is just to the side of the finger pad (see Fig. 4.8B), which has more blood vessels and fewer nerve endings. Avoid steadying the finger against a hard surface.

Collect blood sample in appropriate specimen container.

Apply pressure to puncture site with a dry, sterile gauze pad until bleeding stops.

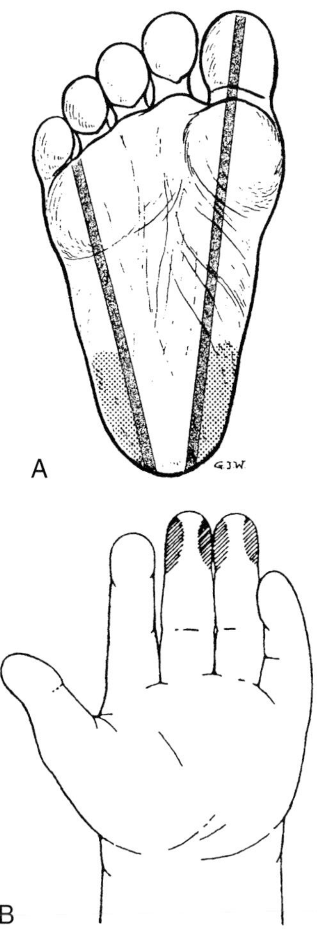

FIG. **4.8** (A) Puncture sites (shaded areas) on infant's heel. (B) Puncture sites on fingers. (B, From Smith DP, Wong DL. *Comprehensive Child and Family Nursing Skills*. St Louis: Mosby; 1991.)

Vein

Apply tourniquet; alternative tourniquet for neonate is a rubber band.

Visualize or palpate vein.

Insert needle with bevel up; a slight pop may be felt when entering a child's vein; in small and preterm infants this may not occur.

Withdraw required amount of blood, and place in appropriate container.

Release tourniquet.

Withdraw needle from site, and apply dry, sterile gauze or cotton ball to site with firm pressure until bleeding stops. If an antecubital site is used, keep arm extended to reduce bruising.

Artery

Arterial blood samples from punctures are painful and often cause crying and breath holding, which affect the accuracy of blood gas values (decreased PaO_2). Provide pain intervention with buffered lidocaine, and for infants use sucrose before stick.

Arterial punctures may be performed using the radial, brachial, or femoral arteries.

Palpate artery for puncture.

Perform Allen test to determine the adequacy of collateral circulation prior to radial puncture:

- Elevate extremity distal to puncture site, and blanch by squeezing gently (e.g., making a fist); two arteries supplying blood flow to the extremity (radial and ulnar arteries of the wrist) are then occluded.
- Lower extremity, and remove pressure from one artery (ulnar); color return to the blanched extremity in less than 5 seconds indicates adequate collateral circulation.

Prepare area for puncture with an antiseptic agent.

Insert needle at a 60- to 90-degree angle.

Withdraw required amount of blood into syringe (or specimen container, as appropriate).

Withdraw needle, and apply pressure to site with a dry, sterile gauze pad for 5 to 10 minutes until bleeding stops. NOTE: Pressure must be applied at the site to prevent a hematoma.

Place specimen in heparinized syringe after removing bubbles from the syringe.

Place specimen on ice if it will not be processed immediately.

Procedures Related to Administration of Medications

General Guidelines

Approaches to Pediatric Patients

Children's reactions to treatments are affected by the following:

- Developmental characteristics, such as physical abilities and cognitive capabilities
- Environmental influences
- Past experiences
- Current relationship with the nurse
- Perception of the present situation

Expect success: use a positive approach.

Provide an explanation appropriate to the child's developmental level.

Allow the child choices whenever they exist.

Be honest with the child.

Involve the child in the treatment in order to gain cooperation.

Allow the child the opportunity to express his or her feelings.

Hold and comfort the child after medication administration.

Praise the child for doing his or her best.

Provide distraction for a frightened or uncooperative child.
Spend some time with the child after administering the medication.
Let the child know that he or she is accepted as a person of value. (See also section on preparing children for procedures.)

Safety Precautions

Take a drug allergy history.
Check the following five R's for correctness:
- Right drug
- Right dosage
- Right time
- Right route
- Right child (Always check identification band and use two patient identifiers.)

Double-check drug and dosage with another nurse.
Always double-check the following:
- Antiarrhythmics (e.g., Digoxin)
- Insulin
- Anticoagulants (e.g., Heparin)
- Blood
- Chemotherapy
- Cardiotoxic drugs

Some institutions also double-check the following:
- Vasopressors
- Opioids (narcotics)
- Sedatives

Identify the child using two patient identifiers (e.g., patient name and medical record or birth date; neither can be a room number). Compare the same two identifiers to the medication label and order.
Be aware of drug-drug or drug-food interactions.
Document all drugs administered.
Monitor child for side effects.
Be prepared for serious side effects (e.g., respiratory depression, anaphylaxis).
Dispose of any plastic covers that may be on the ends of syringes. These covers are small enough to be aspirated by young children.
Measure liquid medications with a syringe or other specific medication dropper or calibrated spoon; instruct families to not use household teaspoons or tablespoons.

Family Education: Medication Administration

In addition to the General Principles of Family Education, families need to know the following:
- Amount of the drug to be given
- Length of time to be administered
- Time(s) to give the drug; assist family in scheduling the time for administration around the family routine.
- Positioning
- Administration procedure
- Postadministration care
- Safe storage of drug (Safety Alert)
- What to do and whom to contact if any side effects occur

SAFETY ALERT FOR HOME CARE

Do not tell children that medications are candy; if the bottle is ever left in a place where it can be reached, a child may take an overdose. Tell the child to take drugs only from parents or other special people, such as grandparents, babysitters, or nurses. Store all drugs in a safe place such as a locked cabinet. The storage area should be cool and dry. Bathrooms are usually too warm and moist for storing tablets or capsules. Always keep drugs in the original container, with the childproof cap tightly closed. Place drugs that need to be refrigerated on a high shelf toward the back of the refrigerator, not in the door.

Oral Administration

1. Follow safety precautions for administration.
2. Select appropriate vehicle, for example, calibrated cup, oral medication syringe, dropper, measuring spoon, or nipple (Safety Alert).
3. Prepare medication:
   - Measure into appropriate vehicle (Fig. 4.9)
   - Crush tablets (except when contraindicated, e.g., time-released or enteric-coated preparations) for children who will have difficulty swallowing if a liquid medication is unavailable; mix with syrup, juice, and so on (Atraumatic Care box) At home, crushing can be done using two spoons or one spoon and wax paper
   - Capsules should not be opened and sprinkled into food prior to checking with a pharmacist.
   - Avoid mixing medications with essential food items, such as milk and formula.
4. Employ safety precautions in identification and administration (Safety Alert).

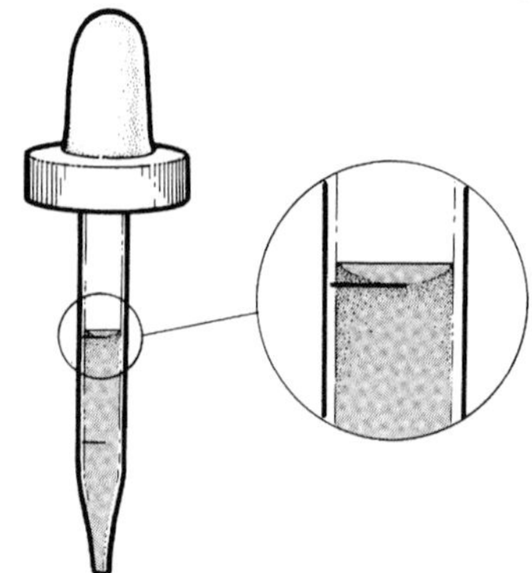

FIG. **4.9** Checking correct amount in a dropper.

ATRAUMATIC CARE

Encouraging a Child's Acceptance of Oral Medications

Give the child a flavored ice pop or a small ice cube to suck to numb the tongue before giving the drug.

Mix the drug with a small amount (about 1 teaspoon) of sweet-tasting substance such as honey (except in infants because of the risk of botulism), flavored syrup, jam, fruit puree, sherbet, or ice cream; avoid essential food items, such as formula or milk, because the child may later refuse to eat or drink them.

Give a chaser of water, juice, soft drink, flavored ice pop, or frozen juice bar after the drug.

If nausea is a problem, give a carbonated beverage poured over finely crushed ice before or immediately after the medication.

When medication has an unpleasant taste, have the child pinch the nose and drink the medicine through a straw. (Much of what we taste is associated with smell.)

Flavorings such as apple, banana, and bubble gum can be added at many pharmacies (e.g., FLAVORx) at a nominal additional cost. Another alternative is to have the pharmacist prepare the drug in a flavored, chewable troche or lozenge.[a]

Infants will suck medicine from a needleless syringe or dropper in small increments (0.25–0.5 mL) at a time. Use a nipple or special pacifier with a reservoir for the drug.

[a]For information about compounding drugs, contact Technical Staff, Professional Compounding Centers of America (PCCA), www.pccarx.com.
Regarding Professional Compounding Centers of America.
Professional Compounding Centers of America dba PCCA—597638—01/27/2021IFDA.

5. Give the medicine to the child in a quiet place so that you will not be disturbed.
6. Tell the child what you are going to do.
7. If needed, hold the infant or young child in your lap. Place whichever of her arms is closer to you behind your back. Firmly hug her other arm and hand with your arm and hand; snuggle her head between your body and your arm (Fig. 4.10). Sometimes you may also want to grasp her legs between yours. Your other hand remains free to give the child the drug.
8. Gently place the dropper or syringe in the child's mouth along the inside of the cheek. Allow the child to suck the liquid from the dropper or syringe. If the child does not suck, squeeze a small amount of the drug at a time. This takes longer, but the child will swallow the medicine and be less likely to spit it out or choke on it.

OR

Place an empty bottle nipple in the child's mouth, add the drug to the nipple, and allow the child to suck the nipple (Fig. 4.11).

OR

Allow the child to sip the drug from the spoon. Make sure that the child takes all of the drug.

9. Rinse the child's mouth with plain water to remove any of the sweetened drug from the gums and teeth. This can be done by wrapping a paper towel around your finger, soaking it in plain water, then swabbing the gums, cheeks, palate, and tongue.

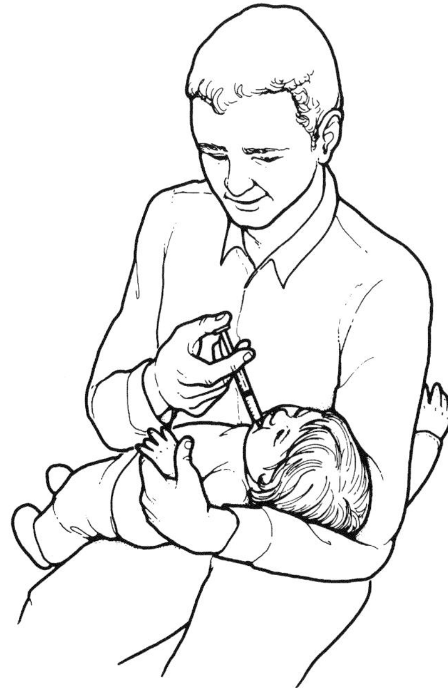

FIG. **4.10** Giving oral medication using a syringe. Note how the child's arms are placed.

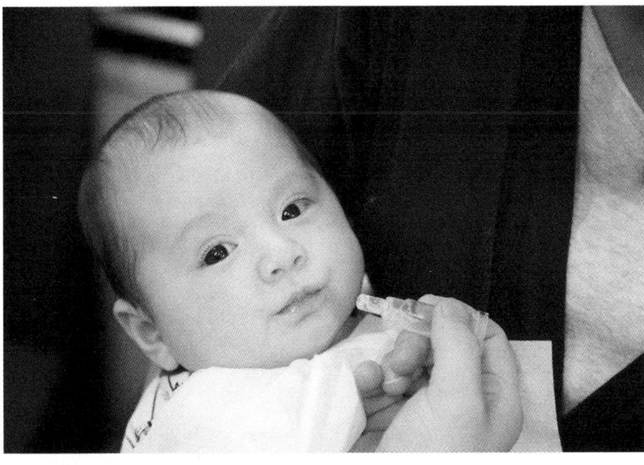

FIG. **4.11** Giving oral medication to an infant.

EVIDENCE-BASED PEDIATRIC NURSING INTERVENTIONS 4

Infants

Hold in a semi-reclining position.

Place oral syringe, measuring spoon, or dropper in mouth well back on the tongue or to the side of the tongue.

Administer slowly to reduce the likelihood of choking or aspiration.

Allow infant to suck medication placed in a nipple.

Older Infant or Toddler

Administer with oral syringe, measuring spoon, or dropper (as with infants).

Use mild or partial restraint with reluctant children.

Do not force actively resistive children because of the danger of aspiration; postpone 20 to 30 minutes, and offer medication again.

Preschool Children

Use straightforward approach.

For reluctant children, use the following:

- Simple persuasion
- Innovative containers
- Reinforcement, such as stars, stickers, or other tangible rewards for compliance

SAFETY ALERT

When a dose is ordered that is outside the usual range, or if there is some question regarding the preparation or the route of administration, the nurse always checks with the practitioner before proceeding with the administration, because the nurse is legally liable for any drug administered.

SAFETY ALERT

Many pediatric medications are given by drops or dropper. A misunderstanding of these terms by parents can result in a potential overdose. In addition, many droppers that come with medications are marked in tenths of cubic centimeters. If a parent were to use a syringe instead of the dropper, 0.4 cc may be thought to be the same as 4 cc. Educate parents about the correct methods for giving medication, and demonstrate the proper techniques.

OTC (over-the-counter) medications manufactured and sold for children often have confusing administration directions, mislabeled dosing devices, and confusing dosage administration directions which could ultimately lead to errors in medication administration. There are inconsistencies among the OTC products in providing standardized measuring units which could easily lead a parent to overdose the child; nonstandardized units of measurement such as tablespoons, drams, cubic centimeters, and fluid ounces.

Nurses working with children are in an excellent position to provide appropriate education to parents and guardians about the administration of OTC medications, proper dosing based on the child's weight, and standardized units of measurement to ensure the safety of medication administration. Because many products do not contain appropriate measuring devices nurses can provide oral medication administration syringes which are calibrated appropriately to prevent dosing errors. In addition, written individualized medication administration instructions for each child in the family and for each medication will prevent confusion and frustration. Discharge instructions should be concisely written and reviewed with the parent prior to discharge.

Family Education: Administering Digoxin at Home

Give digoxin at regular intervals (usually every 12 hours, such as at 8 AM and 8 PM; in some children it may be given every 24 hours).

Plan the times so that the drug is given 1 hour before or 2 hours after feedings.

Use a calendar to mark off each dose that is given; or post a reminder, such as a sign on the refrigerator.

Have the prescription refilled before the medication is completely used.

Do not mix it with other foods, formula, or other fluids, because refusal to consume these results in inaccurate intake of the drug.

If the child has teeth, give water after administering the drug; whenever possible, brush the teeth to prevent tooth decay from the sweetened liquid.

If a dose is missed and more than 4 hours have elapsed, withhold the dose and give the next dose at the regular time; if less than 4 hours have elapsed, give the missed dose.

If the child vomits within 1 hour of receiving the dose, do not give a second dose.

If more than two consecutive doses have been missed, notify the physician or other designated health professional.

Do not increase or double the dose for missed doses.

Avoid administration with herbal preparations such as St. John's wort or Siberian ginseng because these may change the medication's intended effect on the heart.

Notify your child's health practitioner if you need to give the child any over-the-counter medications.

If the child becomes ill with any of the following, notify the physician or other designated health professional immediately:

- Diarrhea
- Nausea
- Vision changes
- Lack of appetite
- Vomiting

Keep digoxin in a safe place, preferably a locked cabinet.

In case of an accidental overdose of digoxin, call the nearest Poison Control Center immediately or the national number: 800-222-1222; the number is usually listed in the front of the telephone directory.

EVIDENCE-BASED PRACTICE

Confirming Nasogastric Tube Placement in Pediatric Patients

Ask the Question

In children, how should the correct placement of nasogastric (NG) tubes be assessed during hospitalization?

Search for the Evidence

Search Strategies

Search selection criteria included English-language, research-based articles, and children and adolescents requiring NG tube placement. Search areas included aspirate, auscultation, and radiology methods, NG tube length prediction methods, age-related height-based methods, and accurate NG tube placement. Searches excluded newborns and preterm infants.

Databases Used

PubMed, Cochrane Collaboration, MDConsult, Joanna Briggs Institute, Agency for Healthcare Research and Quality National Guideline Clearinghouse, TRIP Database Plus, PedsCCM, BestBETS

Critical Appraisal of the Evidence

Studies compared various methods used to evaluate the correct placement of the NG tube.

Accurate Nasogastric Tube Length Measurement

- Children 8 years, 4 months old or younger: Use age-related height-based equation for NG length predictions.
- Children older than 8 years, 4 months old, short stature, or when you cannot obtain accurate height: Use nose-ear–midway to umbilicus (NEMU) (Beckstrand et al., 2007).
- Use of the nose-ear-xyphoid (NEX) method resulted in increased risk of misplaced tubes (Irving et al., 2018).

Radiographs

- Although abdominal x-ray provides confirmation of enteral tube location, the results can sometimes be equivocal. In addition, this method cannot be used for ongoing, frequent placement verification basis due to the risk of radiation exposure to the child (Irving et al., 2018). Alternate methods of verification have evidence-based support in the literature (Emergency Nurses Association, 2019).

Nonradiologic Verification Methods

- A pH of 5 or less supports that the tip of the tube is in the gastric location (Ellett et al., 2005; Gilbertson et al., 2011; Ni et al., 2017; Nyqvist et al., 2005; Society of Pediatric Nurses Clinical Practice Committee et al., 2011).
- A pH greater than 5 does not reliably predict correct distal tip location. This may indicate respiratory or esophageal placement or the presence of medications to suppress acid secretion. Gastric aspirate pH means are statistically significantly lower compared with means from intestinal and respiratory pH aspirates (Ellett et al., 2005; Gilbertson et al, 2011; Society of Pediatric Nurses Clinical Practice Committee et al., 2011).

Visual Inspection of Aspirate

- Visual inspection is less accurate than pH to confirm placement. Aspirate colors are specific to the intended placement location. Gastric contents are clear, off-white, or tan or may be brown-tinged if blood is present. Respiratory secretions may look the same. Intestinal contents are often bile stained, light to dark yellow, or greenish-brown (Society of Pediatric Nurses Clinical Practice Committee et al., 2011).

Enzyme Testing

- Aspirate testing of enzyme levels for bilirubin, pepsin, and trypsin is highly accurate but limited to laboratory assessment (Ellett et al., 2005; Fernandez et al., 2010).

Carbon Dioxide Monitoring

- Carbon dioxide (CO_2) monitoring (capnography or colorimetric capnometry) is as reliable as radiograph for confirmation of gastrointestinal (GI) versus respiratory placement of NG tubes but cannot distinguish between gastric and duodenal placement (Erzincanli et al., 2017; Heidarzadi et al., 2020).

Gastric Auscultation

- Auscultation as a verification tool is not reliable and should not be used without additional methods (Boeykens et al., 2014).
- Although evidence shows auscultation alone is not a reliable confirmatory test, it is still widely used by nurses for evaluation of enteral tube placement (Bourgault et al., 2015; Lyman et al., 2016; Metheny et al., 2012; Northington et al., 2017).
- Using aspirate and nonaspirate NG tube placement verification methods in combination increase the likelihood of accurate NG tube placement to 97%–99%, similar to the chest radiography gold standard of 99% (Ellett et al., 2005; Society of Pediatric Nurses Clinical Practice Committee et al., 2011).

Electromagnetic Device

- An electromagnetic tracing device demonstrated more than 94% accuracy in enteral feeding tubes in a study of both adults and children (Powers et al., 2018); however, the device requires special training and considerable expertise for proper use (Metheny and Meert, 2017) and cannot detect enteral tubes smaller than 8 French (Bourgault et al., 2015; Bryant et al., 2015).

Apply the Evidence: Nursing Implications

- There is **good evidence** with **strong recommendations** (Guyatt et al., 2008) that a combination of verification methods to confirm NG tube placement will reduce the required number of x-rays in children (Society of Pediatric Nurses Clinical Practice Committee et al., 2011). These methods include pH testing and visual inspection of the pH aspirate. There is also good evidence that improving the accuracy of predicting NG tube length before insertion will enhance the precision of successful NG tube placement. Auscultation is used in combination with other NG tube verification methods. Further investigation of additional noninvasive, user-friendly, portable verification methods, including ultrasound and electromagnetic tracer, is warranted (Irving et al., 2018; Powers et al., 2011).

References

Beckstrand J, Cirgin Ellett ML, McDaniel A. Predicting the internal distance to the stomach for positioning nasogastric and orogastric feeding tubes in children. *J Adv Nurs.* 2007;59:274–289.

Boeykens K, Steeman E, Duysburgh I. Reliability of pH measurement and the asucultatory method to confirm the position of a nasogastric tube. *Int J Nurs Stud.* 2014;51:1427–1433.

Bourgault AM, Heath J, Hooper V, et al. Methods used by critical care nurses to verify feeding tube placement in clinical practice. *Crit Care Nurse.* 2015;35(1):e1–e7.

Bryant V, Phang J, Abrams K. Verifying placement of small-bore feeding tubes: electromagnetic device images versus abdominal radiographs. *Am J Crit Care.* 2015;24:525–530.

Ellett ML, Croffie JM, Cohen MD, et al. Gastric tube placement in young children. *Clin Nurs Res.* 2005;14(3):238–252.

Emergency Nurses Association. Clinical practice guideline: gastric tube placement verification. *J Emerg Nurs.* 2019;45(3):306.e1–306.e19.

Erzincanli S, Zaybak A, Guler A. Investigation of the efficacy of colorimetric capnometry method used to verify the correct placement of the nasogastric tube. *Intensive Crit Care Nurs.* 2017;38:46–52.

Fernandez RS, Chau JP, Thompson DR, et al. Accuracy of biochemical markers for predicting nasogastric tube placement in adults—a systematic review of diagnostic studies. *Int J Nurs Stud.* 2010;47(8):1037–1046.

Continued

EVIDENCE-BASED PRACTICE—cont'd

Gilbertson HR, Rogers EJ, Ukoumunne OC. Determination of a practical pH cutoff level for reliable confirmation of nasogastric tube placement. *J Parenter Enteral Nutr.* 2011;35(4):540–544.

Guyatt GH, Oxman AD, Vist GE, et al. GRADE: an emerging consensus on rating quality of evidence and strength of recommendations. *Brit Med J.* 2008;336(7650):924–926.

Heidarzadi E, Jalali R, Hemmatpoor B, et al. The comparison of capnography and epigastric auscultation to assess the accuracy of nasogastric tube placement in intensive care unit patients. *BMC Gastroenterol.* 2020;20(1):196.

Irving SY, Rempel G, Lyman B, et al. Pediatric nasogastric tube placement and verification: Best practice recommendations from the NOVEL project. *Nutr Clin Prac.* 2018;33(6):921–927.

Lyman B, Kemper C, Northington L, et al. Use of temporary enteral access devices in hospitalized neonatal and pediatric patients in the United States. *J Parenter Enteral Nutr.* 2016;40(4):574–580.

Metheny NA, Meert KL. Update on effectiveness of an electromagnetic feeding tube-placement device in detecting respiratory placements. *Am J Crit Care.* 2017;26:157–161.

Metheny NA, Stewart BJ, Mills AC. Blind insertion of feeding tubes in intensive care units: a national survey. *Am J Crit Care.* 2012;21(5):352–360.

Ni MZ, Huddy JR, Priest OH, et al. Selecting pH cut-offs for the safe verification of nasogastric feeding tube placement: a decision analytical modelling approach. *BMJ Open.* 2017;7(11):e018128.

Northington L, Lyman B, Guenter P, et al. Current practices in home management of nasogastric tube placement in pediatric patients: a survey of parents and homecare providers. *J Pediatr Nurs.* 2017;33:46–53.

Nyqvist KH, Sorell A, Ewald U. Litmus tests for verification of feeding tube location in infants: evaluation of their clinical use. *J Clin Nurs.* 2005;14(4):486–495.

Powers J, Luebbehusen M, Aguirre L, et al. Improved safety and efficacy of small-bore feeding tube confirmation using an electromagnetic placement device. *Nutr Clin Pract.* 2018;33(2):268–273.

Powers J, Luebbehusen M, Spitzer T, et al. Verification of an electromagnetic device compared with abdominal radiograph to predict accuracy of feeding tube placement. *J Parenter Enteral Nutr.* 2011;35(4):535–539.

Society of Pediatric Nurses Clinical Practice Committee, Society of Pediatric Nurses Research Committee, Longo MA. Best evidence: nasogastric tube placement verification. *J Pediatr Nurs.* 2011;26(4):373–376.

Nasogastric, Orogastric, or Gastrostomy Tube Administration

Dilute viscous medication or syrup with a small amount of water if possible.

Avoid oily medications because they tend to cling to the sides of the tube.

If administering tablets, crush them to a very fine powder and dissolve the drug in a small amount of warm water.

Never crush enteric-coated or sustained-release tablets or capsules.

Do not mix medication with enteral formula unless fluid is restricted. If adding a drug:

- Check with pharmacist for compatibility.
- Shake formula well, and observe for any physical reaction (e.g., separation, precipitation).
- Label formula container with name of medication, dosage, date, and time infusion started.

Check for correct placement of nasogastric (NG) or orogastric tube.

Attach syringe (with adaptable tip but without plunger) to tube.

Pour medication into syringe.

Unclamp tube and allow medication to flow by gravity.

Adjust height of container to achieve desired flow rate (e.g., increase height for faster flow).

SAFETY ALERT

Sprinkle-type medications should be avoided. However, if there is no other option and the tube is large gauge (18 French or greater), but usually not a Foley catheter, the medication may be given by mixing the sprinkles with a small amount of pureed fruit and thinning with water. The fruit keeps the sprinkles suspended so they do not float to the top. Flush well. This procedure is not recommended for skin-level gastrostomy devices.

As soon as syringe is empty, pour 10 mL of water to flush tubing.

- Amount of water depends on length and gauge of tubing.
- Determine amount before administering any medication by using a syringe to completely fill an unused NG or orogastric tube with water. The amount of flush solution is usually 1½ times this volume.
- With certain drug preparations (e.g., suspensions), more fluid may be needed.

If administering more than one drug at the same time, flush the tube between each medication with clear water.

Clamp tube after flushing, unless tube is left open.

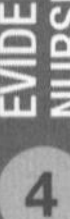

Rectal Administration

Suppository

Medications may need to be administered rectally if the oral route is not available. If half a suppository is to be used, cut it in half lengthwise.

Insertion Procedure

1. Position the child on his or her left side, with the right leg slightly bent.
2. Remove the wrapper from the suppository.
3. Use a gloved index or pinky (fifth) finger to insert the suppository; families may use gloves, finger cots, or plastic wrap at home.
4. Wet the glove or plastic covering and the suppository with warm (not hot) water. Do not use lubricant as it may affect medication absorption.
5. Insert with the apex (pointed end) first; 1 inch into a child's rectum and slightly less for an infant.
6. If the child is too young to help, hold the buttocks together for at least five minutes to prevent the expulsion of the suppository.

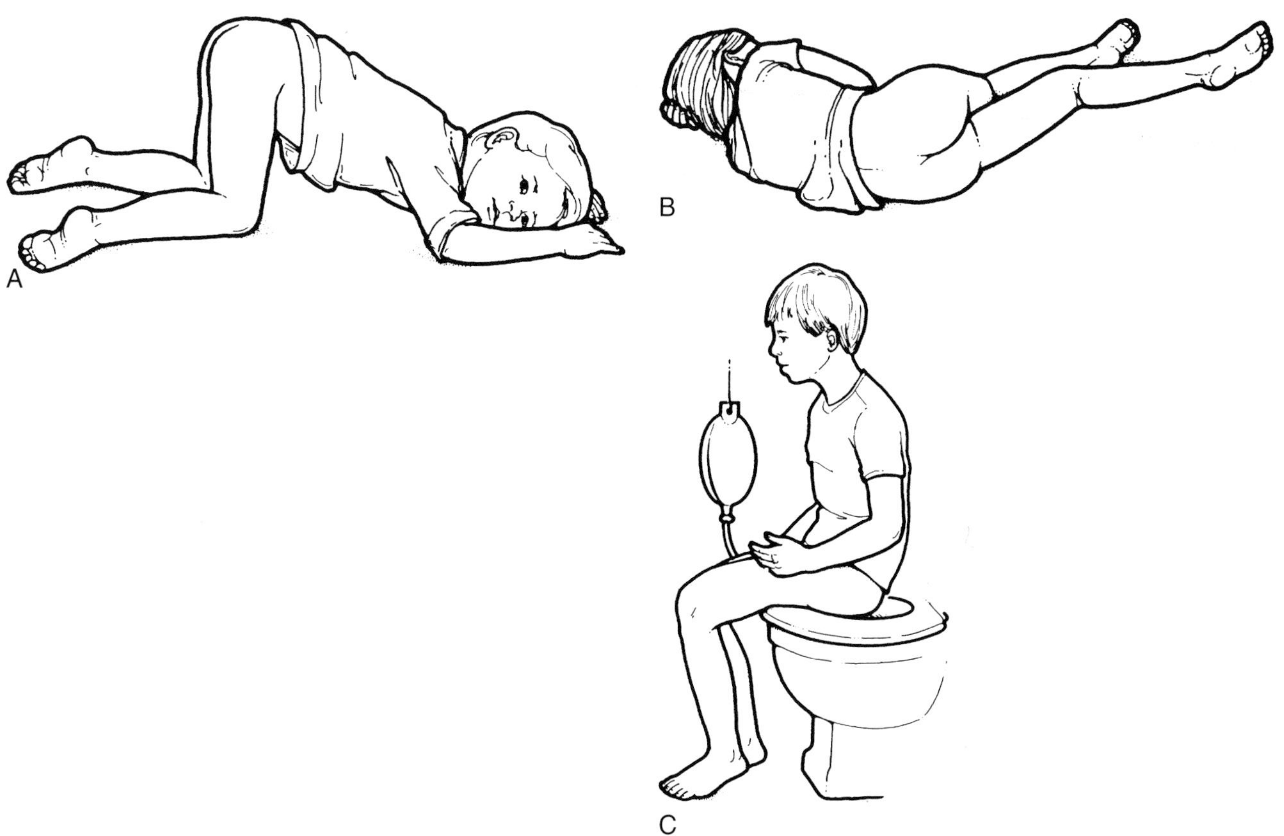

FIG. **4.12** (A) Knee-chest position for receiving an enema. (B) Side-lying position for receiving an enema. (C) Position for receiving an enema on toilet.

Enemas and Constipation

Simple constipation in children should not be treated with enemas but with changes in the child's diet. Increasing the amount of liquids to at least 1 quart each day and the amount of fiber in foods (especially whole grains, bran cereals, fresh vegetables, and fruit with the skin on) should increase the size and number of the child's bowel movements. Fruit juices such as apple, pear, and prune juices contain sorbitol and can prevent or relieve constipation. Oral medications such as mineral oil and polyethylene glycol electrolyte solutions are also effective in relieving constipation. No controlled trials have demonstrated the effectiveness of magnesium hydroxide, magnesium citrate, lactulose, sorbitol, senna, or bisacodyl, but these laxatives are widely thought to be effective. Infants should not be given stimulant laxatives or mineral oil. Glycerin suppositories are effective in infants, and bisacodyl suppositories are used in children. Phosphate soda enemas, saline enemas, or mineral oil enemas are effective. Soap suds, tap water, and magnesium enemas are not recommended because of potential toxicity (North American Society for Pediatric Gastroenterology, Hepatology, and Nutrition, 2006).

Enema Procedure

1. Dilute drug in smallest amount of solution possible.
2. Place the child in one of the following positions:
   - Lying face-down on belly with the knees and hips bent toward the chest (Fig. 4.12A)
   - Lying on the left side with the left leg straight and the right leg bent at the hip and knee and placed comfortably on top of the left leg (see Fig. 4.12B)

GUIDELINES

Administration of Enemas to Children

Age	Amount (mL)	Insertion Distance in Centimeters (Inches)
Infant	120–240	2.5 (1)
2–4 years	240–360	5.0 (2)
4–10 years	360–480	7.5 (3)
11 years	480–720	10.0 (4)

   - Sitting on the potty chair or toilet (see Fig. 4.12C)

1. Place a small amount of lubricant on your finger or on a tissue, and spread the lubricant around the tip of the tube, being careful not to plug the holes with lubricant; prepackaged enema tips are already lubricated.
2. Insert into rectum (Guidelines box). Depending on volume, may use syringe with rubber tubing, enema bottle, or enema bag.
3. If using an enema bag, hold the bottom of the container no more than 4 inches above the child; open the clamp and allow the liquid to flow, holding the tube in place.
4. When the container is empty, remove it.
5. Have the child keep the liquid inside for 3 to 5 minutes. If the child is too young to follow instructions, then hold the buttocks together to keep the liquid inside. For an older child, encourage slow deep breathing, or read a book to take the child's mind off the time.
6. Help the child to the toilet or potty chair, or allow the child to release the liquid into a diaper.

Eye, Ear, and Nose Administration

See Atraumatic Care box.

Eye Medication

Eye drops are administered in the same manner as to adults. Children, however, require additional preparation (Nursing Alert). When both drops and ointment are needed, give the drops first, wait 3 minutes, and then apply the ointment. This allows each drug time to work. When possible, administer eye ointments before bedtime or naptime, because the child's vision will be blurred for a while.

Eye Drop Instillation Procedure

1. Remove any discharge from the eye with a clean tissue. Wipe from nose to ear. If the eye has crusted material around it, wet a washcloth with warm water and place over the eye. After 1 minute, gently wipe the eye from the nose side outward with the washcloth, place it on the eye, and wait again. If you cannot remove the crusting, rewet the washcloth. Continue using the warm, moist washcloth and gently wiping until all the crusting is removed. If both eyes need cleaning, use separate cloths for each eye.

ATRAUMATIC CARE

Oral, Eye, Ear, and Nasal Medication Administration

To administer oral, nasal, ear, or optic medication when only one person is available to restrain the child, use the following procedure:

- Place child supine on flat surface (bed, couch, floor).
- Sit facing child so that child's head is between operator's thighs and child's arms are under operator's legs.
- Place lower legs over child's legs to restrain lower body if necessary.
- To administer oral medication, place small pillow under child's head to reduce risk of aspiration.
- To administer nasal medication, place small pillow under child's shoulders to aid flow of liquid through nasal passages.

2. Position supine with a pillow under the child's shoulders, or a rolled-up towel under his neck so that the head is tilted back and to the same side as the eye to be treated (i.e., right eye, turn head to right; left eye, turn head to left). Eye drops should flow away from the child's nose.
3. Open the medication container.
4. Steady your hand on the child's forehead.
   - Position a bottle so that the drops will fall into the lower eyelid, not directly onto the eyeball.
   - Position an ointment tube at the inner part of the eye near the nose
5. Gently pull down the child's lower eyelid with the other hand by placing gentle downward pressure below the eyelashes (Fig. 4.13).
   - For drops: Tell the child to look up and to the other side (away from the eye into which you are putting the drops). Choose something specific for the child to look at. If the child is young, you can make a game of giving the medication. Tell the child to open his eyes on the count of 3. Then count to 3. When you say 3, apply the medication into the child's eye. Even if the child will not open the eyes on 3, keep him lying down until he decides to open the eyes. The medicine will flow in the eye.
   - For ointment: Squeeze a ribbon of the ointment onto the inside of lower eyelid. Begin at the side of the eye near the nose, and go toward the outer edge of the eye. Avoid touching the eye with the ointment container. Give the tube a half-turn. This helps "cut" the ribbon of medicine.
6. Tell the child to close the eye, then to blink. This helps spread the drug around the eye.
7. Remove any extra drug with a clean tissue, wiping from the nose outward. Putting gentle pressure on the inner corner of the eye for 1 minute prevents any medicine from dripping into the back of the throat and causing an unpleasant taste.
8. If both eyes are to be given the drug, repeat with the other eye.

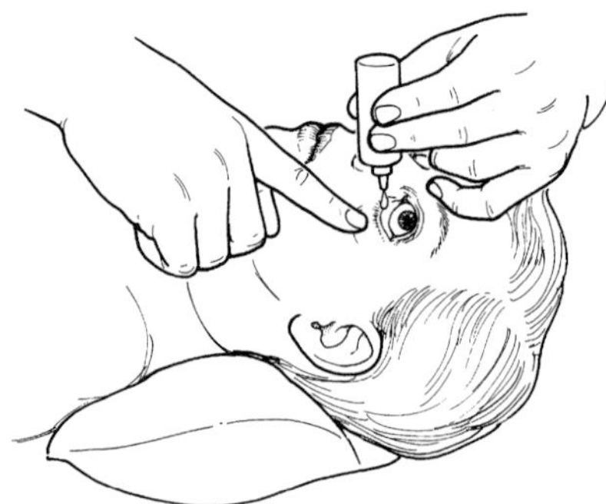

FIG. **4.13** Medication container and hand position for administering eye drops or ointment.

Ear Medication

Depending on the child's age, the pinna is pulled differently.

Ear Medication Instillation Procedure

1. Ear medication may be warmed by placing medication bottle in a container of warm water. Feel a drop to ensure the medication is not uncomfortably cold or hot.
2. Have the child lie on the side opposite the ear into which the medication will be placed (e.g., right ear, on left side).
3. If any drainage is present, remove it with a clean tissue or cotton-tipped applicator. Do not clean any more than the outer ear.
4. Open the bottle of ear drops. Do not let the dropper portion touch anything.
5. Steady your hand by placing your wrist on the child's cheek or head.
6. Straighten the child's ear canal.
   - For children 3 years old and younger, pull the outer ear down and toward the back of the head (Fig. 4.14A).
   - For older children, pull the outer ear up and toward the back (see Fig. 4.14B).

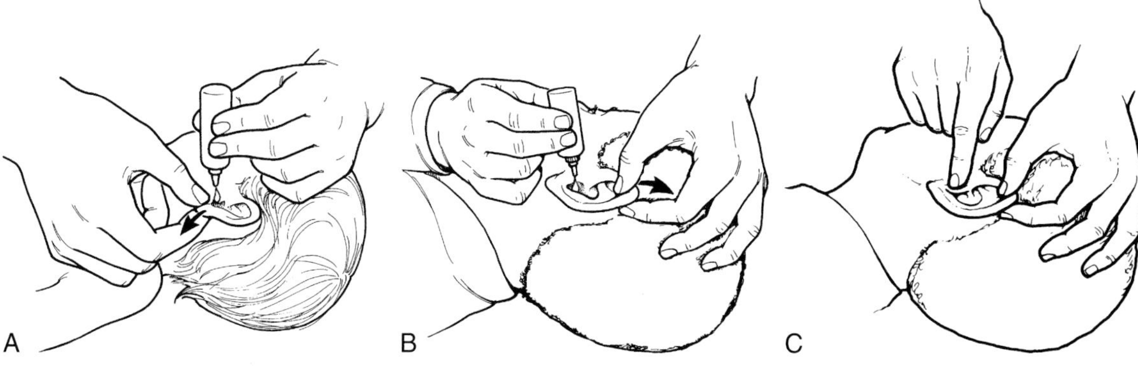

FIG. **4.14** Instilling ear medication. (A) Hand and dropper position for children 3 years old and younger, with earlobe pulled down and back. (B) Hand and dropper position for older children, with earlobe pulled up and back. (C) Rubbing ear to help drug flow to inside of ear.

7. Position the bottle so that the drops will fall against the side of the ear canal.
8. Squeeze the bottle for the right number of drops.
9. Keep the child lying on that side with the medicated ear up for 1 minute. Gently rub the skin in front of the ear (see Fig. 4.14C). This helps the drug flow to the inside of the ear.
10. If any drug has spilled on the skin, wipe the outer ear. A cotton ball can be loosely placed in the ear, but it must be changed each time drops are administered.
11. If both ears need the medication, repeat with the other ear after a one-minute wait.

Nose Drops

Nose drops are administered in the same manner as to adults. Different positions may be used, depending on the child's age.

1. Remove any mucus from the nose with a clean tissue. If the nose has crusted material around it, wet a washcloth with warm water and place this around the nose. Wait about one minute. Gently wipe the nose with the washcloth. If you cannot remove the crusting, rewet the washcloth and again place it around the nose. Continue using the warm, moist washcloth and gently wiping until all of the crusting is removed.
2. Place the child on his back. Tilt the child's head backward by placing a pillow or rolled-up towel under the child's shoulders or letting the head hang over the side of a bed or your lap (Fig. 4.15).

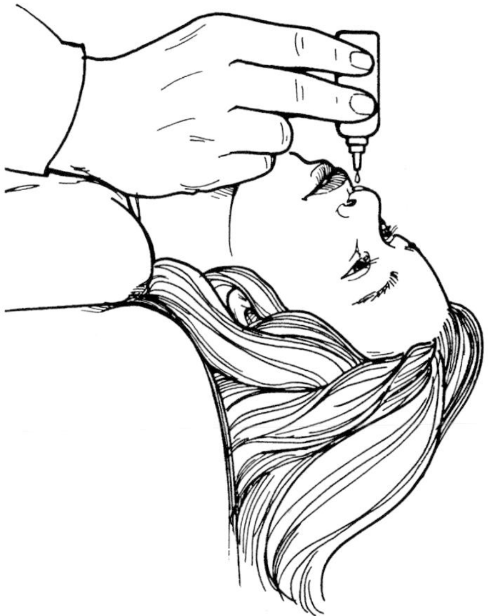

FIG. **4.15** Correct position of child's head and neck for giving nose drops.

3. Place the right number of drops in each side of the nose.
4. Keep the child's head tilted back for at least one minute to prevent gagging or tasting the medication.

Aerosol Therapy

The purpose is the inhalation of a solution in droplet (particle) form for direct deposition in the tracheobronchial tree.

Aerosols consist of liquid medications (e.g., bronchodilators, steroids, mucolytics, decongestants, antibiotics, antiviral agents) suspended in a particulate form in air.

Aerosol generators propelled by air or air-oxygen mixtures generally fall into three categories:

- Small-volume jet nebulizers or handheld nebulizers
- Ultrasonic nebulizers for sterile water or saline aerosol only
- Metered-dose inhalers (MDIs) (sometimes with a "spacer" device that acts as a reservoir and simplifies the use of the inhaler; devices such as the Rotohaler or Turbuhaler eliminate the need for a spacer device and are easier for young children to use)

Deposition of aerosol is maximized by instructing the child to breathe through the mouth with slow, deep inhalations, followed by holding the breath for 5 to 10 seconds, then slow exhalations while in an upright position.

Using an incentive spirometer can help a cooperative child learn this ventilatory pattern.

For infants and young children, activities to produce deep breathing and coughing include feet tapping, tactile stimulation, and crying. The infant must be held upright.

Assessment of breath sounds and work of breathing is performed before and after treatments.

GUIDELINES

Use of a Metered-Dose Inhaler (MDI)

Steps for Checking How Much Medicine Is in the Canister

1. If the canister is new, it is full.
2. If the canister has been used repeatedly, it might be empty. (Check product label to see how many inhalations should be in each canister.)
3. The most accurate way to determine how many doses remain in an MDI is to count and record each actuation as it is used.
4. Many dry powder inhalers have a dose-counting device or dose indicator on the canister to let you know when the canister is empty.
5. Placing dry powder inhalers or MDIs with hydrofluoroalkanes in water will destroy these inhalers.

Steps for Using the Inhaler

1. Remove the cap, and hold inhaler upright.
2. Shake the inhaler.
3. Tilt the head back slightly, take a deep breath, and breathe out slowly.
4. With the inhaler in an upright position, insert the mouthpiece:
   - About 3–4 cm from the mouth (Fig. 4.16A) or
   - Into an aerochamber (see Fig. 4.16B) or
   - Into the mouth, forming an airtight seal between the lips and the mouthpiece (see Fig. 4.16C)
5. At the end of a normal expiration, depress the top of the inhaler canister firmly to release the medication (into either the aerochamber or the mouth), and breathe in slowly (about 3–5 seconds). Relax the pressure on the top of the canister.
6. Hold the breath for 10 s to allow the aerosol medication to reach deeply into the lungs.
7. Remove the inhaler, and breathe out slowly through the nose.
8. Wait 1 minute between puffs (if additional one is needed).

Tips to avoid common inhaler mistakes:

- Breathe out before pressing your inhaler.
- Inhale slowly, evenly, and deeply.
- Breathe in through your mouth, not your nose.
- Press down on your inhaler at the start of inhalation (or within the first second of inhalation).
- Keep inhaling as you press down on inhaler.
- Press your inhaler only once while you are inhaling (one breath for each puff).
- Make sure you breathe in evenly and deeply.

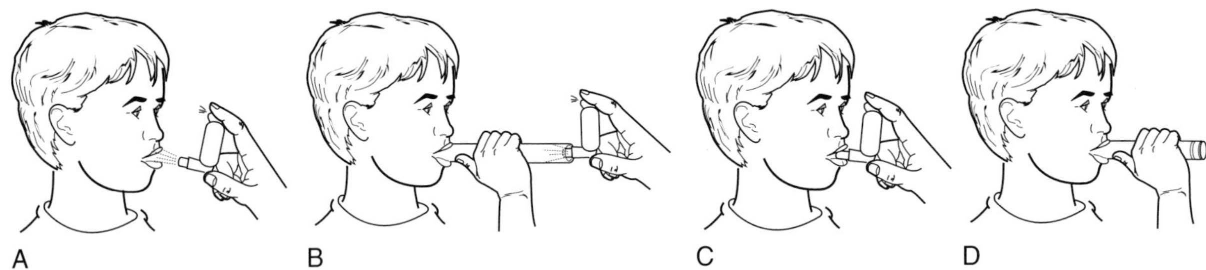

FIG. **4.16** (A) Open mouth with inhaler 3 to 4 cm away. (B) Spacer or aerochamber (recommended especially for young children and for people using corticosteroids). (C) Into the mouth. Do not use for corticosteroids. (D) Inhaled dry powder capsule. (Figures redrawn from the National Asthma Education and Prevention Program.)

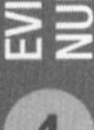

Intramuscular Administration

Explain procedure to child as developmentally appropriate, and provide atraumatic care (Atraumatic Care box).

ATRAUMATIC CARE

Injections

Select a method to anesthetize the puncture site:

- Apply EMLA on site 2½ hours before intramuscular (IM) injection, or apply LMX on site for at least 30 min before injection.
- Use a vapocoolant spray just before injection.
- For young infants, use sucrose before injection.
- Breastfeeding prior to and during the injection.

Prepare site with antiseptic and allow to dry completely before skin is penetrated.

Have medication at room temperature.

Use a new, sharp needle with smallest gauge that permits free flow of the medication and safe penetration of muscle.

Decrease perception of pain:

Reduction of Minor Procedural Pain in Infants

- Distract child with conversation, video, movie, or game on phone, excessive parental reassurance, criticism, or apology increases distress, whereas humor and distraction decrease distress (Bukola and Paula, 2017; Rheel et. al, 2021; Schechter et al., 2007).
- Give child something on which to concentrate (e.g., squeezing a hand or bed rail, pinching own nose, humming, counting, yelling "ouch!").
- Apply pressure at the site with a finger or device.
- Say to child, "If you feel this, tell me to take it out."
- Have child hold a small bandage and place it on puncture site after IM injection is given.

Enlist parents' assistance if they wish to participate and/or assist.

Restrain child only as needed to perform procedure safely. (See restraining methods and therapeutic hugging.)

Insert needle quickly using a dartlike motion.

Avoid tracking any medication through superficial tissues:

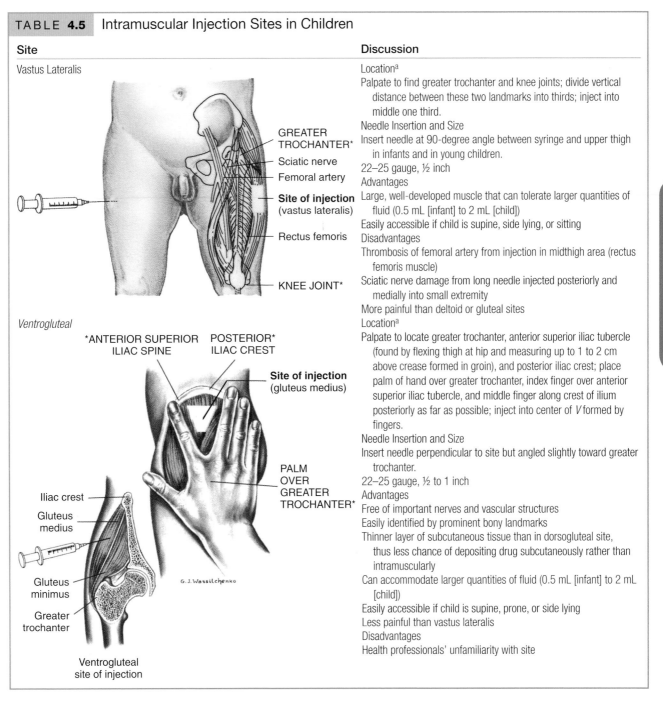

ATRAUMATIC CARE—cont'd

- Replace needle after withdrawing medication, or wipe medication from needle with sterile gauze.
- If withdrawing medication from an ampule, use a needle equipped with a filter that removes glass particles; then use a new, nonfilter needle for injection.
- Use the Z track and/or air-bubble technique as indicated.
- Avoid any depression of the plunger during insertion of the needle.

Place a small bandage on puncture site (unless skin is compromised, e.g., in low-birth-weight infant); with young children decorate bandage by drawing a smiling face or other symbol of acceptance.

Hold and cuddle young child, and encourage parents to comfort child; praise older child.

Use safety precautions in administering medications (see Oral Administration).

Determine the site of injection (Table 4.5); make certain muscle is large enough to accommodate volume and type of medication.

- Older children—Select site as with the adult patient; allow child some choice of site, if feasible.
  - Following are acceptable sites for infants and small or debilitated children (see Safety Alert):
    - Vastus lateralis muscle
    - Ventrogluteal muscle

TABLE 4.5 Intramuscular Injection Sites in Children

Site	Discussion
Vastus Lateralis GREATER TROCHANTER* Sciatic nerve Femoral artery **Site of injection** (vastus lateralis) Rectus femoris KNEE JOINT*	Location[a] Palpate to find greater trochanter and knee joints; divide vertical distance between these two landmarks into thirds; inject into middle one third. Needle Insertion and Size Insert needle at 90-degree angle between syringe and upper thigh in infants and in young children. 22–25 gauge, ½ inch Advantages Large, well-developed muscle that can tolerate larger quantities of fluid (0.5 mL [infant] to 2 mL [child]) Easily accessible if child is supine, side lying, or sitting Disadvantages Thrombosis of femoral artery from injection in midthigh area (rectus femoris muscle) Sciatic nerve damage from long needle injected posteriorly and medially into small extremity More painful than deltoid or gluteal sites
Ventrogluteal *ANTERIOR SUPERIOR ILIAC SPINE POSTERIOR* ILIAC CREST **Site of injection** (gluteus medius) PALM OVER GREATER TROCHANTER* G. J. Wassilchenko Iliac crest Gluteus medius Gluteus minimus Greater trochanter Ventrogluteal site of injection	Location[a] Palpate to locate greater trochanter, anterior superior iliac tubercle (found by flexing thigh at hip and measuring up to 1 to 2 cm above crease formed in groin), and posterior iliac crest; place palm of hand over greater trochanter, index finger over anterior superior iliac tubercle, and middle finger along crest of ilium posteriorly as far as possible; inject into center of *V* formed by fingers. Needle Insertion and Size Insert needle perpendicular to site but angled slightly toward greater trochanter. 22–25 gauge, ½ to 1 inch Advantages Free of important nerves and vascular structures Easily identified by prominent bony landmarks Thinner layer of subcutaneous tissue than in dorsogluteal site, thus less chance of depositing drug subcutaneously rather than intramuscularly Can accommodate larger quantities of fluid (0.5 mL [infant] to 2 mL [child]) Easily accessible if child is supine, prone, or side lying Less painful than vastus lateralis Disadvantages Health professionals' unfamiliarity with site

TABLE 4.5 Intramuscular Injection Sites in Children—cont'd

Site	Discussion
Deltoid 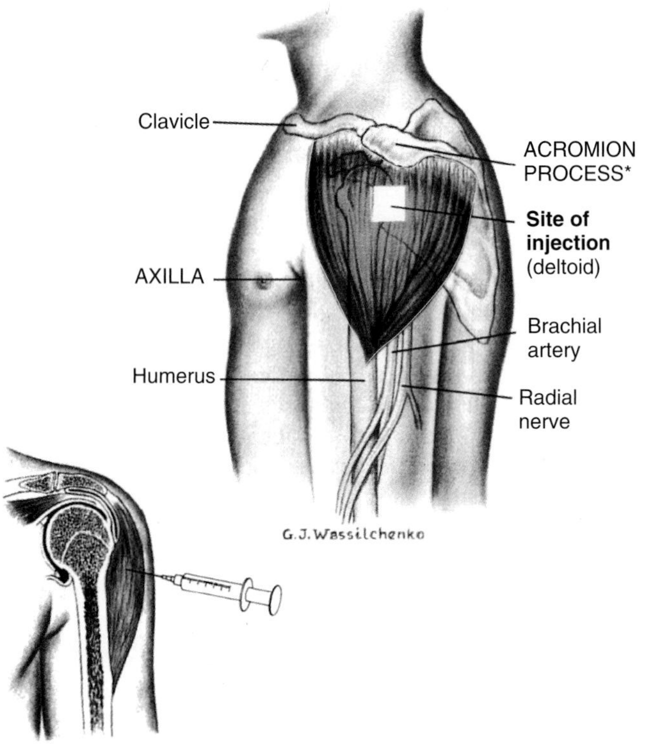	Location[a] Locate acromion process; inject only into upper third of muscle that begins about two fingerbreadths below acromion but is above axilla. Needle Insertion and Size Insert needle perpendicular to site with syringe angled slightly toward elbow. 22-25 gauge, ½ to 1 inch Advantages Faster absorption rates than gluteal sites Easily accessible with minimum removal of clothing Less pain and fewer local side effects from vaccines as compared with vastus lateralis Disadvantages Small muscle mass; only limited amounts of drug can be injected (0.5–1 mL) Small margins of safety with possible damage to radial nerve and axillary nerve (not shown, lies under deltoid at head of humerus)

[a]Locations of landmarks are indicated by asterisks on illustrations.

SAFETY ALERT

Do not use the dorsal gluteal site even in children who are walking.

Select needle and syringe appropriate to the following (Table 4.6):

- Amount of fluid to be administered (syringe size)
- Viscosity of fluid to be administered (needle gauge)
- Amount of tissue to be penetrated (needle length)
- If withdrawing medication from an ampule, use a needle equipped with a filter that removes glass particles; then use a new nonfilter needle for injection. Replace needle after withdrawing medication from a vial.

Maintain aseptic technique, and follow Standard Precautions.

Provide for sufficient help in restraining the child; children are often uncooperative, and their behavior is usually unpredictable.

Prepare area for puncture with antiseptic agent and allow to dry completely.

Administer the medication:

- Expose injection area for unobstructed view of landmarks.
- Select a site where the skin is free of irritation and danger of infection; palpate for and avoid sensitive or hardened areas. With multiple injections, rotate sites.
- Place the child in a lying or sitting position; the child is not allowed to stand for the following reasons:
  - Landmarks are more difficult to assess.
  - Restraint is more difficult.
  - The child may faint and fall.
- Grasp the muscle firmly between the thumb and fingers to isolate and stabilize the muscle for deposition of the drug in its deepest part; in obese children spread the skin with the thumb and index finger to displace subcutaneous tissue and grasp the muscle deeply on each side.
- Insert needle quickly using a dartlike motion.
- Avoid tracking any medication through superficial tissues:
  - Use the Z track and/or air-bubble technique as indicated.
  - Avoid any depression of the plunger during insertion of the needle.
- Inject medication slowly over several seconds.

Remove needle quickly; hold gauze firmly against skin near needle when removing it to avoid pulling on tissue.

Apply firm pressure with dry gauze to the site after injection; massage the site to hasten absorption unless contraindicated (e.g., with iron, or dextran).

Clean area of prepping agent with water to decrease absorption of agent in neonate.

Praise child for cooperation.

Discard syringe and needle in puncture-resistant container near site of use.

Record date, time, dose, drug, and site of injection.

TABLE 4.6 Intramuscular Administration: Location, Needle Length, Gauge, and Fluid Administration Amount

	Location of Injection	Needle Length (inches)	Needle Gauge (G)	Suggested Maximum Amount (mL)[a]
Preterm newborn	Anterolateral thigh	5/8	23–25	0.25–0.5
Term newborn	Anterolateral thigh	5/8	23–25	0.5–1
Infant (1–12 months)	Anterolateral thigh	5/8 – 1	22–25	1
Toddler (13–36 months)	Deltoid	5/8 – 1	22–25	0.5–1
	Anterolateral thigh or ventrogluteal	5/8 – 1 1-1¼	22–25	1–2
Preschool and older children	Deltoid	5/8 – 1	22–25	0.5–1
	Anterolateral thigh or ventrogluteal	1-1¼‡	22–25	2–3
Adolescent	Deltoid	5/8 – 1 1-1½ 1-1¼	22–25	1–1.5 2
	Anterolateral thigh or ventrogluteal	1-1¼ 1-1½	22–25	2–3 2–5

[a]Evaluate size of muscle mass before administration.

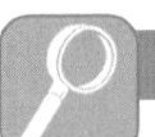

EVIDENCE-BASED PRACTICE

Intramuscular Injections in Infants, Toddlers, and Small Children

Ask the Question

In infants, toddlers, and small children, what is the best site, technique, needle size and gauge, and dosage for intramuscular (IM) injections?

Search the Evidence

Search Strategies

Literature from 1990 to 2018 was reviewed to obtain clinical research studies related to this issue.

Databases Used

CINAHL, PubMed

Critically Analyze the Evidence

Grade criteria: Evidence quality low; recommendation strong (Guyatt et al., 2008)

- The searches reviewed included a range of small studies to systematic reviews of randomized clinical trials.
- Needle Length and Injection Sites

Studies in adults indicate that injection pain can be minimized by deep IM administration since muscle tissue has fewer nerve endings and medications are absorbed faster than those administered subcutaneously (Zuckerman, 2000).

Immunizations such as diphtheria-tetanus–acellular pertussis (DTaP) and hepatitis A and B contain an aluminum adjuvant that, if injected into subcutaneous tissue, increases the incidence of local reactions. Inadvertent injection into subcutaneous tissue may be caused by use of a needle too short to reach IM tissue (Zuckerman, 2000).

- One study found that 4-month-old infants experienced fewer local side effects (redness, tenderness, and swelling) when immunizations were administered into the anterior aspect of the thigh with a 25-mm (1-inch) needle as opposed to the shorter 16-mm (⅝-inch) needle (Diggle and Deeks, 2000).
- Another study comparing needle length and injection method found that a longer needle (25 mm) was preferred for injection when bunching the skin and injecting, whereas a shorter needle (16 mm) was perceived as causing fewer localized reactions when the injection was administered with the skin being held taut (Groswasser et al. 1997). However, the study's conclusions fail to address whether needle lengths were applicable to both the deltoid and vastus lateralis muscles.
- Cook and Murtagh (2002) made ultrasound measurements of the subcutaneous and muscle layer thickness in 57 children ages 2, 4, 6, and 18 months. These researchers concluded that a 16-mm needle was sufficient to penetrate the anterolateral thigh muscle if the needle is inserted at a 90-degree angle without pinching the muscle, whereas thigh measurements demonstrated that a 25-mm needle was necessary to penetrate the muscle when a 45-degree injection technique was employed. This study supports the concept of longer needle length to fully deposit the medication into the muscle.
- In a study by Davenport (2004), needle length proved to be the most significant variable for local reactions in children after injection with 16-mm and 25-mm needles; the 25-mm needle was associated with fewer localized reactions.
- Diggle et al. (2006) likewise found that when long needles (25 mm) were used for infant immunizations, localized vaccine reactions were significantly reduced in comparison to the shorter needles (16 mm).
- A retrospective cohort study of children in the Vaccine Safety Datalink population that included 1.4 million children 12-35

Continued

EVIDENCE-BASED PRACTICE

Intramuscular Injections in Infants, Toddlers, and Small Children—cont'd

months of age and who received 6.0 million IM vaccines that are typically a single agent vaccine(DTaP, inactivated influenza, hepatitis A) over the study period (Jackson et al., 2013). Rate of local reactions after DTaP was higher and vaccinations in the arm increased the risk of a reaction. Injection of the thigh was found to have a lower risk of local reaction to DTaP. Findings support administering IM vaccinations in the thigh for children under 3 years of age.

- A systematic review of randomized- and quasi-randomized controlled trials included 31 studies using GRADE and Cochrane methods evaluated the outcomes of procedural and physical interventions (Taddio et al., 2015), Interventions demonstrating benefit included no aspiration injecting most painful vaccine last, simultaneous injections, vastus lateralis injection, non-nutritive sucking, external vibrating device with cold, and muscle tension.
- A systematic review of several vaccine databases (Cook, 2015) identified vaccine-related complications that were classified in three distinct categories: Nerve Palsies, Musculoskeletal, and Cutaneous. The author identifies four key points in vaccine practice in deltoid intramuscular injection—identification of a safe site for injection; individualizing needle length selection for muscle penetration with standardized injection technique, skin preparation prior to injection, and avoiding aspiration before injection.
- A systematic review (Sisson, 2015) identified six studies relevant to the question of aspiration during intramuscular injections. Findings indicated slower injection with aspiration is more painful than a faster injection without aspiration, and the use of aspiration during intramuscular injection was influenced by how nurses were taught. The author suggests that aspiration is not a necessary part of intramuscular injections, and nursing educators should update their knowledge to advance evidence-based decisions.
- A prospective, descriptive study measured subcutaneous tissue and muscle thickness of anterolateral, deltoid, and ventrogluteal sites to determine the suitability of ventrogluteal site for intramuscular injections (Atay et al., 2017). 120 healthy newborns and toddlers up to 36 months of age and who were scheduled for a radiology appointment were included in the study. Measures included height, weight, head circumference, and ultrasound measure of the IM skin thickness of deltoid, anterolateral and ventrogluteal sites, Results demonstrated that ventrogluteal subcutaneous thickness and muscle layer thickness were higher across all ages. The author concludes that the ventrogluteal site is suitable for IM injections in children aged 0–36 months.
- A Cochrane Systematic Review (Beirne et al., 2018) of needle size for vaccination procedures in children and adolescents included randomized controlled trials of hypodermic needles of any gauge or length to administer vaccines from birth to 24 years. Three trials involving 1135 participants provided data regarding needle sizes. The findings indicate that children immunized with 25-mm needles have fewer severe reactions from DTwP-Hib vaccinations vs infants vaccinated with 16 mm needles. The authors conclude that there was low-quality evidence that wide, long needles may slightly reduce the pain of vaccination.
- The American Academy of Pediatrics (2021) and the Centers for Disease Control and Prevention (2020) recommend that vaccines containing adjuvants such as aluminum (e.g., DTaP, hepatitis A and B, diphtheria-tetanus [DT or Td]) be given deep into the muscle to prevent local reactions. In addition, a 16-mm needle may be adequate for injections in small infants, and a 22- to 25-mm to 1-inch needle can be used in infants 2 months and older. https://www.cdc.gov/vaccines/hcp/admin/downloads/IM-Injection-children.pdf
  Vaccine Administration: Needle Gauge and Length (cdc.gov)
  Vaccine Administration: Intramuscular (IM) injections: Adults 19 years of age and older (cdc.gov)
- The Centers for Disease Control and Prevention (2021) recommends that toddlers receive injections with a 22- to 32-mm to 1 and ¼-inch needle in the deltoid if muscle size is adequate; a minimum of a 25-mm long needle is recommended for anterolateral thigh injection in toddlers www.immunize.org/catg.d/p3085.pdf. Both the American Academy of Pediatrics (2021) and the Centers for Disease Control and Prevention (2020) recommend a 22- to 25- gauge needle for all IM childhood immunizations. The deltoid muscle may be used for immunizations in toddlers, older children, and adolescents.

Apply the Evidence: Nursing Implications

- What is the appropriate muscle in which an IM injection can be administered with the fewest adverse effects in infants and toddlers?
- What is the appropriate needle size based on the infant or toddler's age and weight?
- What is the largest safe amount of medication that can be given to infants and toddlers based on weight and muscle size?
- Based on the evidence in the literature, the recommendation is to continue administering IM injections to children in the anterolateral thigh (up to 12 months old), deltoid (12 months and older), and ventrogluteal site.
- Needle length is an important factor in decreasing local reactions; the length should be adequate to deposit the medication into the muscle for IM injections. Recommendations are for a 25-mm (1-inch) needle in infants, a 25- to 32-mm (1- to 1¼-inch) needle for toddlers, and a 38- to 51-mm (1½- to 2-inch) needle for older children; preterm and small emaciated infants may require a shorter needle (16–25 mm [⅝ to 1 inch]) based on weight and muscle mass size.

References

Atay S, Yilmaz Kurt F, Akkaya G, et al. Investigation of suitability of ventrogluteal site for intramuscular injections in children aged 36 months and under. *J Spec Pediatr Nurs.* 2017;22(4):e12187.

Beirne PV, Hennessy S, Cadogan SL, et al. Needle size for vaccination procedures in children and adolescents. *Cochrane Database Syst Rev.* 2018;8(8):Cd010720.

Cook IF. Best vaccination practice and medically attended injection site events following deltoid intramuscular injection. *Hum Vaccin Immunother.* 2015;11(5):1184–1191.

Cook IF, Murtagh J. Needle length required for intramuscular vaccination of infants and toddlers: an ultrasonographic study. *Austral Fam Phys.* 2002;31(3):295–297.

Davenport JM. A systematic review to ascertain whether the standard needle is more effective than a longer or wider needle in reducing the incidence of local reaction in children receiving primary immunization. *J Adv Nurs.* 2004;46(1):66–77.

Diggle L, Deeks JJ, Pollard AJ. Effect of needle size on immunogenicity and reactogenecity of vaccines in infants: randomized controlled trial. *BMJ.* 2006;333(7568):571.

Guyatt GH, Oxman AD, Vist GE, et al. GRADE: an emerging consensus on rating quality of evidence and strength of recommendations. *BMJ.* 2008;336(7650):924–926.

Jackson LA, Peterson D, Nelson JC, et al. Vaccination site and risk of local reactions in children 1 through 6 years of age. *Pediatrics.* 2013;131(2):283–289.

Sisson H. Aspirating during the intramuscular injection procedure: a systematic literature review. *J Clin Nurs.* 2015;24(17–18):2368–2375.

Taddio A, Shah V, McMurtry CM, et al. Procedural and physical interventions for vaccine injections: systematic review of randomized controlled trials and quasi-randomized controlled trials. *Clin J Pain.* 2015;31(10 suppl):S20–S37.

Subcutaneous and Intradermal Administration

Obtain necessary equipment.

Explain procedure to child as developmentally appropriate, and provide atraumatic care. (See Atraumatic Care box.)

Maintain an aseptic technique, and follow Standard Precautions.

Any site may be used where there are relatively few sensory nerve endings and large blood vessels and bones are relatively deep.

Suggested sites:

- Center third of lateral aspect of upper arm
- Abdomen
- Center third of anterior thigh
- (Avoid the medial side of arm or leg, where skin is more sensitive.)

After injection:

- Clean area of prepping agent with water to decrease absorption of agent in neonate.
- Praise child for cooperation.
- Discard syringe and needle in puncture-resistant container near site of use.
- Record date, time, dose, drug, and site of injection.

Needle Size and Insertion

Use 26- to 30-gauge needle; change needle before skin puncture if it pierced a rubber stopper on a vial.

Prepare area for puncture with an antiseptic agent. Inject small volumes (up to 0.5 mL).

Subcutaneous Administration

Using a dartlike motion, insert needle at a 90-degree angle (Fig. 4.17). (Some practitioners use a 45-degree angle on children with little subcutaneous tissue or those who are dehydrated. However, the benefit of using the 45-degree angle rather than the 90-degree angle remains controversial.)

Inject medication slowly without tracking through tissues.

Intradermal Administration

Spread skin site with thumb and index finger if needed for easier penetration.

Insert needle with bevel up and parallel to skin.

Inject medication slowly.

Use of Indwelling Catheter (Insuflon) for Subcutaneous Administration of Insulin

Small indwelling catheter is placed in the subcutaneous tissues.

The average indwelling time is 3 to 5 days.

The catheter is most often inserted in the abdomen, but the buttocks and other areas can also be used. Topical anesthetic cream is recommended before insertion.

Needles 10 mm or shorter should be used for injecting to avoid penetration of the tubing of the catheter.

Using indwelling catheters for up to 4 to 5 days does not affect the absorption of insulin.

The long-term (measured by HbA1c) and short-term glucose control (measured by blood glucose profiles and insulin levels) is not altered.

The dead space of the catheter is about 0.5 unit of U100, so it may be necessary to give 0.5 units extra with the first dose after insertion if the child uses small doses.

Family Education: Safe Disposal of Needles and Lancets

The growing number of persons being cared for in home settings has increased the amount of medical waste that communities must properly dispose of to prevent accidental needlesticks and the spread of diseases such as hepatitis and

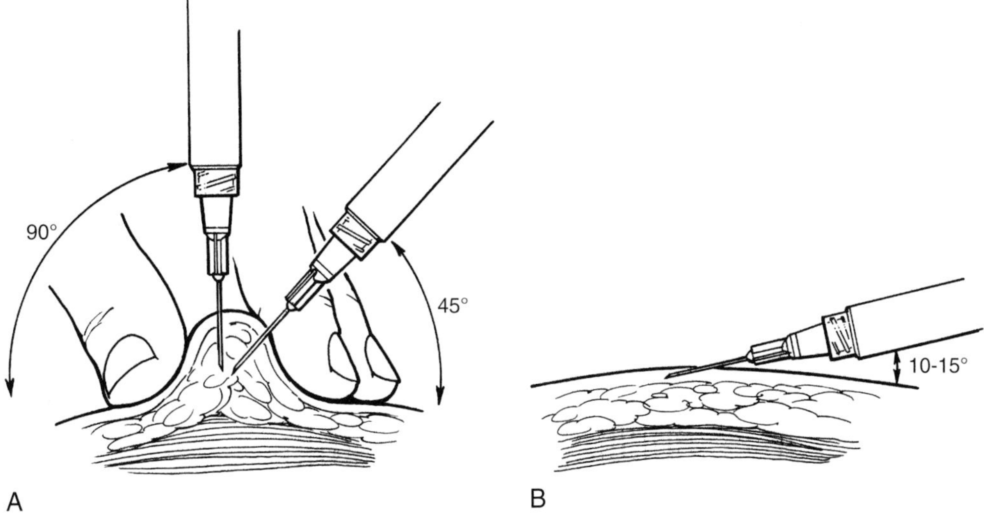

FIG. **4.17** Comparison of the angles of insertion for injections. (A) Subcutaneous (90 degrees or 45 degrees). (B) Intradermal (10 to 15 degrees).

human immunodeficiency virus. Many states have programs to assist with the disposal of sharps such as needles and lancets to prevent environmental contamination and accidental mishaps involving needle exposures. Contact one of the resources listed below to obtain further information about needle disposal in your state, or discuss the proper disposal of sharp medical equipment with your local home care agency.

If your state or community does not have programs for safe needle disposal, an option is to place sharps such as needles or lancets in a rigid container such as a bleach bottle or aluminum coffee can. Place the lid on the container to prevent accidental needle exposure. Once the container is about three-quarters full and ready to be discarded, you may add to it a liquid mixture such as cement or plaster to harden the contents and prevent needle exposure. Special devices that break off the needle into a rigid container are also available in some communities.

Additional information is available at Coalition for Safe Community Needle Disposal, 800-643-1643, www.safeneedldisposal.org; and Environmental Protection Agency, www.epa.gov/osw/nonhaz/industrial/medical/disposal.htm.

Intravenous Administration

SASH is one way to remember several key steps in IV medication administration: Saline-Administer medication-saline-Heparin, if indicated.

Inspect insertion site to make certain the catheter is secure.

Assess the status of IV infusion to determine that it is functioning properly; this may be done by flushing the line with Saline or flushing and then aspirating a blood return.

Dilute the drug in an amount of solution according to the following:

- Compatibility with infusion fluids or other IV medications child is receiving
- Size of the child
- Size of the vein being used for infusion
- Length of time over which the drug is to be administered (e.g., 30 minutes, 1 hour, 2 hours)
- Rate at which the drug is to be infused
- Strength of the drug or the degree to which it is toxic to subcutaneous tissues
- Need for fluid restriction

Administer the medication

Medication is not completely administered until solution in tubing has infused also (amount of solution depends on tubing length and diameter). Flush the tubing with saline to clear the tubing of the medication.

If the line is a dormant or intermittent line that does not have fluids continuously infusing, heparin may be indicated to ensure patency; see Evidence-Based Practice box and Table 4.7.

COMMUNITY FOCUS
Preventing Intravenous Site Infection

With the increasing use of intravenous (IV) therapy in the community, preventing infection is essential. The most effective ways to prevent infection at an IV site are to cleanse hands and wear gloves when inserting an IV catheter. Proper education of the patient and family regarding signs and symptoms of an infected IV site can help prevent infections from going unnoticed.

TABLE 4.7 IV Catheter Flushes for Lines Without Continuous Fluid Infusions

Peripheral lines (Heplock/Saline locks)	Normal saline[a] after medications or every 8 h for dormant lines; Instill 2½ times tubing volume
	24 g catheters: Normal saline[a] or heparin 2 units/mL 2 mL
Midline	Heparin 10 units/mL; 3 mL in a 10-mL syringe[b] after medications or every 8 h if dormant
	Newborns: Heparin 1–2 units/mL to run continuously at ordered rate
External central line (nonimplanted, nontunneled, tunneled, or peripherally inserted central catheter [PICC])	Heparin 10 units/mL; 3 mL in a 10-mL syringe[b] after medications or once daily if dormant
	Newborns: Heparin 2 units/mL; 2–3 mL after medications or to check line patency OR heparin 1–2 units/mL to run continuously at ordered rate
Totally implanted central line (TIVAS, implanted port)	Heparin 10 units/mL; 5 mL after medications or once daily if dormant and accessed. If not accessed, Heparin 100 units/mL; 5 mL every month
Arterial and central venous pressure continuous monitored lines	Heparin 2 units/mL in 55-mL syringe to run continuously at 1 mL/h

[a]Use D_5W when medication is incompatible with saline.
[b]Smaller syringes may be used when flush is delivered by a pump.

EVIDENCE-BASED PRACTICE

Normal Saline or Heparinized Saline Flush Solution in Pediatric Intravenous Lines

Ask the Question

Is there a significant difference in the longevity of peripheral intravenous (IV) intermittent infusion locks in children when normal saline (NS) is used as a flush instead a heparinized saline (HS) solution?

Search for the Evidence

Search Strategies

Selection criteria included evidence during the years 2006–2017 with the following terms: saline versus heparin intermittent flush, children's heparin lock flush, heparin lock patency, peripheral venous catheter in children.

Databases Used

CINAHL, PubMed

Critical Appraisal of the Evidence

- No differences in patency were established in a double-blind prospective randomized study in neonates. NS was deemed preferable to HS in peripheral intravenous (PIV) locks in neonates, in consideration of complications associated with heparin (Arnts et al., 2011).
- Infusion devices flushed with NS lasted longer than those flushed with HS (Cook et al., 2011).
- Peripheral catheters flushed with heparin remained patent longer but were also more likely to develop phlebitis (Tripathi et al., 2008).
- A randomized trial in neonates demonstrated that use of HS for flushing before and after IV antibiotics significantly increased the duration of PIVs when compared to NS flushes (Upadhyay et al., 2015).
- A systematic review of 10 randomized controlled trials in pediatrics found minimal benefit to use of HS as intermittent flush of peripheral catheters compared to NS. The difference was not statistically significant (Kumar et al., 2013).
- Peripheral catheters in children, ages 1–17 years, flushed once every 24 h with NS did not affect patency when compared to flushing with NS every 12 h (Schreiber et al., 2015).
- Either HS or preservative-free NS may be used to flush a PIV line (Arnts et al., 2011; Bellini, 2012; Cook et al., 2011; Infusion Nurses Society, 2021; White et al., 2011).
- After each catheter use, peripheral catheters should be locked with either HS (0.5–10 units/mL) or preservative-free NS, since outcome data remain equivocal (Infusion Nurses Society, 2021).
- Intermittent flushing with NS results in fewer complications, lower cost, and less time compared with continuous infusion (Stok and Wieringa, 2016).
- The Centers for Disease Control and Prevention recommends use of NS for intermittent flushing to avoid complications (O'Grady et al., 2011).
- Switching from HS to NS involves educational and administrative interventions (Cook et al., 2011; Thamlikitkul and Indranoi, 2006).
- NS is more cost effective (Thamlikitkul and Indranoi, 2006).
- NS flush has fewer side effects. HS can be associated with anticoagulation, thrombocytopenia, drug interactions, and hypersensitivity (Arnts et al., 2011).
- NS flushes once a day maintained patency of pediatric PIV locks, resulting in reduced costs and increased patient satisfaction (Schreiber et al., 2015).
- Nurses in Italy tend to use HS with smaller-gauge (24-gauge) catheters when access is less frequent (12 h or more between doses) and when patients are on specific units (hematology/oncology, pediatric surgery, and short-stay units) (Bisogni et al., 2014).

Apply the Evidence: Nursing Implications

- There is **low-quality evidence with a weak recommendation** (Guyatt et al., 2008) for using NS versus HS flush solution in pediatric IV lines. Further research is needed with larger samples of children, especially preterm neonates, using small-gauge catheters (24 gauge) and other gauge catheters flushed with NS and HS as intermittent infusion devices only (no continuous infusions). Variables to be considered include catheter dwell time; medications administered; period between regular flushing and flushing associated with medication administration; pain, erythema, and other localized complications; concentration and amount of HS used; type of needleless connector used (negative pressure, positive pressure, or neutral pressure); flush method (positive-pressure technique vs. no specific technique); reason for IV device removal; and complications associated with either solution. NS is a safe alternative to HS flush in infants and children with intermittent IV locks larger than 24 gauge; smaller neonates may benefit from HS flush (longer dwell time), but the evidence is inconclusive for all weight ranges and gestational ages. Neonates may benefit from a continuous infusion of NS at 5 mL/h to maintain patency.

References

Arnts IJ, Heijnen JA, Wilbers HT, et al. Effectiveness of heparin solution versus normal saline in maintaining patency of intravenous locks in neonates: a double blind randomized controlled study. *J Adv Nurs.* 2011;67(12):2677–2685.

Bellini S. Flushing of intravenous locks in neonates: no evidence that heparin improves patency compared with saline. *Evid Based Nurs.* 2012;15:86–87.

Bisogni S, Guisti F, Ciofi D, et al. Heparin solution for maintaining peripheral venous catheter patency in children: a survey of current practice in Italian pediatric units. *Issues Compr Pediatr Nurs.* 2014;37(2):122–135.

Cook L, Bellini S, Cusson RM. Heparinized saline vs normal saline for maintenance of intravenous access in neonates: an evidence-based practice change. *Adv Neonatal Care.* 2011;11:208–215.

Guyatt GH, Oxman AD, Vist GE, et al. GRADE: an emerging consensus on rating quality of evidence and strength of recommendations. *Br Med J.* 2008;336(7650):924–926.

Infusion Nurses Society. *Policies and Procedures for Infusion Therapy: Neonate to Adolescent.* 3rd ed. South Norwood, MA: The Society; 2021.

Kumar M, Vandermeer B, Bassler D, et al. Low dose heparin use and the patency of peripheral intravenous catheters in children: a systematic review. *Pediatrics.* 2013;131(3):e864–e872.

O'Grady NP, Alexander M, Burns LA, et al. *Guidelines for the Prevention of Intravascular catheter-related Infections.* Atlanta, GA: Healthcare Infection Control Practices Advisory Committee of the Centers for Disease Control and Prevention; 2011.

Schreiber S, Zanchi C, Ronfani L, et al. Normal saline flushes performed once daily maintain peripheral intravenous catheter patency: a randomized controlled trial. *Arch Dis Child.* 2015;100(7):700–703.

Stok D, Wieringa JW. Continuous infusion versus intermittent flushing: maintaining peripheral intravenous access in newborn infants. *J Perinatol.* 2016;36(10):870873.

Thamlikitkul V, Indranoi A. Switching from heparinized saline flush to normal saline flush for maintaining peripheral venous catheter patency. *Int J Quality in Health Care.* 2006;18(3):183185.

Tripathi S, Kaushik V, Singh V. Peripheral IVs: factors affecting complications and patency—a randomized controlled trial. *J Infusion Nurs.* 2008;31(3):182188.

Upadhyay A, Verma KK, Lal P, et al. Heparin for prolonging peripheral intravenous catheter use in neonates: a randomized controlled trial. *J Perinatol.* 2015;35:274–277.

White ML, Crawley J, Rennie EA, et al. Examining the effectiveness of 2 solutions used to flush capped pediatric peripheral intravenous catheters. *J Infus Nurs.* 2011;34:260–270.

Continued

End-of-Life Care Interventions

EVIDENCE-BASED PRACTICE

Pediatric Pain and Symptom Management at the End of Life

Ask the Question

In children, what is the pain and symptom experience at the end of life?

Search the Evidence

Search Strategies

Published studies from 2010 to 2020 were identified and examined. Retrospective descriptive studies characterizing infants' and children's end-of-life experiences through the use of medical record reviews and provider and parental surveys dominated the findings. Most studies examined the symptom experience of the infant or child with cancer.

Database Used

PubMed

Critically Analyze the Evidence

Grade criteria: Evidence quality moderate; recommendation strong (Guyatt et al., 2008).

- Children experience multiple complex, interdependent symptoms over the course of their illness and near the end of life (Requena et al., 2022). Pain, dyspnea, fatigue, loss of motor function, changes in behavior, changes in appearance, not eating, vomiting, cough, diarrhea, mouth sores, sadness, difficulty talking with others about their feelings, fear, and anxiety were the most frequently acknowledged symptoms experienced by most children at the end of life (Feudtner et al., 2021; Baumann et al., 2021; Zernikow et al., 2019; Thomas et al., 2018). Children and their parents reported high distress over pain and symptoms at the end of life. Parents reported the child's pain and suffering as one of the most important factors in deciding to withhold or withdraw their child from life support in the pediatric intensive care unit Bennett and LeBaron, 2019). Health care providers can help alleviate parent's distress by proactively assessing and treating pain and other discomforts.
- Helpful interventions to manage symptoms included physical comfort, time spent with child and family, and pharmacologic agents (Tutelman et al., 2021; Boyden et al., 2021. Morphine, methadone, and fentanyl are common pain medications for complex pain at end of life, and the most common routes of pain medication administration were oral, intravenous, subcutaneous, rectal, and transdermal (Madden et al., 2018; Friedrichsdorf, 2019) Most studies reported a lack of documented symptom assessment and intervention, as well as inadequate symptom management (Feudtner et al., 2021; Requena et al., 2022; Thomas et al., 2018) particularly the psychological symptoms of the dying child Baumann et al., 2021; Boyden et al., 2021; Tutelman et al., 2021

Apply the Evidence: Nursing Implications

- Although the philosophy of palliative care encompasses pain and symptom management for infants and children who may not outlive their disease, the provision of that care to ease physical and psychologic suffering and provide comfort to those who will die continues to lag. Studies show that children experience significant pain and other distressing symptoms at the end of life that are not well managed. Discrepancies in the assessment of infant and child pain and suffering continue to exist between providers and parents. Improvements are needed in the management of pain and symptoms at the end of life for infants and children.

References

Baumann F, Hebert S, Rascher W, et al. Clinical characteristics of the end-of-life phase in children with life-limiting diseases: retrospective study from a single center for pediatric palliative care. *Children (Basel).* 2021;8(6):523.

Bennett RA, LeBaron VT. Parental Perspectives on roles in end-of-life decision making in the pediatric intensive care unit: an integrative review. *J Pediatr Nurs.* 2019;46:18–25.

Boyden JY, Ersek M, Deatrick JA, et al. What do parents value regarding pediatric palliative and hospice care in the home setting? *J Pain Symptom Manage.* 2021;61(1):12–23.

Feudtner C, Nye R, Hill DL, et al. Polysymptomatology in pediatric patients receiving palliative care based on parent-reported data. *JAMA Netw Open.* 2021;4(8):e2119730.

Friedrichsdorf SJ. From tramadol to methadone: opioids in the treatment of pain and dyspnea in pediatric palliative care. *Clin J Pain.* 2019;35(6):501–508.

Guyatt GH, Oxman AD, Vist GE, et al. GRADE: An emerging consensus on rating quality of evidence and strength of recommendations. *British Medical Journal.* 2008;336: 924–926..

Madden K, Mills S, Dibaj S, et al. Methadone as the initial long-acting opioid in children with advanced cancer. *J Palliat Med.* 2018;21(9):1317–1321.

Requena ML, Avery M, Feraco AM, et al. Normalization of symptoms in advanced child cancer: the PediQUEST-Response case study. *J Pain Symptom Manage.* 2022;63(4):548–562.

Thomas R, Phillips M, Hamilton RJ. Pain management in the pediatric palliative care population. *J Nurs Scholarsh.* 2018;50(4):375–382.

Tutelman PR, Lipak KG, Adewumi A, et al. Concerns of parents with children receiving home-based pediatric palliative care. *J Pain Symptom Manage.* 2021;61(4):705–712.

Zernikow B, Szybalski K, Hübner-Möhler B, et al. Specialized pediatric palliative care services for children dying from cancer: a repeated cohort study on the developments of symptom management and quality of care over a 10-year period. *Palliat Med.* 2019;33(3):381–391.

End-of-Life Care Interventions

Communicating With Families of Dying Children

Listen for an "invitation" to talk about the situation.

- "Sometimes I wonder if I am doing the right thing."
- "What have other parents done in this situation?"
- "Do you know of other children who have survived this?"
- "I think the doctor is not telling me everything."

Use open-ended, nonjudgmental questions to explore families' wishes.

- "Can you tell me more about how you are feeling?"
- "What questions do you (or your child) have that I can have answered for you?"
- "What are your concerns (or worries, fears) right now?"
- "What is important to you (your child, your family) at this time?"

Common Symptoms Experienced by Dying Children

Pain

Visceral
Bone
Neuropathic

Gastrointestinal

Anorexia
Nausea and vomiting
Constipation
Diarrhea

Genitourinary

Urinary tract infections
Urinary retention

Hematologic

Anemia
Bleeding

Respiratory

Cough
Congestion
Shortness of breath
Wheezing

Central Nervous System

Fevers and chills
Sleep disturbance
Restlessness, agitation
Seizures

Integumentary

Dry skin
Rash, itching
Pressure sores
Edema

Emotional

Fear
Anxiety
Depression

Physical Signs of Approaching Death

Increased sleeping
Loss of sensation and movement in the lower extremities, progressing toward the upper body
Sensation of heat, although body feels cool
Mottling of skin
Loss of senses:

- Tactile sensation decreases
- Sensitive to light
- Hearing is last sense to fail

Confusion, loss of consciousness, slurred speech
Muscle weakness
Decreased urination, more concentrated urine
Loss of bowel and bladder control
Decreased appetite and thirst
Difficulty swallowing
Change in respiratory pattern:

- Cheyne-Stokes respirations (waxing and waning of depth of breathing with regular periods of apnea)
- "Death rattle" (noisy chest sounds from accumulation of pulmonary and pharyngeal secretions)

GUIDELINES

Supporting Grieving Families

General

Stay with the family; sit quietly if they prefer not to talk; cry with them if desired.
Accept the family's grief reactions; avoid judgmental statements (e.g., "You should be feeling better by now").
Avoid offering rationalizations for the child's death (e.g., "You should be glad your child isn't suffering anymore").
Avoid artificial consolation (e.g., "I know how you feel," or "You are still young enough to have another baby").
Deal openly with feelings such as guilt, anger, and loss of self-esteem.
Focus on feelings by using a feeling word in the statement (e.g., "You're still feeling all the pain of losing a child").
Refer the family to an appropriate self-help group or for professional help if needed.

At the Time of Death

Reassure the family that everything possible is being done for the child, if they wish lifesaving interventions.
Do everything possible to ensure the child's comfort, especially relief of pain.
Provide the child and family the opportunity to review special experiences or memories in their lives.
Express personal feelings of loss or frustration (e.g., "We will miss him so much," or "We tried everything; we feel so sorry that we couldn't save him").
Provide information that the family requests, and be honest.
Respect the emotional needs of family members, such as siblings, who may need brief respites from the dying child.
Make every effort to arrange for family members, especially parents, to be with the child at the moment of death, if they wish to be present.
Allow the family to stay with the dead child for as long as they wish and to rock, hold, or bathe the child.
Provide practical help when possible, such as collecting the child's belongings.
Arrange for spiritual support, such as clergy; pray with the family if no one else can stay with them.

After the Death

Attend the funeral or visitation if there was a special closeness with the family.
Initiate and maintain contact (e.g., sending cards, telephoning, inviting them back to the unit, or making a home visit).
Refer to the dead child by name; discuss shared memories with the family.
Discourage the use of drugs or alcohol as a method of escaping grief.
Encourage all family members to communicate their feelings rather than remaining silent to avoid upsetting another member.
Emphasize that grieving is a painful process that often takes years to resolve.

Care During the Terminal Phase

Physical Support

Provide frequent mouth care to prevent drying, cracking, and bleeding of lips and mucous membranes.
Maintain good hygiene by giving bed baths and using skin lotion as tolerated.
Continue necessary medications to manage symptoms and maintain comfort using IV (if access is easily established) or subcutaneous infusion.
Discontinue unnecessary medications and procedures (e.g., vital signs).
See Table 4.8 for common ethical dilemmas in caring for terminally ill children.

Emotional Support

See Table 4.9.
Encourage family to discuss impending death openly with child and other family members.
Encourage family to continue to speak to child in calm, reassuring voice.
Provide familiar surroundings or objects.
Encourage caregivers to provide one another with periods of respite.
Allow the performance of spiritual and cultural rituals as desired.
Allow family time with child after the death and participation in the preparation of the body if they choose.

Strategies for Intervention With Survivors After Sudden Childhood Death*

Arrival of the Family

Meet the family immediately and escort to a private area.
A health care worker with bereavement training should remain with the family.
Provide information about the extent of illness or injury and treatment efforts (Table 4.10).
If the health care worker must leave the family or if the family requests privacy, return in 15 minutes so the family does not feel forgotten.
Provide tissues and a telephone. Offer coffee, water, and a Bible.

Pronouncement of Death

When available, the family's own physician should inform the family of the child's death.
Alternatively, the physician or nurse should introduce himself or herself and establish calm, reassuring eye contact with the parents.

TABLE 4.8 Common Ethical Dilemmas in Caring for Terminally Ill Children

Rationale for Providing to Patient	Rationale for Withholding from Patient
Pain Control	
Comfort (the primary goal) Improved quality of life Easier dying process if child is pain-free	Side effects of opioids Decreased level of cognition Fear of addiction (unfounded in terminally ill patients)
Chemotherapy or Experimental Therapy	
Prolonged life span Possible increase in quality of life Provision of sense that family has done everything they can to save the child	Decreased blood counts, increased risk of infection, bleeding Side effects of treatment may be painful, uncomfortable
Supplemental Nutrition and Hydration (Intravenous, Nasogastric, Gastrostomy Tube)	
Belief that the child is hungry or thirsty Inability or unwillingness of child to eat Fear that child will "starve" to death Primary role of parent to feed and nourish child Parental guilt	Supplemental feedings beyond what child can ingest may actually cause nausea or vomiting Increase in tumor growth (feeding the tumor) Increase in fluid volume may result in congestive heart failure, increased respiratory secretions, and/or pulmonary congestion, which leads to questions of whether or not to implement diuresis Increased urine output leads to increased risk of skin breakdown if child is incontinent Risk of third spacing More comfortable and natural death Complaint of thirst is associated with dying process, not level of hydration
Resuscitation	
Unwillingness of family to give up Conflicts with cultural or religious beliefs Denial that child is actually going to die	Allowing nature to take its course Family believes child has suffered enough, does not want aggressive intervention Relieves family of responsibility to stop interventions that might prolong life
Autopsy	
Research to help other children Ability to check genetic link	Religious, cultural belief Family emotions Belief that body will be desecrated for funeral viewing (an unfounded fear)

TABLE 4.9 Communicating With Dying Children

Approach	Effective Technique
Discuss at the child's level	Gear information to the child's developmental age, remembering that younger children tend to be concrete thinkers, whereas older children are capable of abstract thought. Begin with the child's experiences: "You've told us how tired you've been lately."
Let the child's questions guide	Begin the conversation with basic information, and let the child's questions direct the conversation.
Provide opportunities for the child to express feelings	Look for clues that child is open to communication. Be accepting of whatever emotion is expressed.
Encourage feedback	Ask the child to summarize what has been heard. This provides the opportunity to clarify misunderstandings.
Use other resources	Use books and movies to encourage dialogue. Ask the child to name the people with whom he or she can discuss problems.
Use the child's natural expressive means to stimulate dialogue	Use books, games, art, play, and music to provide a means of expression.

TABLE 4.10 Communicating Bad News to Families

Approach	Effective Techniques
Provide a setting conducive to communication	Ensure privacy; use appropriate body language; make eye contact. Have parents choose who will attend.
Determine what the family knows	Ask questions (e.g., "What have you made of all this?" or "What were you told?"). Listen to the vocabulary and comprehension of the family. Recognize denial, but do not acknowledge it at this stage.
Determine what the family wants to know	Obtain a clear invitation to share information (if this is what the family wants). Use questions such as, "Are you the sort of person who likes to know every detail, or just the basic facts?"
Give information (aligning and educating)	Start at level of family's comprehension, and use the same vocabulary. Give information slowly, concisely, and in simple language. Avoid medical jargon. Check regularly to be certain that content is understood.
Respond to family's reactions	Acknowledge all reactions and feelings, particularly using the emphatic response technique (identifying emotion, identifying cause of emotion, and responding appropriately). Expect tears, anger, and other strong emotions.
Close	Briefly summarize major areas discussed. Ask parents if they have other important issues to discuss at this time. Make an appointment for the next meeting.

Honest, clear communication that avoids misinterpretation is essential.
Nonverbal communication such as hugging, touching, or remaining with the family in silence may be most empathetic.
Acknowledge the family's guilt, attempt to alleviate it, and deal openly and nonjudgmentally with anger.
Provide information, answer questions, and offer reassurance that everything possible was done for the child.

Viewing the Body

Offer the family the opportunity to see the body; repeat the offer later if they decline.
Before viewing, inform the family of bodily changes they should expect (tubes, injuries, cold skin).
A single staff member should accompany the family but remain inconspicuous.
Offer the opportunity to hold the child.
Allow the family as much time as they need.
Offer parents the opportunity for siblings to view the body.

Formal Concluding Process

Discuss and answer questions concerning autopsy and funeral arrangements; obtain signatures on the body release and autopsy forms.
Provide anticipatory guidance regarding symptoms of grief response and their normalcy.
Provide written materials about grief symptoms.
Escort the family to the exit or to their car if necessary.
Provide a follow-up phone call in 24 to 48 hours to answer questions and provide support.
Provide referral for community health nursing visit.
Provide referrals to local support and resource groups (e.g., bereavement groups, bereavement counselors, SIDS groups, Parents of Murdered Children, Mothers Against Drunk Driving).[b]

Procedures Related to Fluid Balance, Blood Administration, or Nutrition Support

Intravenous Fluid Administration

Characteristics of pediatric administration sets may be as follows:

- Small-gauge catheters (22 to 24 gauge)
- For longer-term administration, consider a midline catheter, peripherally inserted central catheter (PICC), central venous catheter, or implanted port

Sites are as follows:

- Superficial veins of the upper extremities are preferred, then the foot
- Scalp veins (infants)
- A site is chosen that restricts the child's movements as little as possible (e.g., avoid a site over a joint)

- For extremity veins, start with the most distal site, especially if irritating or sclerosing agents are to be used

Maintain integrity of IV site.

Maintain strict asepsis, and follow Standard Precautions.

Use small, padded armboard if IV is inserted at a joint or movement restricts flow.

Provide adequate protection of site.

Observe for signs of infiltration, which may include erythema, pain, edema, blanching, streaking on the skin along the vein, and darkened area at the insertion site.

Change IV tubing and solution at regular intervals (no less than 72 hours) according to the institution's policy.

Electronic infusion pumps are routinely used with infants and children.

Precautions

Assess drip rate by assessing amount infused in a given length of time.

Excess buildup of pressure can occur when the:

- Drip rate is faster than vein can accommodate
- Catheter is out of vein lumen

Procedure for Inserting and Taping a Peripheral Intravenous Catheter

Choose catheter insertion site and an alternative site in case the initial attempt is unsuccessful. A transilluminator can be useful in identifying suitable veins.

Prepare insertion site by applying with friction an antiseptic solution.

Allow solution to dry completely, but do not blow, blot dry, or fan the area.

Put on gloves.

Apply tourniquet when site is ready for catheter insertion.

Stretch the skin taut downward below the point of insertion, upward above the site of insertion, or from underneath level with the point of insertion. This technique helps stabilize veins that roll or move away from the catheter as attempts are made to enter the vein.

Inspect catheter, looking for damage (e.g., bent stylet, shavings on the catheter, frayed catheter tip [follow employer's policy for reporting defective devices]). Look closely at the IV catheter before inserting it, and note that the stylet tip is slightly longer than the catheter. It is necessary to have both pieces inside the vein before the catheter is advanced.

Insert catheter through the skin, bevel up, at a 30-degree angle, and enter the vein. This direct approach is best for large veins and allows the skin and vein to be entered in one step. The indirect approach for smaller veins enables the catheter to enter the vein from the side perpendicularly. It is sometimes helpful with short veins to start the catheter below the intended site and advance through the superficial layers of skin so that the advancement of the catheter in the vein is a shorter distance. In infants or children with very small veins, insert the catheter bevel down, which prevents the needle from puncturing the back wall of the vein and provides an earlier flashback of blood as the vein is entered.

Watch for blood return in the flashback chamber; brands and sizes of safety catheters vary in the way flashback is seen.

Once the flashback is seen, lower the angle between the skin and catheter to 15 degrees. Advance the catheter another 1⁄16 to 1⁄8 inch to ensure that both the stylet and the catheter are inside the vein. Holding the stylet steady, push the catheter off the stylet and into the vein until the catheter hub is situated against the skin at the insertion site. Activate safety mechanism if necessary (some safety catheters are passive and activate automatically), remove the stylet, and discard into sharps container. Apply pressure to catheter within the vein to prevent backflow of blood before attachment of tubing.

Collect blood if ordered. Remove the tourniquet. Flush the IV line with NS to check for patency (ease of flushing fluid, lack of resistance while flushing), complaints of pain, or swelling at the site. If line flushes easily, proceed to secure the catheter to the skin.

Connect the T-connector, J-connector, injection cap, or tubing, and reinforce the connection with a junction securement device (Luer-Lok, clasping device, threaded device) to prevent accidental disconnection and subsequent air embolism or blood loss.

Place transparent dressing across the catheter hub, up to but not including the junction securement device, and surrounding skin.

Further secure the catheter to the skin using tape or adhesive securement devices (e.g., StatLock). Follow manufacturer's directions for adhesive anchors.

Place a ¼- to ½-inch strip of clear tape across the width of the transparent dressing and the catheter hub, but avoid the insertion site. This will serve as an anchor tape strip, and all other tape will be affixed to this strip (tape-on-tape method). This strip will not compromise the transparent dressing properties or interfere with visual inspection of the catheter-skin insertion site.

To stabilize the catheter and junction securement device, attach 1 to 1½ inches of clear tape that is ¼ to ½ inch wide, adhesive side up, to the underneath side of the catheter hub and junction securement device at their connection. Wrap the ends of the tape around the connections, and meet on top to form a V shape (sometimes referred to as a *chevron*); secure the overlapping ends onto the anchor tape strip.

Loop the IV tubing away from the catheter hub and toward the IV fluid source. Secure the looped tubing with a piece of tape on the anchor tape strip. Be certain fingers or toes are visible whenever an extremity is used.

Consider the use of a commercial protective device (e.g., I.V. House) over the catheter hub and looped tubing. Bending one corner of the tape over and onto itself provides a free tab to lift the tape easily for site visualization.

EVIDENCE-BASED PRACTICE

Use of Transillumination Devices in Obtaining Vascular Access

Ask the Question

In children, do transillumination devices decrease the number of attempts needed to obtain vascular access?

Search the Evidence

Search Strategies

Search selection criteria included English-language publications, and research-based articles on children undergoing venipuncture.

Databases Used

PubMed, Cochrane Collaboration, MD Consult, BestBETs

Critically Analyze the Evidence

- **Grade criteria:** Evidence quality low; recommendation weak (Guyatt et al., 2008)
  - Six articles were reviewed regarding the efficacy of transillumination. All concluded that transillumination aids in decreasing the number of access attempts.
- In a seminal work, forty cases were described in which transillumination was used to decrease the number of peripheral intravenous (PIV) attempts. In these patients, small superficial veins that were not previously visualized or palpated were visualized using the transillumination device. Far fewer attempts were needed, and PIV access of infants and obese children was easier for staff (Kuhns et al., 1975).

A sample of 100 infants ages 2–36 months was evaluated for PIV access using a simple otoscope for transillumination. In 40 of the 100 infants, a vein was visible using the otoscope for transillumination. In 23 of these children, transillumination was used after a vein could not be visualized or palpated. In 17 others, one previous attempt to gain PIV access had failed. With transillumination, 39 of 40 PIV attempts were successful on the first attempt. One patient required a second attempt (Goren et al., 2001).

- A systematic review and meta-analysis exploring interventions for peripheral intravenous cannulation of children (PIVC) (Heinrichs et al., 2013) identified seven studies that met inclusion criteria. RCTs included in the meta-analysis were three studies of transillumination, three studies of near-infrared light devices and one study of nitroglycerine ointment. Meta-analysis of the three transilluminator-assisted PIVC demonstrated a lower risk of first-attempt failures compared to traditional PIVC starts. Near-infrared light devices may be helpful in some groups, but evidence is not clear in pediatric patients.
- A systematic review of ultrasound-guided PIVC (Munshey et al., 2020) identified 13 studies for review between 2000 and 2019. Review demonstrated that ultrasound-guided PIV placement shows inconsistent results.
- A systematic review of pediatric PIVC strategies involved 14 randomized controlled studies involving 4539 participants ranging from 15 days of age to 16 years of age (Parker et al., 2017). The reviewers identified 15 studies that met the inclusion criteria. The authors determined that the evidence for US-guided PIVC, transillumination, or nitroglycerine do not demonstrate evidence to recommend their use.

Apply the Evidence: Nursing Implications

- Transillumination may be helpful in PIVC for some children, however, the current evidence does not support regular use. Additional, high-quality studies would contribute to the evidence regarding interventions to assist PIVC procedures in clinical practice.
- Education and practice in this technique are needed for success. Since the veins stand out so clearly with transillumination, they appear more superficial than they are.
- An assistant may be needed to hold the device when using the transilluminator to obtain PIV access.
- The heat and temperature of the transilluminator should be monitored to prevent injury to the patient's skin.
- Appropriate equipment should be used to increase the likelihood of visualization of the vasculature.

References

Goren A, Laufer J, Yativ N, et al. Transillumination of the palm for venipuncture in infants. *Pediatr Emerg Care.* 2001;17(2):130–131.

Guyatt GH, Oxman AD, Vist GE, et al. GRADE: an emerging consensus on rating quality of evidence and strength of recommendations. *BMJ.* 2008;336(7650):924–926.

Heinrichs J, Fritze Z, Klassen T, et al. A systematic review and meta-analysis of new interventions for peripheral intravenous cannulation of children. *Pediatr Emerg Care.* 2013;29(7):858–866.

Kuhns LR, Martin AJ, Gildersleeve S, et al. Intense transillumination for infant venipuncture. *Radiology.* 1975;116(3):734–735.

Munshey F, Parra DA, McDonnell C, et al. Ultrasound-guided techniques for peripheral intravenous placement in children with difficult venous access. *Paediatr Anaesth.* 2020;30(2):108–115.

Parker SIA, Benzies KM, Hayden KA. A systematic review: effectiveness of pediatric peripheral intravenous catheterization strategies. *J Adv Nurs.* 2017;73(7):1570–1582.

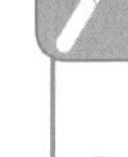

EVIDENCE-BASED PRACTICE

Peripheral Intravenous Catheter Care

Ask the Question

In children, should PIV site replacement be required every 72 hours or when clinically indicated?

Search for Evidence

Search Strategies

Search selection criteria included English-language and research-based publications within the past 20 years on PIV site care.

Databases Used

National Guidelines Clearinghouse (AHQR), Cochrane Collaboration, Joanna Briggs Institute, PubMed, TRIP Database Plus, MD Consult, PedsCCM, BestBETs

Critically Analyze the Evidence

Grade criteria: Evidence quality low to moderate; recommendation strong (Guyatt et al., 2008)

- A multicenter randomized controlled equivalence trial evaluating the duration of peripheral intravenous (PIV) catheter placement (Rickard et al., 2012) recruited 3283 adults with PIV catheter use longer than 4 days. Computer-generated random assignment was between clinically replacing the PIV or third daily routine replacement. Primary outcome was phlebitis during catheterization or within 48 h of removal. Length of catheter insertion for clinical replacement was 99 h versus 70 h for those routinely replaced. Phlebitis rate was 7% in both groups. The authors found that PIVs can be removed as clinically indicated with no increase in risk to patients.
- A descriptive design study used to assess the condition of peripheral IV sites at 72, 96, and greater hours for patients on a medical-surgical unit based on clinical assessment versus length of time since insertion (Helton et al., 2016). Data demonstrated that of 89 PIV sites assessed, no sites demonstrated phlebitis with only one IV showing minimal infiltration. 30 PIV sites maintained patency for 96–200 h; 5 sites were patent at 201–300 h, and four sites were patent at over 300 hours. The authors recommend nurses be empowered to use clinical judgement and use research to answer clinical questions.
- A literature review focused on empirical articles, randomized controlled trials, comparative studies, clinical trials, and reviews (Ansel et al., 2017) of adult patients with regard to short PIV catheter complications (phlebitis, bacteremia, dwell time, cost, and nurses decisions to leave PIV in place. In all reviewed studies, complications of PIVs were low. The author concludes that promoting nursing judgement in clinical assessment of PIV sites increases autonomy in practice and safe clinical practice.
- A Cochrane Database of Systematic Reviews (Webster et al., 2019) included randomized clinical trials (nine studies representing 7412 participants) that compared routine removal of PIV with removal only when clinically indicated. The authors found no difference in rates of catheter-related bloodstream infection, phlebitis, and other problems associated with peripheral catheters. There was uncertainty about rates of local infection when catheters are changed when clinically indicated. Infiltration and catheter blockage are probably reduced with routine catheter change. Cost was reduced when sites were assessed clinically. Evidence was judged to be moderate for most outcomes, particularly due to outcomes being assessed by investigators who were aware of group allocations creating bias.
- A multi-center non-inferiority randomized controlled trial (Vendramim et al., 2020) involving 1319 patients 18 years and over investigated clinically indicated PIV replacement vs routine replacement every 96 hours. Outcome measures included phlebitis, infiltration occlusion, displacement, accidental removal, and bloodstream infection. The study team found that clinically indicated replacement was not inferior to routine replacement.

Apply the Evidence: Nursing Implications

- Data on PIV replacement by clinical assessment or routine replacement is unclear in the pediatric population.
- Adult data suggests that replacing PIVs using nursing clinical assessment is supported by studies demonstrating that there are no significant differences in complications between replacement by clinical assessment or routine replacement.
- In pediatrics, needle pain is a significant issue for children in hospitals and this should be considered when considering routine replacement vs clinical assessment.

References

Ansel B, Boyce M, Embree JL. Extending short peripheral catheter dwell time: a best practice discussion. *J Infus Nurs.* 2017;40(3):143–146.

Guyatt GH, Oxman AD, Vist GE, et al. GRADE: An emerging consensus on rating quality of evidence and strength of recommendations. *British Medical Journal.* 2008;336: 924–926..

Helton J, Hines A, Best J. Peripheral IV site rotation based on clinical assessment vs. length of time since insertion. *Medsurg Nurs.* 2016;25(1):44–49.

Rickard CM, Webster J, Wallis MC, et al. Routine versus clinically indicated replacement of peripheral intravenous catheters: a randomised controlled equivalence trial. *Lancet.* 2012;380(9847):1066–1074.Vendramim P, Avelar AFM, Rickard CM, et al. The RESPECT trial-replacement of peripheral intravenous catheters according to clinical reasons or every 96 hours: a randomized, controlled, non-inferiority trial. *Int J Nurs Stud.* 2020;107:103504.

Webster J, Osborne S, Rickard CM, et al. Clinically-indicated replacement versus routine replacement of peripheral venous catheters. *Cochrane Database Syst Rev.* 2019;1(1):Cd007798.

EVIDENCE-BASED PRACTICE

Frequency of Changing Intravenous Administration Sets

Ask the Question

In children, should intravenous (IV) administration sets be changed at 24, 48, 72, or 96 h to safely prevent patient infection while containing costs?

Search the Evidence

Search Strategies

Search selection criteria included English-language publications within the past 10 years and research-based articles on the frequency of changing IV administration sets.

Databases Used

National Guideline Clearinghouse (AHRQ), Cochrane Collaboration, Joanna Briggs Institute, PubMed, Infusion Nurses Society, Oncology Nurses Society, MD Consult, BestBETs, TRIP Database Plus, PedsCCM

Critically Analyze the Evidence

Grade criteria: Evidence quality moderate; recommendation strong (Guyatt et al., 2008)

- A systematic Cochrane review by Gillies et al. (2005) identified the optimum interval for the routine replacement of IV administration sets when infusate or parenteral nutrition solutions are administered. Data results from 13 randomized or quasi-randomized controlled trials were pooled to compare different time intervals of administration set changes: every 24 h versus 48 h or greater, 48 h versus at least 72 h, and 72 h versus 96 h. Findings revealed no evidence that changing IV administration sets more often than every 96 h reduces the incidence of bloodstream infection. There were no differences in results between patients with central and peripheral catheters and those who did or did not receive parenteral nutrition. For IV administration sets including blood or blood products and lipids, the researchers recommend changing the sets every 24 h.
- The Centers for Disease Control and Prevention (O'Grady et al., 2002) recommends changing IV administration sets for crystalloids at no more than 72-h intervals. Rates of phlebitis were not substantially different for administration sets left in place 96 h compared with 72 h. For tubing used to administer blood and blood products or lipid emulsions, replace tubing within 24 h of starting the infusion.
- The Infusion Nurses Society (2021) and Alexander (2006) recommend replacing continuously infusing IV administration sets no more frequently than every 72 h. Administration sets used intermittently should be changed every 24 h. Secondary piggyback sets may be changed no more frequently than every 72 h when attached to a continuously infusing line; once detached from the primary set, they should be changed at 24 h. Exceptions include sets used with lipids (change at 24 h if continuous or after each unit if intermittently infused) and blood or blood components (change at the end of 4 h if continuous or after each intermittent component). All sets should be changed immediately if contamination is suspected.
- The Oncology Nursing Society (Camp-Sorreli, 2004) recommends replacing IV administration sets every 96 h or with catheter change, except for fluids that enhance microbial growth. Tubing used to administer blood, blood products, lipids, or total parenteral nutrition should be replaced 24 h after initiation of therapy.
- In a systematic review seeking data on the frequency of intravenous tubing change in relation to incidence of sepsis in neonates receiving TPN (Chirinian and Shah, 2012; Kusari et al., 2019) two studies were identified, but neither reported on sepsis as an outcome. The primary outcomes of the reported studies were infusate contamination rather than sepsis. The author concludes that there is insufficient evidence to support or refute decreasing the frequency of IV administration increases the incidence of sepsis.
- A Cochrane Systematic Review (Ullman et al., 2013) sought to identify the optimal timing for intravascular administration set replacement. All randomized controlled trials on the frequency of IV administration set replacement in hospitalized patients were included in the review. A total of 16 studies representing 5001 patients were included in the studies. No evidence suggested that bloodstream infections were more or less likely than with more frequent set changes. There was some evidence that neonatal mortality was increased when receiving parenteral nutrition with less frequent set changes.

Apply the Evidence: Nursing Implications

- Evidence related to IV set change frequency is limited in children. Nurses should consult their institutional policies on IV set changes based on patient-centered care.
- Replace IV administration sets every 96 hours.
- Replace tubing used for lipid emulsions, blood, and blood products every 24 h.
- Replace blood tubing with in-line filters after 2 units or 4 h, whichever comes first.

References

Infusion nursing standards of practice. Alexander M, ed. *J Infus Nurs.* 2006;29(1S):S48–S50.

Camp-Sorreli D, Matey L. *Access Device Guidelines: Recommendations for Nursing Practice and Education.* Pittsburgh: Oncology Nursing Society; 2017.

Chirinian N, Shah V. Does decreasing the frequency of changing intravenous administration sets (>24 h) increase the incidence of sepsis in neonates receiving total parenteral nutrition? *Paediatr Child Health.* 2012;17(9):501–504.

Gillies D, O'Riordan L, Wallen M, et al. Optimal timing for intravenous administration set replacement. *Cochrane Database Syst Rev.* 2005;4:CD003588. pub2. https://doi.org/10.1002/14651858.CD003588.pub2.

Guyatt GH, Oxman AD, Vist GE, et al. GRADE: an emerging consensus on rating quality of evidence and strength of recommendations. *BMJ.* 2008;336(7650):924–926.

Infusion Nurses Society. *Policies and Procedures for Infusion Therapy: Neonate to Adolescent.* 3rd ed. South Norwood, MA: The Society; 2021.

O'Grady N, Alexander M, Dellinger E, others. Guidelines for the prevention of intravascular catheter-related infections. *MMWR Morb Mortal Wkly Rep.* 2002;51(RR-10):1–29.

Ullman AJ, Cooke ML, Gillies D, et al. Optimal timing for intravascular administration set replacement. *Cochrane Database Syst Rev.* 2013;2013(9):Cd003588. https://doi.org/10.1002/14651858.CD003588.pub3.

Hydration

Diarrheal illnesses are a common cause of dehydration in infants and children. Vomiting may precede diarrhea in acute gastroenteritis. Prevention of dehydration may be possible with increased fluid intake early after onset of illness.

Preventing dehydration during diarrheal illnesses

1. Provide more fluids than usual to prevent dehydration: Pedialyte, Gastrolyte, Infalyte, other commercial oral rehydration solution (ORS), or World Health Organization oral rehydration salt packet mixed in 1 L of water.
   - Avoid fluids high in sugar or caffeine: carbonated drinks (non-diet sodas), sports drinks, fruit juices or flavored juice drinks, tea, and coffee.
   - After every loose stool, provide
     - Children younger than 2 years: 50 to 100 mL
     - Children 2 to 10 years: 100 to 200 mL
     - Children older than 10 years: as much as child wants
2. Give the child plenty of food to prevent undernutrition.
   - Breast-feeding should be continued without interruption.
   - Infants taking a cow milk-based formula should continue the full-strength formula.
   - For children old enough to eat, give soft or semisolid foods and offer small, frequent feedings every 3 to 4 hours.
3. Change the plan if the child's diarrhea stops (return to normal diet) or if the child develops signs of dehydration.

Correcting Mild to Moderate Dehydration During Diarrheal Illnesses

1. Provide more fluids than usual; give only rehydration fluids for the first 3 to 4 hours (see above for types to give and to avoid).
2. If the child is vomiting, give the following
   - Children younger than 2 years: 5 mL every 3 to 5 minutes by medication spoon or syringe (without needle)
   - Children over 2 years: 5 to 10 mL every 5 to 10 minutes; increase amount as tolerated.
   - If the child is breast-fed, continue breast-feeding in addition to administering oral rehydration fluids.
3. If the child will drink more than the estimated amount of fluid and is not vomiting, give more.
4. If the child vomits again, wait 10 minutes and then continue giving oral fluid.
5. Reassess at 4 hours. If sufficient rehydration has been achieved, progress to the refeeding diet (Table 4.11). If ORS therapy has failed or if severe dehydration occurs, then boluses of isotonic IV fluid will likely be required. Subsequent IV fluid therapy will typically be administered at 1.5 to 2 times maintenance in order to accomplish sufficient rehydration (Box 4.1).

TABLE 4.11 Foods to Consider for a Child With Gastroenteritis

Foods to Consider	Foods to Keep Away From
1%–2% milk or skim milk; low-fat yogurt; Lactaid milk if suspected lactose intolerance Breast milk, all infant formulas if tolerated (Isomil DF, Lactofree, or Similac Lactose Free if symptoms of lactose intolerance are present); Pediasure or other appropriate supplements	Whole milk and whole milk products; if lactose intolerance is suspected, avoid all regular milk and milk products
Gatorade, oral rehydration solutions such as Pedialyte, Enfalyte, Rehydralyte; diet sodas in limited quantities	Regular soft drinks, caffeine-containing drinks, fruit juices, high sugar–containing drinks.
Low-fat grilled or baked meat, fish, or poultry; boiled or poached eggs Low-fat cheeses Any boiled or baked legumes without added fat; peanut butter in small amounts (<2 Tbsp)	High-fat or fried meats, fish, or poultry; fried eggs High-fat or fried cheeses Peanut butter in large amounts
Low-fat soups and broth with other allowed foods	High-fat creamed soups or chowders
Canned (packed in own juice) peaches, pears, applesauce, bananas	Canned fruit packed in heavy syrup; fruit juices
Most breads or cereals Rice, baked or mashed potatoes, pasta	Donuts, muffins, bran muffins, wheat germ Cereal with nuts, coconut, or granola; bran cereals, high-sugar cereals Fried foods
Angel food cake, vanilla wafers, graham crackers, and other low-fat cookies, cakes, and desserts; diet Jello and sugar-free popsicles in limited quantities	Ice cream, sherbet, pies, popsicles, puddings, chocolate, and other high-fat/high-sugar desserts
Spices, salt, mustard, ketchup, pickles in limited amounts	Highly seasoned foods, sugar, honey, jelly, syrup

BOX 4.1

4 mL/kg/h for first 10 kg of body weight
2 mL/kg/h for second 10 kg of body weight
1 mL/kg/h for each kg over 20 kg

From Johns Hopkins Hospital. The Harriet Lane Handbook. ed 19th ed. St Louis: Elsevier; 201:Holliday-Segar Method.

Family Education: Dehydration and Diarrhea

- Limit exposure to other children (e.g., daycare).
- Encourage continued breastfeeding with infants.
- Use ORS for mild and moderate dehydration.
- Begin refeeding diet once oral fluids are tolerated and sufficient rehydration is achieved.
- Encourage the use of the refeeding diet until symptoms have resolved in 1 to 3 days.
- Advance to regular diet once symptoms have resolved.

Blood Product Administration

Nursing administration of blood components and nursing care of the child receiving blood components are discussed in Tables 4.12 and 4.13.

TABLE 4.12 Blood Components and Nursing Administration

Components and Indications	Dose	Nursing Administration
Packed red blood cells (PRBCs) Symptomatic anemia Renal or liver disease Hemolysis Decreased erythropoiesis Thalassemia major Splenic or liver sequestration	Volume packed RBC = weight (kg) × change in hematocrit (Hct) desired	1. Regulate infusion rate using microaggregate filter via infusion pump at 5 mL/kg/h over 1–2 h (usual rate). Change the filter after 1–2 units of blood are infused or after 4 h. 2. Monitor vital signs before transfusion, 15 min after initiation, and every hour until the end of transfusion.
Whole blood (rarely used) Acute massive blood loss	Volume of whole blood = weight (kg) × change in Hct desired × 2	3. Do not refrigerate blood in the nursing unit. Only the blood bank refrigerator may be used. 4. Ensure that each unit is infused in 4 h or less. If a longer infusion time is needed, the unit must be divided in the blood bank. 5. Do not infuse solutions other than normal saline in the line with RBCs.
Fresh frozen plasma (FFP) Deficiencies of plasma clotting factors in bleeding patients (e.g., disseminated intravascular coagulopathy [DIC]), liver failure, vitamin K deficiency with bleeding, or replacement of antithrombin III (ATIII), protein C, or protein S	10–15 mL/kg (use within 6–24 hours of thawing)	1. Use microaggregate filter over 1–2 h every 12–24 h until hemorrhage stops at a rate of 20 mL/min. 2. Monitor prothrombin time (PT) and partial thromboplastin time (PTT) before and after FFP. 3. Monitor levels of other coagulation factors (e.g., fibrinogen, fibrin split products, D-dimer, ATIII, protein C, and protein S).
Platelets (plt) Active hemorrhage, DIC Thrombocytopenia with bleeding or indicated by clinical status	1 unit/10 kg or 6 units/m^2 intravenously (IV)	1. Regulate infusion rate using 170-μm microaggregate filter at 10 mL/kg/h, IV push or over 1 h or as fast as patient can tolerate. 2. Monitor vital signs before transfusion, 15 min after initiation, and at the end of infusion. 3. Obtain postplatelet count 1–24 hours after infusion.
Granulocytes (rarely used) As an adjunct with other measures in treatment of severe infections in the septic neonate or high-risk patient (e.g., proven bacterial infection in severe neutropenic patient nonresponsive to antibiotic therapy)	10–15 mL/kg IV usually daily ×4 days	1. Monitor vital signs before transfusion, 15 min after initiation, and at the end of transfusion. 2. Premedicate 1 h before transfusion, usually antihistamines, acetaminophen, or steroids. 3. Infuse at slow rate (2–4 h) using 170-μm blood filter within a 24-h period. 4. Minimum of 4–6 h between amphotericin B and granulocyte infusion recommended.

TABLE 4.12 Blood Components and Nursing Administration—cont'd

Components and Indications	Dose	Nursing Administration
Factor VIII (plasma derived or recombinant) Hemophilia A Acquired factor VIII deficiency	1 unit/kg IV of factor VIII = 2% of factor activity 35–50 units/kg IV of factor VIII every 12–24 h	1. Use reconstituted factor within 3 h of mixing. 2. Inject reconstituted factor over 2–5 min. 3. Assess for signs of an adverse reaction such as hives, itchy wheals with redness, tightness in chest, wheezing, low blood pressure, or trouble breathing. Notify health care provider immediately if symptoms are present.
Factor IX (plasma derived or recombinant) Hemophilia B	1 unit/kg IV of factor IX = 1% of factor activity 30–50 units/kg IV every 24 h	
FEIBA (factor eight inhibitor bypass activity) (plasma-derived) Hemophilia A or B with inhibitors (antibodies)	75–100 units/kg IV every 8–24 h (maximum dose 200 units/kg/day	
Factor VII a (recombinant) Hemophilia A or B with inhibitors	90 mcg/kg IV every 2 h (35–120 mcg/kg) dosage range	

TABLE 4.13 Nursing Care of the Child Receiving Blood Transfusions

Complication	Signs and Symptoms	Precautions and Nursing Responsibilities
Immediate Reactions		
Hemolytic Reactions		
Most severe type, but rare Incompatible blood Incompatibility in multiple transfusions	Chills Shaking Fever Pain at needle site and along venous tract Nausea and vomiting Sensation of tightness in chest Red or black urine Headache Flank pain Progressive signs of shock and/or renal failure Often occur within first 15 min	Verify patient identification. Identify donor and recipient blood types and groups before transfusion is begun; verify with another nurse or other practitioner. Transfuse blood slowly for first 15–20 minutes or initial 20% volume of blood; remain with patient. Stop transfusion immediately in event of signs or symptoms, maintain patent intravenous (IV) line, and notify practitioner. Save donor blood to recross-match with patient's blood. Monitor for evidence of shock. Insert urinary catheter, and monitor hourly outputs. Send samples of patient's blood and urine to laboratory for presence of hemoglobin (indicates intravascular hemolysis). Observe for signs of hemorrhage resulting from disseminated intravascular coagulation (DIC). Support medical therapies to reverse shock.
Febrile Reactions		
Most common reaction Leukocyte or platelet antibodies Plasma protein antibodies	Fever Chills Occur within 1–6 h after transfusion	May give acetaminophen for prophylaxis. Leukocyte-poor RBCs are less likely to cause reaction. Stop transfusion immediately; report to practitioner for evaluation.
Allergic Reactions		
Recipient reacts to allergens in donor's blood.	Urticaria Pruritus Flushing Asthmatic wheezing Laryngeal edema	Give antihistamines for prophylaxis to children with tendency toward allergic reactions. Stop transfusion immediately. Administer epinephrine for wheezing or anaphylactic reaction.

Continued

TABLE 4.13 Nursing Care of the Child Receiving Blood Transfusions—cont'd

Complication	Signs and Symptoms	Precautions and Nursing Responsibilities
Circulatory Overload		
Too rapid transfusion (even a small quantity)	Sudden severe headache	Transfuse blood slowly.
Excessive quantity of blood transfused (even slowly)	Precordial pain Tachycardia Dyspnea Rales Cyanosis Dry cough Distended neck veins Hypertension	Prevent overload by using PRBCs or administering divided amounts of blood. Use infusion pump to regulate and maintain flow rate. Stop transfusion immediately if signs of overload. Place child upright with feet in dependent position.
Air Emboli		
May occur when blood is transfused under pressure	Sudden difficulty in breathing Sharp pain in chest Apprehension	Normalize pressure before container is empty when infusing blood under pressure. Clear tubing of air by aspirating air with syringe at nearest Y-connector if air is observed in tubing; disconnect tubing and allow blood to flow until air has escaped only if a Y-connector is not available.
Hypothermia		
	Chills Low temperature Irregular heart rate Possible cardiac arrest	Use approved mechanical blood warmer or electric warming coil to rapidly warm blood; never use microwave oven. Take temperature if patient complains of chills; if subnormal, stop transfusion.
Electrolyte Disturbances		
Hyperkalemia (in massive transfusions or in patients with renal problems)	Nausea, diarrhea Muscular weakness Flaccid paralysis Paresthesia of extremities Bradycardia Apprehension Cardiac arrest	Use washed RBCs or fresh blood if patient is at risk.
Delayed Reactions		
Transmission of Infection		
	Signs of infection (e.g., jaundice) Toxic reaction: high fever, severe headache or substernal pain, hypotension, intense flushing, vomiting/diarrhea	Blood is tested for antibodies to human immunodeficiency virus (HIV), hepatitis C virus, and hepatitis B core antigen; in addition, blood is tested for hepatitis B surface antigen (HBsAg) and alanine aminotransferase (ALT), and a serology test is performed for syphilis; positive units are destroyed; individuals at risk for carrying certain viruses are deferred from donation. Report any sign of infection and, if occurring during transfusion, stop transfusion immediately, send sample for culture and sensitivity tests, and notify physician.
Alloimmunization		
(Antibody formation) Occurs in patients receiving multiple transfusions	Increased risk of hemolytic, febrile, and allergic reactions	Use limited number of donors. Observe carefully for signs of reactions.
Delayed Hemolytic Reaction		
	Destruction of RBCs and fever 2–10 days after transfusion (anemia, jaundice, dark urine)	Observe for posttransfusion anemia and decreasing benefit from successive transfusions.

PRBCs, Packed red blood cells.

Peripherally Inserted Central Catheters

Description

Single or multiple lumen available
Inserted into antecubital fossa and passed through basilic or cephalic vein into superior vena cava (SVC)
Positioning of tip in SVC maximizes hemodilution and reduces likelihood of vessel wall damage, phlebitis, or thrombus formation

Benefits

Do not require operating room placement
Can be inserted by specially trained RNs
Can use small insertion needles
Fast placement

Care Considerations

Sometimes difficult to thread into SVC
Reports of resistance to removal
Not suitable for rapid fluid replacement because of small lumen size
Five- to 10-mL syringe is used for flushing to prevent catheter wall rupture

Long-Term Central Venous Access Devices

Tunneled Catheter (e.g., Hickman/Broviac Catheter)

Description

One or two Dacron cuffs or Vitacuffs (biosynthetic material impregnated with silver ions) on catheter(s) enhance tissue ingrowth.
May have more than one lumen (Fig. 4.18)

Benefits

Reduced risk of bacterial migration after tissue adheres to Dacron cuff or Vitacuff
Easy to use for self-administered infusions

Care Considerations

Requires daily heparin flushes
Must be clamped or have clamp nearby at all times
Must keep exit site dry
Heavy activity restricted until tissue adheres to cuff
Risk of infection still present
Protrudes outside body; susceptible to damage from sharp instruments and may be pulled out; may affect body image
More difficult to repair
Patient and family must learn catheter care

Dressings for Tunneled Catheters

A dressing may not be required to prevent infection for catheters that have been in place for prolonged periods. However, dressings may be used to secure the catheter from dislodgement or breakage. Typically, a clear, transparent dressing will be used that allows visualization of the skin around the tube at least daily.

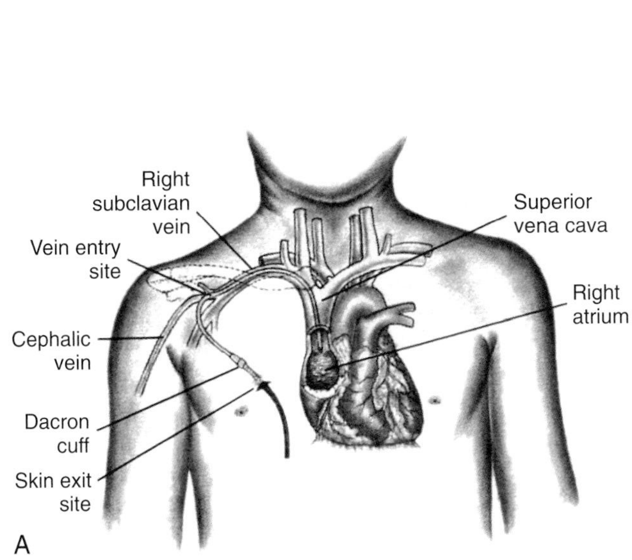

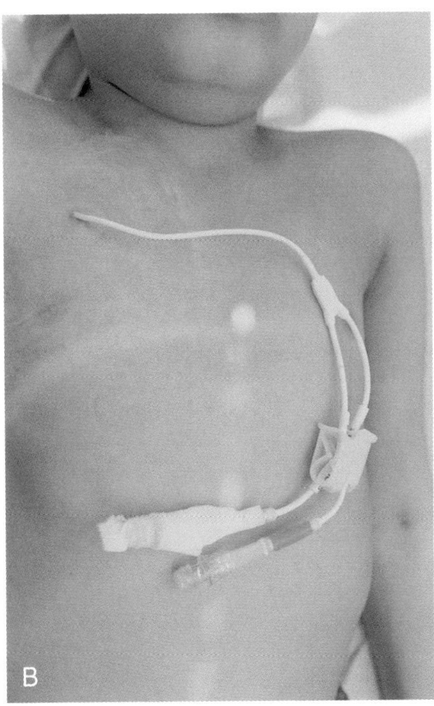

FIG. **4.18** (A) Central venous catheter insertion and exit site. (B) External venous catheter.

Removal of old dressings may be facilitated by applying adhesive remover. Gently peel off one edge of the dressing at a time. Another technique that is more comfortable to some children is to grasp opposite corners and pull them away from each other to stretch and loosen the dressing, then grasp the two remaining corners and pull.

Cleansing technique is specific to the cleanser used. See Evidence-Based Practice: Central Venous Catheter Site Care for a discussion of cleansers. ChloraPrep is applied using a back-and-forth motion and requires at least 30 seconds to dry. Povidone iodine is applied in a circular motion, beginning at the catheter and moving outward; it requires at least two minutes drying time.

The catheter is looped around the entry site and under the dressing (Fig. 4.19). Secure the end of the tube with tape to prevent dangling and dislodgement or damage.

Implanted Ports (e.g., Port-A-Cath, Infusaport, Mediport, Norport)

Description

Totally implantable metal or plastic device that consists of a self-sealing injection port with top or side access with preconnected or attachable silicone catheter that is placed in a large blood vessel

Benefits

Reduced risk of infection
Placed completely under the skin; therefore cannot be pulled out or damaged
Heparinized monthly and after each infusion to maintain patency
Can remain in place for years
No limitations on regular physical activity, including swimming
Dressing needed only when a Huber needle is in place
No or only slight change in body appearance (slight bulge on chest)

Care Considerations

Must pierce skin for access; pain with insertion of needle; can use local anesthetic (EMLA, LMX, buffered lidocaine, or vapocoolant) before accessing port
Special noncoring needle (Huber) with straight or angled design must be used to inject into port (Fig. 4.20).
Hard to manipulate for self-administered infusions
Catheter may dislodge from port, especially if child plays with port site.
Vigorous contact sports generally not allowed
Overlying skin should be protected from irritation by avoiding clothing, straps, and seat belts placing pressure on the port area.

Family Education: Central Venous Catheters

- Signs of infection: fever, chills, pain or redness, site drainage, shortness of breath, chest pain
- Maintaining catheter patency via flushing
- Keep skin dry around the insertion site when bathing using special shower dressings or plastic wrap
- What to do if the catheter breaks (most require clamping; the Groshong does not)
- Site/needle protection during infusions through implanted ports

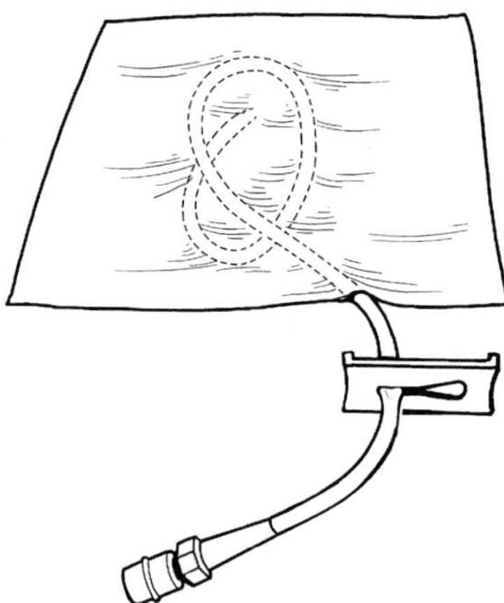

FIG. **4.19** Tunneled catheter dressing.

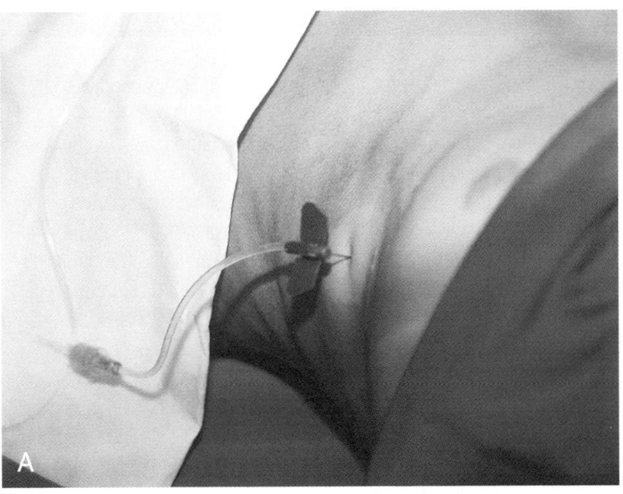

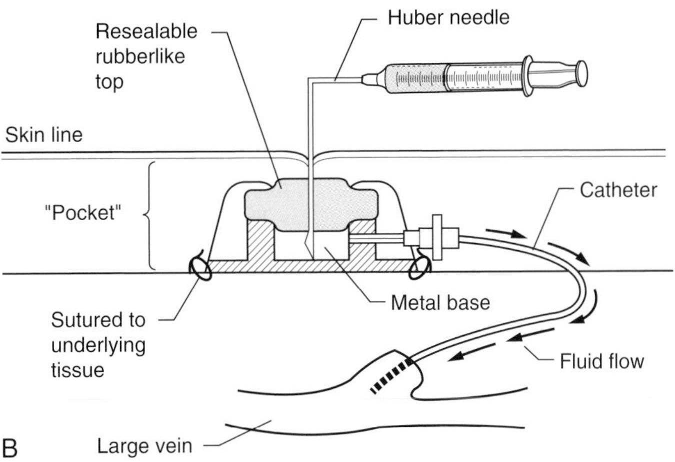

FIG. **4.20** (A) Implanted venous access device with Huber placement. (B) Side view of the implanted port.

EVIDENCE-BASED PRACTICE

Central Venous Catheter Site Care

Ask the Question

In children with central venous catheters (CVC), is chlorhexidine gluconate a more effective antiseptic solution than povidone-iodine in preventing CVC-related site infections and bacteremia?

Search the Evidence

Search Strategies

Search selection criteria included English-language publications within the past 10 years and research-based articles on catheter site care and chlorhexidine.

Databases Used

The National Guideline Clearinghouse (AHRQ), Centers for Disease Control and Prevention (CDC), Cochrane Collaboration, Joanna Briggs Institute, PubMed, Infusion Nurses Society, Oncology Nurses Society, MD Consult, BestBETs, TRIP Database Plus

Critically Analyze the Evidence

Grade criteria: Evidence quality moderate; recommendation strong (Guyatt et al., 2008)

- The CDC (2017) recommends the use of 2% chlorhexidine for disinfecting catheter site before insertion (allow to dry), but tincture of iodine, an iodophor, or 70% alcohol can be used. Iodine needs to remain on the skin for at least 2 minutes or until dry. No recommendations can be made for the use of chlorhexidine in infants younger than 2 months of age. No recommendations can be made regarding the use of topical antibiotic ointments or creams due to the potential to promote fungal infections and antimicrobial resistance. No recommendations are made for the use of impregnated catheters and chlorhexidine sponge dressings to reduce the incidence of infection. Avoid the use of sponges in infants less than 7 days old and less than 26 weeks' gestation. Replace the catheter-site dressing when it becomes damp, loosened, or soiled or when inspection of the site is necessary. Replace dressings used on short-term CVC sites every 2 days for gauze dressings and at least every 7 days for transparent dressings, except in those pediatric patients in whom the risk for dislodging the catheter outweighs the benefit of changing the dressing.
- The Infusion Nurses Society (2021) recommends cleansing the insertion site with an antiseptic solution and allowing to dry completely. Chlorhexidine solution is preferred and applied in a back-and-forth motion for 30 s. If povidone-iodine is used,

Continued

EVIDENCE-BASED PRACTICE—cont'd

allow to remain on the skin for 1.5–2 min to completely dry for adequate cleaning.

- Dress vascular access site with sterile gauze, and cover with sterile transparent dressings. Gauze dressings should be changed every 48 h. Semipermeable transparent dressings should be changed at least every 7 days, and the interval is dependent on the dressing material, age and condition of the patient, infection rate reported by the organization, environmental conditions, and manufacturer's labeled uses and directions.
- The Oncology Nursing Society (Camp-Sorrell and Matey, 2017) finds chlorhexidine for preinsertion and postinsertion site catheter care superior to alcohol and povidone-iodine. No recommendations are made for the use of chlorhexidine sponge dressing. Routine application of antibiotic ointment is not recommended because of the risk of fungal infections and antimicrobial resistance. Gauze dressings should be changed every 48 h. Semipermeable transparent dressings over gauze are treated as gauze dressings and changed every 48 h. Semipermeable transparent dressings should be changed every 5–7 days or more often, as indicated. Five evidence-based systematic reviews were found regarding CVC site care.

- In a nursing evidence-based review by Carson (2004), most studies found chlorhexidine to be superior to povidone-iodine for preventing microbial colonization of the CVC insertion site and catheter tip and for decreasing the risk of local site infection. However, there is still conflicting evidence regarding the efficacy of chlorhexidine versus povidone-iodine for preventing CVC-related bacteremia.
- In a meta-analysis of eight studies by Chaiyakunapruk et al. (2002), chlorhexidine reduced the risk of catheter-related bloodstream infections by 49% compared with povidone-iodine. In a follow-up review (Chaiyakunapruk et al., 2003), the use of chlorhexidine rather than povidone-iodine for site care led to a cost savings of $113 for each catheter used.
- A Cochrane Review of skin antisepsis for reducing CVC-related infections (Lai et al., 2016) reported on twelve studies that contributed data for a total of 3466 CVCs assessed. Participants were mainly adults, and most studies assessed skin antisepsis at insertion and ongoing. Methodologic quality of the studies had a wide variation in risk of bias due to inadequate blinding and incomplete outcome data. The authors found no clear evidence of differences in blood infections in the CVC or need for antibiotics based on cleaning compared to no cleaning. Chlorhexidine may reduce blood infections versus povidone-iodine. Chlorohexidine may also reduce infections within the catheter.
- In a systematic review and meta-analysis, the efficacy of chlorhexidine versus povidone solutions for skin disinfection was assessed (Shi et al., 2019). Ten randomized controlled trials were identified. After meta-analysis, chlorhexidine was significantly better than povidone in preventing catheter-related bloodstream infections. There were no clear differences in skin reactions between the two antiseptics.
    - Five randomized, controlled trials were found comparing chlorhexidine and povidone-iodine in various populations.

Chambers et al. (2005) found that chlorhexidine sponge dressings (Biopatch) reduced the incidence of exit-site or tunnel infections of central venous catheters in adult neutropenic patients.

- In the study conducted by Garland et al. (2001), 705 neonates and infants in the Biopatch group had a substantial decrease in colonized catheter tips compared with the group that used standard dressings but no difference in rates of catheter-related bloodstream infections or bloodstream infections without a source between the two groups. However, Biopatch was associated with localized contact dermatitis in infants of very low birth weight.
- In the study conducted by Langgartner et al. (2004), skin disinfection before CVC insertion and daily with dressing changes with propanol-chlorhexidine followed by povidone-iodine was associated with the lowest rate of microbial catheter colonization.
- In a study conducted by Levy et al., (2005) in a pediatric cardiovascular intensive care unit, patients with chlorhexidine-impregnated CVC dressing (Biopatch) had a significantly reduced risk of CVC colonization compared with patients with transparent dressing alone. Occurrence of catheter-related bloodstream infection was not different in the two groups.
- In a randomized, controlled, prospective study assessing the efficacy of 1% chlorhexidine-gluconate ethanol (CHG-EtOH) and 10% povidone-iodine (PV-I) for skin antisepsis of CVC care (Yamamoto et al., 2014) patients aged 16 years to adulthood receiving hematology treatment via a CVC were randomized to either CHG-EtOH or PV-I. CVC site colonization rates of the groups were 11.9% CHG-EtOH compared to 29.2% PV-I. Catheter-associated bloodstream infections were 0.75 CHG-EtOH to 3.62 PV-I per 1000 catheter days. 1% chlorhexidine-gluconate ethanol was superior to povidone-iodine even with a long duration of CVC use.

Apply the Evidence: Nursing Implications

- Two percent chlorhexidine should be used for catheter site antisepsis.
- Two percent chlorhexidine should be used with caution in premature and low-birth-weight infants.
- Chlorhexidine-impregnated sponges (Biopatch) should be used around the catheter site except in patients older than 2 months of age.

References

Camp-Sorrell D, Matey L. *Access Device Guidelines: Recommendations for Nursing Practice and Education.* Pittsburgh: Oncology Nursing Society; 2017.

Carson S. Chlorhexidine versus povidone-iodine for central venous catheter site care in children. *J Pediatr Nurs.* 2004;19(1):74–80.

Center for Disease Control. *Guidelines for the Prevention of Intravascular Catheter-Related Infections*; 2017. https://www.cdc.gov/infectioncontrol/guidelines/bsi/updates.html. Accessed May 3, 2022.

Chaiyakunapruk N, Veenstra D, Lipsky B, et al. Vascular catheter site care: the clinical and economic benefits of chlorhexidine gluconate compared with povidone iodine. *Clin Infect Dis.* 2003;37(6):764–771.

Chaiyakunapruk N, Veenstra D, Lipsky B, et al. Chlorhexidine compared with povidone-iodine solution for vascular catheter-site care: a meta-analysis. *Ann Intern Med.* 2002;136(11):792–801.

Chambers S, Sanders J, Patton W, et al. Reduction of exit-site infections of tunneled intravascular catheters among neutropenic patients by sustained-release chlorhexidine dressings: results from a prospective randomized controlled trial. *J Hosp Infect.* 2005;61(1):53–61.

Garland J, Alex C, Mueller C, et al. A randomized trial comparing povidone-iodine to a chlorhexidine-impregnated dressing for prevention of central venous catheter infections in neonates. *Pediatrics.* 2001;107(6):1431–1436.

Guyatt GH, Oxman AD, Vist GE, et al. GRADE: an emerging consensus on rating quality of evidence and strength of recommendations. *BMJ.* 2008;336(7650):924–926.

Infusion Nurses Society. *Policies and Procedures for Infusion Therapy: Neonate to Adolescent.* 3rd ed. South Norwood, MA: The Society; 2021.

Lai NM, Lai NA, O'Riordan E, et al. Skin antisepsis for reducing central venous catheter-related infections. *Cochrane Database Syst Rev.* 2016;7(7):Cd010140.

Langgartner J, Linde H, Lehn N, et al. Combined skin disinfection with chlorhexidine/propanol and aqueous povidone-iodine reduces bacterial colonisation of central venous catheters. *Intensive Care Med.* 2004;30(6):1081–1088.

Levy I, Katz J, Solter E, et al. Chlorhexidine-impregnated dressing for prevention of colonization of central venous catheters in infants and children: a randomized controlled study. *Pediatr Infect Dis J.* 2005;24(8):676–679.

Shi Y, Yang N, Zhang L, et al. Chlorhexidine disinfectant can reduce the risk of central venous catheter infection compared with povidone: a meta-analysis. *Am J Infect Control.* 2019;47(10):1255–1262.

Yamamoto N, Kimura H, Misao H, et al. Efficacy of 1.0% chlorhexidine-gluconate ethanol compared with 10% povidone-iodine for long-term central venous catheter care in hematology departments: a prospective study. *Am J Infect Control.* 2014;42(5):574–576.

EVIDENCE-BASED PRACTICE

Obtaining Blood Specimens From Central Venous Catheters in Children

Ask the Question

In children, do blood specimens obtained from central venous catheters using the discard, reinfusion, or push-pull method yield more accurate samples?

Search for Evidence

Search Strategies

Search selection criteria included English-language research-based publications on pediatric blood specimen collection from central venous access.

Databases Used

National Guideline Clearinghouse (AHRQ), Cochrane Collaboration, Joanna Briggs Institute, PubMed, TRIP database Plus, MD Consult, PedsCCM, BestBETs

Critically Analyze the Evidence

Grade criteria: Evidence quality low; recommendation strong (Guyatt et al., 2008)

- Limited scientific research exists that describes the optimal method for drawing blood samples from central venous access devices (CVADs) in the pediatric patient.
- A convenience sample of paired specimens compared blood drawn from central lines via the push-pull method and discard method on 28 pediatric patients ages 6 months to 12 years. Of the 438 pairs of measurements that were compared, 420 or 95.9% were within limits of agreement for hemograms, electrolytes, and glucose. The push-pull method eliminates loss of blood and decreases the number of times the central line is accessed (Barton et al., 2004).
- The Infusion Nurses Society (2021) recommends that the discard method be used when drawing blood samples from CVADs. The discard volume should be 1.5–2 times the fill volume of the CVAD.
- A prospective comparison of blood draws from CVADs using the single syringe push-pull method and the standard of care discard method (Hess and Decker, 2017), All study-related blood collection was completed by two pediatric nurses. Statistical analysis demonstrated differences in lab values between the two methods, however, were not clinically significant and within the standard error measurement. The authors conclude that given the similarity in lab results the push-pull method should be considered for obtaining blood samples to reduce unnecessary blood loss.
- McBride et al. (2018) initiated a standard push-pull protocol for PICU for implementation and evaluation in a 24-bed PICU and 20-bed acute cardiac unit in a southwest children's hospital. Thirty-seven patients aged 2 months to 23 years underwent 88 total blood draws using the push-pull method. Results from the push-pull method and standard samples were analyzed and no significant differences were found between the two methods, and there were no catheter occlusions or infections. The authors conclude that a standard, evidence-based push-pull protocol can be used routinely in the PICU to reduce blood loss and anemia.
- Frey (2003) summarizes the evidence for the practice of all three blood sampling methods. The discard method is the most widely reported, with disadvantages including blood loss, blood exposure risk for clinicians, and the potential to confuse the discard specimen for the blood sample. The reinfusion method does not deplete blood volume but risks blood exposure for the clinician and the potential to reinfuse a contaminated specimen or clots in the discard volume. The push-pull or mixing method demonstrates accuracy for other than coagulation and drug levels and reduces blood loss and clinician exposure risk.

Apply the Evidence: Nursing Implications

- There is limited pediatric research that clearly supports any central line blood sampling method as being superior. All three methods yield accurate results and appear safe. The discard method is the most frequently reported in the literature and benchmarking. However, if there is a concern about blood volume, the push-pull or reinfusion method should be considered.
- If the catheter has multiple lumens, use the distal lumen for laboratory specimen collection.
- Infusions should be stopped and lumens clamped before blood sampling.
- Cleanse the injection cap with an antiseptic agent, and allow to dry before drawing laboratory specimens.
- Attach a syringe or stopcock depending on specimen method selected, to the injection cap, not directly to the catheter hub. The injection cap at the catheter hub should be removed only if blood cultures are drawn.

References

Barton S, Chase T, Latham B, et al. Comparing two methods to obtain blood specimens from pediatric central venous catheters. *J Pediatr Oncol Nurs.* 2004;21(6):320–326.

Frey M. Drawing blood samples from vascular access devices. *J Infus Nurs.* 2003;26(5):285–293.

Guyatt GH, Oxman AD, Vist GE, et al. GRADE: an emerging consensus on rating quality of evidence and strength of recommendations. *BMJ.* 2008;336(7650):924–926.

Hess S, Decker M. Comparison of the single-syringe push-pull technique with the discard technique for obtaining blood samples from pediatric central venous access devices. *J Pediatr Oncol Nurs.* 2017;34(6):381–386.

Infusion Nurses Society. *Policies and Procedures for Infusion Therapy: Neonate to Adolescent.* 3rd ed. South Norwood, MA: The Society; 2021.

McBride C, Miller-Hoover S, Proudfoot JA. A standard push-pull protocol for waste-free sampling in the pediatric intensive care unit. *J Infus Nurs.* 2018;41(3):189–197.

EVIDENCE-BASED PRACTICE

Normal Saline or Heparinized Saline Flush Solution in Pediatric Intravenous Lines

Ask the Question

Is there a significant difference in the longevity of peripheral intravenous (IV) intermittent infusion locks in children when normal saline (NS) is used as a flush instead a heparinized saline (HS) solution?

Search for the Evidence

Search Strategies

Selection criteria included evidence during the years 2006–2017 with the following terms: saline versus heparin intermittent flush, children's heparin lock flush, heparin lock patency, peripheral venous catheter in children.

Databases Used

CINAHL, PubMed

Critical Appraisal of the Evidence

- No differences in patency were established in a double-blind prospective randomized study in neonates. NS was deemed preferable to HS in peripheral intravenous (PIV) locks in neonates, in consideration of complications associated with heparin (Arnts et al., 2011).
- Infusion devices flushed with NS lasted longer than those flushed with HS (Cook et al., 2011).
- Peripheral catheters flushed with heparin remained patent longer but were also more likely to develop phlebitis (Tripathi et al., 2008).
- A randomized trial in neonates demonstrated that use of HS for flushing before and after IV antibiotics significantly increased the duration of PIVs when compared to NS flushes (Upadhyay et al., 2015).
- A systematic review of 10 randomized controlled trials in pediatrics found minimal benefit to use of HS as intermittent flush of peripheral catheters compared to NS. The difference was not statistically significant (Kumar et al., 2013).
- Peripheral catheters in children, ages 1–17 years, flushed once every 24 h with NS did not affect patency when compared to flushing with NS every 12 h (Schreiber et al., 2015).
- Either HS or preservative-free NS may be used to flush a PIV line (Arnts et al., 2011; Bellini, 2012; Cook et al., 2011; Infusion Nurses Society, 2021; White et al., 2011).
- After each catheter use, peripheral catheters should be locked with either HS (0.5 to 10 units/mL) or preservative-free NS, since outcome data remain equivocal (Infusion Nurses Society, 2021).
- Intermittent flushing with NS results in fewer complications, lower cost, and less time compared with continuous infusion (Stok and Wieringa, 2016).
- The Centers for Disease Control and Prevention recommends use of NS for intermittent flushing to avoid complications (O'Grady et al., 2011).
- Switching from HS to NS involves educational and administrative interventions (Cook et al., 2011; Thamlikitkul and Indranoi, 2006).
- NS is more cost-effective (Thamlikitkul and Indranoi, 2006).
- NS flush has fewer side effects. HS can be associated with anticoagulation, thrombocytopenia, drug interactions, and hypersensitivity (Arnts et al., 2011).
- NS flushes once a day maintained patency of pediatric PIV locks, resulting in reduced costs and increased patient satisfaction (Schreiber et al., 2015).
- Nurses in Italy tend to use HS with smaller-gauge (24-gauge) catheters when access is less frequent (12 h or more between doses) and when patients are on specific units (hematology/oncology, pediatric surgery, and short-stay units) (Bisogni et al., 2014).

Apply the Evidence: Nursing Implications

- There is **low-quality evidence with a weak recommendation** (Guyatt et al., 2008) for using NS versus HS flush solution in pediatric IV lines. Further research is needed with larger samples of children, especially preterm neonates, using small-gauge catheters (24 gauge) and other gauge catheters flushed with NS and HS as intermittent infusion devices only (no continuous infusions). Variables to be considered include catheter dwell time; medications administered; period between regular flushing and flushing associated with medication administration; pain, erythema, and other localized complications; concentration and amount of HS used; type of needleless connector used (negative pressure, positive pressure, or neutral pressure); flush method (positive-pressure technique vs. no specific technique); reason for IV device removal; and complications associated with either solution. NS is a safe alternative to HS flush in infants and children with intermittent IV locks larger than 24 gauge; smaller neonates may benefit from HS flush (longer dwell time), but the evidence is inconclusive for all weight ranges and gestational ages. Neonates may benefit from a continuous infusion of NS at 5 mL/h to maintain patency.

References

Arnts IJ, Heijnen JA, Wilbers HT, et al. Effectiveness of heparin solution versus normal saline in maintaining patency of intravenous locks in neonates: a double blind randomized controlled study. *J Adv Nurs.* 2011;67(12):2677–2685.

Bellini S. Flushing of intravenous locks in neonates: no evidence that heparin improves patency compared with saline. *Evid Based Nurs.* 2012;15:86–87.

Bisogni S, Guisti F, Ciofi D, et al. Heparin solution for maintaining peripheral venous catheter patency in children: a survey of current practice in Italian pediatric units. *Iss Compr Pediatr Nurs.* 2014;37(2):122–135.

Cook L, Bellini S, Cusson RM. Heparinized saline vs normal saline for maintenance of intravenous access in neonates: an evidence-based practice change. *Adv Neonatal Care.* 2011;11:208–215.

Guyatt GH, Oxman AD, Vist GE, et al. GRADE: an emerging consensus on rating quality of evidence and strength of recommendations. *Br Med J.* 2008;336(7650):924–926.

Infusion Nurses Society. *Policies and Procedures for Infusion Therapy: Neonate to Adolescent.* 3rd ed. South Norwood, MA: The Society; 2021.

Kumar M, Vandermeer B, Bassler D, et al. Low dose heparin use and the patency of peripheral intravenous catheters in children: a systematic review. *Pediatrics.* 2013;131(3):e864–e872.

O'Grady NP, Alexander M, Burns LA, et al. *Guidelines for the Prevention of Intravascular Catheter-related Infections.* Atlanta, GA: Healthcare Infection Control Practices Advisory Committee of the Centers for Disease Control and Prevention; 2011.

Schreiber S, Zanchi C, Ronfani L, et al. Normal saline flushes performed once daily maintain peripheral intravenous catheter patency: a randomized controlled trial. *Arch Dis Child.* 2015;100(7):700–703.

Stok D, Wieringa JW. Continuous infusion versus intermittent flushing: maintaining peripheral intravenous access in newborn infants. *J Perinatol.* 2016;36(10):870873.

Thamlikitkul V, Indranoi A. Switching from heparinized saline flush to normal saline flush for maintaining peripheral venous catheter patency. *Int J Qual Health Care.* 2006;18(3):183185.

Tripathi S, Kaushik V, Singh V. Peripheral IVs: Factors affecting complications and patency—a randomized controlled trial. *J Infus Nurs.* 2008;31(3):182188.

Upadhyay A, Verma KK, Lal P, et al. Heparin for prolonging peripheral intravenous catheter use in neonates: a randomized controlled trial. *J Perinatol.* 2015;35:274–277.

White ML, Crawley J, Rennie EA, et al. Examining the effectiveness of 2 solutions used to flush capped pediatric peripheral intravenous catheters. *J Infus Nurs.* 2011;34:260–270.

Tube Feeding

The purpose of tube feeding is to supply gastrointestinal feeding for the child who is unable to take nourishment by mouth because of anomalies of the throat or esophagus, impaired swallowing capacity, severe debilitation, respiratory distress, or unconsciousness.

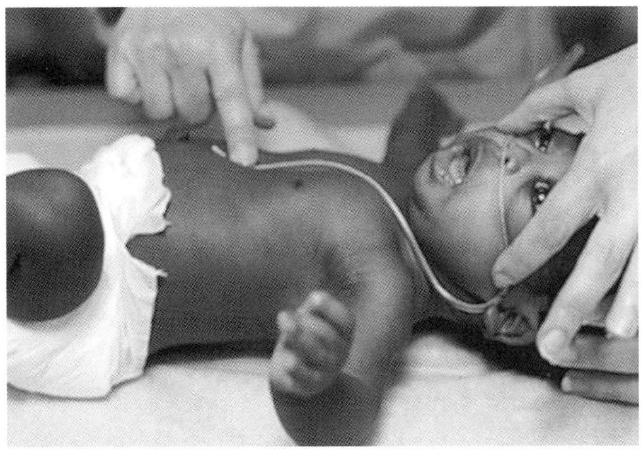

FIG. **4.21** Measuring tube for orogastric feeding from tip of nose to earlobe and to midpoint between end of xiphoid process and umbilicus.

Procedure: Placement of a Nasogastric or Orogastric Tube

1. Place the child supine with the head slightly hyperflexed or in a sniffing position (nose pointed toward ceiling).
2. Measure from tip of nose to earlobe, then to a point midway between the end of the xiphoid process and umbilicus for the approximate length of insertion (Fig. 4.21), and mark the point with a small piece of tape.

NURSING ALERT

Studies evaluating NG/OG tube length in infants and children found that age-specific methods for predicting the distance based on height is a more accurate prediction of the internal distance to the stomach (Beckstrand et al., 2007; Klasner et al., 2002). The morphologic measure most commonly used by clinicians (nose-ear-xiphoid distance) is often too short to locate the entire tube pore span in the stomach. However, the nose-ear-mid xiphoid umbilicus span approached the accuracy of the age-specific prediction equations and is easier to use in a clinical setting. The best option is to adopt the nose-ear-mid xiphoid umbilicus measurement for NG/OG tube length.

1. Lubricate the tube with sterile water or water-soluble lubricant, and insert through one of the nares or the mouth to the predetermined mark. In older infants and children, the tube is passed through the nose and the position alternated between nostrils. An indwelling tube is almost always placed through the nose. Because most young infants are obligatory nose breathers, insertion through the mouth may be used for intermittent gavage feedings because it causes less distress and also helps to stimulate sucking.
   - When using the nose, slip the tube along the base of the nose and direct it straight back toward the occiput.
   - When entering through the mouth, direct the tube toward the back of the throat.
   - If the child is able to swallow on command, synchronize passing the tube with swallowing.
2. Confirm placement by x-ray if available. Document pH and color of aspirate with initial placement and ongoing placement checks (see Evidence-Based Practice box).
3. Stabilize the tube by holding or taping it to the cheek, not to the forehead because of possible damage to the nostril (Fig. 4.22). To assist in maintaining correct placement, measure and record the amount of tubing extending from the nose or mouth to the distal port when the tube is first positioned. Recheck position before each feeding. A hydrocolloid barrier may be placed on the cheeks to protect the skin from tape irritation.

EVIDENCE-BASED PRACTICE

Assessing Correct Placement of Nasogastric or Orogastric Tubes in Children

Confirming Nasogastric Tube Placement in Pediatric Patients

Ask the Question

In children, how should the correct placement of nasogastric (NG) tubes be assessed during hospitalization?

Search for the Evidence

Search Strategies

Search selection criteria included English-language, research-based articles, and children and adolescents requiring NG tube placement. Search areas included aspirate, auscultation, and radiology methods, NG tube length prediction methods, age-related height-based methods, and accurate NG tube placement. Searches excluded newborns and preterm infants.

Databases Used

PubMed, Cochrane Collaboration, MDConsult, Joanna Briggs Institute, Agency for Healthcare Research and Quality National Guideline Clearinghouse, TRIP Database Plus, PedsCCM, BestBETS.

Continued

EVIDENCE-BASED PRACTICE—cont'd

Critical Appraisal of the Evidence

Studies compared various methods used to evaluate the correct placement of the NG tube.

Accurate Nasogastric Tube Length Measurement

- Children 8 years, 4 months old or younger: Use the age-related height-based equation for NG length predictions.
- Children older than 8 years, 4 months old, short stature, or when you cannot obtain accurate height: Use nose-ear–midway to umbilicus (NEMU) (Beckstrand et al., 2007).
- Use of the nose-ear-xyphoid (NEX) method resulted in an increased risk of misplaced tubes (Irving et al., 2018).

Radiographs

- Although abdominal x-ray provides confirmation of enteral tube location, the results can sometimes be equivocal. In addition, this method cannot be used for ongoing, frequent placement verification basis due to the risk of radiation exposure to the child (Irving et al., 2018). Alternate methods of verification have evidence-based support in the literature (Emergency Nurses Association, 2019).

Nonradiologic Verification Methods

- A pH of 5 or less supports that the tip of the tube is in the gastric location (Ellett et al. 2005; Gilbertson et al., 2011; Nyqvist et al., 2005; Society of Pediatric Nurses Clinical Practice Committee et al., 2011; Ni et al., 2017).
- A pH greater than 5 does not reliably predict the correct distal tip location. This may indicate respiratory or esophageal placement or the presence of medications to suppress acid secretion. Gastric aspirate pH means are statistically significantly lower compared with means from intestinal and respiratory pH aspirates (Ellett et al., 2005; Gilbertson et al, 2011; Society of Pediatric Nurses Clinical Practice Committee et al., 2011).

Visual Inspection of Aspirate

- Visual inspection is less accurate than pH to confirm placement. Aspirate colors are specific to the intended placement location. Gastric contents are clear, off-white, or tan or may be brown-tinged if blood is present. Respiratory secretions may look the same. Intestinal contents are often bile stained, light to dark yellow, or greenish-brown (Society of Pediatric Nurses Clinical Practice Committee et al., 2011).

Enzyme Testing

- Aspirate testing of enzyme levels for bilirubin, pepsin, and trypsin is highly accurate but limited to laboratory assessment (Ellett et al., 2005; Fernandez et al., 2010).

Carbon Dioxide Monitoring

- Carbon dioxide (CO_2) monitoring (capnography or colorimetric capnometry) is as reliable as radiograph for confirmation of gastrointestinal (GI) versus respiratory placement of NG tubes but cannot distinguish between gastric and duodenal placement (Erzincanli et al., 2017; Heidarzadi et al., 2020).

Gastric Auscultation

- Auscultation as a verification tool is not reliable and should not be used without additional methods (Boeykens et al., 2014).
- Although evidence shows auscultation alone is not a reliable confirmatory test, it is still widely used by nurses for evaluation of enteral tube placement (Bourgault et al., 2015; Lyman et al., 2016; Metheny et al., 2012; Northington et al., 2017).
- Using aspirate and nonaspirate NG tube placement verification methods in combination increase the likelihood of accurate NG tube placement to 97% to 99%, similar to the chest radiography gold standard of 99% (Ellett et al., 2005; Society of Pediatric Nurses Clinical Practice Committee et al., 2011).

Electromagnetic Device

- An electromagnetic tracing device demonstrated more than 94% accuracy in enteral feeding tubes in a study of both adults and children (Powers et al., 2018); however, the device requires special training and considerable expertise for proper use (Metheny and Meert, 2017) and cannot detect enteral tubes smaller than 8 French (Bourgault et al., 2015; Bryant et al., 2015).

Apply the Evidence: Nursing Implications

- There is **good evidence** with **strong recommendations** (Guyatt et al., 2008) that a combination of verification methods to confirm NG tube placement will reduce the required number of x-rays in children (Society of Pediatric Nurses Clinical Practice Committee et al., 2011). These methods include pH testing and visual inspection of the pH aspirate. There is also good evidence that improving the accuracy of predicting NG tube length before insertion will enhance the precision of successful NG tube placement. Auscultation is used in combination with other NG tube verification methods. Further investigation of additional noninvasive, user-friendly, portable verification methods, including ultrasound and electromagnetic tracer, is warranted (Irving et al., 2018; Powers et al., 2011).

References

Beckstrand J, Cirgin Ellett ML, McDaniel A. Predicting the internal distance to the stomach for positioning nasogastric and orogastric feeding tubes in children. *J Adv Nurs.* 2007;59:274–289.

Boeykens K, Steeman E, Duysburgh I. Reliability of pH measurement and the auscultatory method to confirm the position of a nasogastric tube. *Int J Nurs Stud.* 2014;51:1427–1433.

Bourgault AM, Heath J, Hooper V, et al. Methods used by critical care nurses to verify feeding tube placement in clinical practice. *Critical Care Nurse.* 2015;35(1):e1–e7.

Bryant V, Phang J, Abrams K. Verifying placement of small-bore feeding tubes: electromagnetic device images versus abdominal radiographs. *Am J Crit Care.* 2015;24:525–530.

Ellett ML, Croffie JM, Cohen MD, et al. Gastric tube placement in young children. *Clin Nurs Res.* 2005;14(3):238–252.

Emergency Nurses Association. Clinical practice guideline: gastric tube placement verification. *J Emerg Nurs.* 2019;45(3):306.e1–306.e19.

Erzincanli S, Zaybak A, Guler A. Investigation of the efficacy of colorimetric capnometry method used to verify the correct placement of the nasogastric tube. *Intens Crit Care Nurs.* 2017;38:46–52.

Fernandez RS, Chau JP, Thompson DR, et al. Accuracy of biochemical markers for predicting nasogastric tube placement in adults—a systematic review of diagnostic studies. *Int J Nursing Stud.* 2010;47(8):1037–1046.

Gilbertson HR, Rogers EJ, Ukoumunne OC. Determination of a practical pH cutoff level for reliable confirmation of nasogastric tube placement. *J Parent Enteral Nutr.* 2011;35(4):540–544.

Guyatt GH, Oxman AD, Vist GE, et al. GRADE: an emerging consensus on rating quality of evidence and strength of recommendations. *Br Med J.* 2008;336(7650):924–926.

Heidarzadi E, Jalali R, Hemmatpoor B, et al. The comparison of capnography and epigastric auscultation to assess the accuracy of nasogastric tube placement in intensive care unit patients. *BMC Gastroenterol.* 2020;20(1):196.

Irving SY, Rempel G, Lyman B, et al. Pediatric nasogastric tube placement and verification: best practice recommendations from the NOVEL project. *Nutr Clin Pract.* 2018;33(6):921–927.

Lyman B, Kemper C, Northington L, et al. Use of temporary enteral access devices in hospitalized neonatal and pediatric patients in the United States. *J Parent Enteral Nutr.* 2016;40(4):574–580.

Metheny NA, Meert KL. Update on effectiveness of an electromagnetic feeding tube-placement device in detecting respiratory placements. *Am J Crit Care.* 2017;26:157–161.

Metheny NA, Stewart BJ, Mills AC. Blind insertion of feeding tubes in intensive care units: a national survey. *Am J Crit Care.* 2012;21(5):352–360.

Ni MZ, Huddy JR, Priest OH, et al. Selecting pH cut-offs for the safe verification of nasogastric feeding tube placement: a decision analytical modelling approach. *BMJ Open.* 2017;7(11):e018128.

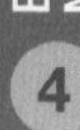

EVIDENCE-BASED PRACTICE—cont'd

Northington L, Lyman B, Guenter P, et al. Current practices in home management of nasogastric tube placement in pediatric patients: a survey of parents and homecare providers. *J Pediatr Nurs.* 2017;33:46–53.

Nyqvist KH, Sorell A, Ewald U. Litmus tests for verification of feeding tube location in infants: evaluation of their clinical use. *J Clin Nurs.* 2005;14(4):486–495.

Powers J, Luebbehusen M, Aguirre L, et al. Improved safety and efficacy of small-bore feeding tube confirmation using an electromagnetic placement device. *Nutr Clin Pract.* 2018;33(2):268–273.

Powers J, Luebbehusen M, Spitzer T, et al. Verification of an electromagnetic device compared with abdominal radiograph to predict accuracy of feeding tube placement. *J Parenter Enteral Nutr.* 2011;35(4):535–539.

Society of Pediatric Nurses Clinical Practice Committee, Society of Pediatric Nurses Research Committee, Longo MA. Best evidence: nasogastric tube placement verification. *J Pediatr Nurs.* 2011;26(4):373–376.

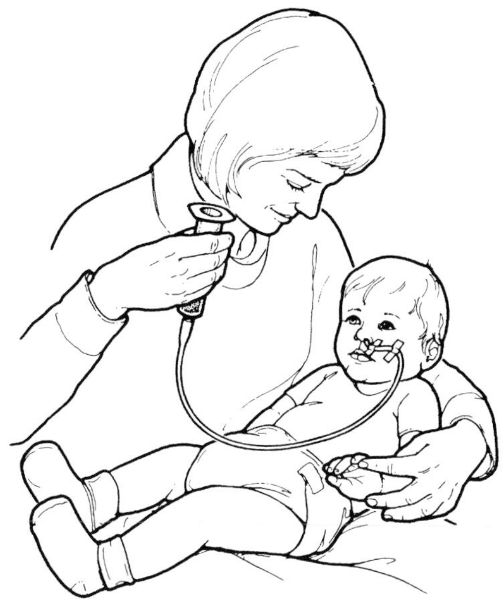

FIG. **4.22** Tube securement.

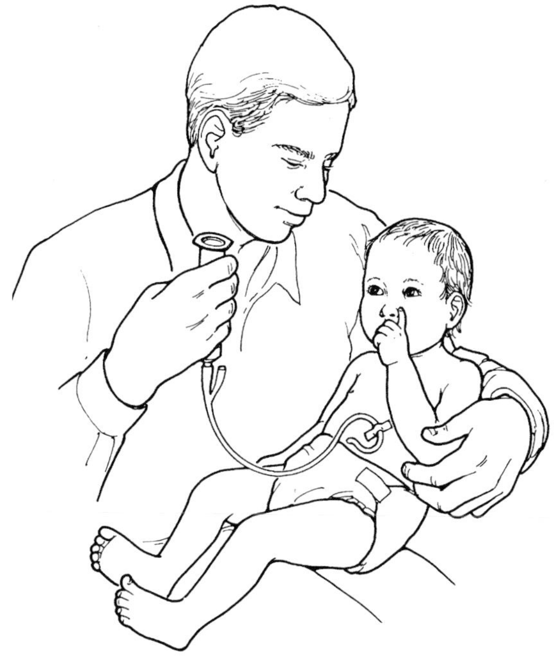

FIG. **4.23** Comforting child during feeding.

Procedure: Feeding through the Tube

1. Verify placement of the tube.
2. Check residual. For most infant feedings, any amount of residual fluid aspirated from the stomach is refed to prevent electrolyte imbalance, and the amount is subtracted from the prescribed amount of feeding. For example, if the infant is to receive 30 and 10 mL is aspirated from the stomach before the feeding, the 10 mL of aspirated stomach contents is refed along with 20 mL of feeding. Another method can be used in children. If residual fluid is more than one-fourth of the last feeding, return the aspirate and recheck in 30 to 60 minutes. When residual fluid is less than one-fourth of the last feeding, give the scheduled feeding. If large amounts of aspirated fluid persist and the child is due for another feeding, notify the practitioner.
3. Warm the formula to room temperature. Do not microwave.
4. Provide a pacifier for infants to suck on during the feeding. Whenever possible, hold the infant or young child during the feeding to associate the comfort of physical contact with the procedure (Fig. 4.23). When this is not possible, place the infant or child supine or slightly toward the right side with head and chest slightly elevated.
   - Use a folded blanket under the head and shoulders for infants and a pillow for small children.
   - Raise the head of the bed for larger children.
   - If possible, allow infant to suck on a pacifier during feeding for association of suck and satiation (feeling satisfied).
5. For feedings delivered by mechanical pump, pour formula into bag or syringe, and prime tubing. Connect to patient and set desired rate.
6. For gravity feedings via syringe, pour formula into the barrel of the syringe attached to the feeding tube. To start the flow, give a gentle push with the plunger, but then remove the plunger and allow the fluid to flow into the stomach by gravity. To prevent nausea and regurgitation, the rate of flow should not exceed 5 mL every 5 to 10 minutes in preterm and very small infants and 10 mL/min in older infants and children. The rate is determined by the diameter of the tubing and the height of the reservoir containing the feeding. The rate is regulated by adjusting the height of the syringe. A typical feeding may take 15 to 30 minutes to complete.
7. Flush the tube with sterile water: 1 or 2 mL for small tubes; 5 to 15 mL or more for large ones.

8. Cap or clamp indwelling tubes to prevent loss of feeding. If the tube is to be removed, first pinch it firmly to prevent escape of fluid as the tube is withdrawn, then withdraw the tube quickly.
9. Position the child with the head elevated about 30 to 45 degrees or on the right side for 30 to 60 minutes in the same manner as following any infant feeding to minimize the possibility of regurgitation and aspiration. If the child's condition permits, bubble the youngster after the feeding.
10. Record the feeding, including the type and amount of residual, the type and amount of formula, and the manner in which it was tolerated. For most infant feedings, any amount of residual fluid aspirated from the stomach is refed to prevent electrolyte imbalance. The amount is subtracted from the prescribed amount of feeding. For example, if the infant or child is to receive 30 mL, and 10 mL is aspirated from the stomach before the feeding, the 10 mL of aspirated stomach contents are refed, plus 20 mL of feeding. Another method in children is that if residual is more than one-fourth of the last feeding, then aspirate is returned and rechecked in 30 to 60 minutes. When residual is less than one-fourth of last feeding, give scheduled feeding. If high aspirates persist and the child is due for another feeding, notify the practitioner.
11. Between feedings, give infants pacifiers to satisfy oral needs.

Nasoduodenal and Nasojejunal Tubes

Children at high risk for regurgitation or aspiration such as those with gastroparesis, mechanical ventilation, or brain injuries may require placement of a postpyloric feeding tube. Insertion of a nasoduodenal or nasojejunal tube is done by a trained practitioner because of the risk of misplacement and the potential for perforation in tubes requiring a stylet. Accurate placement is verified by radiography. Small-bore tubes may easily clog. Flush tube when feeding is interrupted, before and after medication administration, and routinely every 4 hours or as directed by institutional policy. Tube replacement should be considered monthly to ensure optimal tube patency.

Feeding Procedure

Continuous feedings are delivered by mechanical pump to regulate volume and rate. Bolus feeds are contraindicated. Tube displacement is suspected in the child showing signs of feeding intolerance such as vomiting. Stop feedings and notify the practitioner.

Gastrostomy Tubes

The gastrostomy tube is placed with the patient under general anesthesia or percutaneously using an endoscope with the patient under local anesthesia (typically known as percutaneous endoscopic gastrostomy [PEG]). The tube can be a Foley, skin-level wing tip, or mushroom catheter G-button. Skin-level/G-button devices are cosmetically pleasing in appearance (Fig. 4.24), afford increased comfort and mobility to the child, are easy to care for, are fully immersible in water, and have a one-way valve that minimizes reflux and eliminates the need for clamping. Gastrostomy tubes need to be changed periodically.

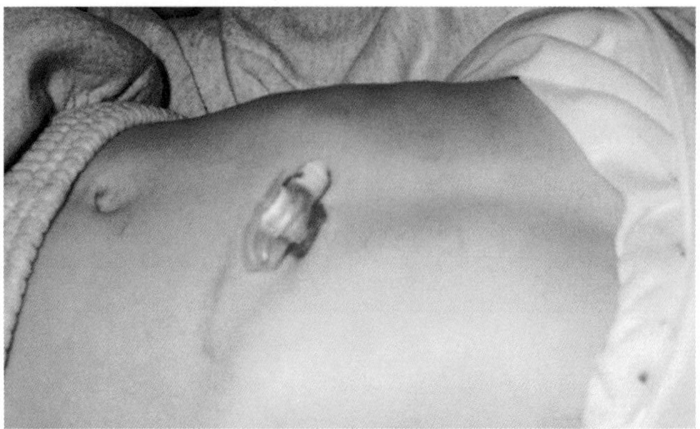

FIG. **4.24** Example of skin-level device (G-button).

To prevent tube clogging, medication tablets should be crushed well and mixed with water or food before instillation. Thick liquids can be mixed with warm water to make them thinner. Periodically, flush devices used for continuous feedings with 5 to 10 mL water.

Clean the skin around the gastrostomy each day with mild soap and water. G-buttons should be turned around in a complete circle to ensure that they are clean and without encrusted formula. Small amounts of leakage (less than 5 mL) may occur upon occasion; continual leaking, leaking large amounts, or skin breakdown around the site should be reported. Skin barriers may be used. Balloon inflation should be checked weekly to ensure that the correct amount of water is in the balloon. Dress the child in loose-fitting clothing that does not press the gastrostomy tube against the skin. Bib-type overalls cover the tube, making it less likely that the child or other children will play with the tube.

Feeding Procedure

Positioning and feeding of water, formula, and pureed foods are carried out in the same manner and rate as NG feedings. A mechanical pump may be used to regulate the volume and rate of feeding. With some skin-level devices that do not lock, the child must remain fairly still, because the tubing may easily disconnect from the device if the child moves. Some devices require a tube other than the feeding tube to be used for stomach decompression; some do not. After feedings, the infant or child is positioned on the right side or in the Fowler position; the tube may be clamped or left open between feedings, depending on the child's condition.

If the skin-level device is used, insert the extension tube (or decompression tube, in some devices) to remove air in the stomach. This will reduce leaking.

If a Foley catheter is used as the gastrostomy tube, very slight tension is applied and the tube securely taped to maintain the balloon at the gastrostomy opening. This prevents leakage of gastric contents and the tube's progression toward the pyloric sphincter, where it may occlude the stomach outlet. As a precaution, the length of the tube should be measured postoperatively and remeasured each shift to be sure it has not slipped. A mark can be made above the skin level to further ensure its placement. Tube holders are available commercially to assist with tube stabilization.

Ostomy Care Procedures

This is a brief overview of ostomy care procedures. Consult a Wound/Ostomy/Continence (WOC) nurse for more information, or see the resource list later in this chapter for additional literature.

Changing Ostomy Pouch

Materials Needed

Ostomy pouch—One- or two-piece pouches of appropriate type and size and indication (fecal ostomy versus urostomy). A urostomy pouch has a spout opening at the bottom and is appropriate for urine and liquid stool. A drainable ostomy pouch has a large opening at the bottom for thicker stool.

Ostomy closure—Disposable closure provided in box of pouches or reusable clamp to close pouch. Some pouches have a built-in closure so that no additional closure is needed.

Ostomy pattern or measuring guide and marker—This can be a paper backing from a previous pouch that was cut out or a measuring guide found in a box of pouches.

Curved ostomy scissors—Can also use manicure scissors if there is not a starter hole in the pouch wafer.

Barrier paste/strips/rings—Caulking pectin barrier that fills in crevices and skin folds to flatten pouching surface or is placed around the stoma to prevent leaking. Stoma paste usually contains alcohol and may sting if skin is irritated; paste strips and rings may not contain alcohol.

Liquid skin barrier—Skin sealant or barrier wipes protect the peristomal skin from epidermal stripping by applying a clear film to the skin and may improve pouch adhesion in high humidity. Many contain alcohol and can sting denuded skin. Use an alcohol-free skin sealant for infants.

Washcloth or soft paper towel—To cleanse skin with warm water. Do not use a baby wipe to cleanse the skin because many of these contain lanolin, which interferes with the pouch adhering.

Mild soap—Use a mild soap that does not contain moisturizers, lotions, or deodorizers, which can leave a film on the skin and interfere with the pouch adhering.

Stoma powder (optional)—Apply only if peristomal skin is broken, reddened, or denuded. Dust off excess amount before pouching, leaving a thin layer of powder. May use a liquid skin barrier to pat over the powder to assist pouch to seal.

Procedure

Place child supine, and empty pouch.

If the pouch is leaking, note where the leak is coming from under the wafer.

Using a warm cloth, gently push down on the child's abdomen and pull up a corner of the pouch. Work your way circumferentially around the stoma, removing the pouch.

Discard the pouch, saving the ostomy closure if it is a plastic reusable type clamp.

Gently cleanse the peristomal skin with warm water and soap if needed. It is normal for the stoma to bleed a little when the cloth rubs against it; this does not hurt the child. Allow area to dry thoroughly.

Assess the stoma for color, edema, retraction, bleeding, and prolapse. Assess the peristomal skin to decide what additional products are needed to treat any sign of irritation.

Measure the stoma with a previous pattern or measuring guide, and place the pattern on the pouch wafer to trace. The stoma opening can be cut off-center to move the pouch away from umbilicus or an incision if needed. Do not cut beyond the cutting guide printed on the pouch wafer. The stoma's measurements may change for up to 6 weeks after surgery.

Cut out the pouch wafer, taking care to lay it over the stoma repeatedly until the wafer fits completely and easily over the stoma without more than ⅛ inch of peristomal skin exposed.

If skin is reddened or denuded, apply stoma powder to dry peristomal skin and dust off excess.

Apply a liquid skin barrier to protect peristomal skin, and let dry.

Peel pouch wafer paper, and apply barrier paste, strips, and rings directly around opening cut out for stoma. A syringe may be used to deliver the stoma paste in a thin bead closely around the opening on an infant or toddler ostomy pouch. Barrier paste and strips may also be placed directly on the child's skin to fill in deep crevices, skin folds, or problematic areas for leakage.

Turn the pouch over, and place the pouch on the skin. Ensure that the skin is clean and dry. If stool has seeped onto the skin, clean off with a moist cloth and let dry. It is helpful to apply the pouch at an angle away from the body with the opening down toward the feet if the child is in diapers. If the child is up walking, the pouch can be placed straight down or angled inward for ease in emptying between the legs into the toilet.

Press the wafer down around the stoma to ensure that it is sealed, and place your hand over the wafer for 1 to 2 minutes to warm it and allow it to melt into the skin. The pouch can also be warmed between the hands before peeling off the paper backing and applying.

Apply the pouch closure, and put supplies away. If using a disposable bendable closure, wrap pouch end around the closure three or four times and bend the ends tightly. If using a plastic reusable clamp, fold end of pouch one time over the smooth end of the clip and snap closed. Save new paper pattern from pouch wafer if needed.

Pouching Tips

Empty the child's pouch when it is ⅓ to ½ full to prevent it from becoming too heavy and pulling off or leaking.

Choose a quiet time to change an infant's ostomy pouch, such as when the infant is sleepy, or have someone hold the infant's hands while the pouch is changed.

Release gas (flatus) build-up in pouch by opening bottom of pouch, or apply filter to pouch. If pouch gets too taut, it may pull away and leak.

Deodorizing ostomy drops and powders may be placed inside the pouch. Do not spray a nonostomy deodorizer inside the pouch, but it can be used in the room away from the child's face.

If the child has a candidal (yeast) rash around the stoma, apply an antifungal powder in place of a stoma powder. Remove pouch every 48 hours, and retreat for 7 to 10 days.

Warm soapy water may be placed inside a small squirt bottle and flushed up inside the pouch to cleanse the pouch of its contents.

Cuffing the bottom of the pouch before emptying the pouch will help keep the ends clean and free of odor. Clean the pouch ends with toilet paper or moist toilet cloths or baby wipes. The pouches are odor-proof.

Pediatric ostomy pouches are designed to adhere for 2 to 3 days. Adult ostomy pouches usually adhere for 5 to 7 days.

Incorporate the child in his or her own care as much as possible, as appropriate for age.

Measure a growing child's stoma weekly or whenever a previous pattern is no longer effective.

Urostomy pouches can be attached to a urinary collection container at night.

Bathing and Hygiene

The child can bathe with the ostomy pouch on or off. If the pouch is left on, ensure that the edges are dried thoroughly when the bathing is finished. If the pouch is taken off, soap and water will not harm the stoma. The stoma may become active during the bath, but to limit this occurrence, bathe 1 hour before or 2 hours after the child eats. Dry the skin thoroughly before replacing the pouch.

Clothing

There are no restrictions regarding types of clothing. The child can wear items that are form-fitting or loose. Tighter clothing that contains Spandex or Lycra and nylons do not harm the stoma nor hinder the stool output. Do make sure belts and elastic waistbands do not rub across the stoma. One-piece bathing suits with skirts are flattering for girls, and one-piece wetsuits work well for boys. Onesies for infants, overalls for toddlers, and one-piece sleepers keep hands away from pouches and prevent pouches from getting pulled off. Place pouch inside diaper to help keep pouch secure and prevent it from catching on clothing or getting pulled off.

Diet and Medications

There are no diet restrictions for an infant. There are no diet restrictions for an older child if he or she has a colostomy.

If an older child has an ileostomy, there are specific foods that are fibrous and difficult to digest that can cause a blockage. Instruct the child to eat slowly and chew well, cut food up into small pieces, and encourage plenty of fluids to help prevent blockages.

Foods that commonly cause blockages include the following:

- Raw fruits and vegetables, especially celery
- Peelings of apples and potatoes
- Meat with casing (bologna, sausage)
- Popcorn
- Seeds in fruit and vegetables
- Peanuts and other nuts

Consult a WOC nurse regarding additional information on foods that cause blockages, how to treat a blockage, and foods that cause excess gas and odors.

Children with an ileostomy are at risk of becoming dehydrated because they do not have a colon to reabsorb water back into the body. Instruct parents on signs and symptoms of dehydration that can occur from diarrhea, vomiting, or sweating and when to call the doctor or go to the emergency room. Encourage plenty of fluids that replenish sodium and potassium, such as ORSs and sports drinks.

Time-released medications may not be absorbed if the child has an ileostomy. Encourage parents to let their pharmacist know that their child has an ileostomy each time they fill a new prescription.

Activities and School

There are no activity restrictions for infants with ostomies. Infants can lie and play on their stomach and can be hugged and held against an adult without concern of harming the stoma. Keep the pouch tucked into a diaper or under clothing so it is not pulled off while the child is crawling.

All activities including swimming and playing sports are generally allowed for children after obtaining a release from the surgeon. A WOC nurse can be consulted for more information about extra protective gear (stoma cups and pouch belts) during contact sports. Waterproof ostomy tape can be used to "picture frame" the edges of the wafer for extra security when swimming or during sports.

Carry extra pouching supplies in a diaper bag, fanny pack, or small backpack, and store them in a cool, dry place. The extra supplies should include a pouch that is already cut out to fit and a plastic bag to dispose of the soiled pouch. Pouches cannot be flushed!

Encourage the family to meet with the school nurse to discuss the child's ostomy. The family should find out if there is a private bathroom at school available for the child to use if the pouch needs to be changed or emptied. Have the child keep an extra change of clothes in a backpack, a school locker, or the nurse's office for emergencies.

Discharge

Ensure that the family has information regarding how to reorder ostomy supplies once the child is discharged from the hospital. The family should reorder pouches when they open the last box so they will not run out of supplies.

Family Education: When to Call for Help With a Colostomy

- Bleeding from stoma more than usual when cleaning stoma
- Bleeding from skin around stoma
- Change in bowel pattern
- Change in size of stoma
- Change in color of stoma
- Temperature above 100.4° F

Family Education: Ostomy Care

In addition to the General Principles of Family Education, families need to know the following:

- Emptying pouch
- Changing pouch
- Skin care
- Clothing
- Activities

Procedures Related to Maintaining Cardiorespiratory Function

Oxygen Therapy

Methods include the use of a mask, hood, nasal cannula, or face tent.

Method is selected on the basis of the following:

- Concentration of inspired oxygen needed
- Ability of the child to cooperate in its use

Oxygen is a drug and is administered only as prescribed by dose.

Concentration is regulated according to the needs of the child.

Oxygen is dry; therefore it must be humidified.

Use the following precautions with an oxygen hood:

- Do not allow oxygen to blow directly on the infant's face.
- Position hood to avoid rubbing against the infant's neck, chin, or shoulders.

Provide comfort and reassurance to the child. Make sure the child is able to see someone nearby.

Invasive and Noninvasive Oxygen Monitoring

An essential goal in managing sick or injured children is to ensure the continuous delivery of adequate oxygen to vital organs. Although lifesaving, oxygen therapy can cause a number of serious sequelae. To monitor oxygen therapy, blood oxygen levels are routinely measured.

Arterial Blood Gas

Direct sampling of the blood's oxygen content (measured as partial pressure of oxygen [PO2]) can be done on blood obtained from an indwelling arterial catheter or from arterial puncture (Atraumatic Care box).

ATRAUMATIC CARE

Blood Gas Monitoring

For continuous monitoring of blood gases, noninvasive measurements are used whenever possible. Oximetry should be used before arterial punctures are performed when information about O_2 saturation is sufficient to evaluate the child's condition.

Arterial blood gases may also be drawn via an umbilical arterial catheter in neonates, and a radial arterial catheter is sometimes used for blood sampling. These arterial catheters have inherent dangers, and sampling for arterial blood gases must follow stringent institutional policy to minimize complications.

Arterial Blood Gas Analysis

Subtle and extreme changes in a patient's status need evaluation by a tool that helps give the "big picture" quickly. Arterial blood gas (ABG) analysis results are rapidly available and provide a baseline to determine a patient's current respiratory and metabolic status and needs.

Interpretation of these variables allows the practitioner to assess the degree to which the patient is able to maintain the most essential of bodily functions: airway and breathing (how well the body provides oxygen to the lungs and eliminates carbon dioxide end-products) and circulation (how well the body carries that oxygen to vital end-organs). Interpretation of ABGs is directed at determining whether the blood pH value—an important determinant of how effectively cellular processes occur—has been affected by a lung problem (respiratory acidosis or alkalosis) or kidney problem (metabolic acidosis or alkalosis).

Blood gases are obtained from an artery either via arterial puncture or from an indwelling arterial line. Ice is used to preserve the blood sample for accurate analysis if it cannot be processed within 15 minutes. Delays in analysis may cause inaccuracies owing to the separation of blood cells from plasma.

Blood gas interpretation is based on assessing the arterial serum levels of the variables in Table 4.14.

Consistent Approach Is Key

In order to make an interpretation based on the individual ABG values, a consistent sequence of steps should be followed:

1. Evaluate pH to determine the presence of acidosis or alkalosis. The lungs and kidneys regulate the hydrogen ion status within the plasma. Alterations in these systems affect the acid-base balance, causing pH changes that affect multiple body systems.
   - Within normal limits (WNL) indicates normal or compensated state
   - Outside normal limits
   - Less than 7.35: Acidosis—Acidosis may cause pulmonary vasoconstriction leading to decreased pulmonary blood flow. Acidosis may also cause vasoconstriction to cerebral blood vessels.
   - Greater than 7.45: Alkalosis—Alkalosis may diminish cellular metabolism, depress myocardial function, and dilate pulmonary blood vessels.
2. Evaluate $PaCO_2$ to assess the alveolar ventilation status. In an uncompensated acidosis or alkalosis, an abnormal $PaCO_2$ level will generally indicate that origin of the pH imbalance is respiratory rather than metabolic.
   - Within normal limits—Adequate ventilation
   - Outside normal limits
     - Greater than 45: Hypercarbia—Hypoventilation leads to an increase in $PaCO_2$, which in turn lowers the pH, resulting in a respiratory acidosis.
     - Less than 30: Hypocarbia—Hyperventilation leads to decreased $PaCO_2$, which in turn raises the pH, resulting in a respiratory alkalosis.
3. Evaluate HCO_3 to assess the effectiveness of renal regulation of blood pH. In an uncompensated acidosis or alkalosis, an abnormal HCO_3 level will generally indicate that origin of the pH imbalance is metabolic rather than respiratory.
   - Within normal limits—Normal renal function
   - Outside normal limits
     - Less than 22: Decreased bicarbonate—Renal mechanisms lead to increased excretion of bicarbonate and a lower serum bicarbonate level. Owing to the absence of normal levels of bicarbonate to buffer serum H+ (acid), the pH lowers and metabolic acidosis is the result.
     - Greater than 29: Increased bicarbonate—Renal mechanisms lead to increased retention of bicarbonate. Owing to the higher levels of bicarbonate, more serum H+ (acid) is buffered, the pH increases and metabolic alkalosis is the result.
4. Look for signs of compensation—With prolonged abnormalities in pH, the body tries to return the pH to normal through respiratory compensation (adjusting $PaCO_2$ levels) or metabolic compensation (adjusting

TABLE 4.14 ABG Values for Interpretation

Interpretation	pH	$PaCO_2$	HCO_3
Normal Values	7.35–7.45	35–45	22–26
Acidosis			
Respiratory	<7.35	>45	WNL
Compensated respiratory	WNL	>45	>29
Metabolic	<7.35	WNL	<22
Compensated metabolic	WNL	<30	<22
Alkalosis			
Respiratory	>7.45	<30	WNL
Compensated respiratory	WNL	<30	<22
Metabolic	>7.45	WNL	>29
Compensated metabolic	WNL	>45	>29

WNL, Within normal limits.

HCO_3 levels). In a compensated acidosis or alkalosis, the pH will be normal, but the $PaCO_2$ and HCO_3 will both be abnormal in the same "direction" (increased or decreased). Table 4.8 may be used to assist with the differentiation of respiratory versus metabolic acid-base imbalances, including the presence of compensation.

5. Evaluate PaO_2 to assess the oxygenation status. It is important to be aware of a patient's specific "normal" values. Patients with certain cardiac or pulmonary conditions may have an "acceptable" PaO_2 that is below normal limits. Assess each patient's unique needs and treat them accordingly.
   - Within normal limits—Adequate oxygenation
   - Outside normal limits
     - 55 to 85: Mild hypoxemia
     - 40 to 55: Moderate hypoxemia
     - Less than 40: Severe hypoxemia

Pulse Oximetry

Measures arterial hemoglobin oxygen saturation (SaO_2) by passage of two different wavelengths of light through blood-perfused tissues to a photodetector. SaO_2 and heart rate are displayed on a digital readout.

Attach sensor to earlobe, finger, or toe (Fig. 4.25); make certain light source and photodetector are in opposition.

Avoid sites with restricted blood flow (e.g., distal to a blood pressure cuff or indwelling arterial catheter).

Secure sensor cord with self-adhering wrap or tape to avoid interference by patient movement. Shield sensor from bright light. Keep extremity warm (e.g., use a sock over foot or hand if extremity is cool).

Avoid IV dyes; green, purple, or black nail polish; nonopaque synthetic nails; and possibly footprint ink, which may cause erroneous readings.

Change placement of sensor every 4 to 8 hours. Inspect skin at sensor site in compromised children, and change sensor more frequently if needed to prevent pressure necrosis.

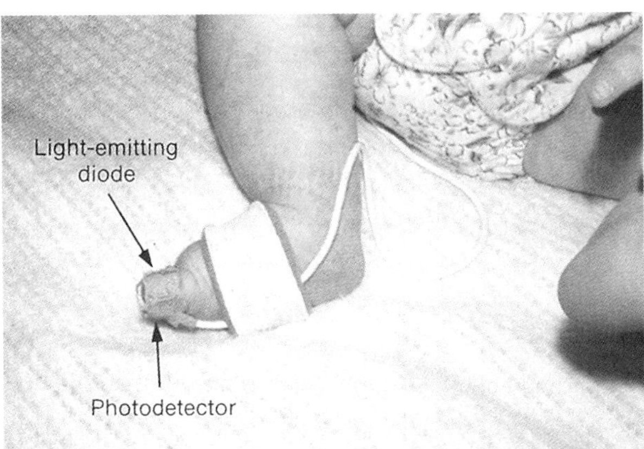

FIG. **4.25** Oximeter sensor on great toe. Note that sensor is positioned with light-emitting diode opposite photodetector. Cord is secured to foot with self-adhering band (not tape) to minimize movement of sensor.

Advantages:
- Noninvasive technique
- No complicated preparation or calibration of sensor
- No special skin care needed
- Convenient sites can be used

Disadvantages:
- Requires peripheral arterial pulsation
- Limited use in hypotension or with vasoconstricting drugs
- Sensor affected by movement (Safety Alert)

SaO_2 is related to PO_2, but the values are not the same. As a rule of thumb, an SaO_2 of:
  - 98% = PO_2 of 100 mm Hg or greater
  - 90% = PO2 of 60 mm Hg
  - 80% = PO_2 of 45 mm Hg
  - 60% = PO_2 of 30 mm Hg
- See Fig. 4.26.
- In general, normal range is 95% to 99%. A consistent SaO2 less than 95% should be investigated, and an SaO_2 of 90% signifies developing hypoxia.

SAFETY ALERT

For the Infant

Attach the sensor securely to the great toe. Do not apply additional tape to the disposable sensors because it can cause a false reading if the sensor becomes disconnected but remains unnoticed. Place a snugly fitting sock over the foot.

For the Child

Attach the sensor securely to the index finger, and tape the cable to the back of the hand.

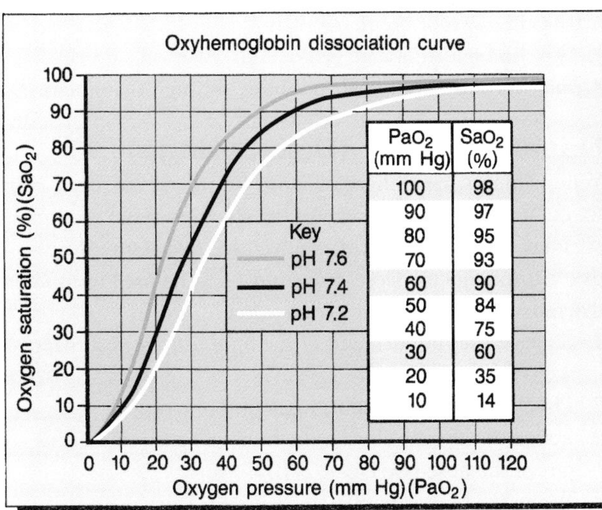

FIG. **4.26** Oxyhemoglobin dissociation curve. Changes in the affinity of hemoglobin for oxygen shift the position of the oxyhemoglobin dissociation curve. Standard curve (middle curve): Assumes normal pH (7.4), temperature, PCO2, and 2,3-DPG levels. Shift to left (left curve): Increases O2 affinity of Hb; decreased pH; and increased temperature, PCO_2, and 2,3-DPG. Shift to right (right curve): Decreases O_2 affinity of Hb; decreased pH, and increased temperature, PCO_2, and 2,3-DPG.

End-Tidal Carbon Dioxide Monitoring

End-tidal carbon dioxide (CO_2) ($ETCO_2$) monitoring measures exhaled carbon dioxide noninvasively. Capnometry provides a numeric display, and capnography provides a graph over time. Continuous capnometry is available in many bedside physiologic monitors as well as stand-alone monitors. $ETCO_2$ differs from pulse oximetry in that it is more sensitive to the mechanics of ventilation rather than oxygenation. Hypoxic episodes can be prevented through the early detection of hypoventilation, apnea, or airway obstruction.

Children who are experiencing an asthma exacerbation, receiving procedural sedation, or who are mechanically ventilated may have $ETCO_2$ monitoring. Special sampling cannulas are used for nonintubated patients, and a small device is placed between the ET tube and the ventilator tubing in intubated patients. While $ETCO_2$ monitoring is not a substitute for arterial blood gases, it does have the information of providing ventilation information continuously and noninvasively. Normal $ETCO_2$ values are 30 to 43 mm Hg, which is slightly lower than normal arterial PCO_2 of 35 to 45 mm Hg. During CPR, $ETCO_2$ values consistently less than 15 mm Hg indicate ineffective compressions or excessive ventilation. Changes in wave form and numeric display follow changes in ventilation by a very few seconds and precede changes in respiratory rate, skin color, and pulse oximetry values.

For years, disposable colorimetric $ETCO_2$ detectors have been used to assess ET tube placement. A color change with each exhaled breath when there is adequate systemic perfusion indicates that the tube is in the lungs. These devices do not provide numbers or graphic representation and do not provide the same early detection of hypoventilation as the continuous quantitative monitors.

Additional uses of $ETCO_2$ monitoring have limited supporting research. While wave form analysis does not yet have standardized nomenclature, some clinicians utilize the angles of the waveform coupled with the quantitative value of $ETCO_2$ to classify the severity of asthma exacerbations.

When there is a change in the $ETCO_2$ value or waveform, assess the patient quickly for adequate airway, breathing, and circulation. Sedated patients may be hypoventilating and need stimulation. Intubated patients may need suctioning, have self-extubated or dislodged the tube, or have equipment failure/disconnection. Asthmatic patients may have a worsening condition. Problems with the $ETCO_2$ monitoring system can include a kink in the sample line or disconnection. In general, check the patient first, then the equipment.

Suctioning

Indications for suctioning include the following:

- The child is having difficulty breathing.
- The child appears very restless.
- The child has difficulty eating or sucking.
- The child's color becomes paler.
- The child's nostrils flare (spread out).
- You hear the sound of air bubbling through the mucus.

Nasal Aspirator (Bulb Syringe)

Young infants are obligatory nose breathers and need clear nares. Young children may also benefit from nasal suctioning at times. The aspirator can remove excessive runny mucus or dry, crusted mucus. Nose drops must first be used to moisten dry mucus; saline nose drops are safest.

1. Squeeze the rounded end of the bulb to remove air (Fig. 4.27A).
2. Place the tip of the bulb snugly into one nostril.
3. Let go of the bulb slowly; the bulb will suck the mucus out of the nose (see Fig. 4.27B).
4. When the bulb is reinflated, remove it from the nose.
5. Squeeze the bulb into a tissue to get rid of the mucus.
6. Repeat steps 1 through 5 for the other side of the nose.
7. Repeat this process as often as needed to keep the nose clear.
8. When used in the home, clean the nasal aspirator by filling it with tap water. Then squeeze the bulb to remove the water and the mucus. Refill the bulb with water and boil for 10 minutes. Let the bulb cool, and squeeze out the water before using it again.

Nasopharyngeal Suctioning

Equipment

Suction regulator or machine with tubing
Suction catheters
Saline or water (cool)
Clean container for rinsing catheter

Procedure

1. Turn on the suction regulator/machine.
2. Open the suction catheter package, put on gloves, and connect the catheter to the suction regulator/machine.
3. Measure the tube for the insertion distance. Place the tip of the catheter at the child's earlobe, and mark the distance to the tip of the child's nose. Hold the catheter at this mark.
4. Wet the tip of the catheter by placing the tip of the catheter in the sterile saline, and place your thumb over the opening to obtain suction.
5. Tell the child to take a deep breath.
6. With your thumb off the opening (no suction), insert the suction catheter in one nostril up to the measured distance.
7. Place your thumb on the suction port to obtain suction.
8. Rotate or twist the catheter as you remove it with a slow steady motion. Both inserting the catheter and suctioning

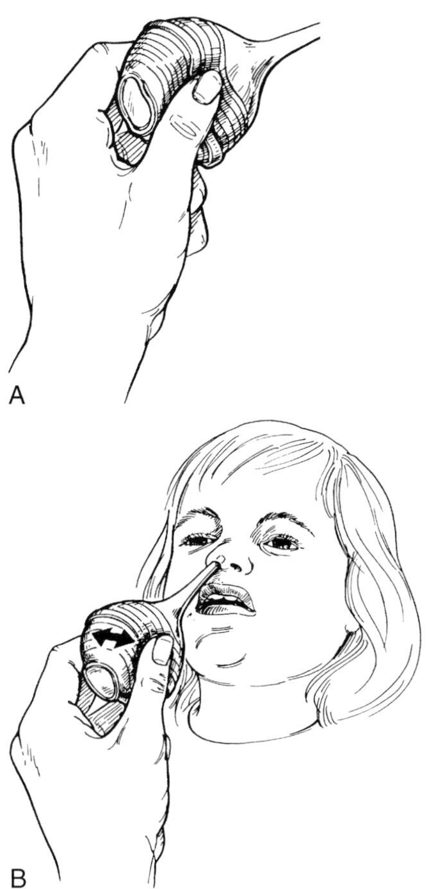

FIG. **4.27** (A) Squeezing nasal aspirator to remove air. (B) Releasing grasp to suck mucus from nose.

should take no longer than 5 seconds. Remember, the child may not breathe while you are suctioning.

9. Look at the mucus. Check the color, smell, and consistency for any change.
10. Rinse the suction catheter in sterile saline or water with your thumb on the suction port.
11. Allow the child to take a few deep breaths.
12. Repeat steps 5 through 10 up to two times if needed (for large amounts of mucus), then repeat for the other nostril.
13. After suctioning the nose, you can use the same catheter to clear the child's mouth up to three times if needed.

Tracheostomy Care

A tracheostomy is a surgical opening in the trachea between the second and fourth tracheal rings (Fig. 4.28). Congenital or acquired structural defects, such as subglottic stenosis, tracheomalacia, and vocal cord paralysis, account for many long-term tracheostomies. A tracheostomy may be required in an emergency situation for epiglottitis, croup, or foreign body aspiration. These tracheostomies remain in place for a short time. An infant or child requiring long-term ventilatory support may also have a tracheostomy.

Pediatric tracheostomy tubes are usually made of plastic or Silastic (Fig. 4.29). The most common types are the Hollinger, Jackson, Aberdeen, and Shiley tubes. These tubes are constructed with a more acute angle than adult tubes, and they soften at body temperature, conforming to the contours of the trachea. Because these materials resist the formation of crusted respiratory secretions, they are made without an inner cannula. Some children require a metal tracheostomy tube (usually made of sterling silver or stainless steel), which contains an inner cannula. The principal advantages of metal tubes are their nonreactivity and decreased chance of an allergic reaction. Tracheostomy tubes are secured using either a Velcro tube holder or twill tape ties; twill tape is more prone to abrading the neck and takes longer to secure.

Tracheostomy Suctioning

The practice of instilling sterile saline in the tracheostomy tube before suctioning is not supported by research and is no longer recommended by many institutions. Suctioning should require no more than 5 seconds. Counting 1, one thousand, 2, one thousand, 3, one thousand, and so on while suctioning is a simple means of monitoring the time. Without a safeguard, the airway may be obstructed for too long. Hyperventilating

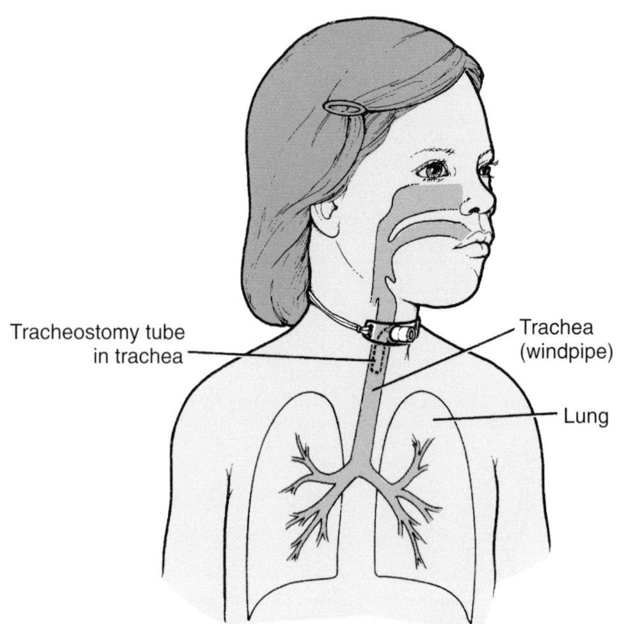

FIG. **4.28** Secured tracheostomy tube.

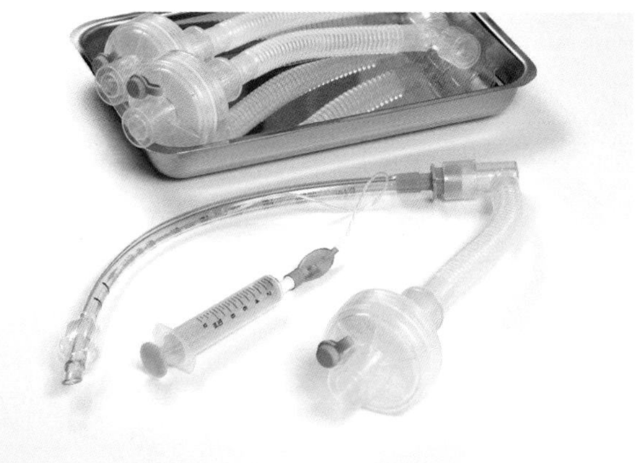

FIG. **4.29** Pediatric tracheostomy tube and obturator.

the child with 100% O_2 before and after suctioning (using a bag-valve-mask or increasing the FiO_2 ventilator setting) is also performed to prevent hypoxia. Closed tracheal suctioning systems that allow for uninterrupted O_2 delivery may also be used. In a closed suction system, a suction catheter is directly attached to the ventilator tubing. This system has several advantages. First, there is no need to disconnect the patient from the ventilator, which allows for better oxygenation. Second, the suction catheter is enclosed in a plastic sheath, which reduces the risk of exposure to the patient's secretions.

In the acute care setting, aseptic technique is used during care of the tracheostomy. Secondary infection is a major concern because the air entering the lower airway bypasses the natural defenses of the upper airway. Standard Precautions are recommended, and the nurse should wear gloves during the suctioning procedure, although a sterile glove is needed only on the hand touching the catheter. It is recommended that the nurse follows institution protocols for the use of nonsterile and sterile gloves during suctioning. Use a new sterile suction catheter and sterile gloves each time in the acute care setting. In the home care setting, nonsterile gloves may be worn, and the suction catheter may be rinsed with water internally and cleansed with alcohol on the external surface.

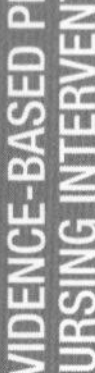

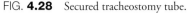

EVIDENCE-BASED PRACTICE

Translating Evidence Into Practice
Normal Saline Instillation Before Endotracheal or Tracheostomy Suctioning: Helpful or Harmful?

Ask the Question

In intubated children and those with a tracheostomy, is normal saline (NS) instillation before suctioning helpful or harmful?

Search for the Evidence

Search Strategies

All English-language literature from 1980 to 2013 was searched.

Databases Used

PubMed, Cochrane Collaboration, MDConsult, BestBETs, PedsCCM

Critically Analyze the Evidence

There is **moderate evidence** with a **strong recommendation** (Balshem et al. 2011).

- Instillation of NS before endotracheal (ET) tube suctioning has been used for years to loosen and dilute secretions, lubricate the suction catheter, and promote cough. In recent years, the possible adverse effects of this procedure have been explored. Adult historic, landmark studies have found decreased oxygen saturation, increased frequency of nosocomial pneumonia, and increased intracranial pressure after instillation of NS before suctioning (Ackerman, 1993; Ackerman and Gugerty, 1990; Bostick and Wendelgass, 1987; Hagler and Traver, 1994; Kinlock, 1999; O'Neal et al., 2001, Reynolds et al. 1990).
- Two of the first research studies evaluating the effect of NS instillation before suctioning in neonates found no deleterious effects. Shorten et al. (1991) found no significant differences in oxygenation, heart rate, or blood pressure before or after suctioning in a group of 27 intubated neonates.
- In a second study of nine neonates acting as their own controls, no adverse effects on lung mechanics were found after NS instillation and suctioning (Beeram and Dhanireddy, 1992).
- A study evaluating the effects of NS instillation before suctioning in children found results similar to those in the previously published adult studies. Ridling et al. (2003) evaluated the effects of NS instillation before suctioning in a group of 24 critically ill children, ages 10 weeks to 14 years old (level 1 evidence). A total of 104 suctioning episodes were analyzed. Children experienced significantly greater oxygen desaturation after suctioning if NS was instilled. Sedigheh and Hossein (2011) also found that instillation of NS before suctioning can cause an adverse effect on oxygen saturation. Another study by Zahran and Abd El-Razik (2011) found a significant increase in arterial carbon dioxide ($PaCO_2$) after suctioning and a reduction in oxygen tension and arterial oxygen saturation (SaO_2) 5 minutes after suctioning. The authors advocate to educate caregivers to avoid using saline to liquefy secretions

EVIDENCE-BASED PRACTICE—cont'd

before suctioning and recommend adequate hydration and humidification, as well as the use of mucolytics.

- The American Thoracic Society states that routine use of NS is not recommended and that adequate humidification should be maintained (Sherman et al., 2000).
- Gardner and Shirland (2009) evaluated 10 studies on the effects of instilling NS in intubated neonates and concluded that the evidence does not support routine instillation of NS; however, the evidence indicating the adverse effect of NS instillation is abundant. Morrow and Argent (2008) suggest that despite evidence indicating the detriment of the use of saline for suctioning in adults, evidence is lacking in the pediatric population. They conclude, however, that saline should not be routinely used for suctioning infants and children.
- Wang et al. (2017) evaluated five studies on the effects of instilling NS before suctioning in 337 intubated pediatric patients in the intensive care unit. Oxygen saturations remained significantly higher in groups without NS instillation, whereas blood pressure and heart rate did not significantly vary. Overall, the authors conclude that there is no benefit to instilling NS prior to suctioning for pediatric patients.

Apply the Evidence: Nursing Implications

- Studies support the contention that the adverse effects of NS instillation before suctioning in children are similar to those found in adults. This technique causes a significant reduction in oxygen saturation that can last up to 2 min after suctioning. The evidence does not support the use of NS instillation before ET suctioning in children.

References

Ackerman MH. The effect of saline lavage prior to suctioning. *Am J Crit Care.* 1993;2(4):326–330.

Ackerman MH, Gugerty B. The effect of normal saline bolus instillation in artificial airways. *J Soc Otorhinolaryngol Head-Neck Nurses.* 1990;8:14–17.

Balshem H, Helfand M, Schunemann HJ, et al. GRADE guidelines: rating the quality of evidence. *J Clin Epidemiol.* 2011;64(4):401–406.

Beeram MR, Dhanireddy R. Effects of saline instillation during tracheal suction on lung mechanics in newborn infants. *J Perinatol.* 1992;12(2):120–123.

Bostick J, Wendelgass ST. Normal saline instillation as part of the suctioning procedure: effects of PaO2 and amount of secretions. *Heart Lung.* 1987;16(5):532–537.

Gardner DL, Shirland L. Evidence-based guideline for suctioning the intubated neonate and infant. *Neonatal Netw.* 2009;28(5):281–302.

Hagler DA, Traver GA. Endotracheal saline and suction catheters: sources of lower airway contamination. *Am J Crit Care.* 1994;3(6):444–447.

Kinlock D. Instillation of normal saline during endotracheal suctioning: effects on mixed venous oxygen saturation. *Am J Crit Care.* 1999;8(4):231–240.

Morrow BM, Argent AC. A comprehensive review of pediatric endotracheal suctioning: effects, indications, and clinical practice. *Ped Crit Care Med.* 2008;9(5):465–477.

O'Neal PV, Grap MJ, Thompson C, et al. Level of dyspnoea experienced in mechanically ventilated adults with and without saline instillation prior to endotracheal suctioning. *Intensive Crit Care Nurs.* 2001;17(6):356–363.

Reynolds P, Hoffman LA, Schlichtig R, et al. Effects of normal saline instillation on secretion volume, dynamic compliance, and oxygen saturation (abstract). *Am Rev Respir Dis.* 1990;141:A574.

Ridling DA, Martin LD, Bratton SL. Endotracheal suctioning with or without instillation of isotonic sodium chloride in critically ill children. *Am J Crit Care.* 2003;12(3):212–219.

Sedigheh I, Hossein R. Normal saline instillation with suctioning and its effect on oxygen saturation, heart rate, and cardiac rhythm. *Int J Nurs Education.* 2011;3(1):42.

Sherman JM, Davis S, Albamonte-Petrick S, et al. Care of the child with a chronic tracheostomy. This official statement of the American Thoracic Society was adopted by the ATS Board of Directors, July 1999. *Am J Respir Crit Care Med.* 2000;161(1):297–308.

Shorten DR, Byrne PJ, Jones RL. Infant responses to saline instillations and endotracheal suctioning. *J Obstet Gynecol Neonatal Nurs.* 1991;20(6):464–469.

Wang CH, Tsai JC, Chen SF, et al. Normal saline instillation before suctioning: a meta-analysis of randomized controlled trials. *Aust Crit Care.* 2017;30(5):260–265.

Zahran EM, Abd El-Razik AA. Tracheal suctioning with versus without saline instillation. *J Am Sci.* 2011;7(8):23–32.

Suction Catheter Length

Traditional technique for suctioning ET or tracheostomy tubes recommends advancing a suction catheter into the tube until it meets resistance, then withdrawing it slightly and applying suction. However, studies indicate that this approach causes trauma to the tracheobronchial wall. This trauma can be avoided by inserting the catheter and advancing it to the premeasured depth of just to the tip (especially in infants) or no more than 0.5 cm beyond the (Fig. 4.30).

Calibrated catheters are easier to use for premeasured suctioning technique, but unmarked catheters can also be used. To measure the length for catheter insertion, place the catheter near a sample ET or tracheostomy tube (same size as child's tube), with the end of the catheter at the correct position. Grasp the catheter with a sterile-gloved hand to mark the length, and insert the catheter until the hand reaches the stoma.

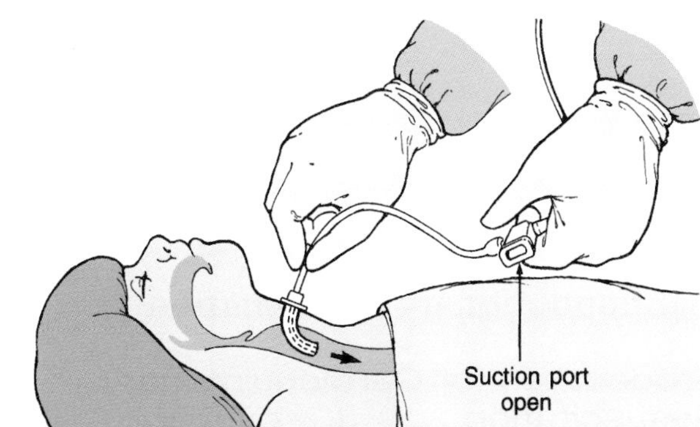

FIG. **4.30** Tracheostomy suction catheter insertion. Note that catheter is inserted just to the end of the tracheostomy tube.

Changing the Tracheostomy Tube

Tracheostomy tubes are changed monthly or when a mucus plug is suspected of obstructing airflow and cannot be cleared by suctioning.

Non-emergent changes should be done 2 to 3 hours after meals to avoid any chance of the child vomiting. Assess the skin around the tracheostomy for any redness, swelling, cuts, or bruises.

Procedure for Changing the Tracheostomy Tube

1. Place the child in an infant seat or sitting upright.
2. If the child is unable to help, have someone hold the child's arms while the tube is being changed.
3. Suction the tracheostomy until it is clear.
4. Remove the old tracheostomy tube holder or ties.

5. Remove the tracheostomy tube.
6. Quickly check the skin.
7. Quickly dip the clean tracheostomy tube in sterile saline, and shake to remove excess water.
8. Insert the clean tracheostomy tube (with or without an obturator) into the opening (stoma).
9. Remove obturator if used.
10. Secure the tracheostomy tube. If ties requiring a knot are used, change the position of the knot each time the tube or ties are changed. Make sure that the holder is snug enough to let you put only one finger underneath.
11. If you are unable to put the new tube in, reposition the child's neck, dip the tube into the saline, and try again. If you still cannot get the tube in, seek additional help. If the child is having difficulty breathing, begin rescue breathing if necessary.

Skin Care

Keep the area around the tracheostomy clean and dry to prevent skin irritation and infection. Wash the skin with soap and water, and dry well. Change the tracheostomy tube holder each day or if it becomes wet or dirty. Dressings should of a material free of lint (e.g., gauze or foam) and fenestrated (preslit); cutting the dressing will allow fraying and unraveling. Lint can be irritating to the stoma and may enter the respiratory tract. Dressings, if used, should be changed when soiled and when routine skin care is performed.

Do not apply any ointments or other medications on the skin unless specifically ordered. Barrier creams or ointments (e.g., Desitin, Vaseline, Ilex) or barrier wafers, wipes, or dressings (e.g., Cavilon No Sting barrier film, AllKare Protective Barrier Wipe, Stomahesive Skin Barrier, Coloplast Skin Barrier) can be used to protect the skin around the tube if leaking occurs.

Safety

Careful adult supervision is needed when the child is near water. Tub baths can be given, but be careful not to allow water into the tracheostomy. Swimming and boating must be avoided; however, the child can use a wading pool with supervision.

Any smoke, aerosol sprays, powder, or dust can irritate the lining of the child's trachea. Therefore the child should not be in the same room with anyone who is smoking or where aerosol sprays (e.g., hairspray, antiperspirants) are being used. Strong cleaning liquids such as ammonia are also irritating. Hair from animals that shed can clog the child's trachea. Avoid stuffed animals and toys with small parts that can be removed and put into the tracheostomy by a curious child.

All the people who provide care for the child must be aware of how to suction the tracheostomy. Anyone caring for the child alone must also know cardiopulmonary resuscitation (CPR).

Family Education: Traveling Outside the Home with a Tracheostomy

Keep the following supplies in a to-go bag that is ready at all times for when you are outside the house:

- Suction catheters, suction source, a mucus trap that can be used when the suction machine is not available
- Sterile saline
- Water-soluble lubricant
- Tracheostomy tube of current size with tube holder or ties attached, tracheostomy tube one size smaller, extra ties
- Towel or blanket for shoulder roll
- Scissors
- Ambu bag
- Emergency phone numbers, brief description of medical history

In hot, dry, or cold weather or on very windy days, wrap a handkerchief or scarf around the child's neck since inspired air is no longer warmed, moistened, or filters through the nose and mouth prior to entering the lungs.

Cardiopulmonary Resuscitation

Procedures for Cardiopulmonary Resuscitation

Methods of CPR for health care workers are discussed in Fig. 4.31. The American Heart Association (AHA, 2020), places emphasis on faster and deeper chest compression and a sequence of Chest compressions, Airway, and Breathing (C-A-B). Continuous end-tidal carbon dioxide monitoring (via a change in color, numeric value, or waveform) is recommended for confirming tracheal tube placement, monitoring the quality of CPR, and detecting spontaneous circulation. Automated external defibrillators (AEDs) are supported for infant use if a manual defibrillator is not immediately available. A summary of basic life support maneuvers for infants, children, and adults are shown in Table 4.15. Medications used during CPR in children are summarized in Table 4.16.

Airway obstruction procedures are initiated for infants and children who are awake and alert but not making any sounds or cries, appear to be choking, have a dusky color or bluish lips, have high-pitched noisy breathing, or make the choking sign of clutching the neck with both hands. Should the infant or child become unconscious, begin CPR. Each time the rescuer opens the airway, check to see if a foreign object can be visualized; if seen, attempt to remove with a finger sweep. Fig. 4.32 shows procedures for airway obstruction.

Postrescuscitation Stabilization

Preserving brain function, avoiding secondary organ injury, and treating the underlying cause are the goals of post-resuscitation care.

- Continue supplemental oxygen to maintain an arterial oxyhemoglobin saturation ≥94% but less than 100%; mechanically ventilate if significant respiratory compromise.
- Medicate for pain and agitation.
- Monitor respiratory and cardiovascular function. Continuous quantitative capnography is recommended for intubated patients.
- Replace intraosseous access (if used) with venous access.
- Maintain cardiac output with vasoactive medications.
- Brain function preservation efforts include normal ventilatory rate (not hyperventilation), aggressive seizure management, and temperature control. Therapeutic hypothermia may be considered for pediatric patients who remain unresponsive after resuscitation from cardiac arrest; fever is aggressively treated due to its adverse effects on ischemic brain injury.

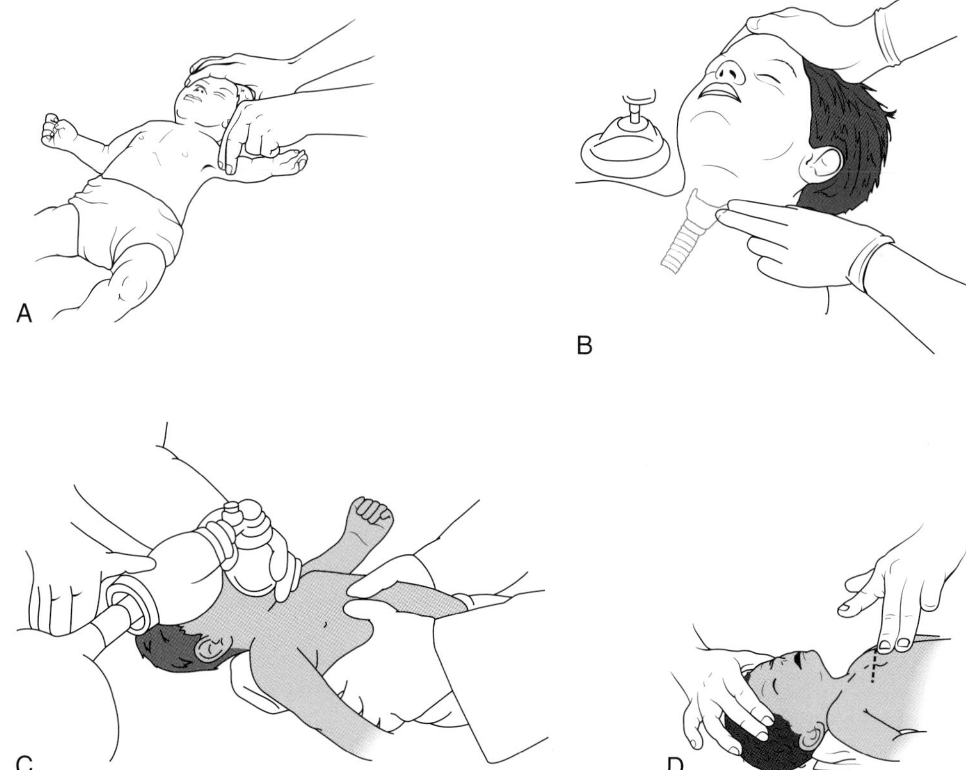

FIG. **4.31** Cardiopulmonary resuscitation guidelines. (A) Locating and palpating the brachial pulse. (B) Locating and palpating the carotid artery pulse. (C) Two-rescuer chest compression technique in infant. (D) One-rescuer chest compression technique in infant.

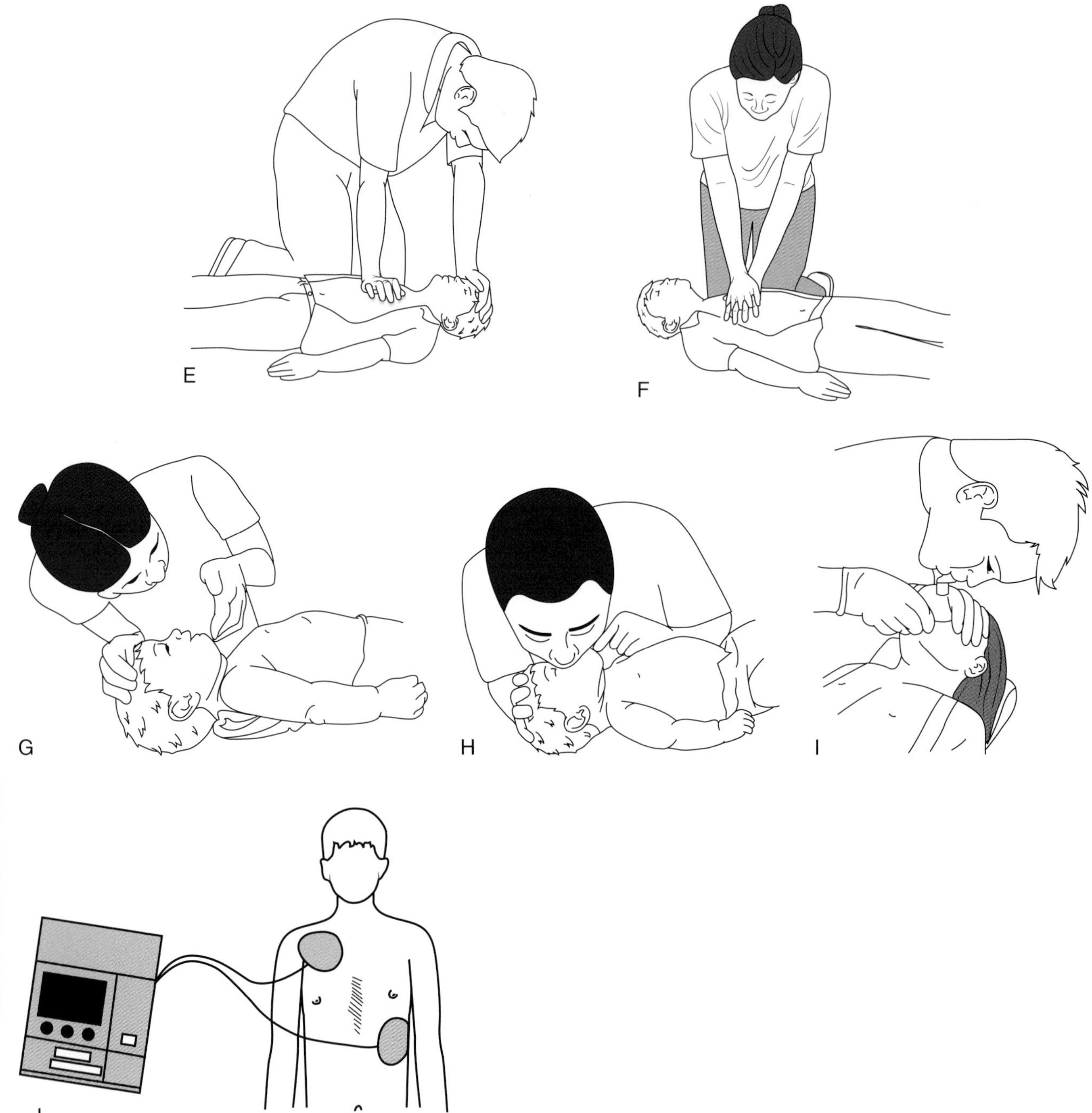

FIG. **4.31, Cont'd** (E) One-handed chest compressions in a child. (F) Two-handed chest compressions in a child or adult. (G) Open airway and check breathing. (H) Mouth-to-mouth-and-nose breathing for an infant. (I) Mouth-to-barrier breathing for child; mask covers nose and mouth. (J) Placement of the automated external defibrillator on a child.

TABLE 4.15 Summary of Basic Life Support Maneuvers for Infants, Children, and Adults [a,b,c]

Component	RECOMMENDATIONS Adults	Children	Infants
Recognition	Unresponsive (for all ages)		
	No breathing or no normal breathing (i.e., only gasping)	No breathing or only gasping	
	No pulse palpated within 10 s for all ages (HCP only)		
CPR sequence	C-A-B		
Compression rate	At least 100/min		
Compression depth	At least 2 inches (5 cm)	At least ½ AP diameter About 2 inches (5 cm)	At least AP diameter About 1½ inches (4 cm)
Chest wall recoil	Allow complete recoil between compressions HCPs rotate compressors every 2 min		
Compression interruptions	Minimize interruptions in chest compressions Attempt to limit interruptions to <10 s		
Airway	Head tilt–chin lift (HCP suspected trauma: jaw thrust)		
Compression-to-ventilation ratio (until advanced airway placed)	30:2 1 or 2 rescuers	30:2 Single rescuer 15:2 2 HCP rescuers	
Ventilations: when rescuer untrained or trained and not proficient	Compressions only		
Ventilations with advanced airway (HCP)	1 breath every 6–8 s (8–10 breaths/min) Asynchronous with chest compressions About 1 s per breath Visible chest rise		
Defibrillation	Attach and use AED as soon as available. Minimize interruptions in chest compressions before and after shock; resume CPR beginning with compressions immediately after each shock.		

[a]From Highlights of the 2020 American Heart Association guidelines for CPR and ECC available at https://professional.heart.org/en/guidelines-and-statements/guidelines-and-statements-search.
[b]Excluding the newly born, in whom the etiology of an arrest is nearly always asphyxial.
[c]Newborn/neonatal information not included.
AED, Automated external defibrillator; *AP*, anterior-posterior; *CPR*, cardiopulmonary resuscitation; *HCP*, healthcare provider.
From the American Heart Association. *2020 Guidelines for Pediatric Basic and Advanced life Support.* Dallas, TX: American Heart Association.

TABLE 4.16 Drugs for Pediatric Cardiopulmonary Resuscitation

Drug and Dose	Action	Implication
Epinephrine HCl[a] IV/IO: 0.01 mg/kg (1:10,000) Maximum single dose: 1 mg Endotracheal tube (ET): 0.1 mg/kg (1:1000)	Adrenergic Acts on both alpha- and beta-receptor sites, especially heart and vascular and other smooth muscle	Most useful drug in cardiac arrest Disappears rapidly from bloodstream after injection; instill 5 mL saline after ET administration May produce renal vessel constriction and decreased urine formation
Atropine sulfate[a] 0.02 mg/kg/dose Minimum dose: 0.1 mg Maximum single dose: infants and children, 0.5 mg; adolescents, 1 mg	Anticholinergic-parasympatholytic Increases cardiac output, heart rate by blocking vagal stimulation in heart	Used to treat bradycardia caused by increased vagal tone or cholinergic drug toxicity Always provide adequate ventilation, and monitor oxygen saturation Produces pupillary dilation, which constricts with light

Continued

EVIDENCE-BASED PEDIATRIC NURSING INTERVENTIONS 4

TABLE **4.16** Drugs for Pediatric Cardiopulmonary Resuscitation—cont'd

Drug and Dose	Action	Implication
Calcium chloride 10% 20 mg/kg IV/IO 0.2 mg/kg/dose q 10 min	Electrolyte replacement Needed for maintenance of normal cardiac contractility	Not routinely recommended. Used only for hypocalcemia, calcium blocker overdose, hyperkalemia, or hypermagnesemia Administer slowly; very sclerosing; administer in central vein Incompatible with phosphate solutions
Lidocaine HCl[a] 1 mg/kg/dose	Antidysrhythmic Inhibits nerve impulses from sensory nerves	Used for ventricular arrhythmias only
Amiodarone IV: 5 mg/kg over 30 min followed by continuous infusion Start at 5 mcg/kg/min May increase to maximum 10 mcg/kg/min	Antidysrhythmic agent Inhibits adrenergic stimulation; prolongs action potential and refractory period in myocardial tissues; decreased atrioventricular (AV) conduction and sinus node function	Recommended as first choice for shock-refractory or recurrent ventricular fibrillation or pulseless ventricular tachycardia Contraindicated in severe sinus node dysfunction, marked sinus bradycardia, second- and third-degree AV block Monitor ECG and blood pressure
Adenosine 0.1–0.2 mg/kg as a rapid IV bolus Maximum single initial dose: 6–12 mg (given over 1–2 s) May repeat administration: double initial dose (maximum dose = 12 mg) Follow with ≥5 mL normal saline flush	Antidysrhythmic, for supraventricular tachycardia Causes temporary block through AV node and interrupts reentry circuits	Administer by rapid IV push followed by saline flush May cause transient bradycardia
Naloxone (Narcan)[a] 0.1 mg/kg/dose[b] May repeat q 2–3 min	Reverses respiratory arrest caused by excessive opiate administration	Evaluate level of pain after administration because analgesic effects of opioids are reversed with large doses of naloxone
Magnesium sulfate 25–50 mg/kg IV/IO Maximum: 2 g	Inhibits calcium channels and causes smooth muscle relaxation	Given by rapid IV infusion for suspected hypomagnesemia Have calcium gluconate (IV) available as antidote
Infusions		
Epinephrine HCl infusion 0.05 mcg/kg/min	Adrenergic See above	Titrated to desired hemodynamic effect
Dopamine HCl infusion 2 mcg/kg/min	Agonist Acts on alpha receptors, causing vasoconstriction Increases cardiac output	Titrated to desired hemodynamic response
Dobutamine HCl infusion 2 mcg/kg/min	Adrenergic direct-acting β_2-agonist Increases contractility and heart rate	Titrated to desired hemodynamic response Little vasoconstriction, even at high rates
Lidocaine HCl infusion 20–50 mcg/kg/min	Antidysrhythmic Increases electrical stimulation threshold of ventricle	See above Lower infusion dose used in shock

Calculate drugs on actual body weight for nonobese pediatric patients. In obese patients, use ideal body weight, estimated from length to avoid drug toxicity.
[a]These drugs may be administered via ET tube if IV/IO is not available; IV/IO is the preferred route.
[b]Dose of naloxone to reverse respiratory depression:
- Children <20 kg: 0.1 mg/kg IV or IO (maximum 2 mg per dose) except neonates¥
- Children over 20 kg: 2 mg IV or IO

(From Yin, S. Opioid intoxication in children and adolescents: Rapid overview of emergency management. Up To Date. January 4, 2023.)
ECG, Electrocardiogram; *IO,* intraosseous; *IV,* intravenous.

4 EVIDENCE-BASED PEDIATRIC NURSING INTERVENTIONS

EVIDENCE-BASED PRACTICE

Family Presence during Resuscitation of a Child

Ask the Question

Is family presence at the resuscitation of a child perceived by the family and medical team as a positive event?

Search the Evidence

Search Strategies

The literature between 2000 and 2020 was searched to obtain information regarding the presence of family members during the resuscitation of a child family member.

Databases Used

PubMed, CINAHL, Professional Organization Websites

Critically Analyze the Evidence

Grade criteria: Evidence quality moderate; recommendation strong (Moreland, 2005)

- A systematic review of the literature on parental presence during invasive procedures cardiopulmonary resuscitation (IP-CPR) published between 1995 and 2012 was conducted according to the PRISMA model (McAlvin and Carew-Lyons, 2014). Six articles met criteria for review and thematic analysis was used to summarize finding. Results were identified around key topics—being present, satisfaction with experience, and coping. With regard to being present, parents expressed desire to be present during IP-CPR. Parents reported that they should be given the option to decide about whether or not to be present; they felt that their presence was helpful to the child, themselves and medical team. Parents specifically noted physical contact with the child was valuable.

With regard to satisfaction with presence during IP-CPR, 94%–100% of parents voiced willingness to be present if circumstances led to another event. Importantly, parents they were able to advocate and participate in decision-making, and that their presence helped them understand the seriousness of their child's illness and efforts made to help their child. Lastly, parental coping was helped by being present and those who were not present reported imagining the worst, experiencing distress and uncertainty. Parents who were present had less distress and coped better after the event. The authors concluded that family presence is beneficial to parents and aids in coping.

- An observational mixed-methods study using structured interview/focus groups across three level 1 trauma centers interviewed 126 family members with 25 also participating in focus groups (O'Connell et al., 2017). Outcome measures included a family present survey, family not present survey, and family present/not present focus groups. Findings indicated that being present was positive for families. They reported providing emotional support to their child and health information to the medical team. Presence allowed families to advocate for their child, understand their conditions and provide comfort. All families believed the choice to be present or not was theirs, but contingent on their bedside behavior.
- A systematic, qualitative, integrative review (Stewart, 2019) posed the research question "what is the parents experience while present during resuscitation?" The review involved nine studies and selection, attrition and reporting bias were assessed using the Cochrane Risk of Bias tool. All studies in the review had a low risk for bias. The investigator identified four themes—conflicting emotion, need for communication and support, being physically present as comforting, and reactions to the experience. Findings demonstrated that despite the frightening and stressful experience, it is overshadowed by the intense need to be present. They understand the work of the medical team and do not want to get in the way. Lastly, even when resuscitation was not successful, parents benefited from being present in the last moments of their child's life.
- In a systematic review of the literature focused on understanding family presence during pediatric and neonatal resuscitation (Dainty et al., 2021). The PICO question for this review was 'in children with cardiac arrest, in any setting, does family presence during resuscitation result in improved patient outcomes, family-centered outcomes, and health care provider-centered outcomes. The review yielded 38 papers that employed a wide range of methodologies, making the risks of selection bias increased in the majority of articles. Findings are discussed related to parental/family experience and opinion, health care provider experience and opinion, and neonatal studies during resuscitation after birth. With regard to parental opinion, the majority of parents prefer to be offered the option to be present, as it provided comfort for the child, helped the grief process, and understand what was happening to their child. Parents in the neonatal group had more polarized views on being present, and in particular, fathers experience was unique as they were often more focused on their partner than the resuscitation. Health care provider opinions varied across studies, many voiced hypothetical concerns but had no evidence related to their concerns. Providers with more experience with family presence during resuscitation had a more positive view of the process. Lastly—differences in providers' experience were based on the stage of the providers' careers.
- An observational cohort study of 252 hospitals in the US representing 41,568 patients with cardiac arrest to assess patterns of care at hospitals with and without a Family Presence During Resuscitation (FPDR) policy (Goldberger et al., 2015). Primary outcomes included return of spontaneous circulation and survival to discharge. There were no significant differences in facilities between hospital with and without FPDR policy. There was a small, borderline significant decrease in time to defibrillation at hospitals with an FPDR policy compared to those without. Outcomes of resuscitation quality, interventions, and potential resuscitation systems errors did not differ between hospitals. These findings suggest that the presence of FPDR policies may not affect resuscitation care.
- A narrative review of critical care nurses' views on FPDR identified 12 studies that met inclusion criteria focused on critical care nurses' experiences and support of FPDR in adult and pediatric patients (Walker and Gavin, 2019). Twelve studies were identified to meet criteria for review. Analysis identified several topics related to nurses' experience with FPDR, support of FPDR, perceived effects of FPDR on resuscitation teams, the resuscitation event, and family members. The data from nurses demonstrated a negative view of FPDR and cited several concerns regarding harmful effects on the team and family. The author concludes that there was a noticeable absence of compliance with recommended guidelines and suggests development of unit protocols or policy to assist decision making.
- Lastly, a qualitative study of FPDR during team-based pediatric resuscitation simulation in a skills lab that included the presence of an actor playing the role of a distressed parent (Deacon et al., 2020). Video-recorded debriefing sessions occurred after each

Continued

EVIDENCE-BASED PRACTICE—cont'd

simulation. Seventy-four providers participated in the simulations and debriefs, revealing five factors related to FPDR in a simulation setting—resuscitation environment, affective responses, cognitive responses, behavioral responses, and team dynamics. Analysis identified concerns about parent questions during the event that affected teams attention to tasks; reported concerns related to the parent wanting to be close to the child, making the resuscitation event more difficult to handle, in addition to concerns about the parents' well-being, which led to the team recognizing the need for a team member to take on a 'parent management role. Lastly, team dynamics and closed-loop communications were challenged when the presence of the parent added additional questions that distracted the team. The author presents four recommendations based on findings—(1) creating guidelines to dedicated a support person dedicated to managing the parent at all times, (2) develop further strategies to better manage FPDR, (3) teams should be educated and trained in managing FPDR, and (4) teams should be trained ineffective overall team skills to decrease error and improve patient safety.

Tinsley et al. (2008) conducted 40 interviews of guardians or parents who were present during the child's resuscitation in a PICU. Seventy-one percent of the parents/guardians surveyed felt that their presence during the resuscitation comforted the child, while 67% of the parents/guardians expressed that their presence helped them adjust to the loss of the child. This study is unique in that all of the children resuscitated died 6 months before the interview.

The American Heart Association (Goldberger, 2015) recommends that providers offer families the option to remain with their loved one during resuscitation. Likewise, the PALS (pediatric advanced life support) Provider Manual (AHA, 2020) supports the presence of family during the child's CPR with the presence of a family support facilitator.

Summary of Findings

- Studies included in this review demonstrate that family members overwhelmingly prefer the option to choose to be with their child/family member during resuscitation
- Parents/family members that are present during resuscitation find the experience helpful in providing comfort to their child, provide important information to medical teams, help them understand what is happening to their child/family member, and feel that everything was done for their child/family member, and the experience helped with grief after a death.
- Several studies addressed provider experiences with FPDR, primarily focused on concerns for the family members during the resuscitation event, as well as the management of the resuscitation event. Based on the studies reviewed, there is no evidence to support excluding family members during a child's resuscitation
- Further research is needed to strengthen the evidence for family presence in childhood resuscitation events.

Apply the Evidence: Nursing Implications

- The presence of family at the resuscitation of a child can be beneficial for the child and family
- Giving the family the option of being present during a pediatric resuscitation may help the family be a part of the decision-making process and help achieve closure in the event of the child's death.
- Health care workers should encourage family presence during resuscitation when appropriate.
- Protocols for family presence during resuscitation should be developed and implemented in institutions where children and families are served.

References

Dainty KN, Atkins DL, Breckwoldt J, et al. Family presence during resuscitation in paediatric and neonatal cardiac arrest: a systematic review. *Resuscitation.* 2021;162:20–34. https://doi.org/10.1016/j.resuscitation.2021.01.017.

Deacon A, O'Neill T, Delaloye N, et al. A qualitative exploration of the impact of a distressed family member on pediatric resuscitation teams. *Hosp Pediatr.* 2020;10(9):758–766. https://doi.org/10.1542/hpeds.2020-0173.

Goldberger ZD, Nallamothu BK, Nichol G, et al. Policies allowing family presence during resuscitation and patterns of care during in-hospital cardiac arrest. *Circ Cardiovasc Qual Outcomes.* 2015;8(3):226–234. https://doi.org/10.1161/circoutcomes.114.001272.

McAlvin SS, Carew-Lyons A. Family presence during resuscitation and invasive procedures in pediatric critical care: a systematic review. *Am J Crit Care.* 2014;23(6):477–484; quiz 485. https://doi.org/10.4037/ajcc2014922.

Moreland P. Family presence during invasive procedures and resuscitation in the emergency department: a review of the literature. *J Emerg Nurs.* 2005;31(1):58–72.

O'Connell K, Fritzeen J, Guzzetta CE, et al. Family presence during trauma resuscitation: family members' attitudes, behaviors, and experiences. *Am J Crit Care.* 2017;26(3):229–239. https://doi.org/10.4037/ajcc2017503.

Stewart SA. Parents' experience when present during a child's resuscitation: an integrative review. *West J Nurs Res.* 2019;41(9):1282–1305. https://doi.org/10.1177/0193945918822479.

Tinsley C, Hill B, Shah J, et al. Experience of families during cardiopulmonary resuscitation in a pediatric intensive care unit. *Pediatrics.* 2008;122(4):e799–e804.

Walker W, Gavin C. Family presence during resuscitation: a narrative review of the practices and views of critical care nurses. *Intens Crit Care Nurs.* 2019;53:15–22. https://doi.org/10.1016/j.iccn.2019.04.007.

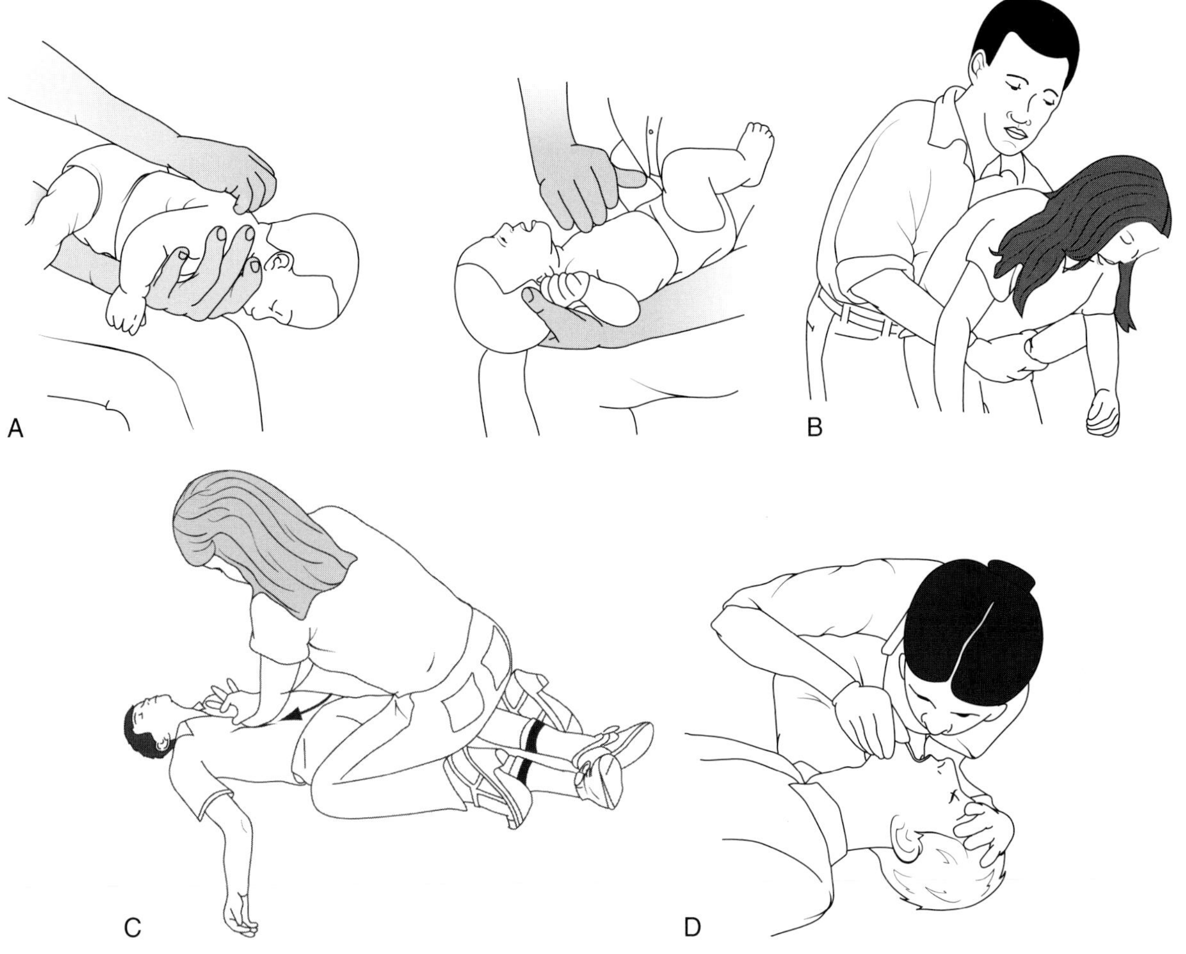

FIG. **4.32** Procedures for airway obstruction. (A) Relief of choking in the infant. Left, Back slaps. Right, Chest thrusts. (B) Abdominal thrusts in standing choking child. (C) Abdominal thrusts in supine choking child. (D) Open airway and look for object.

Intubation Procedures

Rapid Sequence Intubation

Rapid sequence intubation (RSI) is commonly performed in pediatric (and some neonatal) patients to induce an unconscious, neuromuscular blocked condition to avoid the use of positive pressure ventilation and the risk of possible aspiration (Bottor, 2009). Atropine, fentanyl, and vecuronium or rocuronium are drugs commonly used during RSI. In neonates, endotracheal intubation is often a stressful event, and hypoxia and pain are commonly associated with routine intubation; RSI in neonates may serve to prevent such adverse events (Bottor, 2009).

Indications for Intubation

Respiratory failure or arrest, agonal or gasping respirations, apnea

Upper airway obstruction

Significant increase in work of breathing, use of accessory muscles

Potential for developing partial or complete airway obstruction—respiratory effort with no breath sounds, facial trauma, and inhalation injuries

Potential for or actual loss of airway protection, increased risk for aspiration

Anticipated need for mechanical ventilation related to chest trauma, shock, increased intracranial pressure (ICP)

Hypoxemia despite supplemental oxygen

Inadequate ventilation

Intubation Procedure

Gather supplies needed for intubation.

- Suction, large bore tonsil tip or Yankauer, and sterile suction catheter
- ET tube of appropriate size plus 0.5 mm larger and 0.5 mm smaller. Length-based charts are most reliable for determining appropriate ET size. Estimation formulas for children greater than 2 years of age are as follows:
  - Uncuffed ET tube size in mm = (age in years/4) + 4
  - Cuffed ET tube size in mm = (age in years/4) + 3.5
- Stylet to fit the selected ET
- Laryngoscope and blade
- Light source (ensure that it is functioning)
- Bag and mask

- Oxygen source
- Adhesive tape and skin barrier or securement device
- End-tidal carbon dioxide detector
- NG tube and catheter tip syringe
- Gloves and eye protection for universal precautions
- Emergency CPR equipment including medications
- RSI medications

Monitor cardiac rhythm, heart rate, and pulse oximetry continuously with audible tones.

Preoxygenate with 100% oxygen using appropriately sized bag and mask.

Administer RSI medications.

- Sedative, if conscious
- Short-acting muscle relaxant
- Muscarinic anticholinergic

Assist with intubation by providing supplies and monitoring patient.

Verify placement by at least one clinical sign and at least one confirmatory technology:

- Visualization of bilateral chest expansion
- Auscultation over the epigastrium (breath sounds should not be heard) and the lung fields bilaterally in the axillary region (breath sounds should be equal and adequate)
- Water vapor in the tube (helpful; not definitive)
- Color change on end-tidal carbon dioxide detector during exhalation after at least 3 to 6 breaths or waveform/value verification with continuous capnography
- Chest radiograph

Apply protective skin barrier, and secure ET tube with tape or securement device.

Insert NG tube, and verify placement.

Ongoing Assessment

Chest rise and fall, symmetry

Bilateral breath sounds

Pulse oximetry

End-tidal carbon dioxide

Vital signs

- Heart rate too fast or too slow is a possible indication of hypoxemia, air leak, or low cardiac output.
- Hypotension or hypertension may be indicative of hypoxemia or hypovolemia.

Capillary refill and skin color

Level of consciousness

Intake and output

Blood gas

ET tube stabilization and patency

Skin integrity

If sudden deterioration of an intubated patient occurs, consider the following (DOPE):

Displacement—tube is not in trachea or has moved into a bronchus (right mainstream most common)

Obstruction—secretions or kinking of the tube

Pneumothorax—chest trauma, barotraumas, or non-compliant lung disease

Equipment failure—check oxygen source, ambu bag, and ventilator

Verify placement again during each transport and when patients are moved to different beds.

Patient Comfort and Safety Procedures

Skin Integrity

Reposition at least every 2 hours, as patient condition tolerates.

Apply a hydrocolloid barrier to protect facial cheeks.

Place gel pillows under pressure points such as occiput, heels, elbows, and shoulders.

Allow no tubes, lines, wires, or wrinkles in bedding under patient.

Provide meticulous skin care.

Comfort

Provide analgesia and sedation as needed.

Use a system for communication including sign boards, pointing, opening and closing eyes.

Provide oral care every 2 hours.

Safety

Use soft restraints if necessary to maintain a critical airway.

Continuously assess for complications:

- Tube dislodgment caused by position change, agitation, or transport
- Tube occlusion caused by excessive secretions or biting on ET tube
- Pneumothorax or other air leaks
- Equipment failure or disconnection from ventilator

Procedures to Prevent Ventilator-Associated Pneumonia

Use aggressive hand hygiene.

Provide enteral nutrition to decrease the risk of bacterial translocation.

Minimize aspiration potential with enteral feeds.

Elevate the head of the bed between 30 and 45 degrees unless contraindicated.

Routinely verify the appropriate placement of the feeding tube.

Routinely assess the patient's intestinal motility (e.g., by auscultating for bowel sounds and measuring residual gastric volume or abdominal girth), and adjust the rate and volume of enteral feeding to avoid regurgitation.

Use postpyloric (duodenal or jejunal) feeding in high-risk patients (decreased gag reflex, delayed gastric emptying, gastroesophageal reflux, severe bronchospasm).

Provide aggressive oral care every 2 hours with an approved oral care regimen.

To prevent the aspiration of pooled secretions, suction hypopharynx before suctioning the ET tube, before repositioning the ET tube, and before repositioning the patient.

- Use closed endotracheal suctioning.

- Do not instill saline.

Prevent ventilator circuits' condensate from entering ET tube or in-line medication nebulizers.
Use orotracheal or orogastric tubes to prevent nosocomial sinusitis.
If cuffed ET tubes are used, inflate them to maintain cuff pressure no greater than 20 cm H_2O.
Provide peptic ulcer prophylaxis, as ordered.
Avoid neuromuscular blockade.
Assess readiness to extubate daily.

- Underlying condition improved
- Hemodynamically stable
- Able to clear and maintain secretions
- Mechanical support no longer necessary

Extubation Procedure

Assess level of consciousness and ability to maintain a patent airway by mobilizing pulmonary secretions through effective coughing.
Maintain nothing by mouth (NPO) status 4 hours before extubation.
Preoxygenate.
Place patient in a semi-Fowler position.
Suction the ET tube and the oropharynx. Suction down to the cuff when using a cuffed ET tube.
Remove tape or ET tube securement device.
If cuff is present, deflate and ask the patient to cough if developmentally appropriate.
Remove ET tube.
Provide oxygen via facemask or nasal cannula.
Perform chest x-ray examination after extubation as ordered.
Monitor for postextubation respiratory distress, which could develop within minutes or hours after extubation:

- Unstable vital signs
- Desaturations
- Stridor
- Hoarseness
- Increased work of breathing

Pericardiocentesis

Pericardiocentesis is a procedure performed to remove the fluid of a pericardial effusion (PCE). A PCE is an accumulation of fluid in the pericardial space that surrounds the heart. Therapeutic indications for pericardiocentesis include the relief of cardiac tamponade or the prevention of cardiac compression by a moderate to large PCE. Pericardiocentesis is also performed to assist in diagnosis of neoplasms, rheumatologic conditions, and infections.

Sedatives and analgesics are administered before the procedure. The xyphoid area is prepped with antiseptic, a needle is introduced into the pericardial space by a physician, and the catheter is then placed. Pericardial fluid is aspirated via the catheter until most of the fluid has been evacuated. The catheter is then secured to the skin with sutures, and the drainage bag is attached. In emergent situations, a 60-mL Luer-Lok syringe attached to a stopcock and an 18-gauge Angiocath may be used to tap the pericardial space and aspirate fluid (Fig. 4.33).

Preparation for Procedure

Gather supplies. Many institutions stock prepackaged pericardiocentesis kits that will include the supplies needed for the procedure. Be familiar with these kits so that items not included can be obtained from floor stock supplies.

- Sterile gloves, mask, gown, and cap
- Sterile drapes and towels
- Sterile gauze (variety of sizes)
- Sterile drainage bag
- Sterile saline flush
- Sterile specimen container
- Skin antiseptic, per hospital policy
- Three- or four-way stopcock
- Luer-Lok syringes in a variety of sizes (10, 15, 30, 60 mL)
- Straight or pigtail catheter with side holes (request style and size from physician)
- 18-gauge needle (6 inches long) or 18-gauge Angiocath (physician preference)
- 1% or 2% lidocaine for local anesthesia
- Suture material (physician preference)
- Scalpel blade
- Fluid for volume resuscitation as needed
- Emergency equipment nearby

Ensure that the patient has well-functioning venous access.
Administer pain and sedation medication as ordered.
Attach patient to monitoring equipment (electrocardiogram [ECG] at a minimum).

Procedural Support

Position the patient with the head of the bed elevated 30 to 45 degrees.
Assist physician with preparation of the sterile field as directed.
Provide sterile supplies to the physician as directed.
Monitor airway, breathing, circulation, and cardiac rhythm throughout the procedure.
Send specimens to the laboratory as ordered. Ask the physician before discarding fluid.
Place dressing over catheter insertion site per hospital policy.
Obtain chest radiograph to confirm placement of catheter.

After the Procedure

Ensure that daily chest radiographs are scheduled to monitor placement of the pericardial drain.
Assess for signs and symptoms of infection around the catheter insertion site throughout the duration of pericardial drain placement.
Assess drainage for color, consistency, and quantity. If quantity of drainage significantly decreases, assess area around the insertion site for drainage.
Notify the physician of any changes in quality or quantity of drainage.

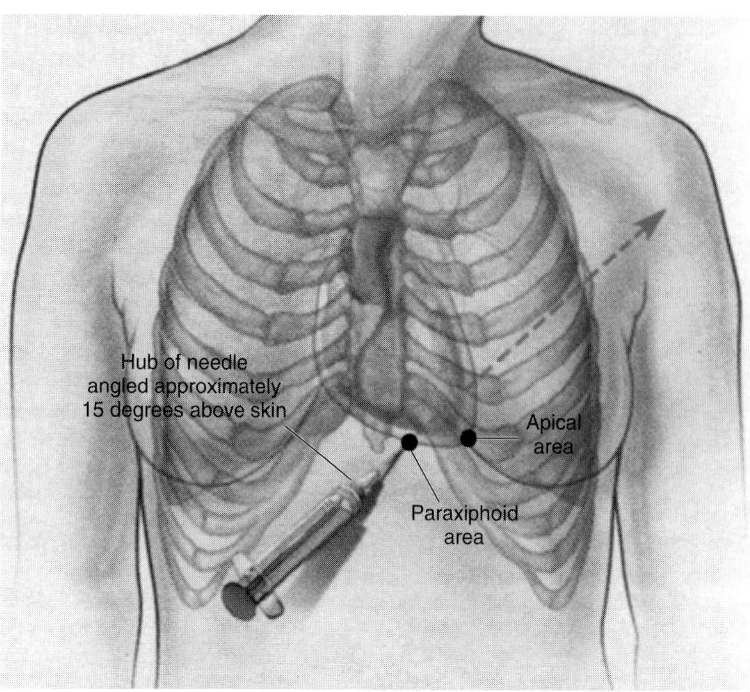

FIG. **4.33** Pericardiocentesis.

Chest Tube Procedures

A chest tube is placed to remove fluid or air from the pleural or pericardial space. Chest tube drainage systems collect air and fluid while inhibiting backflow into the pleural or pericardial space. Indications for chest tube placement include pneumothorax, hemothorax, chylothorax, empyema, pleural or PCE, and prevention of accumulation of fluid in the pleural and pericardial space after cardiothoracic surgery. Nursing responsibilities include assisting with chest tube placement, managing chest tubes, and assisting with chest tube removal.

Chest Tube Insertion

Before procedure, assess hematologic and coagulation studies for any risk of bleeding during the procedure. Notify the physician of abnormal findings.

Gather supplies.

- Appropriately sized chest tube with or without trocar, as desired by inserter
- Disposable chest drainage system (pediatric or adult size)
- Connecting tubing
- Vacuum suction
- Skin antiseptic such as chlorhexidine or povidone-iodine, per hospital policy
- Scalpel, blade, suture, needle driver, clamps
- 1% or 2% lidocaine for local anesthesia
- Selection of syringes and needles
- Tape
- Sterile gloves, mask, gown, and cap
- Sterile drapes and towels
- Sterile gauze (variety of sizes)
- Sterile specimen container
- Sterile water

Attach monitoring equipment (pulse oximeter at a minimum) to patient.

Administer pain and sedation medications as ordered.

Follow Universal Protocol for Preventing Wrong Site, Wrong Procedure, Wrong Person Surgery (Time-Out Procedure) as guided by hospital policy.

Prepare drainage system with sterile water as described in package insert (some systems may not require this step).

Monitor airway, breathing, and circulation throughout the procedure.

Once the chest tube is inserted and secured, hand the physician the drainage system tubing while keeping the open end sterile. The physician will join the chest tube to the drainage system with the patient tube connector. Secure tubing so it does not become disconnected.

If suction is required, use connection tubing to join the drainage system to a wall suction adapter, and adjust suction on drainage system as ordered (usually −10 to −20 cm H2O). There should be gentle, continuous bubbling in the suction control chamber.

Place occlusive dressing over chest tube insertion site per hospital policy. Note date, time, and your initials on the dressing. If gauze is used, use presplit gauze; "homemade" split gauze may leave loose threads in the wound.

Ensure that the drainage system is positioned below the patient's chest.

Obtain a chest radiograph to confirm placement of the chest tube. Ensure that daily chest radiographs are scheduled to monitor placement of the chest tube as well as the resolution of the pneumothorax or effusion.

Chest Drainage System Management

Disposable chest drainage systems typically consist of three chambers next to one another in one drainage unit (Fig. 4.34). The fluid collection chamber collects drainage from the patient's pleural or pericardial space. The water seal chamber is directly connected to the fluid collection chamber and acts as a one-way valve, protecting patients from air returning to the pleural or pericardial space. The suction chamber may be a dry suction or calibrated water chamber. It is connected to external vacuum suction set to the amount of suction ordered and controls the amount of suction patients experience.

Closely monitor the patient's cardiorespiratory status.

Provide adequate analgesia.

Secure the drainage system to the floor or bed.

Ensure that all connections are tight.

Keep drainage tubing free of dependent loops.

Assess for blood clots and fibrin strands in tubes with sanguineous or serosanguineous drainage, and ensure that there are no obstructions to drainage in the tube. Maintain chest tube clearance per hospital policy. Milking or stripping of chest tubes is not recommended for chest tube clearance because of the high negative intrathoracic pressure that is created. However, there are special circumstances that warrant chest tube clearance with these methods, such as maintaining chest tube patency while a patient is bleeding. Notify the physician immediately if chest tube obstruction is suspected.

Generally, chest tubes should not be clamped. However, it may be necessary to clamp a chest tube when exchanging the collection chamber or to determine the site of an air leak.

Assess the drainage in the collection chamber.

- Type (sanguineous, serosanguineous, serous, chylous, empyemic), color, amount, consistency. If there is a marked decrease in the amount of drainage, assess for drainage around the chest tube insertion site.
- Notify the physician of any changes in the quantity or quality of drainage.
- If 3 mL/kg/h or greater of sanguineous drainage occurs for 2 to 3 consecutive hours after cardiothoracic surgery, it may indicate active hemorrhaging and warrants immediate attention of the physician.
- If the collection chamber is almost full, exchange existing drainage system with a new one per manufacturer's instructions using sterile technique.

Assess the suction control chamber.

- Ensure that the prescribed amount of suction is being applied to the patient.
- Assess the water seal chamber.
- Water level is at 2 cm. If the water column is too high, the flow of air from the chest may be impeded. To lower the water column, depress the manual vent on the back of the unit until the water level reaches 2 cm. Do not depress the filtered manual vent when the suction is not functioning or connected.
- Bubbling in the water seal chamber is normal if the chest tube was placed to evacuate a pneumothorax.

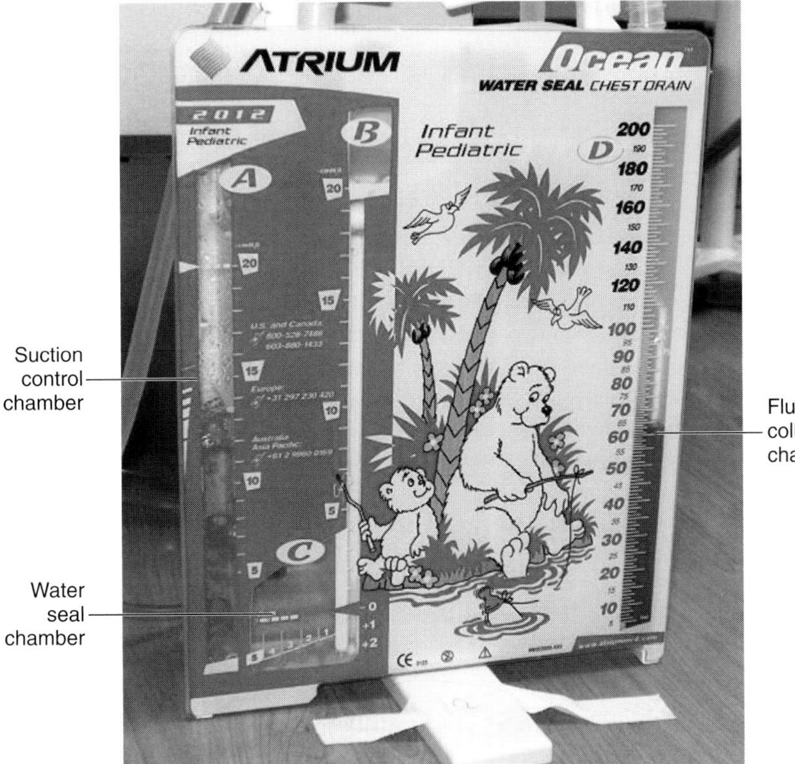

FIG. **4.34** Chest tube drainage system.

The bubbling will stop when the pneumothorax has resolved.
- If evacuation of a pneumothorax was not the indication for placement of the chest tube, bubbling in the water seal chamber may be the result of a break in the chest drainage system. Identify the break in the system by briefly clamping the system between the drainage unit and the patient. When the clamp is placed between the unit and the break in the system, the bubbling will stop. Tighten any loose connections. If the air leak is suspected to be at the patient's chest wall, notify the physician.
- Fluctuations may be seen in the water column because of changes in intrathoracic pressure. Substantial fluctuations may reflect changes in a patient's respiratory status.
- Assess and maintain the chest tube insertion site.
- Change dressing and perform site care per hospital policy. Typically a minimal, occlusive dressing is applied.
- Ensure that chest tube sutures are intact.
- Dressing should be clean, dry, and intact.
- Assess skin for signs and symptoms of infection or skin breakdown.
- Palpate for the presence of subcutaneous air.

Encourage patient ambulation. Secure chest tube drainage system to prevent chest tube dislodgment from patient or disconnection from drainage system.

Obtain samples from the chest tube per hospital infection control policy.

Prepare a syringe with a 20-gauge (or smaller) needle.

Form a temporary dependent loop, and, using aseptic technique, insert the needle at an angle into the dependent loop.

Aspirate amount of drainage required.

Chest Tube Removal

Administer additional pain medication before removal.

Gather supplies: gloves, suture removal kit, sterile gauze (2 × 2 or 4 × 4), and tape.

Assist in removal of the chest tube. The chest tube is removed on patient exhalation to prevent a pneumothorax.

Apply dressing, and perform site care per hospital policy.

Obtain a chest radiograph as ordered to confirm that a pneumothorax has not occurred after chest tube removal.

Closely monitor patient's respiratory status.

Cardioversion Procedures

Supraventricular tachycardia (SVT) is the most common tachydysrhythmia in children. SVT is a rapid, regular rhythm of over 200 beats per minute. Because cardiac output is a product of heart rate and stroke volume, prolonged SVT can cause hemodynamic compromise. Signs and symptoms of SVT in infants include irritability, poor feeding, sweating, and pallor. Older children may complain of dizziness, chest pain, or a feeling that their heart is racing.

Whenever SVT is suspected, assess the adequacy of the patient's airway and ventilatory effort. Check for a pulse. If the patient does not have a pulse or adequate respirations, proceed with CPR. If a patient does have a pulse, assess the patient's perfusion. Notify the physician if SVT is suspected. Choosing the appropriate type of treatment depends on an accurate evaluation of the patient's cardiac output and hemodynamic status.

The treatment of SVT is cardioversion, or converting an abnormal heart rhythm into a normal one. A physician should be present for all forms of cardioversion. There are three types of cardioversion:

- Mechanical refers to the use of vagal maneuvers such as ice to the face, one-sided carotid massage, or Valsalva maneuvers
- Chemical refers to the use of medications
- Electrical refers to the use of electrical energy delivered to a patient to convert the tachydysrhythmia to a normal rhythm.

If the patient has adequate perfusion, anticipate the need for a 12-lead ECG and pediatric cardiology consult (if available). Proceed with mechanical cardioversion, then chemical, if needed. Elective synchronized cardioversion may also be required.

If the patient has poor perfusion, mechanical cardioversion may be attempted but should not delay treatment. Chemical cardioversion may be attempted if reliable IV access in a large vein, such as antecubital, is immediately available. Electrical cardioversion should be employed if reliable IV access is not available or chemical cardioversion is unsuccessful. Administer sedation or analgesia before chemical or electrical cardioversion.

Mechanical Cardioversion

Administer oxygen.

Attach an ECG monitor and pulse oximeter to the patient.

Vagal maneuvers such as ice to the face, one-sided carotid massage, and the Valsalva maneuver may be attempted to cardiovert the patient.

Ice to the face is the most effective vagal maneuver. Place crushed ice in a glove or bag and apply to the patient's face for 10 to 15 seconds, being careful not to obstruct the nose or mouth. If a Valsalva maneuver is desired, one method is to have the child blow into an occluded straw.

Assess the patient's cardiac rhythm, breathing, pulse, and perfusion.

If cardioversion is unsuccessful and the patient remains stable with adequate perfusion, additional attempts at mechanical cardioversion may be considered before advancing to chemical cardioversion.

Chemical Cardioversion

Adenosine is the drug of choice for chemical conversion of SVT. It works by blocking electrical conduction through the AV node. To be effective, adenosine must be delivered rapidly because it is metabolized quickly in the bloodstream. Verapamil is an alternative in older children, but not infants, Procainamide or amiodarone may be considered for refractory SVT.

Administer oxygen.

Attach the ECG monitor component of a defibrillator to the patient. Also attach a pulse oximeter.

Check patency of IV, or start IV in large vein, such as antecubital.

Have several syringes of saline flush available.

Prepare the dose of adenosine based on the patient's weight.

Rapidly administer adenosine using two syringes connected to a T-connector or stopcock; give adenosine rapidly with one syringe, and immediately flush with 5 mL of NS with the other.

Assess the patient's cardiac rhythm, breathing, pulse, and perfusion.

Because adenosine blocks conduction through the AV node, patients may have asystole for 1 to 2 seconds after adenosine administration. Closely monitor the patient; if asystole does not resolve, proceed with CPR.

Electrical Cardioversion

Electrical cardioversion for SVT is synchronized. This means that the electrical impulses delivered to the patient are coordinated with the patient's own rhythm. This is very important because delivering electrical impulses that are not synchronized can cause the patient to develop a more dangerous dysrhythmia. Ensure that the "sync mode" is always used.

Administer oxygen, as ordered.

Attach the ECG monitor of a defibrillator to the patient. Attach a pulse oximeter to the patient.

Place appropriately sized pads or paddles on the patient.

Select the sync mode.

Set the appropriate amount of energy to be delivered. The starting dose is 0.5 to 1 joules/kg.

Deliver energy to the patient.

Assess the patient's cardiac rhythm, breathing, pulse, and perfusion.

Advance to 2 J/kg if the first dose is ineffective.

Assess the patient's cardiac rhythm, breathing, pulse, and perfusion.

Throughout all cardioversion procedures, monitor the patient's airway, breathing, and circulation. Continuously monitor the patient's heart rhythm. Intervene with CPR if warranted at any point.

Procedures Related to Maintaining Neurologic Function

Increased Intracranial Pressure Management

A neurologic pressure monitoring system is used to measure ICP. Causes of increased ICP include accidental and abusive head trauma, hydrocephalus, tumor, edema, and subarachnoid or other intracranial hemorrhage. The system may be used to alleviate increased ICP by draining cerebral spinal fluid (CSF) from the ventricular system. A decrease in cerebral oxygen delivery related to hypotension, hypoxemia, cerebral edema, intracranial hypertension, or abnormalities in cerebral blood flow may precipitate a secondary injury. General nursing care activities and environmental stimuli can present a challenge to the patient with increased ICP. If ICP is increasing, then further nursing activities should be delayed if possible. Care must be individualized based on the patient's responses. The optimal rest period is at least 1 hour between nursing care interventions.

Positioning

Maintain neutral or midline head and neck alignment.

Elevate the head of bed (HOB) 15 to 30 degrees to promote venous drainage.

Closely evaluate the effect of HOB elevation on ICP, cerebral perfusion pressure (CPP), and mean arterial pressure (MAP).

Avoid extreme hip flexion, as this can increase intraabdominal pressure and restrict movement of the diaphragm and impede respiratory effort.

Reposition the patient by using the logrolling technique.

Endotracheal Suctioning

Preoxygenate per intensive care unit (ICU) routine. Use of hyperventilation is controversial, can reduce cerebral blood flow to ischemic levels, and may cause loss of autoregulation.

Premedicate as ordered. Adequate sedation may prevent movement and coughing during suctioning and prevent decreases in CPP.

Administer lidocaine intravenously or via endotracheal tube to attenuate possible ICP increases that occur with endotracheal suctioning.

Limit each pass of the suction catheter to 10 seconds or less.

Temperature

Maintain normothermia (37°C). Core temperatures greater than 37.5°C are associated with increased cerebral metabolic rate, increased oxygen consumption, and increased ICP.

Moderate hypothermia is reserved for children with refractory intracranial hypertension that is not responsive to traditional therapies.

Sedation and Neuromuscular Blocking Agents

Use of sedatives and analgesics should be based on the patient's ICP and response to the sedation being administered. Protocols vary from institution to institution.

Cautious use of neuromuscular blocking agents is recommended. Neuromuscular assessment is altered (with the exception of pupillary response) with the use of neuromuscular blockade, sedation, and analgesia. This is an important consideration when assessing the patient's ICP response and neurologic status. Continuous electroencephalographic (EEG) monitoring may be indicated for patients at risk for seizures and receiving neuromuscular blocking agents. The risk for ventilator-acquired pneumonia is also increased with the use of neuromuscular blocking agents.

When neuromuscular blocking agents are used, sedation and analgesia should always be used.

Eye care should be implemented to prevent corneal abrasions. Polyethylene covers (e.g., Glad wrap) are most effective; ointments and drops are more effective than nothing at all.

Touch and Family Visitation

ICP does not generally increase significantly or decrease with family presence or with physical touch.

Nursing Essentials

Normal Intracranial Pressure Ranges

ICP: 0 to 15 mm Hg or 0 to 20 mm H_2O

CPP represents the pressure drop between the arterial pressure and the venous pressure. Normal CPP is not delineated in the pediatric population. The thought is that if CPP is greater than 50 mm Hg, then there is adequate cerebral perfusion; if CPP is less than 40 mm Hg, cerebral perfusion is compromised. CPP is calculated by subtracting the ICP from the MAP: CPP = MAP − ICP.

Hemodynamic Monitoring

Arterial line—necessary for consistent blood pressure monitoring and obtaining MAP for calculation of CPP.

Central venous left atrium line—necessary for monitoring of central venous pressure (CVP).

Pulmonary artery pressure monitoring—if indicated.

Patient and Family Preparation

Placement of ICP monitoring systems may be performed at the bedside or in the operating room.

Family should be aware that the patient may remain intubated for an extended period of time if the neurologic status is compromised.

Explain the monitor and the waveforms and that the patient will be continually monitored for increased ICP.

Intracranial Pressure Monitoring Systems

Fluid-coupled systems—An intraventricular catheter (IVC) is placed in the anterior horn of the lateral ventricle; this is the most accurate and reliable method of monitoring. This system allows for CSF drainage and measurement of ICP when attached to an external fluid-filled transducer (not simultaneously). Must be zeroed to atmosphere and maintained at a fixed point such as the foramen of Monroe.

Fiberoptic—Placed in intraventricular, intraparenchymal, subarachnoid, and subdural spaces. These catheters are light-sending and light-receiving systems and respond to the movement of a diaphragm at the tip of the catheter. Zeroed to atmospheric pressure just before insertion. No leveling or rezeroing is necessary because the transducer is located in the catheter tip.

Internal strain gauge or microchip transducer—Placed in intraparenchymal, subarachnoid, and subdural spaces. A miniature strain-gauge pressure sensor is positioned at the tip of the catheter; when pressure is exerted, an electrical signal is generated and pressure is measured. Catheter is zeroed to atmosphere before insertion and never rezeroed after the catheter is inserted.

External Ventricular Drain Procedures

Children with external ventricular drains (EVDs) may be hospitalized in an ICU, step-down unit, or acute care floor. EVDs are used to temporarily control ICP by draining CSF from the ventricles, most often in shunt infections, brain tumors, and intracranial bleeds. The drainage is dependent on gravity, and the level of the flow chamber determines the amount of CSF flow. Proper positioning, maintenance of patency, infection prevention, and patient monitoring are important aspects of care.

Positioning of External Ventricular Drains

Raising the flow chamber too high results in decreased CSF flow into the external reservoir and increased ICP. Positioning a flow chamber too low will result in too much drainage of CSF and potential collapse of the ventricles. The zero reference point is the foramen of Monro, usually aligned with the external auditory canal. The level of the flow chamber is prescribed by a physician. A level and measure is then used to set the collection device at the prescribed height, often 20 cm H2O. Physicians will lower a chamber to increase drainage and reduce ICP and raise the height as the patient's condition improves. The drain will be removed when normal ICPs have been sustained and a temporary condition has resolved. Internal ventriculoperitoneal shunts are placed when hydrocephaly continues, infection clears, and protein amounts are low enough to maintain shunt tubing patency.

Patency of External Ventricular Drains

Keep the tubing free from kinks. Observe for oscillation of CSF in the tubing. Do not milk or strip EVD tubing. Keep the air filter on the collection chamber dry. Change the bag when three-quarters full using aseptic technique.

Infection Prevention: External Ventricular Drain Dressing Changes

Dressings are not used by all practitioners. There is limited evidence on the infection rates of EVDs with and without the use of dressings. When dressings are used, they should be changed when damp, loose, or soiled. Report damp dressings caused by CSF leak immediately. Dressing change frequency is established by each institution.

Clamp ventriculostomy drainage system.

Allow the child to choose a position of comfort as long as head control and sterility of supplies and dressing area can be maintained.

Open sterile dressing kit using sterile technique. Prepare sterile supplies on sterile drape.

Put on clean gloves. Remove all components of the dressing.

Assess insertion site for redness, edema, drainage from site, and intact sutures.

Remove clean gloves, perform hand hygiene, and put on sterile gloves.

Clean skin around ventriculostomy insertion site. Start at the insertion site, making concentric circles around the ventriculostomy 3 inches in diameter. Conclude by cleaning the length of the tubing that was coiled, if applicable. Repeat two times.

A 1-inch antimicrobial disc may be placed around drain at insertion site.

Using forceps, place 2 × 2 split gauze on ventriculostomy with catheter between the split. Place 2 × 2 gauze over split gauze.

Carefully coil remainder of catheter, if applicable, on top of 2 × 2 gauze. Prevent pressure ulcers by padding hub of catheter with additional 2 × 2 gauze.

Place 2 × 2 gauze on top of coiled ventriculostomy tubing. Place 4-inch clear occlusive dressing on top of gauze dressing.

Remove sterile gloves.

Position the patient for comfort. Ensure that the collection chamber is at the level ordered, and unclamp ventriculostomy drainage system.

Patient Monitoring

Record CSF drainage. Report excessive drainage or a sudden cessation in drainage immediately. Document color, and report any changes in color (milky, cloudy, blood-tinged).

Monitor neurologic status including verbal, motor, and pupillary assessments hourly.

Abnormal findings include irritability, confusion, lethargy, headache, and vomiting. Changes in blood pressure (increased), heart rate (decreased), respiratory pattern (periods of apnea), and pupils (dilated, sluggish, or nonreactive) are later signs of increased ICP.

Patient Activity or Clamping of the External Ventricular Drain System

Nurses should assist the child with all position changes and ensure the proper height of the collection chamber at all times the tubing is unclamped.

Clamp for short periods of time, not to exceed 30 minutes. Clamping is generally done to allow position changes, during transport to other areas of the hospital, and during patient ambulation.

Seizure Precautions

The extent of precautions depends on type, severity, and frequency of seizures. They may include the following:

- Side rails raised when child is sleeping or resting.
- Side rails and other hard objects padded.
- Waterproof mattress or pad on bed or crib.
- Suction and oxygen set up in room.

Family Education: Safety With Seizures

- Swimming with a companion.
- Showers preferred; bathing only with close supervision.
- Use of protective helmet and padding during bicycle riding, skateboarding, or skating.
- Medical identification with child at all times.
- May not operate hazardous machinery or equipment or drive a vehicle unless seizure free for designated period (varies by state).

Pediatric Coma Rating Scale

Several scales have been devised in an attempt to standardize the description and interpretation of the degree of depressed consciousness. The most popular of these is the Glasgow Coma Scale (GCS), which consists of a three-part assessment: eye opening, verbal response, and motor response. A pediatric version incorporates developmental principles into the assessment of verbal and motor responses and can be used for infants and children age 6 months and older. In children younger than age 5 years, speech is understood to be any sound at all, even crying. A person with an unaltered level of consciousness would score the highest, 15; a score of 8 or below is generally accepted as a definition of coma; the lowest score, 3, indicates deep coma or death.

REFERENCES

American Heart Association. *American Heart Association guidelines for CPR and ECC.* Dallas, Texas: American Heart Association; 2020.

Baranoski S, Ayello E. *Wound Care Essentials: Practice Principles.* Philadelphia: Lippincott Williams & Wilkins; 2004.

Beckstrand J, Ellett MLC, McDaniel A. Predicting internal distance to the stomach for positioning NG and OG feeding tubes in children. *J Adv Nurs.* 2007;59(3):274–289.

Benbow M. Exploring the concept of moist wound healing and its application in practice. *Br J Nurs.* 2008;17(15):S4. S6, S8 passim.

Bottor L. Rapid sequence intubation in the neonate. *Adv Neonat Care.* 2009;9(3):111–117.

Bukola IM, Paula D. The Effectiveness of Distraction as Procedural Pain Management Technique in Pediatric Oncology Patients: A Meta-analysis and Systematic Review. *J Pain Symptom Manage.* 2017;54(4):589–600.

Bryant R. *Acute and Chronic Wounds: Nursing Management.* ed 2. St Louis: Elsevier; 2020.

Fernandez R, Griffiths R, Ussia C. Water for wound cleansing. *In Cochrane Database Syst Rev 2002.* 2002. Issue 4. Article No. CD003861.

Kilbane BJ. Images in emergency medicine. Knotting of a urinary catheter. *Ann Emerg Med.* 2009;53(5):e3–4.

King A, Stellar JJ, Blevins A, et al. Dressings and Products in Pediatric Wound Care. *Adv Wound Care (New Rochelle).* 2014;3(4):324–334.

Klasner AE, Luke DA, Scalzo AJ. Pediatric orogastric and nasogastric tubes: A new formula evaluated. *Ann Emerg Med.* 2002;39(3):268–272.

Kusari A, Han AM, Virgen CA, Matiz C, et al. Evidence-based skin care in preterm infants. *Pediatr Dermatol.* 2019;36(1):16–23.

Levison J, Wojtulewicz J. Adventitious knot formation complicating catheterization of the infant bladder. *J Paediatr Child Health.* 2004;40(8):493–494.

Lodha A, Ly L, Brindle M, Daneman A, et al. Intraurethral knot in a very-low-birth-weight infant: Radiological recognition, surgical management and prevention. *Pediatr Radiol.* 2005;35(7):713–716.

Moore ZEH, Cowman S. Wound cleansing for pressure ulcers. *In Cochrane Database Syst Rev.* 2005. Issue 4. Article No. CD004983.

North American Society for Pediatric Gastroenterology, Hepatology, and Nutrition. Evaluation and treatment of constipation in children: Recommendations of the North American Society for Pediatric Gastroenterology, Hepatology, and Nutrition. *J Pediatr Gastroenterol Nutr.* 2006;43(4):e1–e13.

Nuutila K, Eriksson E. Moist Wound Healing with Commonly Available Dressings. *Adv Wound Care (New Rochelle).* 2021;10(12):685–698.

Rheel E, Ickmans K, Caes L, Vervoort T. The Impact of Parental Pain-attending and Non-pain-attending Responses on Child Pain Behavior in the Context of Cancer-related Painful Procedures: The Moderating Role of Parental Self-oriented Distress. *Clin J Pain.* 2021;37(3):177–185.

Schechter NL, Zempsky WT, Cohen LL, et al. Pain reduction during pediatric immunizations: Evidence-based review and recommendations. *Pediatrics.* 2007;119(5):e1184–1198.

Turner TW. Intravesical catheter knotting: An uncommon complication of urinary catheterization. *Pediatr Emerg Care.* 2004;20(2):115–117.

Next-Generation NCLEX® Examination–Style Unfolding Case Studies

Symbol ▶ indicates material that may be photocopied and distributed to families.

Unfolding Case Studies

Care at the End of Life

Day 1, 8:00 a.m.

1. A 9-year-old boy has paravertebral fibrosarcoma of the right lumbosacral area, complicated by paraplegia, urine retention, constipation, and neuropathic pain. He has a 5-month history of progressive lower back pain and swelling and paralysis of the lower limbs. The patient received and responded well to chemotherapy and radiotherapy, with a 40% regression in his tumor. However, the patient continued to suffer severe "burning/piercing" pain in the lower extremities, especially when the limbs are moved. He continues to require oral analgesics daily and remains bedridden with weakness of the lower extremities. Because of the clinically poor response and poor long-term prognosis, a decision was made by him and his family to focus on comfort and consult palliative care. Plans are for him to be discharged on hospice care once the pain is managed.

The nursing admission assessment reveals the following results. Select the assessment findings that need further follow-up. **Select all that apply.**

A. Temperature = 98.6°F (37.0°C)
B. Blood pressure (BP) = 100/58 mmHg
C. Heart rate = 124 beats/min
D. Respirations = 16 breaths/min
E. Visual pain score 8/10
F. Persistent localized pain in the vertebrae or lumbar region
G. Burning/piercing pain in the lower extremities or neuropathic pain
H. Swelling around the lower lumbar area
I. Numbness of the lower extremities due to pressure exerted on nerves
J. Capillary refill less than 3 seconds in left finger
K. Weight = 60 lbs (27.2 kg)

Day 1, 8:30 a.m.

2. Pain is not being controlled by low-dose oral pain medications and opioids, and the plan is to begin intravenous (IV) pain medications to control his pain. Since it is unclear from the history exactly how much morphine has been given and at what intervals throughout the day, the plan is to use a standard starting dose of IV morphine.

Choose the most likely options for the information missing from the statements below by selecting from the lists of options provided.

An appropriate standard starting dose of IV morphine to administer is __________1__________. This may be given every 10 minutes for three doses until pain relief is achieved, then scheduled every __________2__________ hours.

Option 1	Option 2
1–2 mg/kg	4 h
0.1–0.2 mg/kg	15 min
0.5–1.0 mg/kg	2 h
0.1–1 mg/kg	6 h
1.0–2.0 mg/kg	10 min

Day 1, 9:15 a.m.

3. IV morphine was started, and the pain assessment revealed a score of 3/10. Because this patient is 9 years old, consideration must be given to the type of pain assessment tool that is most appropriate for a child this age. What specifically would the nurse consider when completing a pain assessment of this 9-year-old? **Select all that apply.**

A. Self-report should be used
B. Observe the child's behavior
C. Evaluate how the patient responds
D. Use an infant scale since he is in a great deal of pain
E. Use a verbal intensity scale (less, moderate, or severe pain)
F. Assess pain once a shift and do not disrupt sleep
G. If the child is in a great deal of pain, use the Wong-Baker FACES Pain Rating Scale

Day 1, 10:00 a.m.

4. The patient is resting comfortably with both parents at his side. The IV morphine dose is relieving the pain. Further discussion with the mother reveals that the child is also taking gabapentin orally due to the burning/piercing pain

in his lower extremities. She states that since starting on this medication the burning sensations have resolved. The nurse reports this to the medical team, and oral gabapentin is ordered. What potential complications are prevented by the nursing actions listed below?

Indicate which nursing action number listed in the far-left column is appropriate for the potential complication listed in the middle column. Place the number in the far-right column. Note that NOT all nursing actions will be used.

Nursing Action	Potential Complication	Nursing Action for Complication
1. Administer morphine safely. Observe the patient for excessive sedation and respiratory depression.	To reduce unfounded fears	
2. Monitor for side effects of morphine: decreased respiratory rate, urinary retention, constipation, and pruritus.	To prevent unwanted side effects that may cause additional discomfort	
3. Educate parents on the safety and effectiveness of the pain-relieving medications.	To ensure optimal pain relief	
4. Reassess the pain level after administering pain medication. Assess within 1 h of oral morphine and 30 min after IV administration.	To prevent adverse effects and overdose	
5. Recognize when pain is not well controlled on morphine.	To ensure satisfactory pain relief	
6. Provide appropriate bowel regimen and monitor urine output.		
7. Provide distraction and counseling to assure parents that everything possible is being done.		

Two Days Later, 9:00 a.m.

5. The parents and child want to go home and want to manage the pain with oral medications. Since the current dose of morphine provides adequate relief, a plan for pain management on discharge is made to switch to oral morphine. The most recent nursing assessment reveals the following:

- Temperature = 98.6°F (37°C)
- BP = 104/60 mmHg
- Heart rate = 76 beats/min
- Respirations = 16 breaths/min
- Visual pain score 2/10
- No burning/piercing pain in the lower extremities or neuropathic pain
- Swelling remains around the lower lumbar area

The nurse discusses proper administration of the pain medications at home. His regimen will include both oral morphine and gabapentin.

For each nursing action, use an X to indicate whether it was Effective (helped to meet expected quality patient outcomes) or Ineffective (did not help to meet expected quality patient outcomes)

Nursing Action	Effective	Ineffective
Assure parents that the IV morphine dose can be the same dose they administer at home.		
Instruct parents to continue around-the-clock medications at home.		
Encourage parents to communicate any signs of pain; observe patient for nonverbal signs of pain.		
A home bowel regimen should be included in the discharge teaching.		
Stress with the parents that escalating doses will not be needed, and that tolerance to pain medications never occur in children.		
Discuss appropriate nonpharmacologic options that can relieve pain.		

12:00 Noon

6. The nurse, while obtaining vital signs, notes that the patient looks more withdrawn. He no longer talks to the nursing staff and the parents answer all assessment questions. The mother also notices this and asks the nurse why her son is no longer talking to others. She states he seems to be shutting himself off from the world and wants to know if this is what children do when they are dying. The mother confides to the nurse that she is scared to take him home and asks how the hospice nurse will be of support to her during her son's last days. How would the nurse respond to her question? **Select all that apply.**
   A. "The hospice nurse will stay with you in your house until your child dies."
   B. "The hospice nurse will focus on providing comfort for your child."
   C. "The hospice nurse will keep you informed of what is happening to your child."
   D. "The hospice nurse will bring your child to the hospital if he gets worse."
   E. "The hospice nurse will focus on minimizing pain experienced by your child."
   F. "The hospice nurse will begin antibiotics if your child has fever."
   G. "The hospice nurse will answer any questions you have."

The Child With Chronic Kidney Disease

Day 1, 9:00 a.m.

1. A 9-year-old girl who has a history of chronic pyelonephritis has increased symptoms. Over the past several months, she has experienced increased fatigue and lack of appetite, is unable to participate in physical activities, and appears pale and listless. Her parents took her to the pediatrician, who on examination found signs and symptoms of weight loss, facial puffiness, bone and joint pain, and dryness of the skin. She told the pediatrician she was having headaches. With the child's history of chronic pyelonephritis, she was immediately referred to a pediatric nephrologist. The nurse in the pediatric nephrology clinic performs a complete history and physical examination and finds the following data. Select the history and physical assessment findings that require follow-up by the nurse. **Select all that apply.**
   A. Nausea
   B. Pallor
   C. Headache
   D. Facial edema
   E. Increased fatigue
   F. Pulse 90 beats/min
   G. Muscle cramps
   H. Height = 128 cm (25% for height)
   I. BP = 128/90 mmHg
   J. Weight = 55 lb (24.9 kg)
   K. Respirations = 20 breaths/min
   L. Temperature 98.4°F (36.9°C)
   M. Dryness and itchiness of the skin

Day 1, 10:00 a.m.

2. Chronic kidney disease (CKD) occurs when the diseased kidneys can no longer maintain the normal chemical structure of blood fluids, and chronic pyelonephritis can cause CKD. The pediatric nephrologist confirms that this young girl has CKD. What are the most appropriate nursing actions for a child with CKD?

Indicate which nursing action listed in the far-left column is appropriate to prevent the potential complication of CKD listed in the middle column. Indicate the nursing action number in the far-right column. Note that ONLY one nursing action can be used for each potential postoperative complication and that NOT all nursing actions will be used.

Nursing Action	Potential Complication	Nursing Action to Prevent Complication
1. Close monitoring of the patient's status. Follow clinical and laboratory findings. Blood studies included complete blood count (CBC), electrolytes, and kidney status.	Waste products accumulate	
2. Observe for evidence of accumulated waste products.	Increased excretory kidney demands	

Nursing Action	Potential Complication	Nursing Action to Prevent Complication
3. Provide dietary instructions for foods that reduce excretory demands on kidneys and provide sufficient calories and protein for growth.	Changes in kidney status go unrecognized	
4. Limit phosphorus, salt, and potassium as prescribed.	Growth failure unrecognized	
5. Monitor growth closely since short stature is a significant side effect.	Accumulation of minerals	
6. Monitor cardiovascular status, including BP measurement.	Renal bone disease	
7. Minimize renal bone disease by maintaining optimal calcium, phosphorus, intact parathyroid hormone levels, and acid–base balance.		
8. Monitor for anemia. Child may require school accommodations and rest periods due to fatigue.		
9. Identify patient and family stressors that may accompany a diagnosis of CKD.		

Thirty Days Later, 9:00 a.m.

3. A 9-year-old girl diagnosed with CKD is now being followed by a nephrology specialty team and has returned to the clinic for her monthly evaluation. The nurse performing the assessment finds Susie's BP elevated and notices the child's skin is pale and sallow in appearance. The child tells the nurse that she has been really tired lately and her headaches have returned. She also says her feet are more swollen than usual. Which **immediate** steps would be taken to further evaluate the kidney status? **Select all that apply.**
   A. Check complete blood count (CBC).
   B. Check electrolyte status.
   C. Check kidney function.
   D. Check liver function.
   E. Perform lumbar puncture.
   F. Document weight, height, and BP.
   G. Compare vital signs and weight to previous visit.
   H. Evaluate patient adherence to medication and dietary recommendations.
4. The laboratory tests are ordered, and results are found below. Which findings require immediate follow-up? **Select all that apply.**
   A. Hematocrit, 29%
   B. Hemoglobin, 9.8 gm/dL
   C. Platelets, 150,000/mm^3
   D. Potassium, 4.9 mmol/L
   E. Sodium, 139 mmol/L
   F. Phosphorus, 5.4 mmol/L
   G. Serum creatinine, 1.9 mg/dL
   H. White blood count (WBC), 8500/mm^3
   I. Blood urea nitrogen (BUN), 25 mg/dL
   J. Urinalysis, elevated protein and hematuria
   K. Glomerular function rate (GFR), 45 mL/min/1.73 m^2

Thirty Days Later, 11:00 a.m.

5. A 9-year-old girl diagnosed with CKD is now being followed by a nephrology specialty team. There is concern that the kidney status may be deteriorating based on the history and physical examination. Based on the abnormal history, physical and laboratory findings, what are the most appropriate dietary management strategies at this time? **Select all that apply.**
   A. Restrict sodium intake.
   B. Restrict foods high in sugar.
   C. Reduce foods high in calories.
   D. Limit protein to the reference daily intake for age.
   E. Reduce milk intake to correct sodium-glucose imbalance.
   F. Give oral medications to decrease creatinine gastrointestinal absorption.
   G. Provide sufficient calories and protein for growth while limiting excretory demands on the kidneys.

Thirty Days Later, 1:00 p.m.

6. The nurse is meeting with the child and family to discuss CKD and what to observe for at home. The mother confides she is extremely scared that she will miss something, and symptoms will worsen without her recognizing them. She states, "I did not even realize her BP was up and her kidneys were worse. How will I know

when they are abnormal at home?" The nurse spends time reviewing the most important concerns to look for at home. The mother and child also meet with the dietician to review important things to remember about the diet. Which statements by the mother indicate that the health teaching was effective? **Select all that apply.**

A. "My child will need to restrict her total calories each day to under 1500 a day."
B. "My child's kidneys do not work to extract wastes from her body and we have to be careful about her diet."
C. "Her protein intake will be limited to the reference daily intake for her age and outlined by the dietician."
D. "I will need to call the health care team if I notice more swelling in her arms and feet and if she develops frequent headaches at home."
E. "Frequent rest periods can help my child have more energy since she is anemic."
F. "Since her BP is elevated, I will follow the guidelines for medication administration and sodium restriction discussed with me by the dietician."

The Child With Appendicitis

Day 1, 11:00 a.m.

1. A 10-year-old girl has a 2-day history of generalized periumbilical pain and anorexia. Today she developed a fever and vomiting, so her parents took her to the clinic. On review of the history, physical examination, and laboratory results, the nurse notes the findings below. Select findings that require follow-up by the nurse. **Select all that apply.**
   A. Weight 70 lb (32 kg)
   B. Hemoglobin = 13.8 g/dL
   C. Platelets = 252,000/mm^3
   D. C-reactive protein (CRP) of 40 mg/dL
   E. Pain intensifies with any activity or deep breathing
   F. Oral temperature of 102°F (38.9°C)
   G. Pulse of 80 beats/min and BP is 108/74 mm/Hg
   H. Abdominal pain midway between the anterior superior iliac crest and umbilicus
   I. WBC count of 21,000/mm^3, 79% bands, 14% lymphocytes, 6% eosinophils

2. Based on the case presented in the question above, choose the most likely options for the information missing from the statements below by selecting from the lists of options provided. Based on the child's assessment data, the nurse determines that the laboratory findings reflect the probable presence of __________1__________. The __________2__________ is elevated and her periumbilical pain, along with other symptoms, is most likely due to __________3__________.

Options for 1	Options for 2	Options for 3
Anemia	BP of 108/74	Ruptured kidney
Pain	Pulse of 80	Acute abdomen
Bleeding	CRP	Influenza
Infection	Hemoglobin	Urinary Tract Infection
Heart failure	Platelets	Vomiting
Cancer	Serum sodium	Anxiety

Day 1, 11:30 a.m.

A 10-year-old girl who has a 2-day history of generalized periumbilical pain and anorexia. Today she developed a fever and vomiting, so her parents took her to her pediatrician. On review of the history, physical examination, and laboratory results, the nurse notes the following:

- Oral temperature of 102°F (38.9°C)
- Pulse of 80 beats/min and BP is 108/74 mm/Hg
  - Abdominal pain midway between the anterior superior iliac crest and umbilicus
- Pain intensifies with any activity or deep breathing
- WBC count of 21,000/mm^3, 79% bands, 14% lymphocytes, 6% eosinophils
- CRP of 18 mg/dL
- Hemoglobin = 13.8 g/dL
- Platelets = 252,000/mm^3
- Weight 70 lb (32 kg)

3. The pediatrician examines the child and highly suspects appendicitis. A CT scan of the abdomen has been prescribed and the child is placed on NPO status. When planning care for this child, which **priority** symptoms would the nurse consider most immediate at this time? **Select all that apply.**
   A. Pain
   B. Anemia
   C. Infection
   D. Vomiting
   E. Weight loss
   F. Dehydration
   G. Constipation
   H. Hyperthermia
   I. Rupture of the appendix

A 10-year-old girl who has a 2-day history of generalized periumbilical pain and anorexia. Today she developed a fever and vomiting, so her parents took her to her pediatrician. On review of the history, physical examination, and laboratory results, the nurse notes the following:

- Oral temperature of 102°F (38.9°C)
- Pulse of 80 beats/min and BP is 108/74 mm/Hg
- Abdominal pain midway between the anterior superior iliac crest and umbilicus
- Pain intensifies with any activity or deep breathing
- WBC count of 21,000/mm^3, 79% bands, 14% lymphocytes, 6% eosinophils
- CRP of 18 mg/dL
- Hemoglobin = 13.8 g/dL
- Platelets = 252,000/mm^3
- Weight 70 lb (32 kg)

Day 1, 12:00 Noon

Results of the CT scan demonstrate a ruptured appendix. The child is being prepared for surgery. The nurse performing the assessment finds her temperature is 102°F (38.9°C). The child reports that the pain had initially resolved but now reports increasing pain (rated 9 out of 10 on a 1 to 10 pain intensity scale) and nausea.

Day 1, 2:00 p.m.

The child undergoes surgery for an appendectomy. She is transferred to the pediatric unit from the recovery room and the nurse plans care.

4. Indicate which nursing action listed in the far-left column is appropriate for the potential postoperative complication following appendectomy listed in the middle column. **Indicate the nursing action number in the far-right column. Note that ONLY one nursing action can be used for each potential postoperative complication and that NOT all nursing actions will be used.**

Nursing Action	Potential Postoperative Complication	Nursing Action for Postoperative Complication
1. Administer pain medications.	Inflammation at the wound site	
2. Initiate IV fluids and assess intake and output (I&O).	Electrolyte imbalance	
3. Assess temperature and report elevation.	Fluid deficit	
4. Administer antiemetics.	Pain	
5. Administer IV sodium heparin.	Nausea and vomiting	
6. Draw blood as scheduled and evaluate results.	Infection	
7. Report changes in vital signs, behavior, and level of consciousness.	Fever	
8. Administer IV antibiotics.		
9. Administer a blood transfusion.		
10. Observe wound site.		

Day 3, 9:00 a.m.

5. The child is recovering well following surgery. The nurse performing the assessment finds her oral temperature is 98.6°F (37°C). The child reports that the pain is a 1 out of 10 on a 10-point pain intensity scale). She has no nausea or vomiting. **For each nursing action, use an X to indicate whether it was Effective (helped to meet expected quality patient outcomes) or Ineffective (did not help to meet expected quality patient outcomes).**

Nursing Action	Effective	Ineffective
Observe no signs of infection.		
Pain is controlled.		
No complaints of nausea or vomiting, and a regular diet is tolerated.		
Temperature remains in the normal range.		
Child spending all of the time in bed.		

Day 5, 10:00 a.m.

6. The child has recovered and is ready for discharge and the nurse is providing essential education to the parents and child for care at home. **Use an X for the health teaching statement below that is Indicated (appropriate or necessary) or Contraindicated (could be harmful).**

Health Teaching	Indicated	Contraindicated
"Take your child's temperature if she feels warm and call the surgeon if she has a fever over 101° F."		
"Give ibuprofen every 6 hours for the next 5 days."		
"Inspect the surgical incision every day for increased redness, heat, or drainage; if present, call the surgeon immediately."		
Ask the parents, "What are your concerns regarding your daughter's care at home?"		
"Apply a topical antibiotic to the surgical wound for the next week."		

The Child With Acute Respiratory Tract Illness

Day 1, 8:00 a.m.

1. A 7-month-old infant girl is being evaluated in the emergency department (ED) for fever and cough. Mom reports over the past 2 days that she has not been as active as usual and is eating less. She started coughing during the night and, upon awakening, had a temperature of 103°F (39.4°C). The mother states her infant is "*breathing fast and she doesn't seem to be getting enough air.*" The nurse performs a complete history and assessment and finds the following. **Select the assessment findings that require follow-up by the nurse. Select all that apply.**
   A. Nasal flaring
   B. Decreased appetite
   C. Skin color—pallor
   D. Irritable and restless
   E. Pulse = 164 beats/min
   F. Retractions visualized
   G. Respiration = 42 breaths/min
   H. SaO_2 on pulse oximeter 88%
   I. BP = 100/60 mmHg
   J. Rhonchi and fine crackles in left lung
   K. Axillary temperature = 102.4°F (39.1°C)
2. The nurse understands that common conditions affect the bronchi in children. The nurse plans care knowing which findings are **most likely** to be noted. **Choose the most likely options for the information missing from the table below by selecting from the lists of options provided.**

Diagnosis	Characteristics	Treatment
Asthma	Wheezing, cough, labored respirations	Inhaled corticosteroids, bronchodilators
Bronchitis	2	Cough suppressants
1	Labored respirations, poor feeding, cough tachypnea, retractions, flaring nares, fever	3

Options for 1	Options for 2	Options for 3
Pneumonia	Persistent dry, hacking cough worse at night, more productive in 2–3 days	Inhaled corticosteroids, antibiotics
Bronchiolitis	Retractions, labored respirations	Allergen and "triggers control"
Emphysema	Poor feeding, inability to sleep, gastrointestinal symptoms	Supplemental oxygen, fluid intake, suctioning as needed
Wheezing	Seizures, altered consciousness, inability to focus	Long-term anti-inflammatory medications

Day 1, 3:00 p.m.

The infant has been diagnosed with bronchiolitis, and laboratory results confirm it is caused by respiratory syncytial virus (RSV). The infant is resting comfortably on oxygen therapy and receiving IV antibiotics and fluids. The nursing assessment reveals the following:

- Axillary temperature = 99.0°F (37.2°C)
- Pulse = 92 beats/min
- Respiration = 24 breaths/min
- SpO_2 on pulse oximeter 97% room air
- BP = 102/54 mmHg
- No retractions visualized
- No nasal flaring
- Rhonchi and fine crackles in left lung
- Skin color—no pallor noted
- Sleeping

3. **Choose the most likely options for the information missing from the statements below by selecting from the lists of options provided.** The nurse realizes that bronchiolitis is the most common infectious disease of the _____1_____ airways. RSV affects the _______2_______ cells of the respiratory tract. The respiratory illness usually begins with an upper respiratory infection (URI) after an incubation of about ____3____ days.

Options for 1	Options for 2	Options for 3
Upper	Skin	1–2
Middle	Epithelial	2–3
Lower	Blood	5–8
Extreme	Muscle	10–14
Left	Nasal	14–18
Right	Bone	21–24

4. What are the most appropriate immediate nursing interventions for this infant with acute respiratory tract illness? **Indicate which nursing action number listed in the far-left column is appropriate for the potential complication listed in the middle column. Place the number in the far-right column. Note that NOT all nursing actions will be used.**

Nursing Action	Potential Complication	Nursing Action for Complication
1. Position infant for maximum ventilation and airway patency.	Inability to identify alterations in temperature, respiratory status, or circulation and need for additional interventions is missed	
2. Monitor vital signs, including temperature and respiratory, cardiac, and oxygen status.	Nasal mucosal membrane drying	
3. Provide humidified oxygen as indicated.	Fever	
4. Suction airway (nares, mouth, nasopharynx) as indicated.	Bronchial constriction and decreased ventilation	
5. Provide gentle chest percussion and chest physiotherapy (CPT) as indicated.	Secretions causing lack of airway patency	
6. Administer antipyretics as indicated.	Infection	
7. Administer bronchodilators as indicated.	Spread of infection	
8. Administer antibiotics if indicated.	Dehydration or fluid overload	
9. Obtain specimens (e.g., secretions, blood) as indicated.		
10. Maintain appropriate precautions such as Standard Precautions, droplet isolation, and frequent hand washing.		
11. Monitor hydration status through strict intake and output and daily weights.		
12. Implement comfort measures such as allowing parent presence, parent holding infant, and comfort item such as favorite blanket or stuffed animal.		

Day 2, 9:00 a.m.

5. The infant remains hospitalized and the nurse caring for the infant performs the change of shift assessment. Which of the assessment findings support discharge of the infant to home? **Select all that apply.**
   A. SaO_2 of 97% on room air.
   B. Axillary temperature = 102.4°F (39.1°C)
   C. Respiratory rate 24 breaths/ min
   D. Oral intake 100 mL/24 hours
   E. Minimal nasal secretions in past 24 hours
   F. Lungs clear to auscultation

Day 3, 10:00 a.m.

6. The infant has been afebrile for 24 hours and has an SpO_2 of 98% on room air. She is now taking oral fluids and there is no longer any nasal discharge. The nurse prepares for discharge teaching and evaluates how prepared the parents are for taking the infant home. **Use an X for the health teaching evaluation below that is Indicated (appropriate or necessary) or Contraindicated (could be harmful).**

Health Teaching Evaluation	Indicated	Contraindicated
Parents able to verbalize definition and characteristics of acute respiratory tract infection.		
Parents able to verbalize treatment, including medication and interventions that promote ventilation and airway clearance.		
Parents can identify discharge medications, including antipyretics, bronchodilators, and antibiotics as prescribed.		
Parents want to purchase a pulse oximeter before taking the infant home so they can constantly monitor the oxygen level.		
Parents feel that keeping the infant supine will assist with any nasal secretions the infant may have.		

The Child With Acute Asthma Exacerbation

Day 1, 10:00 a.m.

1. A 15-year-old male presents to the ED with a history of asthma and symptoms that are not resolving with his current rescue medications. His asthma symptoms have been controlled with use of a long-acting inhaler twice daily, but an increase in seasonal allergies and a recent URI have caused an exacerbation of his symptoms. The patient rarely uses his peak expiratory flow meter (PEFM); instead, he waits until his symptoms become severe before starting to use his rescue medications. The nurse completes a history and physical assessment and finds the following. **Select the assessment findings that require follow-up by the nurse. Select all that apply.**
   A. Temperature = 98.6°F (37°C)
   B. Heart Rate = 114 beats/min
   C. Respirations = 28 breaths/min
   D. SpO_2 = 88% on room air
   E. BP = 110/64 mmHg
   F. Wheezing auscultated in both lungs
   G. Unable to lie down on the stretcher
   H. PEFM results are less than 50% of baseline
2. Based on these findings, what are the most important subjective and objective data that should be considered as the defining characteristics of an acute asthma exacerbation? **Select all that apply.**
   A. Dyspnea
   B. Moist cough
   C. Shortness of breath
   D. High BP
   E. Increased respiratory rate
   F. Profuse thick secretions
   G. Chest tightness or chest pain
   H. Use of accessory muscles (retractions)
   I. Diminished breath sounds and/or adventitious breath sounds (wheezing)

Day 1, 10:15 a.m.

3. A 15-year-old male with a history of asthma is in the ED for immediate treatment. The physician has examined the patient and written orders. Which nursing interventions are of **highest priority** for this adolescent with an asthma exacerbation? **Use an X to indicate whether the nursing actions listed below are Emergent (appropriate or immediately necessary) or Not Emergent (not appropriate or not immediately necessary) for the patient's care at this time.**

Nursing Action	Emergent	Not Emergent
Administer humidified oxygen to keep the oxygen saturation (SpO_2) above 90%.		
Administer methylprednisolone per the physician order.		
Administer albuterol per hospital protocol.		
Place the patient in a comfortable standing, sitting upright, or learning forward position.		
Discuss possible allergens in the home that might have triggered the attack.		
Review how to use the metered dose inhaler.		

4. Indicate which nursing action number listed in the far-left column is most appropriate for each potential complication listed in the middle column. **Place the number in the far-right column. Note that not all actions will be used.**

Nursing Action	Potential Complication	Nursing Action to Prevent Complication
1. Allow patient to assume position of comfort.	To minimize drying of nasal mucous membranes	
2. Administer rescue medications (as prescribed) that can include inhalers, nebulization, and/or oral or IV steroids.	To prevent airway obstruction	
3. Administer humidified oxygen to maintain oxygen saturation (SaO_2) above 90%.	Decreased patient's awareness of factors that exacerbate asthma	
4. Assess patient's response to rescue medications.	To prevent constricted airways and decreased air exchange	
5. Assist patient in recognizing factors that trigger asthma symptoms.	Lack of awareness of need for more aggressive interventions	
6. Assure respirations will be easy and nonlabored at a rate within normal limits for age.		
7. Teach the patient how to use the PEFM.		
8. Evaluate the use of the PEFM.		

Day 2, 11:00 a.m.

5. A 15-year-old male with a history of asthma was admitted yesterday for acute asthmatic care. He has responded well to treatment and will be discharged. The nurse will be discussing discharge plans that are essential aspects of asthma care and prevention. What would the nurse include in the teaching plan? **Select all that apply.**
   A. Avoiding smoke and other irritants
   B. Avoiding Tylenol containing products
   C. Encouraging daily albuterol use
   D. Identifying early signs of an asthma exacerbation
   E. Identifying specific asthmatic triggers in the environment
   F. Reviewing home medications, dosing, and precautions
   G. Recommending physical exercise and mental training
   H. Avoiding exposure to excessive cold, wind, and other extremes of weather

Day 2, 2:00 p.m.

6. A 15-year-old male with a history of asthma who is in the ED for immediate treatment. He has responded well to treatment and no longer needs oxygen and plans are being discussed for discharge. Since there is a history of this adolescent not using the PEFM, the nurse will meet with him and his mother to review how to use the PEFM. The nurse realizes that the adolescent and his mother must understand how to interpret the peak expiratory flow rates using the PEFM. **Choose the most likely options for the information missing from the statements below by selecting from the lists of options provided.** The PEFR measures the maximum _____1_____ that can be forcefully exhaled in _____2_______. Asthma is under reasonably good control when the PEFR indicates _____3_____ of the patient's personal best value is obtained. This value is established by obtaining a PEFR over a _____4___ period of time.

Options for 1	Options for 2	Options for 3	Options for 4
Flow of air	5 s	80%–100%	4–5 weeks
Flow of oxygen	10 s	50%–70%	2–3 weeks
Flow of water	1 s	60%–80%	1–2 days

The Child With Coarctation of the Aorta

Day 1, 8:00 a.m. Hospitalization

1. The nurse is caring for a 3-week-old male with congenital heart disease (CHD). At birth, he initially showed no signs or symptoms, but within the second week of life he developed symptoms of heart failure (HF). He was found to have coarctation of the aorta and is now under the care of the cardiology team and scheduled for surgery. The infant is experiencing increased signs of HF and was hospitalized early this morning. His care is focused on preventing further symptoms before he goes to surgery. What are the most important signs of HF that the nurse would look for in this infant? **Select all that apply.**
   A. Edema
   B. Tachypnea
   C. Weight loss
   D. Tachycardia
   E. Hypotension
   F. Warm extremities
   G. Feeding difficulty
   H. Slow peripheral pulses
   I. Prolonged capillary refill, longer than 2 or 3 seconds
   J. Ineffective peripheral circulation, cool extremities
2. The nurse reviews the history of this 3-week-old infant and reads that he is diagnosed with coarctation of the aorta. The nurse realizes that the symptoms experienced by the infant are caused by this congenital disorder. **Choose the most likely options for the information missing from the statements below by selecting from the lists of options provided.** Coarctation of the aorta is described as the _____1_____ of the aortic arch that results in _______2_______ cardiac output. A classic finding is _____3____ pulses in the arms and _______4_______ femoral pulses.

Options for 1	Options for 2	Options for 3 and 4
Widening	Increased	Bounding
Absence	Decreased	Widening
Narrowing	Lack of	Weak or absent
Crossing	Absent	Narrowing
Absence	Complex	Unstable

Day 1, 2:00 p.m. Hospitalization

3. Surgery is planned for tomorrow. The infant's BP is 120/70 mmHg, and the pulses in his arms are 220 beats/min and bounding. You find weak femoral pulses at 40 beats/min and his extremities are cool to touch. His breathing is at 36 breaths/min, and no nasal flaring or intercostal retractions are noted at this time. His color is pale without mottling. The infant is not on mechanical ventilation at this time. What are **priority** nursing actions? **Use an X to indicate which nursing actions listed below are Emergent (appropriate or immediately necessary) or Not Emergent (not appropriate or not immediately necessary) for the patient's care at this time.**

Nursing Action	Emergent	Not Emergent
Frequently assess and record heart rate, respiratory rate, BP, and any signs or symptoms of decreased cardiac output.		
Administer cardiac drugs on schedule. Assess and record any side effects or any signs and symptoms of toxicity. Follow hospital protocol for administration.		
Administer cool humidified oxygen to increase available oxygen during inspiration.		
Change the infant's position every 2 h to prevent skin breakdown.		
Keep accurate record of intake and output.		
Weigh infant on same scale at same time of day.		
Maintain a 3-h feeding schedule.		
Restrict fluids if the intake and output is unbalanced.		

Day 1, 4:00 p.m.

4. The nurse continues to closely observe the infant since there are obvious signs of HF related to the congenital defect. **Indicate which nursing action listed in the far-left column is appropriate for each potential complication listed in the middle column. Indicate the nursing action number in the far-right column. Note that NOT all actions will be used.**

Nursing Action	Potential Complication	Nursing Action to Prevent Complication
1. Assess and record heart rate, respiratory rate, BP, and any signs or symptoms of altered cardiac output every 2–4 h.	Decreased urinary output is a symptom of HF and could go unnoticed	
2. Administer cardiac drugs on schedule. Assess and record any side effects or any signs and symptoms of toxicity. Follow hospital protocol for administration.	Undetected changes in vital signs and infant's physical status that reflect altered cardiac output and high BP	
3. Keep accurate record of intake and output.	Excess water and salt because fluid retention commonly occurs with HF	
4. Weigh infant on same scale at same time of day as previously. Document results and compare to previous weight.	Dangers inherent in failure to administer cardiac drugs as prescribed and to perform careful assessment before administration	
5. Administer diuretics on schedule. Assess and record effectiveness and any side effects noted.		
6. Offer small, frequent feedings to infant's tolerance.		
7. Organize nursing care to allow infant uninterrupted rest.		

Day 5 Hospitalization, 3 Days Post-Surgery

5. The infant underwent surgery 3 days ago. Resection of the coarcted portion of the aorta was performed. Cardiopulmonary bypass was not required due to this defect being outside the heart and pericardium. The infant is in stable condition. The nurse is performing a change of shift assessment of the infant. What assessment findings demonstrate that the infant is stable at this time? **Select all that apply.**
   A. Color pink
   B. Lack of edema
   C. Successful feeding
   D. Heart rate 120 beats/min
   E. Skin warm to touch
   F. Weight gain (0.5 kg/day)
   G. Respiratory 48 breaths/min
   H. Lack of distended neck veins
   I. Strong and equal peripheral pulses
   J. Brisk capillary refill within 5 seconds
   K. Adequate urinary output (1 to 2 mL/kg/h)

Day of Discharge

6. The infant has recovered well from surgery with no complications. The nurse is preparing for discharge and notes that both parents are nervous and afraid of taking their infant home. What education would the nurse provide to the family at this time? **Use an X for the health teaching evaluation below that is Indicated (appropriate or necessary), or Contraindicated (could be harmful).**

Health Teaching	Indicated	Contraindicated
Discuss the characteristics of Coarctation of the Aorta (COA) and the surgery done to repair the obstructive defect.		
Review the infant's daily care, including medication administration.		
Review signs and symptoms that could be of concern (fever, blue skin color, poor eating).		
Inform parents to purchase a pulse oximeter before taking the infant home so they can constantly monitor the oxygen level.		
Keep the infant supine at all times to assist with blood flow.		
Give parents the opportunity to express their fears and concerns.		

The Child With Sickle Cell Anemia

Day 1, 9:00 a.m.

1. A 12-year-old male with sickle cell anemia (homozygous sickle cell disease [HgbSS]) is being seen in the ED for increasing pain over the past 2 days. The mother is giving him the pain medications as prescribed by the hematology team, but she feels that his pain is getting worse. Which assessment findings require follow-up by the nurse? **Select all that apply.**
   A. Pulse oximetry 96%
   B. Hematocrit = 34%
   C. Pulse = 112 beats/min
   D. Hemoglobin = 10.6 g/dL
   E. Respiration = 24 breaths/min
   F. Abdomen tender to palpation
   G. 8/10 on the number pain scale
   H. BP = 102/50 mmHg
   I. Total serum bilirubin = 0.3 mg/dL
   J. Oral temperature = 100.4°F (38°C)
   K. Weight = 40 kg

2. **Review the question above. Choose the most likely options for the information missing from the statements below by selecting from the lists of options provided.** As a result of this child's diagnosis of sickle cell disease, the nurse is aware, based on the assessment findings, that the child may be experiencing __________1__________. This is caused by __________2__________.

Options for 1	Options for 2
Aplastic crisis	High BP
Sequestration crisis	Ischemia
Acute chest syndrome	Bleeding
Vasoocclusive crisis	Infection
Hyperhemolytic crisis	Diminished red blood cell production
Cerebral vascular accident	Decreased serum sodium

Day 1, 9:30 a.m.

3. The hematologist arrives to examine the child. At this time, the child has findings that are consistent with a vasoocclusive crisis (VOC). When planning care for this child, which **priority** interventions would the nurse consider at this time? **Select all that apply.**
   A. Hydration
   B. Antibiotics
   C. Strict bedrest
   D. Pain medication
   E. Pain assessment
   F. Blood transfusion
   G. Oxygen therapy

Day 1, 10:00 a.m.

4. In the last hour an IV dose of morphine (0.1 mg/kg) was given every 10 minutes for three doses. The numeric pain score of 7/10 is assessed after these initial doses. A decision is made to start both morphine and ketorolac since the pain was not relieved after three doses of IV morphine. The morphine is changed to patient-controlled analgesia (PCA). Ketorolac 1 mg/kg for the first dose, then 0.5 mg/kg/dose (maximum of 30 mg/dose) IV every 6 hours also is started. IV fluids at 1½ maintenance rate are administered. What are the **most appropriate** nursing interventions for this child with SCD experiencing pain who is now receiving morphine by PCA and IV Ketorolac? **Indicate which nursing action listed in the far-left column is appropriate for each potential complication listed in the middle column. Indicate the nursing action number in the far-right column. Note that ONLY one nursing action can be used for each potential complication and that NOT all nursing actions will be used.**

Nursing Action	Potential Complication	Nursing Action for Complication
1. Discuss schedule of medication around the clock with parents.	Uncontrolled pain	
2. Encourage high level of fluid intake.	Breakthrough pain	
3. Recognize that various analgesics, including opioids and medication schedules, may need to be tried.	To avoid needless suffering because of unfounded fears	
4. Reassure child and family that analgesics, including opioids, are medically indicated; that high doses may be needed; and that children rarely become addicted.	To prevent vasoconstriction that may enhance sickling with cold applications	
5. Apply heat application or massage to affected area. Avoid applying cold compresses.	Dehydration	
6. Provide protein shake with each meal.		
7. Weigh the child each morning with the same scale.		

Day 1, 2:00 p.m.

5. The patient is now resting comfortably, having been admitted to the pediatric unit. His mother is at the bedside and the last numeric pain assessment reveals his level of pain at 3/10. These are the PCA doses used: Loading dose of 0.1 mg/kg (maximum 8 mg); basal rate of 0.01 mg/kg and intermittent dose 0.035 mg/kg (maximum 8 mg) with the interval lockout at approximately 10 minutes. A 4-hour limit of 0.5 mg/kg is set. His weight is 40 kg. **Based on these PCA loading doses above, choose the most likely options for the information missing from the table by selecting from the list of options provided.**

Loading Dose	Basal Rate	Intermittent Dose	Interval Lockout
1	2	3	4

Options for 1	Options for 2	Options for 3	Options for 4
6	0.4	2.2	5 min
4	0.2	1.8	6 min
8	0.8	1.4	8 min
2	0.9	1.2	10 min

Day 1, 7:00 p.m.

A 12-year-old male with sickle cell anemia (HgbSS) was seen this morning in the ED for increasing pain over the past 2 days. He is admitted for pain management and is on IV Morphine and Ketorolac. His pain assessment is 2/10 on the numeric scale. Assessment findings at the nurse's change of shift at 7 p.m. reveal:

- Oral temperature = 99.0°F (37.2°C)
- Pulse = 60 beats/min
- Respiration = 16 breaths/min
- BP = 100/48 mmHg
- Weight = 89 lb (40 kg)
- Abdomen slightly tender to palpation
- 2/10 on the number pain scale
- Pulse oximetry 98%

6. The patient is resting comfortably and the nurse at the end of her shift is assessing important nursing actions for the care of this child. **For each nursing action, use an X to indicate whether it was Effective (helped to meet expected quality) or Ineffective (did not meet expected quality).**

Nursing Action	Effective	Ineffective
Administer morphine and ketorolac safely.		
Monitor for side effects of morphine; assess respiratory status closely and prevent constipation.		
Monitor for side effects of ketorolac; assess for bleeding (gastrointestinal [GI] or renal) closely.		
Educate parents on the safety and effectiveness of IV morphine and ketorolac when using them at home.		
Reassess the child's pain level once a shift after administering morphine and ketorolac.		
Recognize that various analgesics and doses may need to be tried.		

NEXT-GENERATION NCLEX® EXAMINATION STYLE UNFOLDING CASE STUDIES 5

The Child With Acute Lymphoblastic Leukemia

Day 1, 8:00 a.m.

1. A 7-year-old male developed bilateral neck swelling 1 month ago and is being seen in the ED. His mother had taken him to a nearby health center twice because the swelling is increasing in size; oral antibiotics were prescribed. Two-weeks later, he now has hoarseness when speaking and his mother also reports that he is sleeping most of the time. On presentation to the hospital this morning, the CBC revealed a hemoglobin of 6.0 g/dL, WBC of 85,000/mm^3 and a platelet count of 60,000/mm^3. On examination, the child has bilateral parotid

gland enlargement, submental nodes and axillary nodes, and hepatomegaly approximately 6 cm below the right subcostal margin. Leukemia is suspected and the child is admitted for further evaluation. Based on the list below, what are the most common signs and symptoms of leukemia the nurse would look for? **Select all that apply.**

A. Fever
B. Seizure
C. Fatigue
D. Infection
E. Bone pain
F. Short stature
G. Shortness of breath
H. Lymphadenopathy
I. Hepatosplenomegaly
J. Bruising and bleeding

Day 1, 8:00 a.m. Continued

2. It is important for the nurse to be aware of pathophysiology associated with the signs and symptoms of childhood leukemia. Symptoms are caused by bone marrow dysfunction that causes the rapidly proliferating leukemia cells to depress bone marrow production of the formed elements of the blood.

Choose the most likely options for the information missing from the table below by selecting from the lists of options provided.

Symptom	Pathophysiology	Assessment Finding
Anemia	2	Pale, tired, listless
Infection	Decreased production of WBCs	3
1	Decreased production of platelets	Nosebleed, bruising
Bone pain	Increased pressure	Unable to bear weight on legs

Option 1	Option 2	Option 3
Seizure	Decreased production of RBCs	Lack of appetite and weight loss
Blindness	Increased production of plasma cells	Headache and seizure
Hemorrhage	Decreased production of CNS fluid	Enlarged spleen
Hearing loss	Increased production of bilirubin	Fever and infection

Day 1, 4:00 p.m.

3. This afternoon a diagnostic work-up was completed and the child underwent a bone marrow aspiration and biopsy. Flow cytometry revealed 70% B-cell leukemia blast cells and the diagnosis of acute lymphoblastic leukemia (ALL) is confirmed. He is to start chemotherapy tomorrow as part of the initial therapy for ALL. The child's WBC is extremely high, 85,000/mm^3 this morning, and he is at risk for tumor lysis syndrome.

Choose the most likely options for the information missing from the statements below by selecting from the lists of options provided.

Children who present with a high WBC caused by leukemia are at risk for __________1__________ abnormalities that are a direct result of the _________2_________ release of intracellular contents during the __________3______________ of malignant cells, in this child's case-leukemia cells.

Options for 1	Options for 2	Options for 3
Cardiac	Rapid	Production
Cellular	Slow	Growth
Metabolic	Intermittent	Lysis
Neurologic	Prolonged	Mitosis

Day 1, 5:00 p.m.

4. A 7-year-old male was diagnosed with acute lymphocytic leukemia and has done well overnight. He continues on IV fluids and medication to reduce uric acid formation and prevent tumor lysis syndrome. He is due to start chemotherapy today and will undergo a lumbar puncture with intrathecal chemotherapy administered to prevent invasion of leukemia cells into the CNS. The nurse is preparing the child and family for the lumbar puncture procedure.

For each nursing action, use an X to indicate whether it was Effective (helped to meet expected quality patient outcomes), or Ineffective (did not help to meet expected quality patient outcomes).

Nursing Action	Effective	Ineffective
Explain the procedure to the patient and family and obtain informed consent.		
Monitor vital signs during the procedure (pulse rate, oxygen saturation, respirations, BP).		
Administer a bolus of IV fluids before the procedure begins.		
Administer sedation during the procedure to provide optimal comfort and to minimize pain.		
Provide comfort and reassure the patient and family throughout the procedure.		
Watch for signs of bleeding from the puncture site.		

Day 2, 8:00 a.m.

5. A 7-year-old male was diagnosed today with acute lymphocytic leukemia confirmed by bone marrow examination and a complete diagnostic work up. He will begin chemotherapy tomorrow. Orders are written for preventing tumor lysis syndrome since his WBC is 85,000 mm^3. Which of the following actions would the nurse take? **Select all that apply.**
   A. Restrict IV fluids
   B. Monitor WBC
   C. Check urine pH with each void
   D. Administer aggressive IV fluids
   E. Monitor serum chemistries frequently
   F. Maintain strict record of intake and output
   G. Administer medication to prevent HF
   H. Administer medication to reduce uric acid formation

Day 5, 8:00 a.m.

6. A 7-year-old male was diagnosed with acute lymphocytic leukemia 5 days ago and has no complications from starting chemotherapy. He remains afebrile and the blood count today reveals a hemoglobin of 8.0 g/dL, WBC of $10{,}000/mm^3$ and a platelet count of $65{,}000/mm^3$. Packed red blood cells were given on day 3 due to decreasing hemoglobin. The WBC count has decreased dramatically from $85{,}000/mm^3$ to $10{,}000/mm^3$. Chemistries are without evidence of tumor lysis syndrome.

   Plans are for the child to be discharged in the next 2 days if he does not develop fever and there are no signs of tumor lysis. The nurse begins preparing the child and family for discharge.

   Indicate which nursing action listed in the far-left column is appropriate for potential complications following the start of leukemia treatment listed in the middle column. Indicate the nursing action number in the far-right column.

   Note that ONLY one nursing action can be used for each potential complication and that NOT all nursing actions will be used.

Nursing Action	Potential Complication	Nursing Action to Prevent Complication
1. Explain the disease course of treatment and adverse effects to the family.	Skin as an entry point for infection	
2. Teach the patient and family ways to prevent infection through hand washing, bathing frequently, and not using cups and utensils used by another person.	Lack of recognition of infection	
3. Teach the family how to recognize symptoms of infection such as fever, chills, cough, and sore throat and report these to the health care worker immediately.	Lack of understanding of leukemia treatment	
4. Provide skin care to patient by keeping the skin and perianal area clean and apply mild lotion.	Mouth ulceration	
5. Provide a high-protein and high-calorie diet.	Lack of knowledge on how to prevent infection in the home	
6. Provide adequate hydration and encourage a high-fiber diet and stool softeners.	Bleeding	

Nursing Action	Potential Complication	Nursing Action to Prevent Complication
7. Educate family and patient on how to recognize and report abnormal bleeding through bruising and petechiae.		
8. Provide frequent mouth care and saline rinses and check for ulcers in the mouth and gum swelling.		
9. Instruct patient and family to avoid contact sports.		

The Child With Seizures

Day 1, 10:00 a.m.

1. A 7-year-old boy who was playing during physical education class at school when he suddenly stopped his activity, stared into space, repetitively moved his left arm up and down, and smacked his lips. After approximately 1 minute, he stopped the behavior and was drowsy but responsive to his environment. He had no memory of the event. He was accompanied by his teacher to the school nurse for further assessment. While waiting for the parents to arrive, what are the most important subjective and objective data that the nurse would document? **Select all that apply from the boy and from the person who observed the seizure.**

   From the boy:

   A. Aura
   B. Sensory phenomena that the child can describe during the event (i.e., ability to hear)
   C. Postictal feelings (i.e., confusion, inability to speak, amnesia, headache, sleepiness)

   From the person who observed the seizure:

   D. Duration of seizure
   E. Time of onset of seizure
   F. Other students who have the same symptoms
   G. Change in level of consciousness (LOC) before, during, and after the seizure
   H. Movements (ask for demonstration of the seizure rather than relying on verbal description)

Day 1, 11:30 a.m.

2. The child is seen in the ED after the mother picked him up from school. The physician wants to observe the child while tests results are pending. Blood work and an electroencephalogram (EEG) were done. **Indicate which nursing action listed in the far-left column is appropriate to prevent the potential complication following a seizure listed in the middle column. Indicate the nursing action number in the far-right column. Note that ONLY one nursing action can be used for each potential complication and that NOT all nursing actions will be used.**

Nursing Action	Potential Complication	Nursing Action to Prevent Complication
1. Monitor time (onset and duration), movements, and LOC during seizure.	Child experiences anxiety and fear	
2. If child is at risk of falling, ease child to floor. Prevent child from hitting head on objects. Do not attempt to restrain child or use force.	An accurate description of the seizure is not obtained	
3. During seizure, place child in a side-lying position on a flat surface such as floor. Do not put anything in child's mouth.	Parents unable to cope with the diagnosis and management of their son	
4. Stay with the child and reassure the child when awakening from seizure.	Physical harm occurs	
5. Involve child and parents in discussion of fears, anxieties, and resources and support options available to patient and family.	Aspiration can occur	
	Lack of description of the postictal state	
	Further seizures occur	

One Week Later, 11:00 a.m.

3. A 7-year-old boy who was playing during physical education class at school a week ago had a seizure. The work-up revealed an abnormal EEG and the physical examination and clinical history supported the decision to begin anticonvulsant therapy with a single medication. This morning he has another seizure while playing with his siblings in the backyard. His brother ran inside to get help and his mother ran outside to see him staring into space with his head turned to the side and his left arm moving rhythmically up and down. This activity stopped for a few seconds and then started again. His mother called for emergency assistance (911), and he was transported to the hospital. Which of the signs and symptoms experienced by this 7-year-old child would the nurse expect to find with a focal seizure? **Select all that apply.**
   A. Automatisms
   B. Aura experienced
   C. Mental disorientation
   D. Postictal impairment
   E. Lasted less than a minute
   F. Occurs multiple times a day
   G. Seizure lasted for 45 minutes

One Week Later, 11:30 a.m.

4. The child was transferred by ambulance to the hospital. He had not regained consciousness during the transport. Choose the most likely options for the information missing from the statements below by selecting from the lists of options provided.

Since the child is not regaining a premorbid LOC between seizures is concerning and meets criteria for a diagnosis of __________1__________. The child's __________2__________ should be monitored closely, and supportive measures (i.e., cardiopulmonary resuscitation) should be initiated as indicated. Simple, effective, and safe treatments for home or prehospital management of prolonged seizures and impending status epilepticus include __________3__________ midazolam and rectal diazepam.

Options for 1	Options for 2	Options for 3
Simple partial seizure	BP	Intrathecal
Complex partial seizure	Seizure activity	IV
Status epilepticus	Circulation, airway, and breathing (CAB)	Rectal
Absence seizure	Blood levels	Buccal

One Week Later, 1:00 p.m.

5. The child is admitted to the hospital after the seizure was stopped in the ED by administering IV lorazepam. The child has gained consciousness and is being monitored closely with his parents at the bedside. He is undergoing a comprehensive neurological examination with neuroimaging studies. The child had no history of signs of infection or head trauma. **For each nursing action, use an X to indicate whether it was Effective (helped to meet expected patient outcomes) or Ineffective (did not help to meet expected patient outcomes).**

Nursing Action	Effective	Ineffective
Monitor circulation, airway, and breathing closely.		
Ensure antiepileptic drugs are being administered as directed.		
Monitor and record characteristics, onset, and duration of any new seizures, including motor effects, alterations in consciousness, and postictal state.		
Attempt to stop the seizure if one occurs again; keep the child upright.		
Do not place anything in child's mouth during the seizure.		
Place child in a side-lying position; suction the oral cavity and posterior oropharynx as needed.		
Observe for hyperthermia, hypertension, and respiratory depression.		

Three Days Later, 11:00 a.m.

6. The child is stabilized and has completed the comprehensive neurological evaluation. The evaluation revealed no definitive etiology for the seizures. However, the EEG remains abnormal and the MRI study was also abnormal. He will remain on seizure medications at home and be followed by the neurology team. The child's parents are anxious and upset and concerned about taking their son home. The nurse caring for him is to begin discharge teaching today. What are the most important aspects of home care to discuss with his parents at this time? **Select all that apply.**
   A. Have the child wear a helmet to school.
   B. Have child wear medical identification.
   C. Arrange for a class presentation to all students to help with observation while at school.
   D. Educate family about characteristics of seizures, including aura, seizure activity, and postictal state.
   E. Educate family about safety precautions before and during a seizure, including side-lying positioning, padding area if needed, and not placing items in mouth or attempting to stop the seizure.
   F. Educate family about medication administration, including scheduled and as necessary (prn) medications and potential side effects of medications.
   G. Arrange for social worker to meet with family to assess emotional and financial needs.
   H. Consider consultation with child life specialist to assist with education of school personnel and classmates.
   I. Have eyes-on supervision when swimming in pools and an adult within arm's reach in natural bodies of water.
   J. Use protective helmet and padding during bicycle riding, skateboarding, and in-line skating.

The Child With Diabetes Mellitus

Day 1, 1:00 pm

1. An 8-year-old who has been healthy has lost weight in the past 2 weeks. His mother noticed that he is getting up several times during the night to go to the bathroom. He was drinking a great deal more in the past week, and she thought that was the reason for needing to use the bathroom. However, today he has a headache and is too tired to go to school. She also notices that he has wet the bed during the night. She becomes alarmed and cal0s the pediatrician for an appointment the next day. She has a brother with diabetes and thinks that the symptoms are similar to her brother's problems when he was first diagnosed as a child. The next day at the pediatrician's office the nurse performs a history and assessment. Which findings in the child's history and assessment findings would require the nurse to **immediately** investigate further? **Select all that apply.**
   A. Tiredness
   B. Headache
   C. Increased thirst
   D. Increased urination
   E. Wetting the bed at night
   F. Oral temperature 98.8 F
   G. Pulse 60 beats per minute
   H. Blood pressure= 94/60 mmHg
   I. Respirations 20 breaths per minute

Day 1, 2:30 pm

2. At the pediatrician's office, several tests are completed, and results are listed below.
   - Random blood glucose = 230 mg/dl
   - Hemoglobin (hgb) a1c level = 10.5%.
   - Hematocrit = 35%
   - Platelets = 250,000/mm^3
   - White blood cells = 8,000/mm^3
   - Urine dip test is positive for glucose and ketones

   He is admitted to the hospital for further evaluation to establish a diagnosis.

Choose the most likely options for the information missing from the statements below by selecting from the lists of options provided.

Based on the child's history and physical assessment, along with laboratory findings, the nurse suspects a diagnosis of __________1__________ because his __________2__________ and __________2__________ are high. His symptoms may be caused by an increased concentration of __________3__________ in the bloodstream.

Options for 1	Options for 2	Options for 3
Diabetes mellitus	platelets	Insulin
Addison disease	hematocrit	Glucose
Cushing syndrome	blood glucose	Potassium
Hyperparathyroidism	A1c level	Calcium
Pituitary hyperfunction	white blood cells	Sodium

Day 2, 12:00 noon

3. An 8-year-old who has been healthy has lost weight in the past 2 weeks. His mother noticed that he is getting up several times during the night to go to the bathroom. He was drinking a great deal more in the past week, and she thought that was the reason for needing to use the bathroom. However, today he has a headache and is too tired to go to school. She also notices that he has wet the bed during the night. She becomes alarmed and calls the pediatrician for an appointment the next day. She has a brother with diabetes and thinks that the symptoms are similar to her brother's problems when he was first diagnosed as a child.

He was admitted yesterday for further evaluation. To obtain a fasting blood glucose he was given nothing to eat or drink but water for 8 hours before the test this morning. Laboratory results from this AM include the following:

- 8 hour fasting glucose level =145 mg/dl
- Oral Glucose tolerance test (OGTT)= 240 mg/dl in 2 hr sample
- Urine dip test is positive for glucose and ketones
- Hgb A1C level = 10.5%

1. He has met the criteria for the diagnosis of type 1 diabetes mellitus. He will start with a twice-daily insulin regimen combining a rapid-acting (regular) insulin with an intermediate-acting (neutral protamine Hagedorn [NPH]/Lente) insulin. The nurse meets with the mother and patient to begin insulin therapy teaching. The mother asks why two types of insulin are needed. What are the **most appropriate** responses for the nurse to provide to help the mother and child understand about types of insulin? **Select all that apply.**

A. "Rapid-acting insulin peaks in about 30-90 minutes and may last about 5 hours."
B. "Short-acting insulin reaches the blood in about 5 minutes and peaks in about an hour."
C. "Extended insulin takes 4 hours to start working and can stay in the blood for up to 14 hours."
D. "Intermediate-acting insulin peaks in about 4-14 hours and can stay in the blood for 14-20 hours."
E. "Long-acting insulin takes 6-14 hours to start working and can stay in the blood for up to 24 hours."
F. "The types of insulin are based on how soon they start working, when the insulin works the hardest and how long it lasts."

Day 2, 4:30 pm

4. The insulin injections are ordered to be given at least 30 minutes before breakfast. The second one will be given 30 minutes before dinner. Even though the patient will start off receiving insulin twice daily, he will still need to check his blood glucose before meals and at bedtime. Based on his age, his glucose goal range before meals should be 90 to 180 mg/dl and at bedtime should be 100 to 180 mg/dl. The nurse is planning the teaching session and is preparing to give an injection of insulin before dinner after checking his blood glucose level. She will demonstrate to the child and parents how to administer the medication with this injection and discuss important aspects of insulin administration at home.

Indicate which nursing action listed in the far-left column is appropriate for each potential complication listed in the middle column. Indicate the nursing action number in the far-right column.

Note that ONLY one nursing action can be used for each potential complication and that NOT all nursing actions will be used.

Nursing Action	Potential Complication	Nursing Action for Complication
1. Obtain blood glucose level before meals and at bedtime.	Normal blood glucose level is not maintained	
2. Administer insulin as prescribed.	Appropriate dose of insulin is not administered	
3. Monitor urine glucose before each meal.	Appropriate type of insulin is not administered	
4. Use aseptic techniques when preparing and administering insulin.	Infection occurs	
5. Store insulin in the freezer to preserve the medication.	Absorption of insulin is impaired	
6. Understand the action of insulin: differences in composition, time of onset, and duration of action for the various preparations.		
7. Rotate insulin injection sites.		
8. Give less insulin before physical activity		

Day 3, 8:00 am

5. Before breakfast, the blood glucose was checked by the mother with guidance from the nurse. The mother administers the insulin into his left thigh; the patient wanted to have his mother give the insulin the first few times so that he can observe. An hour later the nurse is called to the bed site because he feels funny and his head hurts. He is dizzy when he stands, and his hands are shaking. The parents tell the nurse he did not eat breakfast because he is hoping to be discharged and wanted to eat on the way home.

For each nursing action, use an X to indicate whether it was Effective (helped to meet expected quality patient outcomes) or Ineffective (did not help to meet expected quality patient outcomes).

Nursing Action	Effective	Ineffective
Immediately administer cup of fruit juice or a glass of nonfat or 1% milk.		
Check blood glucose after 15 minutes.		
Give a starch-protein snack.		
Start intravenous fluids with glucose.		
Give parents instructions regarding signs and symptoms of hypoglycemia versus hyperglycemia.		
Teach parents how to administer intramuscular glucagon if unresponsive, unconscious, or seizing.		
Place the child on a portable insulin infusion pump.		

Day 3, 3:00 pm

6. The patient experienced hypoglycemia this morning after receiving the morning insulin injection. He did not eat breakfast after the injection. The nurse will use this experience to continue teaching the parents and child about how to monitor and manage his diabetes. What are the **most important** teaching topics for the nurse to include at this time? **Select all that apply.**
   A. "Signs of hyperglycemia or high blood sugar include fever, headache, seizures, and cough."
   B. "The blood sugar should be maintained within a target range of 90 to 180 mg/dl during the day."
   C. "Signs of hypoglycemia or low blood sugar include headache, dizziness, shaking, sweating and the pulse is fast."
   D. "Your child should no longer participate in any sports of physical activity that would cause his blood glucose to fall."
   E. "Learning how to plan meals, understanding specific good groups and making good food choices will be an important part of managing his diabetes."
   F. "The health care provider should be contacted when your child has fever for 2 days, vomiting and diarrhea, is unable to keep fluids down, and his glucose levels are above the target range."

A Child With a Fracture and Cast

Day 1, 10:00 a.m.

1. A 12-year-old boy is in the Emergency Center after falling off his skateboard. He tumbled forward off the board and fell on his right side with his right leg collapsing underneath him while using his right hand to resist the fall. The mother called 911 because the child was screaming in pain. At the scene, the child was conscious but continued to cry in pain. The Emergency Medical Technician (EMT) gave the child pain medication and started IV fluids when in route to the hospital. Due to the lacerations noted on the head, the child's spine was immobilized. He has a swollen, painful lower leg, bruised right lower arm, and swollen hand. He has lacerations on the forehead and cheeks from the fall. The nurse in the Emergency Center documents the following assessment findings. **Select the assessment findings that require follow-up by the nurse. Select all that apply.**
   A. Temperature = 98.4°F
   B. Pulse = 130 beats/min
   C. Respirations = 28 breaths/min
   D. BP = 128/80 mm Hg
   E. Drowsy but arouses easily
   F. Swelling of the right hand
   G. Swelling and bruising of the right lower leg
   H. Reports pain at 6/10 on a 0–10 pain scale

I. Voided 100 mL clear yellow urine

2. Based on the assessment findings above, **choose the most likely options for the information missing from the statements below by selecting from the lists of options provided.**

The nurse determines that the vital sign findings could be an emergency sign of ___________1___________ and should be further assessed immediately. The client's drowsiness is a concern and could be caused by _________2_________. Immobilization of the spine was performed by the EMT because of concern for ___________3_____________.

Options for 1	Options for 2	Options for 3
Nausea	Pain medication	Spinal cord damage
Brain injury	IV fluids	Right leg swelling
Vomiting	Trauma to the head	Headaches
Anxiety	Riding in the ambulance	Nausea
Stress from surgery	Fear	Seizures
Urinary tract infection	Lack of sleep	Venous access

Day 1, 2:00 p.m.

3. A 12-year-old boy is in the Emergency Center after falling off his skateboard. He tumbled off the board and fell on his right side with his right leg collapsing underneath him while using his right hand to resist the fall. A CT scan was done to assess for head injury and was normal with no evidence of concussion. X-rays of the right lower leg confirm a complete, closed fracture of the tibia with an intact fibula. The right arm and hand x-rays reveal soft tissue swelling with no fractures, but there are dislocated proximal interphalangeal joints on the second and third fingers of the right hand.

Upon reassessment, he complains of headache and pain in his right arm and leg. He undergoes a closed reduction on the two fingers under sedation in the Emergency Center. Following the procedure the fingers are buddy-taped for stability. A cast is placed on the right lower leg, and he is hospitalized overnight for observation and pain management.

When planning care for this patient, which **priority** actions would the nurse implement at this time? **Select all that apply.**

A. Administer pain medications
B. Assess pulses distal to the fracture site
C. Assess for paresthesia proximal to the fracture site
D. Keep the lower right limb below heart level
E. Apply cold to the right lower limb and right hand as tolerated
F. Assess for edema in the right lower extremity
G. Assess for erythema in the right lower extremity
H. Perform right hand range of motion exercises every 4 hours
I. Assess capillary refill in the right lower extremity

Day 1, 6:00 p.m.

4. A 12-year-old boy has a fracture of the right tibia after falling of his skateboard and is now in a lower leg cast. He has dislocated the proximal interphalangeal joints on the second and third fingers as well and is hospitalized overnight for observation and pain management. The evening nurses perform an assessment and find the following:

- Temperature = 99.2°F
- Pulse = 120 breaths/min
- BP = 128/80 mmHg
- Respirations = 26 breaths/min
- Increased pain in right lower extremity
- Undetected peripheral pulse in right lower extremity
- Capillary refill 6 seconds in right lower extremity
- Swelling noted below the cast on the right extremity

Use an X for the nursing actions below that are <u>Indicated</u> (appropriate or necessary) or <u>Contraindicated</u> (could be harmful) at this time.

Nursing Action	Indicated	Contraindicated
"Apply a cold compact to right lower leg."		
"Notify the medical team immediately."		
"Control pain."		
"Move the patient to a chair for better circulation."		
"Place the left leg above the heart."		
"Continue to assess peripheral pulse and capillary refill."		
"Inspect skin for color changes proximal to the cast."		

Day 1, 9:00 p.m.

5. A 12-year-old boy has a fracture of the right tibia after falling of his skateboard and is now in a cast. He has dislocated the proximal interphalangeal joints on the second and third fingers as well and is hospitalized overnight for observation and pain management. The nurse is concerned about her assessment findings and asked the medical team to immediately evaluate the child. The cast was removed to assess for compartment syndrome and within a few minutes the following assessment is found:

- Decreased pain in right lower extremity
- Peripheral pulse 70 beats/min in right lower extremity
- Less than 3 seconds capillary refill in right lower extremity

Indicate with nursing action listed in the far-left column is most appropriate for each potential complication that could result from a bone fracture.

Note that NOT all actions will be used.

Nursing Action	Potential Complications	Appropriate Nursing Action for Complication
1. Observe for pain, pallor, pulselessness, paresthesia, and paralysis.	Circulatory impairment	
2. Observe for altered sensation when sensory testing with touch and pinprick.	Compartment syndrome	
3. Observe for peripheral pulses.	Nerve compression	
4. Observe for fever and drainage from the site.	Pulmonary emboli	
5. Observe for signs of urinary retention.	Uncontrolled pain	
6. Assess for dyspnea, keep head of bed elevated and administer oxygen. Note this is a medical emergency.		
7. Frequently assess pain using a pain rating scale.		

Day 3, 3:00 p.m.

6. A 12-year-old boy has a fracture of the right tibia after falling of his skateboard and is now in a cast again since yesterday morning when a new one was placed. He was experiencing increased pain, decreased peripheral pulses and decreased capillary refill within hours of the first cast being placed. He did well yesterday after another cast was placed with no further complications, and the nurse is preparing him and his family for discharge.

Which of the following responses by the nurse are appropriate for discharge teaching? Select all that apply.

A. "Your child can swim in a pool but should avoid the river or ocean."
B. "Encourage frequent rest periods for a few days at home."
C. "His right leg can be elevated on pillows for more comfort."
D. Cover the cast at all times with waterproof tape and plastic."
E. "Observe the toes for any evidence of swelling or discoloration."
F. "Look at the skin at the cast edges to make sure it is not irritated or red."
G. Check your child's pulses in all extremities every 4 hours during the day."

A Child With Cerebral Palsy

Day 1, 9:00 a.m.

1. A 4-month-old male infant is seen in the pediatrician's office for routine follow-up. The infant was born prematurely at 33 weeks' gestation and weighed 2300 g at birth. There was a twin who died at birth. There was intrauterine exposure to maternal chorioamnionitis documented in the medical record. The nurse documents the following history and physical assessment findings. **Select the assessment findings that require follow up by the nurse. Select all that apply**.
   A. Tongue thrust
   B. Hands fisted
   C. Tonic neck reflex present
   D. Pulse = 85 beats/min
   E. Temperature = 98.4°F.
   F. Primitive infant reflexes present
   G. Respirations = 28 breaths/min
   H. Awakens during the night for feeding
   I. Mother notes feeding difficulties and poor sucking
   J. Rigid and unbending at the hip and knee joints
2. Based on the assessment findings above, **choose the most likely options for the information missing from the statements below by selecting from the lists of options provided.**

   The nurse determines that the history and assessment findings could be signs of __________1__________ and should be further assessed. The birth history reveals _________2_________ that is a risk factor for this disorder. __________3____________ is a diagnostic tool that is now recommended for a child suspected of this disorder.

Options for 1	Options for 2	Options for 3
Infantile seizures	Poor feeding	Lumbar puncture
Traumatic brain injury	Prematurity	Neuroimaging
Cerebral palsy	Trauma to the head	Blood lead level
Myelomeningocele	Sleep disruption	Echocardiogram
Diabetes	Constipation	Chest X-ray
Urinary tract infection	Nystagmus	Venous blood gas

Day 8, 10:00 a.m.

3. A week later the infant and parents are seen in the pediatric neurology specialty clinic for further evaluation. The specialty team begins by performing a careful history and assessment. The birth history and examination in the pediatrician's office a week ago cause concerns that the child may have cerebral palsy. The nurse on the specialty team performs a complete assessment and focuses on specific physical characteristics that increase suspicion of the diagnosis.

   Which clinical manifestations listed below are **priority** items that the nurse would develop a plan of care for this infant at this time? **Select all that apply.**
   A. Abnormal postures
   B. Reflex abnormalities
   C. Sleeping during the day
   D. Alteration of muscle tone
   E. Opening both eyes to voices
   F. Crying at night when hungry
   G. Abnormal motor performance
   H. Delayed gross motor development

Day 14, 9:00 a.m.

4. The infant completes a comprehensive diagnostic evaluation by the multidisciplinary neurology team. While the diagnosis can be difficult to confirm at an early age, the persistence of primitive reflexes confirms the diagnosis of cerebral palsy. The nurse working with the neurology team is to begin teaching the parents how to care for the child at home.

Use an X for the nursing actions below that are Indicated (appropriate or necessary) or Contraindicated (could be harmful) at this time.

Nursing Action	Indicated	Contraindicated
"Your infant may have difficulty keeping his head upright. Let me show you some ways to support his head."		
"Notify the medical team immediately if your infant begins to vomit."		
"If your infant has difficulty feeding and swallowing, I can show you some ways that might help."		
"Keep your infant in an upright position at all times. You can use pillows to prop him up."		
"Your infant may need nutritional supplements. I will have the nutritionist meet with you to discuss this."		
"Because of your child's disease, he should not receive his immunizations."		
"I will show you how to look at your infant's skin to make sure there is no breakdown."		

Day 30, 9:00 a.m.

5. The infant is now 5 months of age and returns to the neurology specialty clinic for follow-up. The mother notes the infant is having increasing difficulty feeding because he thrusts his tongue out. He still cannot hold his head upright. She states he is more "floppy" than he was a month ago and when she tries to pull him into a sitting position, he extends his entire body and does not bend at the hips or knees. She is having more problems trying to diaper the infant. The infant has stools every 2 to 3 days that are hard.

Indicate which nursing action listed in the far-left column is most appropriate for each potential complication that could result from a bone fracture.

Note that NOT all actions will be used.

Nursing Action	Potential Complications	Appropriate Nursing Action for Complication
1. Teach parents how to diaper the infant, clean the perianal area, and observe for signs of skin breakdown.	Inadequate nutrition	
2. Teach parents how to observe for fever and administer antibiotics.	Lack of support for parents	
3. Discuss nutrition needs with nutritionist to provide suggestions to promote adequate caloric intake.	Skin breakdown	
4. Discuss parent concerns and fears and offer support available in the community and nationally.	Bodily harm	
5. Teach parents how to observe for signs of urinary retention.	Communicable illnesses	
6. Discuss measures to promote safety in the home environment and prevent falls, and safe transport in a vehicle.		
7. Discuss the importance of the infant receiving immunizations to prevent common childhood illnesses.		

One Year Later, 10:00 a.m.

6. The child with cerebral palsy is now 1 year old and returns to the neurology specialty clinic for follow-up. He has a gastrostomy (G) tube for supplementing regular feedings to promote weight gain. The mother asks for advice on ways she can support her child at home. She says that she is having difficulty with the G tube clogging and is not sure she is doing the physical exercises correctly.

Which of the following responses by the nurse are appropriate during this visit? Select all that apply.

A. "I recommend you stop using the G tube for medications since it is clogging."
B. "Passive range of motion exercises will not help your child at this young age. We will start those exercises in a few years."
C. "I recommend you do not try to perform any physical exercises that include stretching his muscles at home since you might hurt him."
D. "I will ask the pharmacist to give us ideas on how to best dissolve or crush the pills before administering them through the G tube."
E. "I recommend you work with your child to promote oral feeding. I will show you how to promote jaw control when feeding your child."
F. "Because your child is at risk for infection, take your child's temperature and pulse every 4 hours while awake. Let me show you how to take his pulse."
G. "It sounds like you are doing a good job using the G tube. I can show you how to prevent clogging which can often occur after pills are given through it."
H. "The exercise program includes stretching that consists of passive, active, and resistive movements to specific muscle groups. I will have the physical therapist review the exercises with you."

Unfolding Case Studies Answer Key

Care at the End of Life

1. **C, E, F, G, H, I**

Rationales: Findings requiring further follow-up are related to pain this boy is experiencing because of a paravertebral fibrosarcoma of the right lumbosacral area. The visual pain score of 8/10 is a measure of persistent pain experienced as burning/piercing pain in the lower extremities or neuropathic pain, swelling around the lower lumbar area, and numbness of the lower extremities. Heart rate is increased above normal findings for a school-age child. Other vital signs are normal including capillary refill. The weight for age is not a concern.

2.

Option 1	Option 2
1–2 mg/kg	**4 h**
0.1–0.2 mg/kg	15 min
0.5–1.0 mg/kg	2 h
0.1–1 mg/kg	6 h
1.0–2.0 mg/kg	10 min

Rationales: The history reveals the child has been on oral pain medication, but it is unclear exactly how much oral opioids have been given. Because of this, the standard starting IV dose will be used which is 0.1 to 0.2 mg/kg. After three doses are given initially, the medication is scheduled for every 4 hours.

3. **A, B, C, E, G**

Rationales: Routine reassessment of pain is essential for this child and, if possible, self-report should be used. Nursing observation regarding how the child responds to the medication and his behavior after receiving it is important to determine if the child is receiving enough pain medication. A variety of pain scales can be used for a 9-year-old including verbal report scales or the simple FACES scale. It is not appropriate to use an infant scale. Pain should be assessed more than once a shift so that proper pain management can occur as needed.

4.

Nursing Action	Potential Complication	Nursing Action for Complication
1. Administer morphine safely. Observe the patient for excessive sedation and respiratory depression.	To reduce unfounded fears	3
2. Monitor for side effects of morphine: decreased respiratory rate, urinary retention, constipation, and pruritus.	To prevent unwanted side effects that may cause additional discomfort	2
3. Educate parents on the safety and effectiveness of the pain-relieving medications.	To ensure optimal pain relief	4
4. Reassess the pain level after administering pain medication. Assess within 1 hour of oral morphine and 30 min after IV administration.	To prevent adverse effects and overdose	1
5. Recognize when pain is not well controlled on morphine.	To ensure satisfactory pain relief	5
6. Provide appropriate bowel regimen and monitor urine output.		
7. Provide distraction and counseling to assure parents that everything possible is being done.		

Rationales: When using multiple medications to manage pain, it is important to monitor side effects for each medication. When morphine is administered, the patient should be closely observed for excessive sedation and respiratory depression. Pain should be reassessed after administration—within 1 hour of oral morphine and 30 minutes after IV morphine administration. This helps the nurse recognize when pain is not being well-controlled. Parents must be educated on the safety and effectiveness of the pain-relieving medications.

5.

Nursing Action	Effective	Ineffective
Assure parents that the IV morphine dose can be the same dose they administer at home.		X
Instruct parents to continue around-the-clock medications at home.	X	
Encourage parents to communicate any signs of pain; observe patient for nonverbal signs of pain.	X	
A home bowel regimen should be included in the discharge teaching.	X	
Instruct parents to talk to other family members about their feelings toward pain management.		
Stress with the parents that escalating doses will not be needed, and that tolerance to pain medications never occur in children.		X
Discuss appropriate nonpharmacologic options that can relieve pain.	X	

Rationales: For pain medication in a child with cancer it is essential for parents to understand that they must continue the medications around the clock. If they do not do so, the child will experience breakthrough pain that can be severe. They must also be aware that the IV and oral dosing is different. Teaching parents how to assess pain in a child with cancer is important since it can help them effectively manage pain. Parents may need to escalate doses as the cancer progresses and pain medication tolerance can occur in children. Include discussion on constipation as a common side effect of opioids and assist with a home bowel regimen. Nonpharmacologic options also should be taught.

6. **B, C, E, G**

Rationales: It is frightening for the family, especially parents, to face the death of a child at home. The introduction of a new health care provider—the hospice nurse—also causes anxiety since many families have developed strong relationships with the health care team caring for the child with cancer. The nurse would respond by focusing on the child's needs for comfort and pain management. Assuring the mother that the hospice nurse will keep them informed of what is happening and will answer any questions they have is important. The nurse should not tell the mother that the hospice nurse will take the child to the hospital or start antibiotics since this may not be part of the end-of-life care plan.

The Child With Chronic Kidney Disease

1. **A, B, C, D, E, G, I, M**

Rationales: Pallor, headache, facial edema, fatigue, muscle cramping, and nausea are common symptoms associated with kidney disease. The child's BP is elevated based on the child's age and height (see growth charts on the CDC website and BP levels on the back cover). Skin dryness and itchiness are commonly reported. In this case study, vital signs are normal for age; height is in the 25th percentile for age, and weight is just below the 25th percentile for age.

2.

Nursing Action	Potential Complication	Nursing Action to Prevent Complication
1. Close monitoring of the patient's status. Follow clinical and laboratory findings. Blood studies included CBC, electrolytes, and kidney status.	Waste products accumulate	2
2. Observe for evidence of accumulated waste products.	Increased excretory kidney demands	3
3. Provide dietary instructions for foods that reduce excretory demands on kidneys and provide sufficient calories and protein for growth.	Changes in kidney status go unrecognized	1
4. Limit phosphorus, salt, and potassium as prescribed.	Growth failure unrecognized	5

Nursing Action	Potential Complication	Nursing Action to Prevent Complication
5. Monitor growth closely since short stature is a significant side effect.	Accumulation of minerals	4
6. Monitor cardiovascular status, including BP measurement.	Renal bone disease	7
7. Minimize renal bone disease by maintaining optimal calcium, phosphorus, and intact parathyroid hormone levels, and acid–base balance.		
8. Monitor for anemia. Child may require school accommodations and rest periods due to fatigue.		
9. Identify patient and family stressors that may accompany a diagnosis of CKD.		

Rationales: Essential nursing actions focus on identifying changes in kidney status that result in the accumulation of waste products and minerals. Clinical and laboratory findings would be followed closely: blood studies include CBC, electrolytes, and kidney function. The nurse would spend time emphasizing dietary instructions for foods that reduce excretory demands on kidneys and provide sufficient calories and protein for growth. Phosphorus, salt, and potassium may be limited. The nurse would closely monitor the child's growth since short stature is a significant side effect. Actions to minimize renal bone disease by maintaining optimal calcium, phosphorus, and intact parathyroid hormone levels, and acid–base balance would be implemented.

3. **A, B, C, F, G, H**

Rationales: The case study reflects that the child is experiencing increased symptoms of kidney disease and that the kidney disease may be worsening. The child's kidney function, electrolyte status, and CBC should be immediately assessed. Damaged kidneys cause retention of waste products, and serum creatinine and BUN levels are increased. Sodium and potassium can be increased, and metabolic acidosis can occur. Calcium and phosphorus disturbances also occur. Anemia is common. Careful assessment of the child's weight, height, and vital signs should be compared to the previous visit. Review of adherence to medications and dietary recommendations is also important.

4. **A, B, G, I, J, K**

Rationales: As discussed in the answer to 3, there are many laboratory results that confirm worsening of CKD. In this case study, the child is anemic based on the hemoglobin and hematocrit level. Laboratory studies confirm kidney abnormalities with an increase in serum creatinine, BUN, and GFR. The urine analysis also indicated elevated protein and hematuria that are signs of CKD. The child's potassium, sodium, and phosphorus are not a concern at this time.

5. **A, D, G**

Rationales: Dietary management for children with CKD focuses on providing sufficient calories and protein for growth, while limiting excretory demands on the kidneys. This is accomplished by limiting protein to the recommended daily allowance. While sodium is not always restricted, because this child has increased edema and elevated BP, it would be recommended. Sugar restrictions, milk intake reduction, and use of oral medications to decreased GI absorption are not used for CKD management. Dietary management is focused on providing enough calories to promote growth and development while minimizing excretory demands on the kidneys; decreasing foods high in calories is not therapeutic.

6. **B, C, D, E, F**

Rationales: The nurse would begin by first reviewing why the child is experiencing symptoms and how CKD causes them. Emphasizing the need for limited oral intake such as protein and other minerals provides concrete information for the mother. Discussing specific symptoms, why they are occurring, and what the mother should do about them (e.g., when to call the health care team) provide her with specific interventions that can be essential for this child.

The Child With Appendicitis

1. **D, E, F, H, I**

Rationales: The following findings need to be further explored as they are common signs and symptoms found in a child with appendicitis. These include fever and an elevated CRP—note CRP elevation is nonspecific and noted in many inflammatory and acute illnesses. An elevated WBC count with increased bands is a general sign of infection. Abdominal pain midway between the anterior superior iliac crest and umbilicus and pain that intensifies with any activity or deep breathing is also a concern. The child's weight, pulse, BP, hemoglobin, and platelet count is not abnormal.

2.

Options for 1	Options for 2	Options for 3
Anemia	BP of 108/74	Ruptured kidney
Pain	Pulse of 80	**Acute abdomen**
Bleeding	**CRP**	Influenza
Infection	Hemoglobin	Urinary Tract Infection
HF	Platelets	Vomiting
Cancer	Serum sodium	Anxiety

Rationales: An increased WBC count and increased CRP is a sign of possible infection, although many illnesses can cause this increase. The location of pain in this child warrants close observation since it may be indicative of an acute abdomen that is exemplified by acute abdominal pain.

3. **A, C, D, F, H, I**

Rationales: Immediate intervention should focus on the child's pain and risk of rupture of the appendix that would cause infection. An elevated temperature indicates hyperthermia may also indicate infection. Vomiting is a concern because it can quickly lead to dehydration. Anemia, weight loss, and constipation are symptoms that should be evaluated but they do not need immediate attention.

4.

Nursing Action	Potential Postoperative Complication	Nursing Action for Postoperative Complication
1. Administer pain medications.	Inflammation at the wound site	10
2. Initiate IV fluids and assess intake and output (I&O).	Electrolyte imbalance	6
3. Assess temperature and report elevation.	Fluid deficit	2
4. Administer antiemetics.	Pain	1
5. Administer IV sodium heparin.	Nausea and vomiting	4
6. Draw blood as scheduled and evaluate results.	Infection	8
7. Report changes in vital signs, behavior, and LOC.	Fever	3
8. Administer IV antibiotics.		
9. Administer a blood transfusion.		
10. Observe wound site.		

Rationales: Since the appendix is ruptured, a major concern is risk of infection. IV antibiotics are administered, and vital signs are taken to observe for fever. IV fluids are given to prevent electrolyte imbalance and dehydration and pain is assessed and medications administered as needed post-surgery. The surgical wound should be observed for signs of inflammation that include redness, warmth, swelling, and tenderness.

5.

Nursing Action	Effective	Ineffective
Observe no signs of infection.	X	
Pain is controlled.	X	
No complaints of nausea or vomiting and a regular diet is tolerated.	X	
Temperature remains in the normal range	X	
Child spending all of the time in bed.		X

Rationales: Expected quality patient outcomes post appendectomy include no signs of infection, pain controlled, absence of fever, and no nausea or vomiting. The child is able to take oral fluids and solid foods. The child should be ambulating and sitting in a chair, not spending all of the time in bed.

6.

Health Teaching	Indicated	Contraindicated
"Take your child's temperature if she feels warm and call the surgeon if she has a fever over 101°F."	X	
"Give ibuprofen every 6 h for the next 5 days."		X
"Inspect the surgical incision every day for increased redness, heat, or drainage; if present, call the surgeon immediately."	X	
Ask the parents, "What are your concerns regarding your daughter's care at home?"	X	
"Apply a topical antibiotic to the surgical wound for the next week."		X

Rationales: A major concern following surgery for a ruptured appendix is infection. Parents should be instructed to take the child's temperature if she feels warm and call the surgeon if over 101°F. Parents should be taught to inspect the surgical incision and to call if there is redness, warmth, or drainage at the site. The nurse also should take time to listen to the parent's concerns before discharge. There is no need to give ibuprofen around the clock for 5 days or apply a topic antibiotic to the wound for 7 days. The child should be expected to return to normal activities of daily living as she recovers and not be allowed to watch movies all day long.

The Child With Acute Respiratory Tract Illness

1. **A, B, C, D, E, F, G, H, J, K**

Rationales: There are numerous physical assessment findings that require immediate follow-up. The infant has respiratory compromise based on these symptoms: nasal flaring, retractions, increased respirations, rhonchi and fine crackles in the lung, and a decreased SaO_2 saturation. Other concerns include an elevated temperature, increased pulse, irritability and restlessness, and decreased appetite. The BP is normal for age.

2.

Options for 1	Options for 2	Options for 3
Pneumonia	**Persistent dry, hacking cough worse at night, more productive in 2–3 days**	Inhaled corticosteroids, antibiotics
Bronchiolitis	Retractions, labored respirations	Allergen and "triggers control"
Emphysema	Poor feeding, inability to sleep, gastrointestinal symptoms	**Supplemental oxygen, fluid intake, suctioning as needed**
Wheezing	Seizures, altered consciousness, inability to focus	Long-term anti-inflammatory medications

Rationales: Infants with bronchiolitis present with labored respirations, poor feeding, cough, tachypnea, retractions, and flaring nares similar to the infant in this case study. Treatment for bronchiolitis includes supplemental oxygen, fluid intake, and suctioning as needed. Bronchitis usually presents as a persistent dry, hacking cough that is worse at night and becomes more productive in 2 to 3 days.

3.

Options for 1	Options for 2	Options for 3
Upper	Skin	1–2
Middle	**Epithelial**	2–3
Lower	Blood	**2–8**
Extreme	Muscle	10–14
Left	Nasal	14–18
Right	Bone	40-43

Rationales: Bronchiolitis is an acute viral infection with maximum effect in the lower respiratory tract at the bronchiolar level. RSV is the most common cause of bronchiolitis in children and affects the epithelial cells of the respiratory tract and usually begins after an incubation of about 2 to 8 days.

4.

Nursing Action	Potential Complication	Nursing Action for Complication
1. Position infant for maximum ventilation and airway patency.	Inability to identify alterations in temperature, respiratory status or circulation, and need for additional interventions is missed	2
2. Monitor vital signs, including temperature and respiratory, cardiac, and oxygen status.	Nasal mucosal membrane drying	3
3. Provide humidified oxygen as indicated.	Fever	6
4. Suction airway (nares, mouth, nasopharynx) as indicated.	Bronchial constriction and decreased ventilation	7
5. Provide gentle chest percussion and chest physiotherapy (CPT) as indicated.	Secretions causing lack of airway patency	4
6. Administer antipyretics as indicated.	Infection	8
7. Administer bronchodilators as indicated.	Spread of infection	10
8. Administer antibiotics if indicated.	Dehydration or fluid overload	11

Nursing Action	Potential Complication	Nursing Action for Complication
9. Obtain specimens (e.g., secretions, blood) as indicated.		
10. Maintain appropriate precautions such as Standard Precautions, droplet isolation, and frequent hand washing.		
11. Monitor hydration status through strict intake and output and daily weights.		
12. Implement comfort measures such as allowing parent presence, parent holding infant, and comfort item such as favorite blanket or stuffed animal.		

Rationales: The nurse would closely monitor vital signs, including temperature and respiratory, cardiac, and oxygen status. To support airway patency, humidified oxygen as needed is used and airways are suctioned. Medications may include antipyretics if fever is present, bronchodilators and antibiotics as indicated. Hydration status is closely monitored, and fluids are given if needed. It is essential for appropriate precautions to be implemented to prevent spread of the illness such as Standard Precautions, droplet isolation, and frequent hand washing.

5. **A, C, E, F**

Rationales: The infant has a normal SaO_2 on room air, respirations are normal for age, there are minimal nasal secretions, and the lungs are clear. These all are signs that this infant is recovering. The temperature elevation and minimal oral intake over the past day are concerning and warrant further assessment. The child may need to remain in the hospital longer.

6.

Health Teaching Evaluation	Indicated	Contraindicated
Parents able to verbalize definition and characteristics of acute respiratory tract infection.	X	
Parents able to verbalize treatment, including medication and interventions that promote ventilation and airway clearance.	X	
Parents can identify discharge medications, including antipyretics, bronchodilators, and antibiotics as prescribed.	X	
Parents want to purchase a pulse oximeter before taking the infant home so they can constantly monitor the oxygen level.		X
Parents feel that keeping the infant supine will assist with any nasal secretions the infant may have.		X

Rationales: The infant no longer has a fever and is taking oral fluids well. She is ready for discharge. Important health teaching points include the parents being able to verbalize the definition and characteristics of an acute respiratory tract infection. They should be able to identify discharge medications—how and when they should be administered. Other measures to promote ventilation and airway clearance should be discussed, such as administering saline drops into the nares and suctioning with a bulb syringe. There is no need to purchase a pulse oximeter. Keeping the infant supine is not recommended and will not assist with nasal secretions.

The Child With Acute Asthma Exacerbation

1. **B, C, D, F, G, H**

Rationales: This adolescent's heart rate and respirations are elevated. His SpO_2 and PEFM results are lower than normal. A peak expiratory flow rate of 50% indicates that asthma is not well controlled, and an acute exacerbation may be present. A normal SpO_2 level ranges from 95% to 100%. He is having difficulty breathing when lying down and wheezing is noted in both lungs. His BP is normal for age.

2. **A, C, E, G, H, I**

Rationales: Asthma episodes are associated with airflow limitation or obstruction that are reversible either spontaneously or with treatment. Acute inflammation causes an increase in bronchial hyperresponsiveness to a variety of stimuli. Airflow obstruction and limitation result in dyspnea, shortness of breath, and increased respiratory rate. Chest tightness and even pain is experienced, and the use of accessory muscles observed as retractions is seen. There are diminished breath sounds heard. Moist cough, high BP, and sections are not observed in acute asthma episodes.

3.

Nursing Action	Emergent	Not Emergent
Administer humidified oxygen to keep the oxygen saturation (SpO_2) above 90%.	X	
Administer methylprednisolone per the physician order.	X	
Administer albuterol per hospital protocol.	X	
Place the patient in a comfortable standing, sitting upright, or learning forward position.	X	
Discuss possible allergens in the home that might have triggered the attack.		X
Review how to use the metered dose inhaler.		X

Rationales: The goal for acute care of this teenager is to calm their anxiety while initiating immediate medical care. Humidified oxygen is given to keep the oxygen saturation (SpO_2) above 90%. Methylprednisolone and albuterol are given to relieve respiratory distress. Measures to promote comfort in breathing may include placing the teenager in a comfortable standing, sitting upright, or learning forward position. An acute asthma episode is not the time to discuss ways to prevent an asthma attack in the future or to discuss managing their asthma by using a metered dose inhaler.

4.

Nursing Action	Potential Complication	Nursing Action to Prevent Complication
1. Allow patient to assume position of comfort.	To minimize drying of nasal mucous membranes	3
2. Administer rescue medications (as prescribed) that can include inhalers, nebulization, and/or oral or IV steroids.	To prevent airway obstruction	1
3. Administer humidified oxygen to maintain oxygen saturation (SaO_2) above 90%.	Decreased patient's awareness of factors that exacerbate asthma	5
4. Assess patient's response to rescue medications.	To prevent constricted airways and decreased air exchange	2
5. Assist patient in recognizing factors that trigger asthma symptoms.	Lack of awareness of need for more aggressive interventions	4
6. Assure respirations will be easy and nonlabored at a rate within normal limits for age.		
7. Teach the patient how to use the PEFM.		
8. Evaluate the use of the PEFM.		

Rationales: Humidified oxygen is given to minimize drying of nasal mucous membranes and maintain oxygen saturation (SaO_2) above 90%. Rescue medications can include inhalers, nebulization, and/or oral or IV steroids to treat airway constriction and improve air exchange. Allowing the teenager to sit in a comfortable position, no matter what it may be, helps to prevent airway obstruction. After the acute asthma episode, it would be important to talk about recognizing factors that trigger his asthma symptoms to help him identify problems early.

5. **A, D, E, F, H**

Rationales: Important areas of teaching that may prevent acute asthma episodes include identifying early signs of an asthma exacerbation and what asthma triggers may be present in the environment. Discussion on avoiding smoke, exposure to excessive cold, wind, and other extremes of weather, as well as other environmental irritants, is important to cover. Taking Tylenol is not an issue and albuterol is not routinely administered every day. Physical exercise and training are important healthy habits but are not specific acute asthma episode interventions. Discussion could include exercise-induced bronchospasm events and how to prevent them.

6.

Options for 1	Options for 2	Options for 3	Options for 4
Flow of air	5 s	**80%–100%**	4–5 weeks
Flow of oxygen	10 s	50%–70%	**2–3 weeks**
Flow of water	**1 s**	60%–80%	1–2 days

Rationales: Discharge preparation following an acute asthma episode provides a good opportunity to reinforce how to use the PEFM. The PEFM measures the maximum flow of air that can be forcefully exhaled in 1 second and is measured in liters per minute. Each child/adolescent should establish their own personal best values during a 2- to 3-week period when the asthma is stable. The PEFR is recorded twice a day to obtain the personal best value. This result is used to determine the severity of asthma when symptoms are present.

The Child With Coarctation of the Aorta

1. **A, B, D, E, G, I, J**

Rationales: Signs and symptoms of HF can be divided into three groups: (1) impaired myocardial function, (2) pulmonary congestion, and (3) systemic venous congestion. Common signs of HF include tachypnea and tachycardia at rest, feeding intolerance, edema caused by fluid retention, prolonged capillary refill, hypotension, and cool extremities. HF does not cause weight loss, but weight gain is common due to fluid retention.

2.

Options for 1	Options for 2	Options for 3 and 4
Widening	Increased	**Bounding = 3**
Absence	**Decreased**	Widening
Narrowing	Lack of	**Weak or absent = 4**
Crossing	Absent	Narrowing
Absence	Complex	Unstable

Rationales: Coarctation of the aorta is caused by localized narrowing near the insertion of the ductus arteriosus, which results in decreased pressure distal to the obstruction (body and lower extremities). There may be high BP and bounding pulses in the arms, weak or absent femoral pulses, and cool lower extremities with lower BP.

3.

Nursing Action	Emergent	Not Emergent
Frequently assess and record heart rate, respiratory rate, BP, and any signs or symptoms of decreased cardiac output.	X	
Administer cardiac drugs on schedule. Assess and record any side effects or any signs and symptoms of toxicity. Follow hospital protocol for administration.	X	
Administer cool humidified oxygen to increase available oxygen during inspiration.	X	
Change the infant's position every 2 h to prevent skin breakdown.		X
Keep accurate record of intake and output.	X	
Weigh infant on same scale at same time of day.		X
Maintain a 3-h feeding schedule.		X
Restrict fluids if the intake and output is unbalanced.		X

Rationales: Emergent priority nursing actions prior to heart surgery should focus on keeping the infant as stable as possible. The nurse would assess and record heart rate, respiratory rate, BP, and any signs or symptoms of decreased cardiac output. Medications would be administered as ordered and an accurate record of intake and output would be documented to make sure fluid overload does not occur. While changing the infant's position every few hours is important it is not emergent along with concern for weighing the infant on the same scale at the same time and restricting fluids on the day before surgery.

4.

Nursing Action	Potential Complication	Nursing Action to Prevent Complication
1. Assess and record heart rate, respiratory rate, BP, and any signs or symptoms of altered cardiac output every 2–4 h.	Decreased urinary output is a symptom of HF and could go unnoticed	3
2. Administer cardiac drugs on schedule. Assess and record any side effects or any signs and symptoms of toxicity. Follow hospital protocol for administration.	Undetected changes in vital signs and infant's physical status that reflect altered cardiac output and high BP	1
3. Keep accurate record of intake and output.	Excess water and salt because fluid retention commonly occurs with HF	5
4. Weigh infant on same scale at same time of day as previously. Document results and compare to previous weight.	Dangers inherent in failure to administer cardiac drugs as prescribed and to perform careful assessment before administration	2
5. Administer diuretics on schedule. Assess and record effectiveness and any side effects noted.		

Nursing Action	Potential Complication	Nursing Action to Prevent Complication
6. Offer small, frequent feedings to infant's tolerance. 7. Organize nursing care to allow infant uninterrupted rest.		

Rationales: Essential nursing actions prior to heart surgery for this infant are discussed in question 3. Careful observation of the infant's vital signs assesses altered cardiac output and high BP. Decreased urinary output is a symptom of HF and could go unnoticed since excessive water and salt retention commonly occurs if input and output is not closely observed. The nurse would understand the dangers inherent in failure to administer cardiac drugs as prescribed and to perform careful assessment before administration.

5. **A, B, C, D, E, H, I**

Rationales: Three days after heart surgery the infant should be demonstrating signs of adequate blood flow through the heart since the narrowing within the aorta has been repaired. Signs of normal blood perfusion include normal skin color that is warm to touch, strong and equal pulses in all extremities, lack of distended neck veins with no presence of edema, and a normal heart rate for age. The normal heart rate for a 3-week-old infant ranges from 100 to 150 beats/min. An important indicator is the infant's ability to feed; since he is no longer in respiratory distress, he should have no difficulty sucking.

6.

Health Teaching	Indicated	Contraindicated
Discuss the characteristics of COA and the surgery done to repair the obstructive defect.	X	
Review the infant's daily care, including medication administration.	X	
Review signs and symptoms that could be of concern (fever, blue skin color, poor eating).	X	
Inform parents to purchase a pulse oximeter before taking the infant home so they can constantly monitor the oxygen level.		X
Keep the infant supine at all times to assist with blood flow.		X
Give parents the opportunity to express their fears and concerns.	X	

Rationales: The nurse would play a major role in parent education that should minimize their fears and concerns for discharge to home. The nurse would begin with making sure the family understands the defect and why it was repaired. Common signs and symptoms of HF that could be of concern should be presented (e.g., fever, blue skin color, poor eating). The infant's daily schedule for medications should be discussed with parents, demonstrating an understanding of when, how much, and how to administer medications. The nurse would observe the parent administering medication before discharge. Parents would have opportunities to discuss any fears or concerns during the education session. Pulse oximeter measurements are not needed in the home and the infant would not be placed in a supine position since this does not influence blood flow.

The Child With Sickle Cell Anemia

1. **C, E, F, G, J**

Rationales: The boy's temperature, pulse, and respirations are increased in this case study. Pain in children with sickle cell disease often causes an elevation in vital signs. The pain score is high at 8/10 and the abdomen is tender to palpation. This may be caused by sickle cells sequestering in the abdomen. Pulse oximetry is normal along with serum bilirubin levels. The hemoglobin and hematocrit are lower than normal, but it is important to remember that in children with SCD, because of the rapid turnover of red blood cell due to sickling of erythrocytes, lab results will be lower than normal.

2.

Options for 1	Options for 2
Aplastic crisis	High BP
Sequestration crisis	**Ischemia**
Acute chest syndrome	Bleeding
VOC	Infection
Hyperhemolytic crisis	Diminished red blood cell production
Cerebral vascular accident	Decreased serum sodium

Rationales: VOC is a painful episode caused by ischemia that results in pain. This occurs because the sickled red blood cells clump or block blood flow in a blood vessel. The pain can be generalized or specific to a certain area. In this case study, the child is experiencing abdominal pain from visceral hypoxia.

3. **A, D, E**

Rationales: Acute management of a VOC requires pain assessment and management and hydration. In this case study, there was no indication the child needed blood transfusion or oxygen therapy. Oxygen therapy is of little value unless the patient is hypoxic; it is not effective in reversing red blood cell sickling or reducing pain. Antibiotics are not administered unless there is evidence of an infection since low-grade fever during a crisis can occur. While strict bedrest is not recommended, minimizing energy expenditure during an acute VOC will improve oxygen utilization. Usually it is best to let the child determine their activity tolerance.

4.

Nursing Action	Potential Complication	Nursing Action for Complication
1. Discuss schedule of around-the-clock medication with parents.	Uncontrolled pain	**1**
2. Encourage high level of fluid intake.	Breakthrough pain	**3**
3. Recognize that various analgesics, including opioids and medication schedules, may need to be tried.	To avoid needless suffering because of unfounded fears	**4**
4. Reassure child and family that analgesics, including opioids, are medically indicated, that high doses may be needed, and that children rarely become addicted.	To prevent vasoconstriction that may enhance sickling with cold applications	**5**
5. Apply heat application or massage to affected area. Avoid applying cold compresses.	Dehydration	**2**
6. Provide protein shake with each meal.		
7. Weigh the child each morning with the same scale.		

Rationales: The most important nursing action for a child experiencing a vasoocclusive SCD crisis is to administer pain medications at a dose and route that will provide effective pain relief. It is essential to provide "around the clock" relief using doses needed to relieve the pain, and for the child and family to understand the importance of this approach to pain management. Increased pain medication doses are often needed. Hydration is essential to assist with clearing the clogged vessels and preventing metabolic acidosis because of hypoxia. Some children receive pain relief from heat application or massage, but cold compresses should be avoided because they can enhance vasoconstriction.

5.

Options for 1	Options for 2	Options for 3	Options for 4
6	**0.4**	2.2	5 min
4	0.2	1.8	6 min
8	0.8	**1.4**	8 min
2	0.9	1.2	**10 min**

Rationales: The child's weight of 40 kg and doses would be calculated based on that weight. These are the PCA doses that should be used when starting PCA pain medications: Loading dose of 0.1 mg/kg (maximum 8 mg); basal rate of 0.01 mg/kg and intermittent dose 0.035 mg/kg (maximum 8 mg) with the interval lockout at approximately 10 minutes. For this child the loading dose would be 4 mg, with a basal rate of 0.03 mg and an intermittent dose of 1.4 mg. The interval lockout would occur every 10 minutes.

6.

Nursing Action	Effective	Ineffective
Administer morphine and ketorolac safely.	X	
Monitor for side effects of morphine; assess respiratory status closely and prevent constipation.	X	
Monitor for side effects of ketorolac; assess for bleeding (gastrointestinal [GI] or renal) closely.	X	
Educate parents on the safety and effectiveness of IV morphine and ketorolac when using them at home.		X
Reassess the child's pain level once a shift after administering morphine and ketorolac.		X
Recognize that various analgesics and doses may need to be tried.	X	

Rationales: The case study reveals that pain management is effective in treating this child's pain. Appropriate nursing actions include continuing to administer morphine and ketorolac safely and monitor for side effects: morphine assess respiratory status closely and prevent constipation; ketorolac-assess for bleeding (GI or renal). The nurse would be knowledgeable about various pain medications used to manage SCD VOC and realize different medications and routes may need to be tried. Pain assessment is done more than once a shift and parent education of using both of these agents in the home setting would not be discussed since they would not be used together after discharge.

The Child With Acute Lymphoblastic Leukemia

1. **A, C, D, E, H, I, J**

Rationales: Symptoms experienced by children with leukemia are caused by the rapid production of immature white blood cells, called lymphoblasts, in the bone marrow. This leads to decreased production of other blood cell lines—red blood cells and platelets--and the rapid release of lymphoblasts into the blood stream can invade other organs causing lymphadenopathy and hepatosplenomegaly and bone pain. Since blood cell lines are decreased, there is increased risk of fever and infection due to decreased infection fighting white blood cells. Bruising and bleeding can occur because of a decrease in platelets.

2.

Option 1	Option 2	Option 3
Seizure	**Decreased production of RBCs**	Lack of appetite and weight loss
Blindness	Increased production of plasma cells	Headache and seizure
Hemorrhage	Decreased production of CNS fluid	Enlarged spleen
Hearing loss	Increased production of bilirubin	**Fever and infection**

Rationales: Hemorrhage is caused by a decreased production of platelets in a child with ALL. Anemia, caused by a decreased production of red blood cells, causes symptoms or fatigue, listlessness, and paleness. Fever and infection result from a decreased production of white blood cells that fight infection.

3.

Options for 1	Options for 2	Options for 3
Cardiac	**Rapid**	Production
Cellular	Slow	Growth
Metabolic	Intermittent	**Lysis**
Neurologic	Prolonged	Mitosis

Rationales: This child's WBC is 85,000/mm,[3] which is extremely high (normal range = 4500 to 13,500/mm^3). Because of this, there is increased risk for metabolic abnormalities caused by lymphocyte lysis (death) that results in the release of intracellular contents that must be removed from the body.

4.

Nursing Action	Effective	Ineffective
Explain the procedure to the patient and family and obtain informed consent.	X	
Monitor vital signs during the procedure (pulse rate, oxygen saturation, respirations, BP).	X	
Administer a bolus of IV fluids before the procedure begins.		X
Administer sedation during the procedure to provide optimal comfort and minimize pain.	X	
Provide comfort and reassure the patient and family throughout the procedure.	X	
Watch for signs of bleeding from the puncture site.	X	

Rationales: For any invasive procedure a child must undergo, preparation of the child and family is essential. The developmental level of the child must be considered when discussing the procedure. This child is 7 years of age and will understand concrete statements about what is going to happen. Effective nursing actions are to discuss how the sedation will be given and what the child will experience during the procedure. The nurse would discuss the comfort and support that will be provided during and after the procedure. For a child receiving sedation, the nurse would monitor vital signs during and after the procedure (pulse rate, oxygen saturation, respirations, BP). The lumbar puncture site would be observed for signs of bleeding or infection. An IV bolus of fluids is not needed.

5. **B, C, D, E, F, H**

Rationales: As discussed in question 3, there is an increased risk for rapid breakdown of leukemia cells (lymphoblasts). This is called acute tumor lysis syndrome. Nursing actions include carefully monitoring the WBC, serum chemistries, urine pH, and urine intake and output to assure the child is excreting the byproducts caused by cell lysis. IV fluids are used to assure the patient is alkalinized and medications to reduce urine acid formation is administered. Fluids are never restricted and medications for HF are not routinely needed.

6.

Nursing Action	Potential Complication	Nursing Action to Prevent Complication
1. Explain the disease course of treatment and adverse effects to the family.	Skin as an entry point for infection	4
2. Teach the patient and family ways to prevent infection through hand washing, bathing frequently, and not using cups and utensils used by another person.	Lack of recognition of infection	3
3. Teach the family how to recognize symptoms of infection such as fever, chills, cough, and sore throat, and to report these to the health care worker immediately.	Lack of understanding of leukemia treatment	1
4. Provide skin care to patient by keeping the skin and perianal area clean and apply mild lotion.	Mouth ulceration	8
5. Provide a high-protein and high-calorie diet.	Lack of knowledge on how to prevent infection in the home	2
6. Provide adequate hydration and encourage a high-fiber diet and stool softeners.	Bleeding	7
7. Educate family and patient on how to recognize and report abnormal bleeding through bruising and petechiae.		
8. Provide frequent mouth care and saline rinses and check for ulcers in the mouth and gum swelling.		
9. Instruct patient and family to avoid contact sports.		

Rationales: The newly diagnosed child with leukemia and the family need to understand the diagnosis and how leukemia is treated. Since the majority of treatment is given in the clinic setting, parents will play a key role in assessing and managing side effects of leukemia treatment. Proper education can prevent major toxicities and side effects from occurring if the child and family know what to anticipate and look for during treatment. Infection prevention is a major emphasis during discharge teaching. Families would be taught specific ways to prevent infection through hand washing, bathing frequently, and not using cups and utensils used by another person. The nurse would discuss how to recognize symptoms of infection such as fever, chills, cough, and sore throat, and how to report these to the health care team. Since the skin is a major site of entry for infection, the nurse would discuss ways to keep the skin clean and free of infection-with emphasis placed on the perianal area. Daily mouth care is emphasized with the nurse teaching parents how to check for ulcers in the mouth and gum swelling. Since the child may experience a low platelet count, the nurses would teach the parents how to look for bleeding by the presence of petechiae, ecchymosis, or nose bleeds and would stress the importance of contacting the health care team if this occurs.

The Child With Seizures

1. **A, B, C, D, E, G, H**

Rationales: Details of the seizure episode, what occurred before, during, and immediately after the event can provide important information to facilitate the diagnosis. Obtaining information from those who observed the seizure as well as what the child remembers are equally important. It is important to elicit the sensory findings and presence of an aura as well as postictal symptoms that occur. Those that observed the seizure can provide details on the time of onset, duration, change in LOC, and movements that occurred during the event. Determining whether other students had similar symptoms is not relevant.

2.

Nursing Action	Potential Complication	Nursing Action to Prevent Complication
1. Monitor time (onset and duration), movements, and LOC during seizure.	Child experiences anxiety and fear	4
2. If child is at risk of falling, ease child to floor. Prevent child from hitting head on objects. Do not attempt to restrain child or use force.	An accurate description of the seizure is not obtained	1
3. During seizure, place child in a side-lying position on a flat surface such as floor. Do not put anything in child's mouth.	Parents unable to cope with the diagnosis and management of their son	5
4. Stay with the child and reassure the child when awakening from seizure.	Physical harm occurs	2
5. Involve child and parents in discussion of fears, anxieties, and resources and support options available to patient and family.	Aspiration can occur	3
	Lack of description of the postictal state	
	Further seizures occur	

Rationales: A major nursing action is to closely observe for further seizure activity. Keeping the child and family calm and preventing harm if another seizure occurs is essential. Remember not to attempt to restrain child or use force if a seizure occurs and prevent the child from falling or hitting his head. Always stay with the child throughout the seizure and provide reassurance that everything is alright when he awakens. Involve the child and parents in discussion of fears, anxieties, and resources and support options available to patient and family.

3. **A, B, C, D, E**

Rationales: Focal seizures with impaired awareness commonly present with sensory phenomena, known as an aura, followed by mental disorientation and automatisms such as localized motor movement. In this child's case it was seen by repetitive movement in the left arm and it lasted only a few seconds. Postictal impairment with confusion is common. These types of seizures rarely occur multiple times a day and last for only a short period of time, also less than a minute.

4.

Options for 1	Options for 2	Options for 3
Simple partial seizure	BP	Intrathecal
Complex partial seizure	Seizure activity	IV
Status epilepticus	**Circulation, airway, and breathing (CAB)**	Rectal
Absence seizure	Blood levels	**Buccal**

Rationales: The child initially presented with a focal seizure with impaired awareness and now the child is not regaining a premorbid LOC between seizures. This is defined as status epilepticus and lasts for more than 30 minutes. A major concern is exhaustion that can lead to respiratory and circulatory failure that could result in death. The goal is to support vital functions and stop the seizure and, when the child presents with status epilepticus outside the hospital setting, buccal midazolam or rectal diazepam are the medications of choice to stop the seizure.

5.

Nursing Action	Effective	Ineffective
Monitor circulation, airway, and breathing closely.	X	
Ensure antiepileptic drugs are being administered as directed.	X	
Monitor and record characteristics, onset, and duration of any new seizures, including motor effects, alterations in consciousness, and postictal state.	X	
Attempt to stop the seizure if one occurs again; keep the child upright.		X
Do not place anything in child's mouth during the seizure.	X	
Place child in a side-lying position; suction the oral cavity and posterior oropharynx as needed.	X	
Observe for hyperthermia, hypertension, and respiratory depression.	X	

Rationales: During a seizure episode the nurse would first assess the child's circulation, airway, and breathing. Specifically, the nurse would evaluate for hyperthermia, hypertension, and respiratory depression. The seizure characteristics, including onset and duration of the seizure, motor effects, alterations in consciousness, and postictal state would be monitored and documented. Antiepileptic drugs are administered as directed. During the seizure, place the child in a side-lying position. Nothing should be placed in the child's mouth, and, if suctioning is required, proceed with caution. Do not attempt to stop the seizure. The hemoglobin and platelet count are not affected by a seizure.

6. **B, D, E, F, G, H, I, J**

Rationales: Discharge teaching would focus on protecting the child from injury should another seizure occur. Educate family about safety precautions before and during a seizure, including side-lying positioning, padding area if needed, and not placing items in mouth or attempting to stop the seizure. Parents should be taught to have eyes-on supervision when swimming in pools and an adult within arm's reach in natural bodies of water. The child should use protective helmet and padding during bicycle riding, skateboarding, and in-line skating. The nurse would educate family about medication administration, including scheduled and as necessary (prn) medications and potential side effects of medications. The nurse would educate family about characteristics of seizures, including aura, seizure activity, and postictal state. Have the child wear medical identification. Consultation with a social worker and child life specialist can provide further support for the family. Wearing a helmet to school is not helpful and creating an environment of normalcy in the school setting will provide much more support than including classmates in unnecessary observations.

The Child With Diabetes Mellitus

1. **A, B, C, D, E**

Rationales: History and assessment findings reveal classic signs and symptoms of juvenile diabetes. Increased thirst and urination, wetting of the bed, headaches, and tiredness are commonly found. The vital signs are normal for age.

2.

Options for 1	Options for 2	Options for 3
Diabetes mellitus	Platelets	Insulin
Addison disease	Hematocrit	**Glucose**
Cushing syndrome	**Blood glucose**	Potassium
Hyperparathyroidism	**A1c level**	Calcium
Pituitary hyperfunction	White blood cells	Sodium

Rationales: This child's blood glucose was 230 mg/dL and A1c level was 10.5%. Both of these laboratory tests are elevated and reveal a diagnosis of diabetes mellitus. Symptoms experienced by this child are caused by an increased level of glucoses in the bloodstream.

3. **A, D, E, F**

Rationales: The nurse would provide accurate information on the types of insulin the child will receive. Essential components of insulin education include the types of insulin, how soon they start working, when the insulin works the hardest, and how long it lasts. To review the various types of insulin, discussion would focus on: (1) rapid-acting insulin peaks in about 30 to 90 minutes and may last about 5 hours; (2) intermediate-acting insulin peaks in about 4 to 14 hours and can stay in the blood for 14 to 20 hours; and (3) long-acting insulin takes 6 to 14 hours to start working and can stay in the blood for up to 24 hours. These two statements are false: (1) short-acting insulin reaches the blood in about 5 minutes and peaks in about an hour, and (2) extended insulin takes 4 hours to start working and can stay in the blood for up to 14 hours.

4.

Nursing Action	Potential Complication	Nursing Action for Complication
1. Obtain blood glucose level before meals and at bedtime.	Normal blood glucose level is not maintained	2
2. Administer insulin as prescribed.	Appropriate dose of insulin is not administered	1
3. Monitor urine glucose before each meal.	Appropriate type of insulin is not administered	6
4. Use aseptic techniques when preparing and administering insulin.	Infection occurs	4
5. Store insulin in the freezer to preserve the medication.	Absorption of insulin is impaired	7
6. Understand the action of insulin: differences in composition, time of onset, and duration of action for the various preparations.		
7. Rotate insulin injection sites.		
8. Give less insulin before physical activity.		

Rationales: Teaching how to appropriately administer insulin in the home to a child requires several areas of focus during the teaching session. First, consider the child's developmental level and readiness to learn. Most 8-year-old children are able to participate in insulin administration. The child and parents must understand how to determine the appropriate dose of insulin to be administered. To accomplish this, the blood glucose level will need to be determined before meals and at bedtime. The child and family will need to know the action of insulin: differences in composition, time of onset, and duration of action for the various preparations. The amount of insulin to be given is based on the blood glucose levels and should be administered using aseptic techniques. Emphasis on rotating the injection sites to maximize absorption of the insulin is included in the discussion.

5.

Nursing Action	Effective	Ineffective
Immediately administer cup of fruit juice or a glass of nonfat or 1% milk.	X	
Check blood glucose after 15 min.	X	
Give a starch-protein snack.	X	
Start IV fluids with glucose.		X
Give parents instructions regarding signs and symptoms of hypoglycemia versus hyperglycemia.	X	
Teach parents how to administer intramuscular glucagon if unresponsive, unconscious, or seizing.	X	
Place the child on a portable insulin infusion pump.		X

Rationales: This is an important teaching moment for the child and family about the importance of eating meals on schedule after insulin is given. The nurse would immediately administer a cup of fruit juice or a glass of nonfat or 1% milk and to check blood glucose after 15 minutes. A starch-protein snack could also be given. This situation provides a teaching moment to give parents and the child instructions regarding signs and symptoms of hypoglycemia versus hyperglycemia. Parents would be taught how to administer intramuscular glucagon if unresponsive, unconscious, or seizing. IV fluids with glucose or using a portable insulin infusion pump are not appropriate or needed.

6. **B, C, E, F**

Rationales: Continued emphasis on how to assess the blood sugar and instructing that his levels should be maintained within a target range of 90 to 180 mg/dL during the day is important. Since hypoglycemia may occur again, a review of the symptoms related to low blood sugar should include headache, dizziness, shaking, sweating, and a fast pulse. Learning how to plan meals, understanding specific good groups, and making good food choices will be an important part of managing his diabetes. Reinforcing when the health care provider should be contacted includes when the child has fever for 2 days, vomiting and diarrhea, is unable to keep fluids down, and his glucose levels are above the target range. The child may participate in sports and be supported in managing his glucose levels when active.

A Child With a Fracture and Cast

1. **B, C, D, F, G, H**

Rationales. The increase in vital signs could indicate a number of things; the most concerning at this time is whether the child experienced head injury from the fall. Pain and anxiety can also cause an increase in vital signs, but the possibility of head injury should be evaluated as soon as possible. The child is drowsy and it could be from the pain medications since he is easily awakened. Swelling on the arm, hand, and leg is from the fall and the pain rating reflects this. He is voiding and temperature is normal.

2.

Options for 1	Options for 2	Options for 3
Nausea	Pain medication	**Spinal cord damage**
Brain injury	IV fluids	Right leg swelling
Vomiting	**Trauma to the head**	Headaches
Anxiety	Riding in the ambulance	Nausea
Stress from surgery	Fear	Seizures
Urinary tract infection	Lack of sleep	Venous access

Rationales: There is concern that the fall could have caused head injury and the nurse analyzes the symptoms to make careful observations. The EMT during transport took precautions to immobilize the spine in case the fall caused significant injury to the spinal cord. Pain medications can cause drowsiness, but the immediate concern is whether the symptoms are from a more severe problem—head injury.

3. **A, B, F, G, I**

Rationales: The nurse begins to prioritize actions based on information from the diagnostic evaluation earlier in the day. The child has no evidence of head trauma so the focus in now on the right arm and leg. Priority actions include pain control, peripheral pulse assessment in the arm and leg distal to the fracture site, and erythema, edema, and capillary refill observations. The leg should never be lower than the heart since this will impair blood flow. Cold compresses at this time are not recommended because they will constrict blood flow.

4.

Nursing Action	Indicated	Contraindicated
"Apply a cold compact to right lower leg."		X
"Notify the medical team immediately."	X	
"Control pain."	X	
"Move the patient to a chair for better circulation."		X
"Place the left leg above the heart."		X
"Continue to assess peripheral pulse and capillary refill."	X	
"Inspect skin for color changes proximal to the cast."	X	

Rationales: The nurse's careful assessment detected changes in the assessment of the child's vital signs and the right lower extremity. The nurse notified the medical team immediately of the changes and continued to assess peripheral pulses, capillary refill, and color changes proximal to the cast. Pain control was essential. Cold compresses, moving the child to a chair, and placing the leg that was not fractured above the heart will provide no benefit, and could cause a great deal of pain and discomfort.

5.

Nursing Action	Potential Complications	Appropriate Nursing Action for Complication
1. Observe for pain, pallor, pulselessness, paresthesia, and paralysis.	Circulatory impairment	3
2. Observe for altered sensation when sensory testing with touch and pinprick.	Compartment syndrome	1
3. Observe for peripheral pulses.	Nerve Compression	2
4. Observe for fever and drainage from the site.	Pulmonary emboli	6
5. Observe for signs of urinary retention.	Uncontrolled pain	7
6. Assess for dyspnea, keep head of bed elevated, and administer oxygen. Note: this is a medical emergency.		
7. Frequently assess pain using a pain rating scale.		

Rationales: The nurse takes action to prevent complications in this child by observing peripheral pulses that could be a sign of circulatory impairment. The evening before, there were concerns of compartment syndrome that presents with pain, pallor, pulselessness, paresthesia, and paralysis; the nurse should continue to observe for these symptoms. Nerve compression is a concern, and altered sensation using sensory testing is assessed. In children who are immobilized for longer periods of time, pulmonary emboli is a concern and patients are closely observed for signs of dyspnea. The head of the bed is elevated, and oxygen is administered; this is a medical emergency. Pain is controlled with frequent assessments being conducted to assure pain control is maintained.

6. **B, C, E, F**

Rationales: The nurse in her discharge teaching discussion advises the parents to encourage frequent rest periods for the first few days at home while the child recovers. Elevation of the right leg can provide comfort and improve blood return. The nurse teaches the parents how to observe the toes for swelling and discoloration. Observing the skin at the cast edges to prevent skin breakdown is also taught. The child should not get the cast wet by swimming and the cast does not need to be covered at all times. The parents would not be advised to check the child's pulses every 4 hours; this is not necessary.

A Child With Cerebral Palsy

1. **A, B, C, F, I, J**

Rationales: The findings on the nursing assessment that are concerning and need follow-up include abnormal clinical manifestations of tongue thrust, hands fisted, tonic neck reflexes, and primitive infant reflexes still present that should be gone by 4 months of age. Difficult feeding with poor sucking and rigid, unbending hip and knee joints are all a concern. The infant's vital signs are normal for age and infants frequently awaken at night at this age.

2.

Options for 1	Options for 2	Options for 3
Infantile seizures	Poor feeding	Lumbar puncture
Traumatic brain injury	**Prematurity**	**Neuroimaging**
Cerebral palsy	Trauma to the head	Blood lead level
Myelomeningocele	Sleep disruption	Echocardiogram
Diabetes	Constipation	Chest x-ray
Urinary tract infection	Nystagmus	Venous blood gas

Rationales: Clinical findings on the history and physical assessment are found in infants with cerebral palsy. There are a number of risk factors associated with cerebral palsy, including prematurity. Neuroimaging is becoming an established diagnostic tool.

3. **A, B, D, G, H**

Rationales: Abnormal assessment findings for the nurse to focus on include the presence of reflex abnormalities, abnormal postures, altered muscle tone, abnormal motor performance, and delayed gross motor development. It is normal to open both eyes to voices and to cry at night when hungry. The nurse would teach the parents how to become involved in physical training to promote motor function in this young infant. Physical therapy is an active member of the infant's multidisciplinary team and works closely with the nurse to teach the parents how to perform daily exercises and develop ways to deal with the infant's decreased muscle tone and abnormal posturing.

4.

Nursing Action	Indicated	Contraindicated
"Your infant may have difficulty keeping his head upright. Let me show you some ways to support his head."	X	
"Notify the medical team immediately if your infant begins to vomit."		X
"If your infant has difficulty feeding and swallowing, I can show you some ways that might help."	X	
"Keep your infant in an upright position at all times. You can use pillows to prop him up."		X
"Your infant may need nutritional supplements. I will have the nutritionist meet with you to discuss this."	X	
"Because of your child's disease, he should not receive his immunizations."		X
"I will show you how to look at your infant's skin to make sure there is no breakdown."	X	

Rationales: A major emphasis for teaching parents how to care for the infant at home focuses on how to support altered muscle tone and abnormal postures that occur in children with cerebral palsy. The family must be taught how to support the infant's head and other muscles such as those used when swallowing. Other important aspects of care include supporting the child's nutrition by educating parents on the need for nutritional supplements. The lack of mobility due to decreased muscle tone increases the risk of skin breakdown and the nurse would teach the parents how to assess the skin for breakdown and how to keep the skin clean and dry. The mother would not be taught to notify the team immediately for vomiting, the infant would not need to be in an upright position at all times, and the infant should receive his childhood immunizations.

5.

Nursing Action	Potential Complications	Appropriate Nursing Action for Complication
1. Teach parents how to diaper the infant, clean the perianal area, and observe for signs of skin breakdown.	Inadequate nutrition	3
2. Teach parents how to observe for fever and administer antibiotics.	Lack of support for parents	4
3. Discuss nutrition needs with nutritionist to provide suggestions to promote adequate caloric intake.	Skin breakdown	1
4. Discuss parent concerns and fears and offer support available in the community and nationally.	Bodily harm	6
5. Teach parents how to observe for signs of urinary retention.	Communicable illnesses	7
6. Discuss measures to promote safety in the home environment and prevent falls, safe transport in a vehicle.		
7. Discuss the importance of the infant receiving immunizations to prevent common childhood illnesses.		

Rationales: Potential complications for an infant with cerebral palsy include inadequate nutrition related to difficulty with feeding and swallowing. Due to the decreased muscle tone, the child may develop skin irritation and breakdown. This can also be related to the difficulty of diapering an infant with cerebral palsy because of abnormal posturing. There is an increased risk of injury in an infant with cerebral palsy, and parents should be taught ways to prevent falls when trying to sit the infant upright, and safe ways to transport the infant in a vehicle should be discussed. The importance of the infant receiving routine communicable illness vaccinations should be stressed during teaching. Parents need extensive support, and time to allow them to discuss their concerns and fears is important for their own well-being.

6. **D, E, G, H**

Rationales: This 1-year-old now requires supplementing feeding and the nurse would first give praise to the parents for all their efforts. Offering to demonstrate tasks such as how to prevent the G tube from clogging, how to dissolve the pills correctly, and how to promote jaw control during feeding are very important nursing actions. Offering to have the physical therapist review the exercises for home therapy is another important nursing action; the more direct-observation opportunities provided to the parents to see how skills are performed, the more confident they will be at home. Telling the parents to take the child's vitals frequently is not appropriate, and recommending the parents not use the G tube is not in the best interest of the child. Telling the parents they might hurt their child if they do physical exercises at home also is detrimental.

Reference Data

Symbol ▶ indicates material that may be photocopied and distributed to families.

Common Laboratory Tests

Blood Chemistries

	Conventional Units	SI Units
Alanine Aminotransferase (ALT)		
0 to <1 year	5–33 U/L	5–33 U/L
1 to <13 years	9–25 U/L	9–25 U/L
13–19 years (male)	9–24 U/L	9–24 U/L
13 to <19 years (female)	8–22 U/L	8–22 U/L
Albumin		
0–14 days	3.3–4.5 g/dL	33–45 g/L
15 days to <1 year	2.8–4.7 g/dL	28–47 g/L
1 to <8 years	3.8–4.7 g/dL	38–47 g/L
8 to <15 years	4.1–4.8 g/dL	41–48 g/L
15 to <19 years (male)	4.1–5.1 g/dL	41–51 g/L
15 to <19 years (female)	4.0–4.9 g/dL	40–49 g/L
Alkaline Phosphatase		
0–14 days	90–273 U/L	90–273 U/L
15 days to <1 year	134–518 U/L	134–518 U/L
1 to <10 years	156–369 U/L	156–369 U/L
10 to <13 years	141–460 U/L	141–460 U/L
13 to <15 years (male)	127–517 U/L	127–517 U/L
13 to <15 years (female)	62–280 U/L	62–280 U/L
15 to <17 years (male)	89–365 U/L	89–365 U/L
15 to <17 years (female)	54–128 U/L	54–128 U/L
17 to <19 years (male)	59–164 U/L	59–164 U/L
17 to <19 years (female)	48–95 U/L	48–95 U/L
Ammonia		
0–14 days	35.8–161.8 mcg/dL	21–95 mcmol/L
15 days to 6 years	27.2–115.8 mcg/dL	16–68 mcmol/L
>6 years	30.7–122.6 mcg/dL	18–72 mcmol/L
Amylase		
0–14 days	3–10 U/L	3–10 U/L
15 days to <13 weeks	2–22 U/L	2–22 U/L
13 weeks to <1 year	3–50 U/L	3–50 U/L
1 year to <19 years	25–101 U/L	25–101 U/L
Antistreptolysin O Titer		
0 to <6 months	0 IU/mL	0 IU/mL
6 months to <1 year	0–30 IU/mL	0–30 IU/mL
1 to <6 years	0–104 IU/mL	0–104 IU/mL
6 to <19 years	0–331 IU/mL	0–331 IU/mL
Aspartate Aminotransferase (AST)		
0–14 days	32–162 U/L	32–162 U/L
15 days to <1 year	20–67 U/L	20–67 U/L
1 to <7 years	21–44 U/L	21–44 U/L
7 to <12 years	18–36 U/L	18–36 U/L
12 to <19 years (male)	14–35 U/L	14–35 U/L
12 to <19 years (female)	13–26 U/L	13–26 U/L

	Conventional Units	SI Units
Bicarbonate		
0–14 days	5–20 mEq/L	5–20 mmol/L
15 days to <1 year	10–24 mEq/L	10–24 mmol/L
1 to <5 years	14–24 mEq/L	14–24 mmol/L
5 to <15 years	17–26 mEq/L	17–26 mmol/L
15 to <19 years (male)	18–28 mEq/L	18–28 mmol/L
15 to <19 years (female)	17–26 mEq/L	17–26 mmol/L
Bilirubin (Total)		
0–14 days	0.19–16.60 mg/dL	3.25–283.92 mcmol/L
15 days to <1 year	0.05–0.68 mg/dL	0.86–11.63 mcmol/L
1 to <9 years	0.05–0.40 mg/dL	0.86–6.84 mcmol/L
9 to <12 years	0.05–0.55 mg/dL	0.86–9.41 mcmol/L
12 to <15 years	0.10–0.70 mg/dL	1.71–11.97 mcmol/L
15 to <19 years	0.10–0.84 mg/dL	1.71–14.37 mcmol/L
Bilirubin (Conjugated)		
0–14 days	0.33–0.71 mg/dL	5.64–12.14 mcmol/L
15 days to <1 year	0.05–0.30 mg/dL	0.86–5.13 mcmol/L
1 to <9 years	0.05–0.20 mg/dL	0.86–3.42 mcmol/L
9 to <13 years	0.05–0.29 mg/dL	0.86–4.96 mcmol/L
13 to <19 years (female)	0.10–0.39 mg/dL	1.71–6.67 mcmol/L
13 to <19 years (male)	0.11–0.42 mg/dL	1.88–7.18 mcmol/L

BLOOD GAS, ARTERIAL (BREATHING ROOM AIR)

	pH	PaO_2 (mmHg)	$PaCO_2$ (mmHg)	HCO_3^- (mEq/L)
Cord blood	7.28 ± 0.05	18.0 ± 6.2	49.2 ± 8.4	14–22
Newborn (birth)	7.11–7.36	8–24	27–40	13–22
5–10 min	7.09–7.30	33–75	27–40	13–22
30 min	7.21–7.38	31–85	27–40	13–22
60 min	7.26–7.49	55–80	27–40	13–22
1 day	7.29–7.45	54–95	27–40	13–22
Child/adult	7.35–7.45	83–108	32–48	20–28

	Conventional Units	SI Units
C-Reactive Protein (High Sensitivity)		
0–14 days	0.3–6.1 mg/L	0.3–6.1 mg/L
15 days to <15 years	0.1–1.0 mg/L	0.1–1.0 mg/L
15 to <19 years	0.1–1.7 mg/L	0.1–1.7 mg/L
Calcium (Ionized)		
0–1 month	3.9–6.0 mg/dL	1.0–1.5 mmol/L
1–6 months	3.7–5.9 mg/dL	0.95–1.5 mmol/L
1–19 years	4.9–5.5 mg/dL	1.22–1.37 mmol/L
Calcium (Total)		
0 to <1 year	8.5–11.0 mg/dL	2.1–2.7 mmol/L
1 year to <19 years	9.2–10.5 mg/dL	2.3–2.6 mmol/L
Carbon Monoxide (Carboxyhemoglobin)		
Nonsmoker	0%–2% of total hemoglobin	
Smoker	0%–9% of total hemoglobin	
Chloride (Serum)		
3–5 years	100–107 mEq/L	100–107 mmol/L
6–11 years	101–107 mEq/L	101–107 mmol/L
12–29 years (male)	101–106 mEq/L	101–106 mmol/L
12–29 years (female)	100–107 mEq/L	100–107 mmol/L

BLOOD GAS, ARTERIAL (BREATHING ROOM AIR)				
	pH	**PaO_2 (mmHg)**	**$PaCO_2$ (mmHg)**	**HCO_3^- (mEq/L)**
Cholesterol				
(See LIPIDS, further on)				
Copper				
6 months–2 years	72–178 mcg/dL		11.3–28.0 mcmol/L	
3–4 years	80–160 mcg/dL		12.6–25.2 mcmol/L	
5–6 years	76–167 mcg/dL		12.0–26.3 mcmol/L	
7–8 years	79–147 mcg/dL		12.4–23.1 mcmol/L	
9–10 years	84–154 mcg/dL		13.2–24.2 mcmol/L	
11–12 years	73–149 mcg/dL		11.5–23.4 mcmol/L	
13–14 years	66–137 mcg/dL		10.4–21.6 mcmol/L	
15–16 years	60–132 mcg/dL		9.4–20.8 mcmol/L	
17–18 years	59–146 mcg/dL		9.3–23.0 mcmol/L	
Creatine Kinase				
6 months to 2 years (male)	50–292 U/L		50–292 U/L	
6 months to 2 years (female)	38–260 U/L		38–260 U/L	
3–5 years (male)	59–296 U/L		59–296 U/L	
3–5 years (female)	42–227 U/L		42–227 U/L	
6–8 years (male)	54–275 U/L		54–275 U/L	
6–8 years (female)	50–231 U/L		50–231 U/L	
9–11 years (male)	55–324 U/L		55–324 U/L	
9–11 years (female)	52–256 U/L		52–256 U/L	
12–14 years (male)	63–407 U/L		63–407 U/L	
12–14 years (female)	45–257 U/L		45–257 U/L	
15–17 years (male)	68–914 U/L		68–914 U/L	
15–17 years (female)	45–458 U/L		45–458 U/L	
Creatinine (Serum) (Enzymatic)				
0–14 days	0.32–0.92 mg/dL		28.29–81.33 mcmol/L	
15 days to <2 years	0.10–0.36 mg/dL		8.84–31.82 mcmol/L	
2 to <5 years	0.20–0.43 mg/dL		17.68–38.01 mcmol/L	
5 to <12 years	0.31–0.61 mg/dL		27.40–53.93 mcmol/L	
12 to <15 years	0.45–0.81 mg/dL		39.78–71.61 mcmol/L	
15 to <19 years (male)	0.62–1.08 mg/dL		54.81–95.47 mcmol/L	
15 to <19 years (female)	0.49–0.84 mg/dL		43.32–74.26 mcmol/L	
Erythrocyte Sedimentation Rate (ESR)				
Child	0–10 mm/h			
Adult male	0–15 mm/h			
Adult female	0–20 mm/h			
Ferritin				
4 to <15 days	100–717 ng/mL		224–1611 pmol/L	
15 days to <6 months	14–647 ng/mL		31–1454 pmol/L	
6 months to <1 year	8–182 ng/mL		19–409 pmol/L	
1 to <5 years	5–100 ng/mL		12–224 pmol/L	
5 to <14 years	14–79 ng/mL		31–177 pmol/L	
14 to <19 years (female)	6–67 ng/mL		12–152 pmol/L	
14 to <16 years (male)	13–83 ng/mL		28–186 pmol/L	
16 to <19 years (male)	11–172 ng/mL		25–386 pmol/L	

BLOOD GAS, ARTERIAL (BREATHING ROOM AIR)

	pH	PaO_2 (mmHg)	$PaCO_2$ (mmHg)	HCO_3^- (mEq/L)
Folate (RBC)				
Deficient	≤3.9 ng/mL		≤8.7 nmol/L	
Indeterminate	4.0–5.8 ng/mL		9.1–13.1 nmol/L	
Normal	≥5.9 ng/mL		≥13.4 nmol/L	
Folate (SERUM)	≥366 ng/mL		≥831 nmol/L	
Gamma-Glutamyl Transferase (GGT)				
0–14 days	23–219 U/L		23–219 U/L	
15 days to <1 year	8–127 U/L		8–127 U/L	
1 to <11 years	6–16 U/L		6–16 U/L	
11 to <19 years	7–21 U/L		7–21 U/L	

Glucose and other tests to Diagnose Diabetes

- Fasting plasma glucose (FPG = no caloric intake for at least 8 h) ≥126 mg/dL
- Oral glucose tolerance test (OGTT) with a 2-h postload plasma glucose of ≥200 mg/dL
- Hemoglobin A_{1c} (HbA_{1c}) ≥6.5%

Haptoglobin				
0–14 days	0–10 mg/dL		0–0.10 g/L	
15 days to <1 year	7–221 mg/dL		0.07–2.21 g/L	
1 to <12 years	7–163 mg/dL		0.07–1.63 g/L	
12 to <19 years	7–179 mg/dL		0.07–1.79 g/L	
Hemoglobin F, % Total Hemoglobin				
0–1 month	45.8–91.7			
2 months	32.7–85.2			
3 months	14.5–73.7			
4 months	4.2–56.9			
5 months	1.0–38.1			
6–8 months	0.9–19.4			
9–12 months	0.6–11.6			
13–23 months	0.0–8.5			
2 years and older	0.0–2.1			
Iron				
0 to <14 years	16–128 mcg/dL		2.8–22.9 mcmol/L	
14–19 years (male)	31–168 mcg/dL		5.5–40.0 mcmol/L	
14–19 years (female)	20–162 mcg/dL		3.5–29.0 mcmol/L	
Lactate				
0–90 days	9–32 mg/dL		1.0–3.5 mmol/L	
3–24 months	9–30 mg/dL		1.0–3.3 mmol/L	
2–18 years	9–22 mg/dL		1.0–2.4 mmol/L	
Lactate Dehydrogenase				
0–14 days	309–1222 U/L		309–1222 U/L	
15 days to <1 year	163–452 U/L		163–452 U/L	
1 to <10 years	192–321 U/L		192–321 U/L	
10 to <15 years (male)	170–283 U/L		170–283 U/L	
10 to <15 years (female)	157–272 U/L		157–272 U/L	
15 to <19 years	130–250 U/L		130–250 U/L	

LEAD SCREENING AND GUIDELINES

If Screening BLL Is: (mcg/dL)	Time Frame of Confirmation of Screening BLL	Follow-Up Testing (After Confirmatory Testing)	Later Follow-Up Testing After BLL Declining
≥5–9	1–3 months	3 months	6–9 months
10–19	1 week to 1 month	1–3 months	3–6 months
20–24	1 week to 1 month	1–3 months	1–3 months
25–44	1 week to 1 month	2 weeks–1 month	1 month
45–59	48 h	*Repeat testing as soon as possible after chelation therapy*	
60–69	24 h		
≥70	Urgently		

BLL, Blood lead level.

LIPASE

0 to <19 years	4.0–39.0 U/L	4.0–39.0 U/L

LIPIDS

	Desirable	Borderline	High[e]
Total cholesterol	<170 mg/dL (4.4 mmol/L)	170–199 mg/dL (4.4–5.2 mmol/L)	≥200 mg/dL (5.2 mmol/L)
LDL	<110 mg/dL (2.8 mmol/L)	110–129 mg/dL (2.8–3.3 mmol/L)	≥130 mg/dL (3.4 mmol/L)
Non-HDL	<120 mg/dL (3.1 mmol/L)	120–144 mg/dL (3.1–3.7 mmol/L)	≥145 mg/dL (3.8 mmol/L)
HDL	>45 mg/dL (1.2 mmol/L)	40–45 mg/dL (1.0–1.2 mmol/L)	≤40 mg/dL (1.0 mmol/L)
Triglycerides (0–9 years)	<75 mg/dL (0.8 mmol/L)	75–99 mg/dL (0.8–1.1 mmol/L)	≥100 mg/dL (1.1 mmol/L)
Triglycerides (10–19 years)	<90 mg/dL (1.0 mmol/L)	90–129 mg/dL (1.0–1.5 mmol/L)	≥130 mg/dL (1.5 mmol/L)

	Conventional Units	SI Units
Magnesium		
0–14 days	1.99–3.94 mg/dL	0.82–1.62 mmol/L
15 days to <1 year	1.97–3.09 mg/dL	0.81–1.27 mmol/L
1 to <19 years	2.09–2.84 mg/dL	0.86–1.17 mmol/L
Osmolality		
0–16 years	271–296 mOsm/kg	271–296 mmol/kg
17 years and older	280–303 mOsm/kg	280–303 mmol/kg
Phosphorus		
0–14 days	5.6–10.5 mg/dL	1.8–3.4 mmol/L
15 days to <1 year	4.8–8.4 mg/dL	1.5–2.7 mmol/L
1 to <5 years	4.3–6.8 mg/dL	1.4–2.2 mmol/L
5 to <13 years	4.1–5.9 mg/dL	1.3–1.9 mmol/L
13 to <16 years (male)	3.5–6.2 mg/dL	1.1–2.0 mmol/L
13 to <16 years (female)	3.2–5.5 mg/dL	1.0–1.8 mmol/L
16 to <19 years	2.9–5.0 mg/dL	0.9–1.6 mmol/L
Porcelain		
Male	5.28–20.15 mg/dL	6.15–20.13 mmol/L
Female	7.20–19.21 mg/dL	7.01–20.15 mmol/L

	Conventional Units	SI Units
Potassium		
Preterm	3.0–6.0 mEq/L	3.0–6.0 mmol/L
Newborn	3.7–5.9 mEq/L	3.7–5.9 mmol/L
Infant	4.1–5.3 mEq/L	4.1–5.3 mmol/L
Child	3.4–4.7 mEq/L	3.4–4.7 mmol/L
Thereafter	3.5–5.1 mEq/L	3.5–5.1 mmol/L
Prealbumin		
0–14 days	2–12 mg/dL	0.02–0.12 g/L
15 days to <1 year	5–24 mg/dL	0.05–0.24 g/L
1 to <5 years	12–23 mg/dL	0.12–0.23 g/L
5 to <13 years	14–26 mg/dL	0.14–0.26 g/L
13 to <16 years	18–31 mg/dL	0.18–0.31 g/L
16 to <19 years (male)	20–35 mg/dL	0.20–0.35 g/L
16 to <19 years (female)	17–33 mg/dL	0.17–0.33 g/L
Rheumatoid Factor		
0–14 days	9.0–17.1 IU/mL	9.0–17.1 IU/mL
15 days to <19 years	0–9.0 IU/mL	0–9.0 IU/mL
Sodium		
3–5 years	135–142 mEq/L	135–142 mmol/L
6–15 years	136–143 mEq/L	136–143 mmol/L
16–49 years (male)	137–143 mEq/L	137–143 mmol/L
16–49 years (female)	137–142 mEq/L	137–142 mmol/L
Total Iron-Binding Capacity (TIBC)		
0–2 months	59–175 mcg/dL	11–31 mcmol/L
3 months to 17 years	250–400 mcg/dL	45–72 mcmol/L
18 years and older	240–450 mcg/dL	43–81 mcmol/L
Total Protein		
0–14 days	5.3–8.3 g/dL	53–83 g/L
15 days to <1 year	4.4–7.1 g/dL	44–71 g/L
1 to <6 years	6.1–7.5 g/dL	61–75 g/L
6 to <9 years	6.4–7.7 g/dL	64–77 g/L
9 to <19 years	6.5–8.1 g/dL	65–81 g/L
Transferrin		
0 to <9 weeks	104–224 mg/dL	1.04–2.24 g/L
9 weeks to <1 year	107–324 mg/dL	1.07–3.24 g/L
1 to <19 years	220–337 mg/dL	2.2–3.37 g/L
Triglycerides		
(See LIPIDS, earlier)		
Urea Nitrogen		
0 to <14 days	2.8–23.0 mg/dL	1.0–8.2 mmol/L
15 days to <1 year	3.4–16.8 mg/dL	1.2–6.0 mmol/L
1 to <10 years	9.0–22.1 mg/dL	3.2–7.9 mmol/L
10 to <19 years (male)	7.3–21 mg/dL	2.6–7.5 mmol/L
10 to <19 years (female)	7.3–19 mg/dL	2.6–6.8 mmol/L
Uric Acid		
0–14 days	2.8–12.7 mg/dL	0.2–0.8 mmol/L
15 days to <1 year	1.6–6.3 mg/dL	0.1–0.4 mmol/L
1 to <12 years	1.8–4.9 mg/dL	0.1–0.3 mmol/L
12 to <19 years (male)	2.6–7.6 mg/dL	0.2–0.5 mmol/L
12 to <19 years (female)	2.6–5.9 mg/dL	0.2–0.4 mmol/L

	Conventional Units	SI Units
Vitamin A (Retinol)		
0 to <1 year	8.0–53.6 mg/dL	0–2 mcmol/L
1 to <11 years	27.5–44.4 mg/dL	1–2 mcmol/L
11 to <16 years	24.9–55.0 mg/dL	1–2 mcmol/L
16 to <19 years	28.7–75.1 mg/dL	1–3 mcmol/L
Vitamin B_1 (Thiamine) RBC	4.5–10.3 mcg/dL	106–242 nmol/L
Vitamin B_2 (Riboflavin)	4–24 mcg/dL	106–638 nmol/L
Vitamin B_{12} (Cobalamin)		
5 days to <1 year	259–1576 pg/mL	191–1163 pmol/L
1 to <9 years	283–1613 pg/mL	209–1190 pmol/L
9 to <14 years	252–1125 pg/mL	186–830 pmol/L
14 to <17 years	244–888 pg/mL	180–655 pmol/L
17 to <19 years	203–811 pg/mL	150–599 pmol/L
Vitamin C (Ascorbic Acid)	0.4–2.0 mg/dL	23–114 mcmol/L
Vitamin D (1,25-Dihydroxy-Vitamin D)		
0 to <1 year	32.1–196.2 pg/mL	77–471 pmol/L
1 to <3 years	47.1–151.2 pg/mL	113–363 pmol/L
3 to <19 years	45.0–102.5 pg/mL	108–246 pmol/L
Vitamin D (25-Hydroxy-Vitamin D)		
Deficient	<12 ng/mL	<30 nmol/L
Insufficient	12–20 ng/mL	30–50 nmol/L
Sufficient[f]	≥20 ng/mL	≥50 nmol/L
Excess	>50–60 ng/mL	>125–150 nmol/L
Vitamin E (α-Tocopherol)		
0 to <1 year	0.2–2.1 mg/dL	5.0–50.0 mcmol/L
1 to <19 years	0.6–1.4 mg/dL	14.5–33.0 mcmol/L
Zinc		
6 months to 2 years	56–125 mcg/dL	8.6–19.1 mcmol/L
3–4 years	60–120 mcg/dL	9.2–18.4 mcmol/L
5–6 years	64–117 mcg/dL	9.8–17.9 mcmol/L
7–8 years	65–125 mcg/dL	9.9–19.1 mcmol/L
9–10 years	66–125 mcg/dL	10.1–19.1 mcmol/L
11–12 years	66–127 mcg/dL	10.1–19.4 mcmol/L
13–14 years	69–124 mcg/dL	10.6–19.0 mcmol/L
15–16 years	62–123 mcg/dL	9.5–18.8 mcmol/L
17–18 years	62–133 mcg/dL	9.5–20.3 mcmol

Modified from Kleinman K, McDaniel L, Molloy M, eds. *The Harriet Lane Handbook.* 22nd ed. Philadelphia: Elsevier; 2020.

Hematology

Age	Hb (g/dL)	HCT (%)	MCV (fL)	MCHC (g/dL RBC)	Reticulocytes	WBCs (×10³/mL)	Platelets (10³/mL)
26–30 weeks gestation	13.4 (11)	41.5 (34.9)	118.2 (106.7)	37.9 (30.6)	—	4.4 (2.7)	254 (180–327)
28 weeks	14.5	45	120	31.0	(5–10)	—	275
32 weeks	15.0	47	118	32.0	(3–10)	—	290
Term (cord)	16.5 (13.5)	51 (42)	108 (98)	33.0 (30.0)	(3–7)	18.1 (9–30)[e]	290
1–3 days	18.5 (14.5)	56 (45)	108 (95)	33.0 (29.0)	(1.8–4.6)	18.9 (9.4–34)	192
2 weeks	16.6 (13.4)	53 (41)	105 (88)	31.4 (28.1)	—	11.4 (5–20)	252
1 month	13.9 (10.7)	44 (33)	101 (91)	31.8 (28.1)	(0.1–1.7)	10.8 (4–19.5)	—
2 months	11.2 (9.4)	35 (28)	95 (84)	31.8 (28.3)	—	—	—
6 months	12.6 (11.1)	36 (31)	76 (68)	35.0 (32.7)	(0.7–2.3)	11.9 (6–17.5)	—
6 months–2 years	12.0 (10.5)	36 (33)	78 (70)	33.0 (30.0)	—	10.6 (6–17)	(150–350)
2–6 years	12.5 (11.5)	37 (34)	81 (75)	34.0 (31.0)	(0.5–1.0)	8.5 (5–15.5)	(150–350)
6–12 years	13.5 (11.5)	40 (35)	86 (77)	34.0 (31.0)	(0.5–1.0)	8.1 (4.5–13.5)	(150–350)
12–18 Years							
Male	14.5 (13)	43 (36)	88 (78)	34.0 (31.0)	(0.5–1.0)	7.8 (4.5–13.5)	(150–350)
Female	14.0 (12)	41 (37)	90 (78)	34.0 (31.0)	(0.5–1.0)	7.8 (4.5–13.5)	(150–350)

Age-Specific Leukocyte Differential

	Total Leukocytes	Neutrophils		Lymphocytes		Monocytes		Eosinophils	
Age	Mean (Range)	Mean (Range)	%	Mean (Range)	%	Mean	%	Mean	%
Birth	18.1 (9–30)	11 (6–26)	61	5.5 (2–11)	31	1.1	6	0.4	2
12 h	22.8 (13–38)	15.5 (6–28)	68	5.5 (2–11)	24	1.2	5	0.5	2
24 h	18.9 (9.4–34)	11.5 (5–21)	61	5.8 (2–11.5)	31	1.1	6	0.5	2
1 week	12.2 (5–21)	5.5 (1.5–10)	45	5.0 (2–17)	41	1.1	9	0.5	4
2 weeks	11.4 (5–20)	4.5 (1–9.5)	40	5.5 (2–17)	48	1.0	9	0.4	3
1 month	10.8 (5–19.5)	3.8 (1–8.5)	35	6.0 (2.5–16.5)	56	0.7	7	0.3	3
6 months	11.9 (6–17.5)	3.8 (1–8.5)	32	7.3 (4–13.5)	61	0.6	5	0.3	3
1 year	11.4 (6–17.5)	3.5 (1.5–8.5)	31	7.0 (4–10.5)	61	0.6	5	0.3	3
2 years	10.6 (6–17)	3.5 (1.5–8.5)	33	6.3 (3–9.5)	59	0.5	5	0.3	3
4 years	9.1 (5.5–15.5)	3.8 (1.5–8.5)	42	4.5 (2–8)	50	0.5	5	0.3	3
6 years	8.5 (5–14.5)	4.3 (1.5–8)	51	3.5 (1.5–7)	42	0.4	5	0.2	3
8 years	8.3 (4.5–13.5)	4.4 (1.5–8)	53	3.3 (1.5–6.8)	39	0.4	4	0.2	2
10 years	8.1 (4.5–13.5)	4.4 (1.5–8.5)	54	3.1 (1.5–6.5)	38	0.4	4	0.2	2
16 years	7.8 (4.5–13.0)	4.4 (1.8–8)	57	2.8 (1.2–5.2)	35	0.4	5	0.2	3
21 years	7.4 (4.5–11.0)	4.4 (1.8–7.7)	59	2.5 (1–4.8)	34	0.3	4	0.2	3

Note: Page numbers followed by "f" refer to illustrations; page numbers followed by "t" refer to tables; page numbers followed by "b" refer to boxes.

C

O

P

R

U

V

W

Y

Z